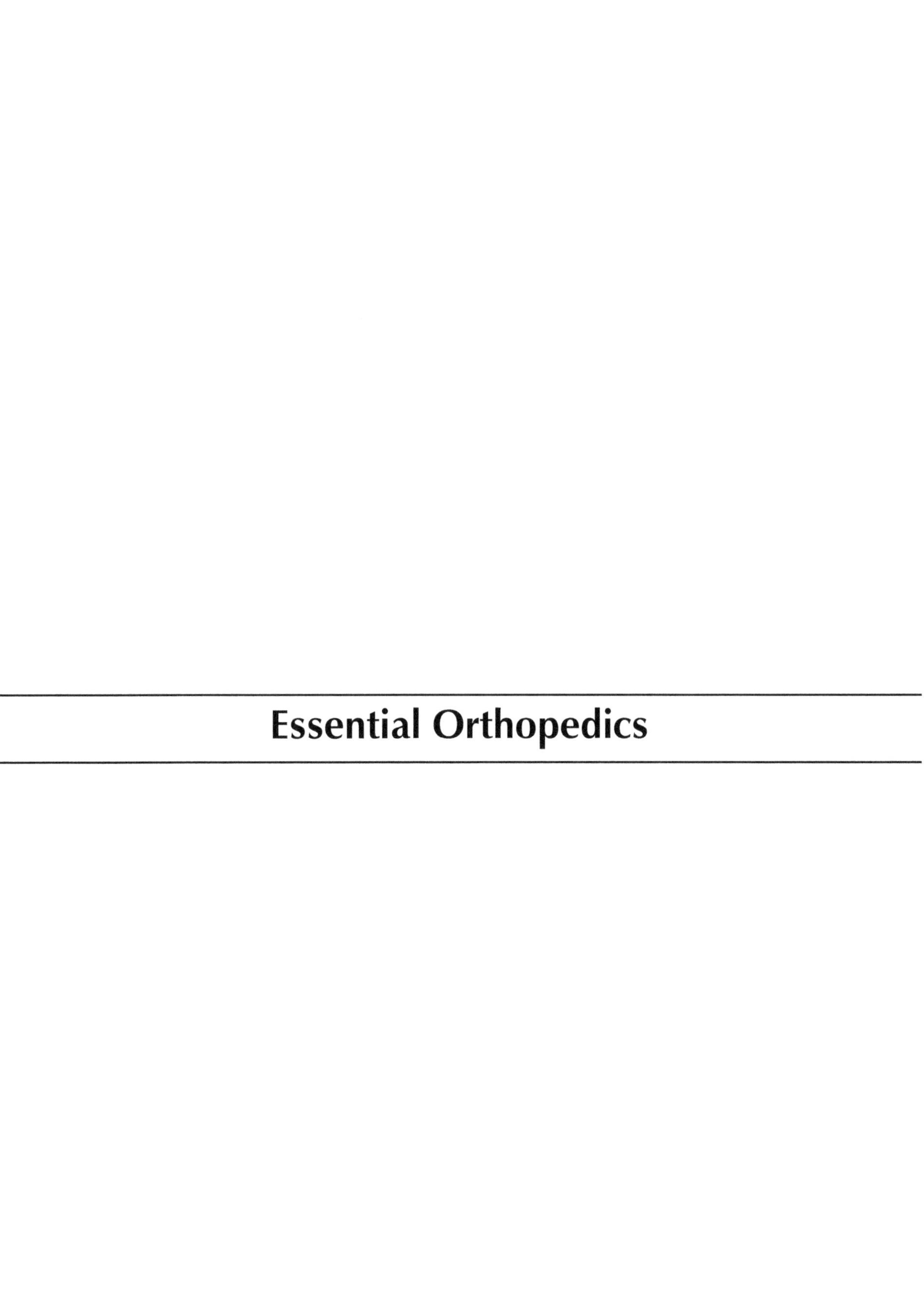

Essential Orthopedics

Essential Orthopedics

Editor: Solomon Willis

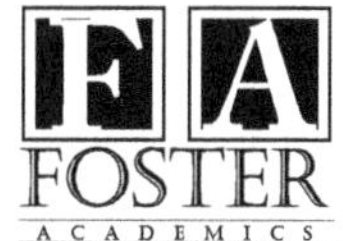

www.fosteracademics.com

www.fosteracademics.com

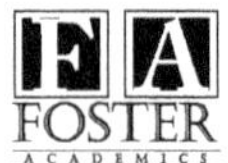

Cataloging-in-Publication Data

Essential orthopedics / edited by Solomon Willis.
p. cm.
Includes bibliographical references and index.
ISBN 978-1-63242-490-7
1. Orthopedics. 2. Musculoskeletal system--Wounds and injuries. 3. Orthopedics--Diagnosis.
I. Willis, Solomon.
RD731 .E87 2017
616.7--dc23

Foster Academics,
118-35 Queens Blvd., Suite 400,
Forest Hills, NY 11375, USA

ISBN 978-1-63242-490-7 (Hardback)

Printed and bound in the United States of America.

Contents

Preface

I am honored to present to you this unique book which encompasses the most up-to-date data in the field. I was extremely pleased to get this opportunity of editing the work of experts from across the globe. I have also written papers in this field and researched the various aspects revolving around the progress of the discipline. I have tried to unify my knowledge along with that of stalwarts from every corner of the world, to produce a text which not only benefits the readers but also facilitates the growth of the field.

Orthopedics is a branch of surgery that concerns itself with the pathophysiology and treatment of the musculoskeletal system. This book on orthopedics deals with the theory and practice of orthopedic practice. Some of the popular disorders treated under this branch are musculoskeletal trauma, spine disorders and injuries, sports injuries, etc. Contents in this book seek to contribute to the vast array of research that has taken place in the field of orthopedics. Most of the topics introduced in this book cover new techniques of diagnosis and treatment under the branch of orthopedics along with their applications. Those with an interest in this field would find this book helpful. It will help the readers in keeping pace with the rapid changes in this area of study.

Finally, I would like to thank all the contributing authors for their valuable time and contributions. This book would not have been possible without their efforts. I would also like to thank my friends and family for their constant support.

Editor

1

Enhancement of Implant Osseointegration by High-Frequency Low-Magnitude Loading

Xiaolei Zhang[1], Antonia Torcasio[2], Katleen Vandamme[1], Toru Ogawa[1,3], G. Harry van Lenthe[2,4], Ignace Naert[1], Joke Duyck[1]*

1 Department of Prosthetic Dentistry, BIOMAT Research Cluster, University of Leuven, Leuven, Belgium, **2** Department of Mechanical Engineering, Division of Biomechanics and Engineering Design, University of Leuven, Leuven, Belgium, **3** Division of Advanced Prosthetic Dentistry, Tohoku University Graduate School of Dentistry, Sendai, Japan, **4** Institute for Biomechanics, ETH Zurich, Zurich, Switzerland

Abstract

Background: Mechanical loading is known to play an important role in bone remodelling. This study aimed to evaluate the effect of high- and low-frequency axial loading, applied directly to the implant, on peri-implant bone healing and implant osseointegration.

Methodology: Titanium implants were bilaterally installed in rat tibiae. For every animal, one implant was loaded (test) while the other one was not (control). The test implants were randomly divided into 8 groups according to 4 loading regimes and 2 experimental periods (1 and 4 weeks). The loaded implants were subject to an axial displacement. Within the high- (HF, 40 Hz) or low-frequency (LF, 8 Hz) loading category, the displacements varied 2-fold and were ranked as low- or high-magnitude (LM, HM), respectively. The strain rate amplitudes were kept constant between the two frequency groups. This resulted in the following 4 loading regimes: 1) HF-LM, 40 Hz-8 μm; 2) HF-HM, 40 Hz-16 μm; 3) LF-LM, 8 Hz-41 μm; 4) LF-HM, 8 Hz-82 μm. The tissue samples were processed for resin embedding and subjected to histological and histomorphometrical analyses. Data were analyzed statistically with the significance set at $p<0.05$.

Principal Findings: After loading for 4 weeks, HF-LM loading (40 Hz-8 μm) induced more bone-to-implant contact (BIC) at the level of the cortex compared to its unloaded control. No significant effect of the four loading regimes on the peri-implant bone fraction (BF) was found in the 2 experimental periods.

Conclusions: The stimulatory effect of immediate implant loading on bone-to-implant contact was only observed in case of high-frequency (40 Hz) low-magnitude (8 μm) loading. The applied load regimes failed to influence the peri-implant bone mass.

Editor: Ryan Keith Roeder, University of Notre Dame, United States of America

Funding: This study was supported by the Research Council of University of Leuven (OT/07/059). The funders had no role in study design, data collection and analysis, decision to publish, or preparation of the manuscript.

Competing Interests: The authors have declared that no competing interests exist.

* E-mail: Joke.Duyck@uz.kuleuven.ac.be

Introduction

Bone tissue is metabolically active in adapting its mass, shape and structure to mechanical stimuli through remodelling. Mechanical loading has been proven to direct the differentiation of mesenchymal stem cells towards the osteoblastic lineage and has therefore been introduced to facilitate fracture healing and to improve bone quality [1,2,3,4]. In animal studies, the anabolic effect of mechanical loading on bone tissue has been evidenced when applied at both high- and low-frequency [2,5].

The effect of mechanical loading on bone regeneration and adaptation also applies to bone around biomaterials, and more specifically around titanium implants [6,7,8]. Findings from *in vivo* studies have shown that force- [9,10,11] or displacement- [7,8,12,13] controlled mechanical loading at low-frequency (<10 Hz), when applied directly onto an implant, can improve bone formation in the peri-implant region and can therefore contribute to implant osseointegration. Recent research also revealed that high-frequency loading (>10 Hz), applied via whole body vibration, can lead to increased bone formation in the peri-implant surroundings and ultimately to an improved osseointegration [14,15,16]. An early investigation revealed a pronounced peri-implant bone response to both high- (20 Hz) and low-frequency (1 Hz) loading [17].

Despite the above notions, further research on the peri-implant tissue response to mechanical loading at high- *versus* low-frequency is warranted due to the variety of animal models and of loading modes (*i.e.* the loading was directly or indirectly applied onto the implant) used in the aforementioned studies [5–11]. Furthermore, the impact of the loading magnitude in high- *versus* low-frequency loading regimes is only partly unraveled. There is evidence that up to a certain limit, the load-induced bone gain is determined by the loading magnitude in a low-frequency regime [18,19,20,21]. In case of high-frequency stimulation, however, the loading magnitude is reported to be less relevant [5,22]. To explore the therapeutic potential of high-frequency mechanical loading in titanium implant healing, it is valuable to fill this knowledge gap and hence to determine appropriate loading strategies.

By use of a rat tibia model and a displacement-controlled loading device, the present study aimed to investigate the influence of controlled mechanical loading, directly applied to the implant and immediately after implant installation, at high- *versus* low-frequency on peri-implant bone (re)modelling and implant osseointegration. It was hypothesized that (i) the peri-implant bone responds to high- and low-frequency loading; and that (ii) this bone response depends on the applied loading magnitude.

Materials and Methods

Ethics Statement

The research protocol was approved by the ethical committee for laboratory animal research of the KU Leuven (P029/2008) and was performed according to the Belgian animal welfare regulations and guidelines.

Animals and Surgical Procedure

Seventy-five male Wistar rats (3 months old) with an average weight of 349.8 g (S.D. ±7.9) were used in the present study. Out of these, 8 rats were used for defining the desired strain magnitude induced by loading (*ex vivo* load calibration). The remaining 67 rats were used for *in vivo* loading. Custom-made cylindrical implants (ø: 2 mm×L: 10 mm) were obtained from titanium rods (99.6% Ti, Goodfellow Cambridge Ltd., Huntingdon, England). The cylindrical endosseous part of the implant was screw-shaped; the percutaneous part was non-threaded hexagonal (Figure 1A). The implants were cleaned in an ultrasonic bath with distilled water and etched with a solution of HF (4%) and HNO_3 (20%), resulting in a roughness value (Ra) of 0.45 μm. Implants were sterilized by high-pressure steam heating at 121°C (15 lb./sq. in.) for 20 minutes prior to surgery. The implants were inserted bi-laterally in the medio-proximal site of the tibia.

Implantation was performed under full anesthesia induced by 2.5% isoflurane inhalation (Isoflurane USPR, Halocarbon, NJ, USA). A longitudinal incision was made on the medial side of the proximal tibia and the bone surface was exposed. Perpendicular to the tibial long axis, a cavity was made by perforating both cortices at low rotational speed under constant saline cooling. A surgical drill, 0.3 mm undersized compared to the implant diameter, was used as the final drill for cavity preparation. The implant was inserted manually into the bone using a custom-fit wrench, the wound was closed with resorbable sutures (Vicryl® 3-0, Ethicon, USA). Part of the implant was non-submerged, resulting in percutaneous protrusion and allowing direct access for loading. At the end of the experiment, the animals were sacrificed by cervical displacement under isoflurane-induced anesthesia.

Ex vivo Strain Gauge Measurement

Ex vivo strain gauge measurements were performed to correlate the loading magnitude (*i.e.* implant displacement) with the resulting peri-implant bone strain. For this purpose, 8 rat hind limbs were excised. After exposure of the medial surface of each tibia, an implant was inserted. The limb was placed on a rotating platform and fixated through clamping at the proximal (knee) and distal (ankle) joint. The position of the platform was determined in such a way that the implant and the loading pin were aligned (Figure 1B). A single element strain gauge (type FLG-02-11, TML, Tokyo Sokki Kenkyujo Co., Ltd., Japan) was glued on the exposed bone surface of the tibia, 1 mm above the implant. The lead wires (type 3WP008, Feteris Components BV, UK) were connected at one end to the strain gauge through bondable terminals (TF-2SS, Feteris Components BV, UK) and at the other end to the acquisition system.

Loading was performed by using a custom-made displacement-controlled device [23]. This loading device consisted of a piezo translator (preloaded closed-loop LVPZT translator, P-841.60, ALT, Best, Netherland), which can induce a displacement of up to 120 μm, and a load cell (XFTC 100-M5M-1000N, FGP Sensors, Les Clayes Sous Bois Cedex, France) with a capacity of 1000 N in tension and 100 N in compression. Strain on the surface of peri-implant cortical bone was recorded during displacement of the implants over 30, 50, 70 and 90 μm at a frequency of 1 Hz. The strain reading system included the acquisition of the signal (SCXI 1314, NI, National Instruments, Austin, Texas, USA), amplification, conditioning (SCXI 1520, National Instruments) and transmission to the PC (SCXI 1600 DAQ module, National Instruments). Labview software (Labview 8.6, National Instruments) provided the necessary interface and read-out. The measurements were repeated 5 times with complete removal of the specimen from the device and repositioning. A linear regression analysis was performed to determine the relationship between the applied displacement (μm) and the resulting strain (με).

In vivo Mechanical Loading

Rats were randomly allocated to 8 groups, corresponding to 4 loading regimes and 2 experimental periods (Table 1). For each animal, one implant was loaded while the implant in the contralateral limb was unloaded. The loading regimes consisted of high- (40 Hz; HF) and low- (8 Hz; LF) frequency protocols. Within each frequency category, the loading magnitude was defined as such that the maximum induced strain in the high-magnitude loading regime was 2-fold the strain occurring in the low-magnitude protocols. The defined loading frequencies and magnitudes resulted in identical maximum strain rate amplitudes for HF-LM and LF-LM, and for HF-HM and LF-HM. Loading was initiated one day post implant installation, and was applied axially (Figure 1B). The load application took 10 minutes per session and was performed 5 times a week for 1 or 4 weeks, respectively. Anesthesia induced by isoflurane inhalation (Isoflurane USPR, Halocarbon, NJ, USA) was applied during the loading.

Specimen Preparation

After sacrifice, the implants and surrounding tissues were isolated and immediately fixed in a $CaCO_3$–buffered formalin solution, dehydrated in an ascending series of ethanol concentration and embedded in polymerized methylmethacrylate resin. The tissue blocks containing the implants were sectioned along the longitudinal direction of the tibia and the implant's axis by a diamond saw (Leica SP1600, Wetzer, Germany). After polishing to a final thickness of 20 to 30 μm (Exakt 400 CS, Exakt Technologies Inc., Germany), the sections were stained with a combination of Stevenel's blue and Von Gieson's picrofuchsin red, visualizing mineralized (red) and non-mineralized (blue) tissues.

Histology and Histomorphometry

Histological observation and histomorphometrical analyses of the sections were performed under a light microscope (Leica Laborlux, Wetzlar, Germany) equipped with a high sensitivity video camera (AxioCam MRc5, Zeiss, Göttingen, Germany). Histomorphometrical analyses were carried out on both the proximal and distal side of the implant, at the cortical and the medullar level. The following parameters were measured by using

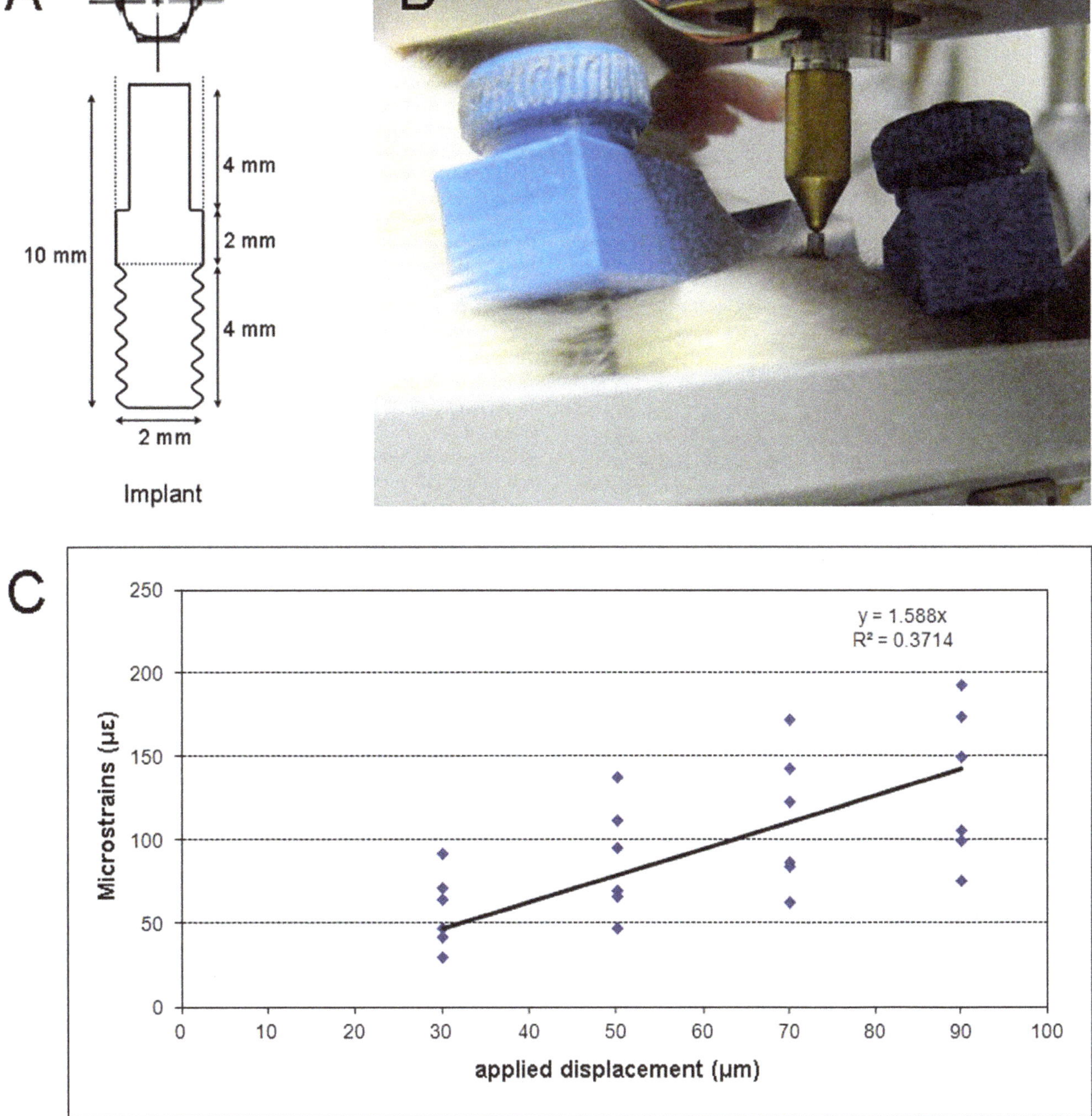

Figure 1. Titanium implants inserted in rat tibiae for *in vivo* loading and *ex vivo* strain gauge measurement. (A) Commercially pure (c.p.) titanium custom-made screw-shaped implant (ISO M2 screw-thread protocol). (B) *In vivo* axial loading applied directly onto the implant. (C) *Ex vivo* strain gauge measurements data on the correlation between the loading magnitude (*i.e.* implant displacement, μm) and the resulting peri-implant strain (με).

an image-analyzing software (Axiovision 4.0, Zeiss, Göttingen, Germany):

- Bone-to-implant contact (BIC, %) = 100 × summation of the lengths of the bone in direct contact with the implant/the implant length from the first till the last bone-to-implant contact.
- Bone fraction (BF, %) = 100 × area occupied by bone/area of the region of interest. Three different regions of interest (ROI) were defined: 0–100 μm (ROI1), 100–500 μm (ROI2) and 500–1000 μm (ROI3) away from the implant surface. The height of all ROI's was defined by the first till the last bone-to-implant contact (Figure 2).

Table 1. The applied loading regimes, the resulting mean strains and estimated strain rate amplitudes in the peri-implant environment, and the number of animals in each group.

	Loading regime		Mean strain and estimated strain rate amplitude		Group size (n)	
	Frequency (Hz)	Magnitude (μm)	Strain (με)	Strain rate amplitude (με/s)	1-week	4-week
HF-LM	40	8	13	520	9	8
HF-HM	40	16	26	1040	8	8
LF-LM	8	41	65	520	9	9
LF-HM	8	82	130	1040	8	8

HF-LM: high-frequency low-magnitude; HF-HM: high-frequency high-magnitude; LF-LM: low-frequency low-magnitude; LF-HM: low-frequency high-magnitude.

Statistical Analysis

Two-way ANOVA followed by Tukey HSD tests was performed to assess the effect of loading and time (*i.e.* the independent variables) on the peri-implant tissue response of BIC (*i.e.* the dependent variable). Three-way ANOVA followed by Tukey HSD tests was performed to assess the effect of loading, time, and region of interest (*i.e.* the independent variables) on the peri-implant tissue response of BF (*i.e.* the dependent variable) (SPSS ver. 13.0, Chicago, IL, USA). Data were reported as mean ± standard error of the mean (SEM). The significance level of $p<0.05$ was acknowledged.

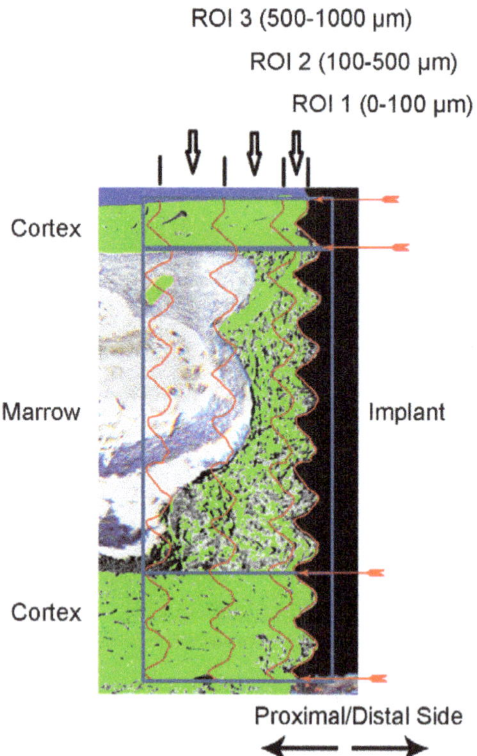

Figure 2. Illustration of the defined regions of interest (ROI) for histomorphometrical analysis of the peri-implant bone. Bone tissue is highlighted in green. The starting and ending points of the cortex and the marrow region that are subject to analysis are indicated by the red arrows. Three ROI's were defined according to their distance relative to the implant surface: 0–100 μm (ROI1), 100–500 μm (ROI2), and 500–1000 μm (ROI3).

Results

Animal and Implant Outcome

Implant surgery and *in vivo* mechanical loading were performed uneventfully for all except 3 implants. A total of 131 samples were obtained, of which 5 were excluded because of peri-implant infection and 3 were lost during histological processing. The remaining 123 samples were successfully processed for histology and histomorphometry.

Ex vivo Strain Gauge Measurement

The measurements on two limbs were not successful due to technical errors; these were not considered for analysis. For the measurements performed on the remaining 6 limbs, the regression between the applied loading displacement (μm) and the resulting strain (με) was determined (Figure 1C). Based on the established correlation, strains of 13 με and 26 με for the HF-LM and HF-HM loading regimes, respectively, were estimated. For the LF-LM and LF-HM loading protocols, strains of 65 με and 130 με respectively were induced for the selected loading magnitudes (Table 1).

Histology

The histological images revealed bicortical bone apposition to the implant for all the loaded and unloaded implants and for both healing periods (Figure 3). After 1 week, woven bone was formed along the implant surface in the medullar cavity, while remodelling occurred at the peri-implant cortex. After 4 weeks, the newly formed bone in the medulla was remodelled into lamellar bone close to the implant surface. Further, the healing of the peri-implant cortex was complete. No obvious differences between loaded and unloaded implant of the four loading regimes could be noticed on the histological sections.

Histomorphometry

Bone-to-implant contact. Out of the 4 assessed loading regimes, only cortical BIC was significantly increased in case of HF-LM (40 Hz-8 μm) loading for 4 weeks, compared to the unloaded control (83.49±2.23% *vs.* 72.44±5.47%; loaded *vs.* unloaded; $p=0.031$, ANOVA) (Figure 4A). No further pronounced loading effect on BIC was detected in the medullar region for the 4 loading regimes (Figure 4B).

Concerning the BIC changes over time, the BIC at the cortical level remained stable ($p>0.05$; ANOVA), whereas a significant increase from 1 to 4 weeks was observed at the medullar level ($p<0.001$; ANOVA). This BIC change was observed in all 4 loading regimes.

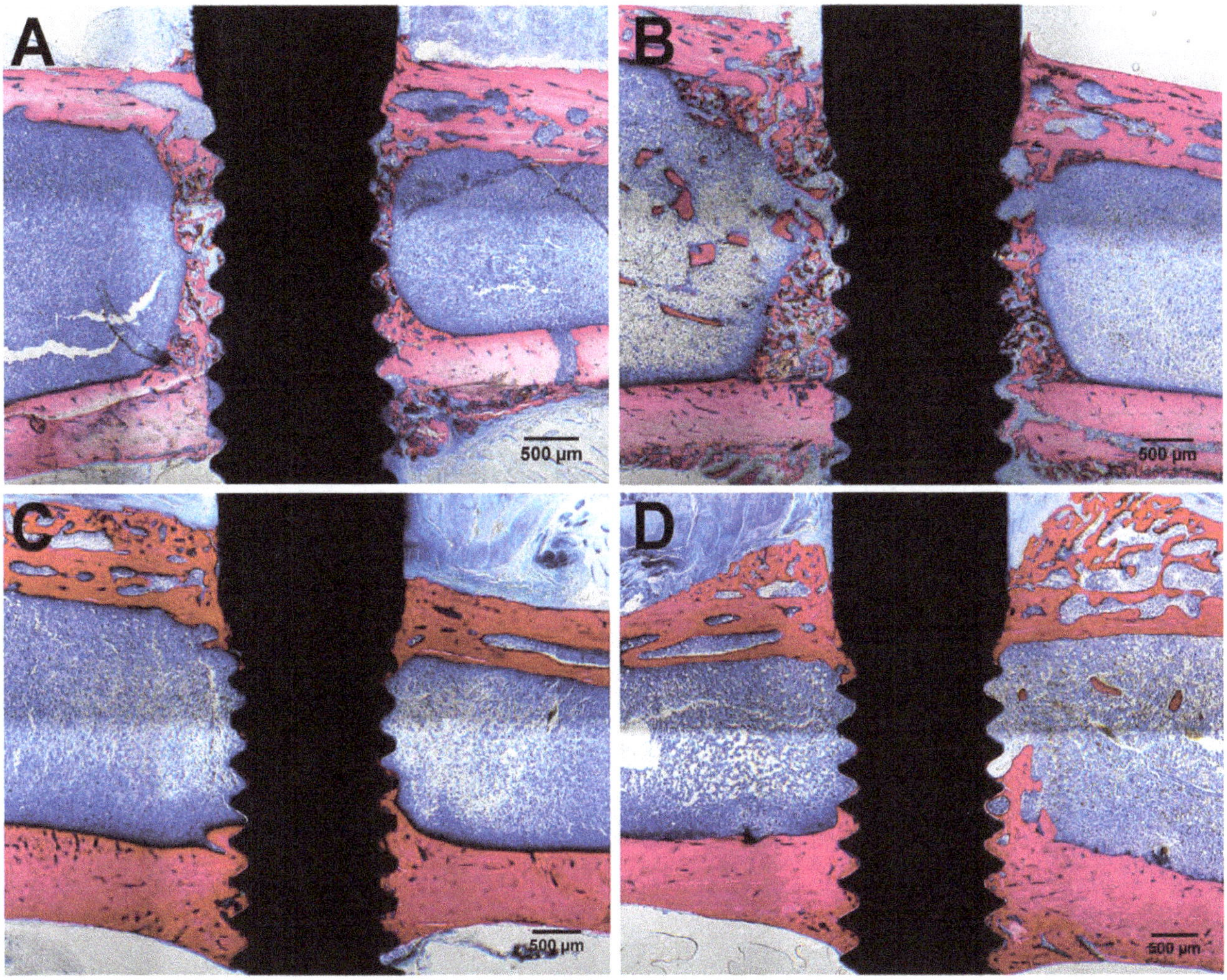

Figure 3. Representative histological sections. Above: for the 1-week experiment, peri-implant bone formation was observed in the medulla around both unloaded (A) and loaded (B) implants. Below: for the 4-week experiment, bone remodeling resulted in a dense bone layer appositioned onto the implant surface in the medullar region for both unloaded (C) and loaded (D) implants.

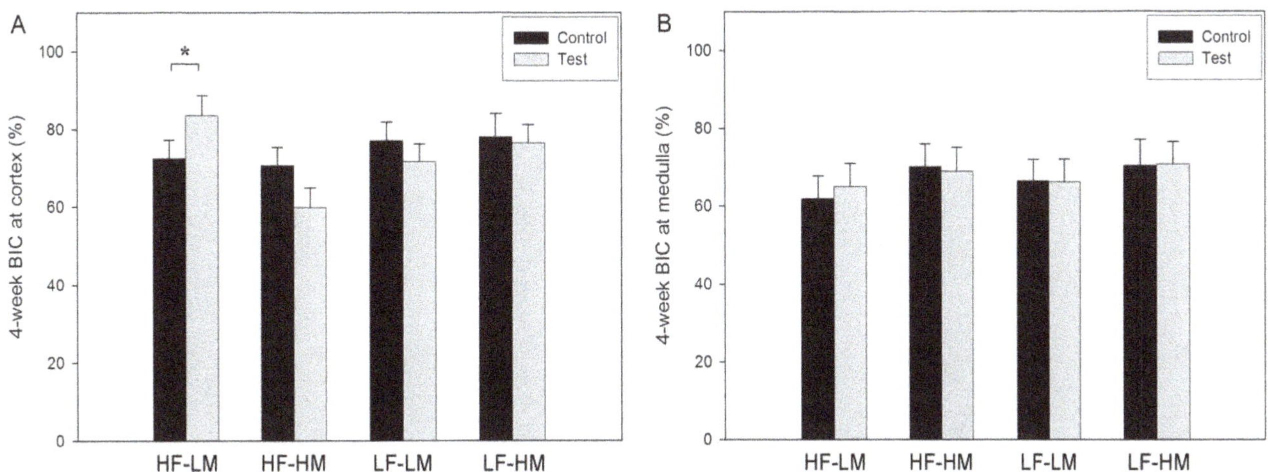

Figure 4. Bone-to-implant contact (BIC) at the cortex (A) and the medulla (B) for the 4-week experiment. Data of the 1-week experiment are not shown as no significant differences were detected (*: $p = 0.031$; ANOVA).

Bone fraction. The comparison between the unloaded and loaded implant revealed that the peri-implant BF of loaded implants did not significantly differ from the BF of the unloaded implants at both cortical and medullar level and for each loading regime.

As neither loading effect nor interactions between loading and time/ROI were detected for the 4 loading regimes, the BF data of the 4 loading regimes were pooled to assess the overall effect of time (*i.e.* the BF evolution over time) and ROI (*i.e.* the BF distribution in peri-implant region).

A significant increase of BF over time was observed at the cortical level ($p<0.001$; ANOVA). Inversely, a significant BF decrease from 1 to 4 weeks was detected at the medullar site ($p<0.001$; ANOVA) (Figure 5).

With regard to the BF distribution in the peri-implant region, again opposing results were found at cortex and medulla. At the cortex, BF significantly increased at further distance from the implant surface (BF in ROI 1<ROI 2<ROI 3, $p<0.001$; ANOVA followed by Tukey HSD). At the medulla, on the other hand, BF significantly decreased with increasing distance from the implant surface (BF in ROI1 >ROI 2>ROI 3) ($p<0.001$; ANOVA followed by Tukey HSD) (Figure 6).

Discussion

In the present study, implant osseointegration was assessed under immediate loading at either high- or low-frequency. It was hypothesized that (i) the peri-implant bone responds to high- and low-frequency loading; and that (ii) the response of the peri-implant bone depends on the applied loading magnitude. The main finding of the present study is that bone-to-implant contact is enhanced after 4 weeks of high-frequency low-magnitude loading. This effect, however, was not observed for the respective loading regime after 1 week of loading, or in case of high-frequency high-magnitude loading, or in case of low-frequency loading. Hence, the first study hypothesis is partly confirmed: a response of the peri-implant bone to direct immediate loading was only found in case of HF loading. At the same time, the suggested role of the loading magnitude (2nd hypothesis) on the peri-implant bone response was confirmed.

According to Frost [24], bone (re)modelling is triggered when the tissue deformation (strain) induced by a low-frequency loading exceeds a certain threshold (*i.e.* 1000 με). On the other hand, when applied at high-frequency, bone can sense and respond to mechanical signals at low magnitudes (*i.e.* from 5 to 10 με) [2,25]. Besides the magnitude of the strain, the strain rate amplitude (defined by both loading magnitude and frequency) is considered to be a determining factor for bone response to mechanical loading [26,27]. In order to define the role of the individual loading parameters (frequency, magnitude – corresponding to the displacement of the loading device, and strain rate amplitude) in immediate implant loading, 4 distinct but comparable loading regimes were defined in this study. The loading parameters were in part chosen based on reports of an anabolic effect of loading on bone [9,10,28]. The *ex vivo* calibration data provided information on which implant displacement was required to achieve a certain peri-implant bone strain. Considering the configuration of the loading device, 40 Hz and 8 Hz were selected as high- and low-frequency respectively. For both frequency categories, the loading magnitude was determined in such a way that identical strain rate amplitudes between the two frequency regimes were obtained. In studies from our group [10,11,28], the peri-implant strain rate amplitude favoring bone formation was found to be 267 με/s to 1600 με/s at low-frequency (3 Hz). In the present study, strain rate amplitudes of 520 με/s and 1040 με/s were achieved by loading magnitudes of 41 μm and 82 μm (leading to strains of 65 με and 130 με) for a low-frequency regime (8 Hz). Accordingly, for high-frequency loading (40 Hz), the estimated strains of 13 με and 26 με induced by loading magnitudes of 8 μm and 16 μm respectively resulted in identical strain rate amplitudes compared with the low-frequency regime. In this way, comparable

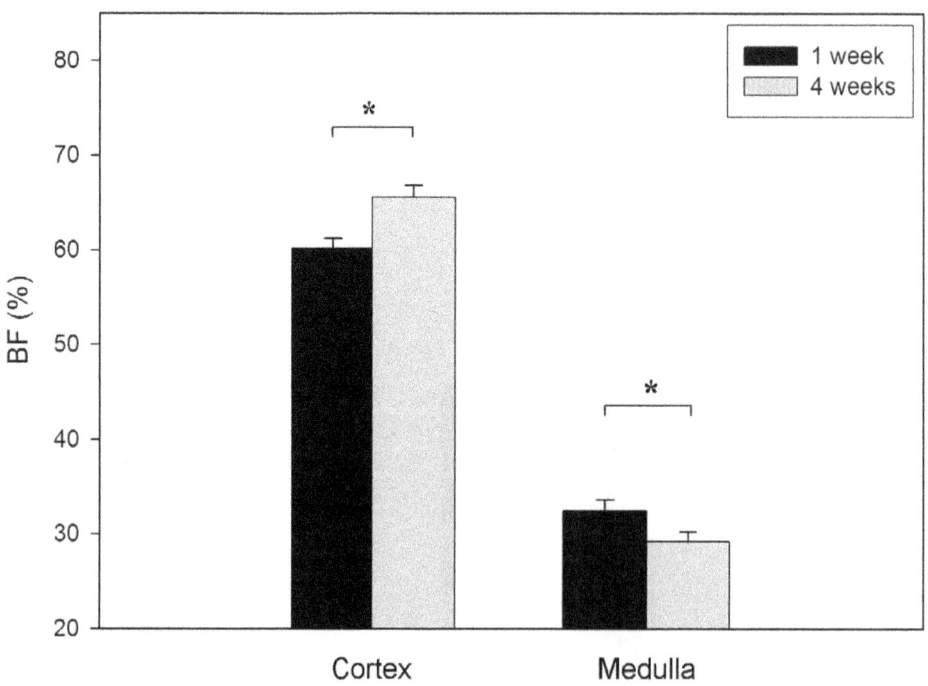

Figure 5. Cortical and medullar bone fraction (BF) evolution from 1 to 4 weeks (*: $p<0.001$; ANOVA).

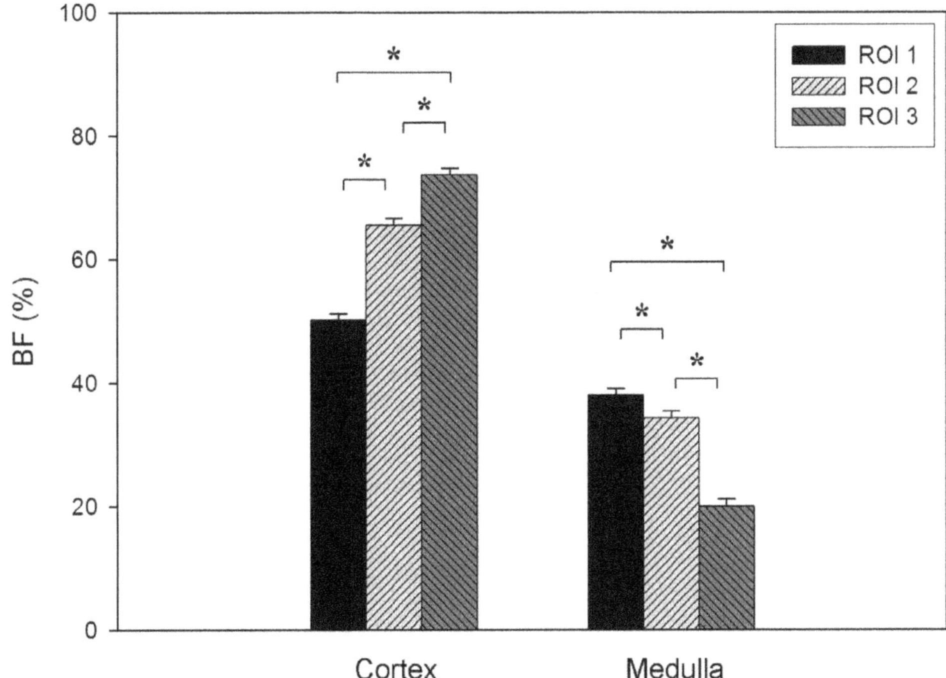

Figure 6. Cortical and medullar bone fraction (BF) distribution in 3 regions of interest (ROI) (*: $p<0.001$; ANOVA followed by Tukey HSD).

strain rate amplitudes, anticipated to be anabolic to the peri-implant bone response, were achieved.

Histological observations revealed a normal healing response after implantation, irrespective of the loading regime. These observations were in line with the histomorphometrical data. At the cortex, bone remodelling led to a bone gain in the peri-implant cortex over time (BF increased from 1 to 4 weeks), while the remodelling did not necessarily influence the direct bone contact with the implant (BIC remained stable over time). Compared to the distant host bone, on the other hand, the bone fraction in the direct implant vicinity remained lower, even after 4 weeks of healing. Histologically, the more prominent presence of blood vessels, playing an active role in bone remodelling, in the implant's vicinity, may explain this lower peri-implant bone fraction. In the peri-implant medullar area – an initially bone-free region – massive woven bone was formed soon after implantation. The formed bone originated from the endosteum of the peri-implant cortex and grew along the implant surface. Subsequent remodelling of this newly formed bone led to less but denser bone, in closer contact with the implant. With regard to the tissue evolution over time in this region, implant osseointegration (quantified as BIC) was found to increase from 1 to 4 weeks, whereas the bone mass (BF) around the implant decreased in the meantime. This is in line with previous findings with the same animal model [15,16].

The anabolic effects of high-frequency loading have been reported in a number of animal studies [5,29,30] and clinical trials [25,31,32]. Only few studies, however, investigated the effect of high-frequency loading on bone surrounding implants. De Smet et al. [28,33] applied high-frequency (30 Hz) loading onto implants 7 days after implantation. They revealed a bone stimulating loading effect in the medullar region. However, no loading effect on implant osseointegration was found. The discrepancy from the findings of the present study (*i.e.* increased cortical osseointegration by HF-LM loading) may owe to the different time of loading. As De Smet *et al.* [28,33] adopted an implant-healing time of 7 days prior to the loading, the impact of loading on the differentiating cells and tissues in peri-implant region can be diminished, compared to the loading initiated one day after implantation.

In another study, applying a high-frequency loading of 40 Hz directly on the implant, failed to improve the osseointegration [34]. In the mentioned study, however, a moment was applied instead of an axial force. Taking into account the detrimental effect of excessive micromotion and shear strains on osseointegration [7], it is logical that, in case of screw-shaped implants, load transfer from the implant to the surrounding tissues is more favorable in case of axial compared to rotational loading.

In the current experiment, HF-LM immediate loading was found to enhance bone-to-implant contact at the peri-implant cortex after loading for 4 weeks. Meanwhile, the high-magnitude loading at the same high-frequency failed to do so. In this respect, low-magnitude loading was better to promote cortical osseointegration. Furthermore, the gain in peri-implant cortical bone mass over time can be attributed to the inherent healing of the host tissue; neither low- nor high-magnitude loading was found to contribute significantly. Similar insignificant findings were observed in the peri-implant medulla. Potential loading effects are likely to be overruled by this active tissue repair and remodeling.

Similar to high-frequency loading, the effect of low-frequency loading on bone adaptation and regeneration has also been acknowledged [2,5]. Well-controlled mechanical loading at low-frequency, when applied directly to the implant, either in an early or immediate loading protocol, can improve bone formation in the peri-implant region and implant osseointegration [7,8,9,12,13]. Relatively small loading displacements were selected for the low-frequency loading regime in the current study. The resultant deformations by the loading were far below the (re)modelling threshold of 1000 $\mu\varepsilon$ recommended by Frost [24]. Although the applied strain rate amplitudes were identical to the ones in high-frequency loadings and considered osteogenic [11,28], no significant effect of low-frequency loading on implant healing was found in the present experiment. The implication might be that (1) to induce a positive bone response to mechanical loading, at least one of the constituting elements of loading (*i.e.* magnitude or frequency) needs to go beyond a certain threshold; (2) after fulfillment of the above condition, the impact of loading element combination (*i.e.* strain rate amplitude) on bone response can be considered.

The exact mechanism of how mechanical loading affects bone is yet unclear. Compared to the high-frequency loading, the host tissue perceiving the low-frequency loading is more dependent on the loading magnitude. When keeping loading frequency and the number of loading events constant, variations in strain magnitude can explain differences in the osteogenic response to the low-frequency loading. *I.e.* the larger the deformations generated in the bone, the greater the increases in bone mass [18,19,20,21]. This can be interpreted with relatively simple models such as the mechanostat [24] and the fluid flow theory [35]. According to the fluid flow theory, the load-induced fluid shear stress acts as the signal activating bone remodelling. The signal acts on osteocytes and cell processes in the lacunar-canalicular system. Therefore, the anabolic effect of low-frequency loading on bone is dependent on the loading magnitude which in turn affects the load-induced strain.

Under the high-frequency regime, the loading can also be sensed by the bone [22,36]. Local strains on the tibia surface have been recorded to be less than 10 $\mu\varepsilon$ in case of whole body vibration [5,37]. Apparently, the induced strain is extremely small, far less than the (re)modelling threshold of 1000 $\mu\varepsilon$ for the low-frequency loading [24]. Therefore, the notion has been called up that the anabolic response of the host tissue to the high-frequency loading was mainly dependent on the loading frequency, rather than the loading magnitude [5,36,38]. Explanations of this dependence were suggested by the theoretical models of You et al. [39] and Han et al. [40]. Their models were based on the facts that (1) osteocyte processes were attached along their length by tethering filaments, and (2) the actin filament bundle in dendritic processes led to a highly polarized cell whose processes were several hundred times stiffer than the osteocyte cell body [40]. Hence, the flow-induced drag on these filaments would produce a tension that could greatly amplify the very small whole tissue strains at the cellular level. By predicting the strain amplification ratio from the tissue to the cell level, they found that this amplification ratio not only increased with loading frequency, but also decreased with loading magnitude [39]. Therefore, under high-frequency loading, low bone strains were amplified most, suggesting a more efficient mechanotransduction due to the cellular perception of the high-frequency signals. This "less is more" phenomenon is also supported by the findings of the high-frequency loadings in the present study.

The frequency referred to as low frequency in this study is in fact higher than 1 to 3 Hz, which is more commonly used as low frequency in other studies. Accordingly, the high strain (130 $\mu\varepsilon$) considered in this study is lower compared to what is usually referred to as high strain [9,10,11,17,41]. Nevertheless, as the loading parameters are interpreted relative to each other in this study, 8 Hz is considered to be the low frequency and 130 $\mu\varepsilon$ is considered as the high strain. Meanwhile, the amount of loading cycles of high- and low-frequency regimes was differing by 5 fold (*i.e.* 24000 *vs.* 4800 cycles for the loading duration of 10 minutes). Considering the above, further research of loading with lower frequency (*e.g.* 1 Hz) and constant loading cycles would be valuable to comprehend the role of high- *vs.* low-frequency loading on peri-implant bone. Another limitation to this study was that the exact mechanical environment at the implant interface remains unknown. More numerical modelling research is needed to identify the detailed mechanics of the bone-to-implant interface.

Although implant therapy is a successful treatment [42], there is room for improvement in case of compromised bone conditions (*e.g.* diabetic, osteoporotic, or irradiated bone). Acceleration of the osseointegration process to allow earlier function of the implant would also be welcomed by the clinical community. Whole body vibration proved its highly significant osteogenic potential around implants [14,15,16], but has the disadvantage that the ruling mechanical conditions in terms of load magnitude and frequency are poorly controlled. This study aimed to overcome this flaw by controlling load magnitude and frequency, but failed to induce such an explicit histological response to the mechanical stimulation compared to whole body vibration. The exact bone-stimulating mechanical environment as in case of whole body vibration could therefore not be mimicked by this direct loading protocol. The closest we get in understanding the local mechanical conditions, is by means of extrapolation of *ex vivo* strain gauge data towards the interface [43] and through numerical modelling [44,45].

In conclusion, the stimulatory effect of immediate implant loading on bone-to-implant contact was only observed in case of high-frequency (40 Hz) low-magnitude (8 μm) loading. The applied load regimes failed to influence the peri-implant bone mass.

Acknowledgments

Sincere gratitude is addressed to Mr. Michel De Cooman (Department of Electrical Engineering, ESAT, KU Leuven) for designing and constructing the loading device.

Author Contributions

Conceived and designed the experiments: XZ JD. Performed the experiments: XZ AT TO. Analyzed the data: XZ AT KV GHL IN JD. Contributed reagents/materials/analysis tools: XZ AT TO KV. Wrote the paper: XZ AT KV TO GHL IN JD.

References

1. Ozcivici E, Luu YK, Rubin CT, Judex S (2010) Low-level vibrations retain bone marrow's osteogenic potential and augment recovery of trabecular bone during reambulation. PLoS One 5: e11178.
2. Ozcivici E, Luu YK, Adler B, Qin YX, Rubin J, et al. (2010) Mechanical signals as anabolic agents in bone. Nat Rev Rheumatol 6: 50–59.
3. Kelly DJ, Jacobs CR (2010) The role of mechanical signals in regulating chondrogenesis and osteogenesis of mesenchymal stem cells. Birth Defects Res C Embryo Today 90: 75–85.
4. Schindeler A, McDonald MM, Bokko P, Little DG (2008) Bone remodeling during fracture repair: The cellular picture. Semin Cell Dev Biol 19: 459–466.
5. Judex S, Lei X, Han D, Rubin C (2007) Low-magnitude mechanical signals that stimulate bone formation in the ovariectomized rat are dependent on the applied frequency but not on the strain magnitude. J Biomech 40: 1333–1339.
6. Isidor F (2006) Influence of forces on peri-implant bone. Clin Oral Implants Res 17 Suppl 2: 8–18.
7. Duyck J, Vandamme K, Geris L, Van Oosterwyck H, De Cooman M, et al. (2006) The influence of micro-motion on the tissue differentiation around immediately loaded cylindrical turned titanium implants. Arch Oral Biol 51:1–9.
8. Duyck J, Slaets E, Sasaguri K, Vandamme K, Naert I (2007) Effect of intermittent loading and surface roughness on peri-implant bone formation in a bone chamber model. J Clin Periodontol 34: 998–1006.
9. De Smet E, Jaecques S, Vandamme K, Vander Sloten J, Naert I (2005) Positive effect of early loading on implant stability in the bi-cortical guinea-pig model. Clin Oral Implants Res 16: 402–407.
10. De Smet E, Jaecques SV, Wevers M, Jansen JA, Jacobs R, et al. (2006) Effect of controlled early implant loading on bone healing and bone mass in guinea pigs, as assessed by micro-CT and histology. Eur J Oral Sci 114: 232–242.

11. De Smet E, Jaecques SV, Jansen JJ, Walboomers F, Vander Sloten J, et al. (2008) Effect of strain at low-frequency loading on peri-implant bone (re)modelling: a guinea-pig experimental study. Clin Oral Implants Res 19: 733–739.
12. Vandamme K, Naert I, Geris L, Vander Sloten J, Puers R, et al. (2007) The effect of micro-motion on the tissue response around immediately loaded roughened titanium implants in the rabbit. Eur J Oral Sci 115: 21–29.
13. Vandamme K, Naert I, Vander Sloten J, Puers R, Duyck J (2008) Effect of implant surface roughness and loading on peri-implant bone formation. J Periodontol 79: 150–157.
14. Akca K, Sarac E, Baysal U, Fanuscu M, Chang TL, et al. (2007) Micro-morphologic changes around biophysically-stimulated titanium implants in ovariectomized rats. Head Face Med 3: 28.
15. Ogawa T, Possemiers T, Zhang X, Naert I, Chaudhari A, et al. (2011) Influence of whole-body vibration time on peri-implant bone healing: a histomorphometrical animal study. J Clin Periodontol 38: 180–185.
16. Ogawa T, Zhang X, Naert I, Vermaelen P, Deroose CM, et al. (2011) The effect of whole-body vibration on peri-implant bone healing in rats. Clin Oral Implants Res 22: 302–307.
17. Rubin CT, McLeod KJ (1994) Promotion of bony ingrowth by frequency-specific, low-amplitude mechanical strain. Clin Orthop Relat Res: 165–174.
18. Cullen DM, Smith RT, Akhter MP (2001) Bone-loading response varies with strain magnitude and cycle number. J Appl Physiol 91: 1971–1976.
19. Mosley JR, March BM, Lynch J, Lanyon LE (1997) Strain magnitude related changes in whole bone architecture in growing rats. Bone 20: 191–198.
20. Gross TS, Srinivasan S, Liu CC, Clemens TL, Bain SD (2002) Noninvasive loading of the murine tibia: an in vivo model for the study of mechanotransduction. J Bone Miner Res 17: 493–501.
21. Torrance AG, Mosley JR, Suswillo RF, Lanyon LE (1994) Noninvasive loading of the rat ulna in vivo induces a strain-related modeling response uncomplicated by trauma or periostal pressure. Calcif Tissue Int 54: 241–247.
22. Garman R, Rubin C, Judex S (2007) Small oscillatory accelerations, independent of matrix deformations, increase osteoblast activity and enhance bone morphology. PLoS One 2: e653.
23. Duyck J, Cooman MD, Puers R, Van Oosterwyck H, Sloten JV, et al. (2004) A repeated sampling bone chamber methodology for the evaluation of tissue differentiation and bone adaptation around titanium implants under controlled mechanical conditions. J Biomech 37: 1819–1822.
24. Frost HM (2004) A 2003 update of bone physiology and Wolff's Law for clinicians. Angle Orthod 74: 3–15.
25. Gilsanz V, Wren TA, Sanchez M, Dorey F, Judex S, et al. (2006) Low-level, high-frequency mechanical signals enhance musculoskeletal development of young women with low BMD. J Bone Miner Res 21: 1464–1474.
26. Goodship AE, Cunningham JL, Kenwright J (1998) Strain rate and timing of stimulation in mechanical modulation of fracture healing. Clin Orthop Relat Res: S105–115.
27. LaMothe JM, Hamilton NH, Zernicke RF (2005) Strain rate influences periosteal adaptation in mature bone. Med Eng Phys 27: 277–284.
28. De Smet E, Jaecques SV, Jansen JJ, Walboomers F, Vander Sloten J, et al. (2007) Effect of constant strain rate, composed of varying amplitude and frequency, of early loading on peri-implant bone (re)modelling. J Clin Periodontol 34: 618–624.
29. Omar H, Shen G, Jones AS, Zoellner H, Petocz P, et al. (2008) Effect of low magnitude and high frequency mechanical stimuli on defects healing in cranial bones. J Oral Maxillofac Surg 66: 1104–1111.
30. Goodship AE, Lawes TJ, Rubin CT (2009) Low-magnitude high-frequency mechanical signals accelerate and augment endochondral bone repair: preliminary evidence of efficacy. J Orthop Res 27: 922–930.
31. Rubin C, Recker R, Cullen D, Ryaby J, McCabe J, et al. (2004) Prevention of postmenopausal bone loss by a low-magnitude, high-frequency mechanical stimuli: a clinical trial assessing compliance, efficacy, and safety. J Bone Miner Res 19: 343–351.
32. Rittweger J, Beller G, Armbrecht G, Mulder E, Buehring B, et al. (2010) Prevention of bone loss during 56 days of strict bed rest by side-alternating resistive vibration exercise. Bone 46: 137–147.
33. De Smet E, Jaecques SV, Wevers M, Sloten JV, Naert IE (2011) Constant Strain Rate and Peri-Implant Bone Modeling: An In Vivo Longitudinal Micro-CT Analysis. Clin Implant Dent Relat Res.
34. Zhang X, Naert I, Van Schoonhoven D, Duyck J (2010) Direct High-Frequency Stimulation of Peri-Implant Rabbit Bone: A Pilot Study. Clin Implant Dent Relat Res.
35. Klein-Nulend J, Bacabac RG, Mullender MG (2005) Mechanobiology of bone tissue. Pathol Biol (Paris) 53: 576–580.
36. Judex S, Rubin CT (2010) Is bone formation induced by high-frequency mechanical signals modulated by muscle activity? J Musculoskelet Neuronal Interact 10: 3–11.
37. Xie L, Jacobson JM, Choi ES, Busa B, Donahue LR, et al. (2006) Low-level mechanical vibrations can influence bone resorption and bone formation in the growing skeleton. Bone 39: 1059–1066.
38. Christiansen BA, Silva MJ (2006) The effect of varying magnitudes of whole-body vibration on several skeletal sites in mice. Ann Biomed Eng 34: 1149–1156.
39. You L, Cowin SC, Schaffler MB, Weinbaum S (2001) A model for strain amplification in the actin cytoskeleton of osteocytes due to fluid drag on pericellular matrix. J Biomech 34: 1375–1386.
40. Han Y, Cowin SC, Schaffler MB, Weinbaum S (2004) Mechanotransduction and strain amplification in osteocyte cell processes. Proc Natl Acad Sci U S A 101: 16689–16694.
41. Zhang X, Vandamme K, Torcasio A, Ogawa T, van Lenthe GH, et al. (2012) In vivo assessment of the effect of controlled high- and low-frequency mechanical loading on peri-implant bone healing. J R Soc Interface.
42. Jemt T, Stenport V, Friberg B (2011) Implant treatment with fixed prostheses in the edentulous maxilla. Part 1: implants and biologic response in two patient cohorts restored between 1986 and 1987 and 15 years later. Int J Prosthodont 24: 345–355.
43. Qin YX, McLeod KJ, Guilak F, Chiang FP, Rubin CT (1996) Correlation of bony ingrowth to the distribution of stress and strain parameters surrounding a porous-coated implant. J Orthop Res 14: 862–870.
44. Torcasio A, Zhang X, Duyck J, van Lenthe GH (2012) 3D characterization of bone strains in the rat tibia loading model. Biomech Model Mechanobiol 11: 403–410.
45. Torcasio A, Zhang X, Van Oosterwyck H, Duyck J, van Lenthe GH (2011) Use of micro-CT-based finite element analysis to accurately quantify peri-implant bone strains: a validation in rat tibiae. Biomech Model Mechanobiol.

2

Focal Adhesion Kinase Plays a Role in Osteoblast Mechanotransduction *In Vitro* but Does Not Affect Load-Induced Bone Formation *In Vivo*

Alesha B. Castillo[1,2,3]*, Jennifer T. Blundo[3,4], Julia C. Chen[4], Kristen L. Lee[4], Nikitha Reddy Yereddi[4], Eugene Jang[4], Shefali Kumar[4], W. Joyce Tang[1], Sarah Zarrin[1], Jae-Beom Kim[2], Christopher R. Jacobs[1,3,4]

1 Department of Rehabilitation Research and Development, Center for Tissue Regeneration, Repair, and Restoration, Veterans Affairs Palo Alto Health Care System, Palo Alto, California, United States of America, **2** Department of Surgery, Stanford University School of Medicine, Stanford, California, United States of America, **3** Department of Mechanical Engineering, Stanford University, Stanford, California, United States of America, **4** Department of Biomedical Engineering, Columbia University, New York, New York, United States of America

Abstract

A healthy skeleton relies on bone's ability to respond to external mechanical forces. The molecular mechanisms by which bone cells sense and convert mechanical stimuli into biochemical signals, a process known as mechanotransduction, are unclear. Focal adhesions play a critical role in cell survival, migration and sensing physical force. Focal adhesion kinase (FAK) is a non-receptor protein tyrosine kinase that controls focal adhesion dynamics and can mediate reparative bone formation *in vivo* and osteoblast mechanotransduction *in vitro*. Based on these data, we hypothesized that FAK plays a role in load-induced bone formation. To test this hypothesis, we performed *in vitro* fluid flow experiments and *in vivo* bone loading studies in FAK−/− clonal lines and conditional FAK knockout mice, respectively. FAK−/− osteoblasts showed an ablated prostaglandin E_2 (PGE_2) response to fluid flow shear. This effect was reversed with the re-expression of wild-type FAK. Re-expression of FAK containing site-specific mutations at Tyr-397 and Tyr-925 phosphorylation sites did not rescue the phenotype, suggesting that these sites are important in osteoblast mechanotransduction. Interestingly, mice in which FAK was conditionally deleted in osteoblasts and osteocytes did not exhibit altered load-induced periosteal bone formation. Together these data suggest that although FAK is important in mechanically-induced signaling in osteoblasts *in vitro*, it is not required for an adaptive response *in vivo*, possibly due to a compensatory mechanism that does not exist in the cell culture system.

Editor: Roger Chammas, Universidade de São Paulo, Brazil

Funding: This work was supported by a Stanford Center on Longevity Postdoctoral Fellowship (ABC) and National Institutes of Health (NIH) grants AR45989 (CRJ) and AR54156 (CRJ). The Stanford Center on Longevity Postdoctoral Fellowship provided salary support for Dr. Alesha Castillo. NIH grants AR45989 and AR54156 provided support for consumables, reagents, cell culture work and animal husbandry. The funders had no role in study design, data collection and analysis, decision to publish, or preparation of the manuscript.

Competing Interests: The authors have declared that no competing interests exist.

* E-mail: alesha.castillo@stanford.edu

Introduction

Mechanical integrity of a healthy skeleton is maintained through the cell-based processes of modeling and remodeling, which are greatly influenced by external physical stimuli. The molecular mechanisms by which skeletal progenitors and bone cells sense and respond to mechanical cues is unclear, but it likely involves activation of force sensitive molecules or "mechanosensors" that, in turn, initiate an intracellular signaling cascade altering cell behavior and function. Focal adhesions are large dynamic complexes that link the extracellular matrix (ECM) through integrin-ECM binding to the intracellular cytoskeleton [1]. Transmembrane integrin heterodimers comprise the core transmembrane component of focal adhesions and bind directly to collagen and fibronectin, among other ECM molecules, via their extracellular domain. Their cytoplasmic tails bind cytoskeletal proteins including talin and paxillin, both of which link directly to the actin cytoskeleton. Indeed, integrins have been shown to be important in load-induced bone formation [2]; however, as integrins do not possess intrinsic enzymatic activity, focal adhesion-mediated signal transduction is carried out by associated molecules that initiate downstream signaling events including tyrosine phosphorylation [3], intracellular calcium release [4] and MAPK activation [5].

Focal adhesion kinase (FAK) is a 125 kD non-receptor tyrosine kinase that regulates focal adhesion dynamics [6,7,8], is required for anchorage-dependent cell survival [9,10], and is important in cell migration, proliferation and survival [11]. The protein structure of FAK includes 3 major domains: the central kinase domain, the N-terminal FERM (protein 4.1, ezrin, radixin and moesin homology) domain, and the C-terminal FRNK (FAK-related-non-kinase) domain, which contains the focal adhesion targeting (FAT) domain. The N-terminal domain contains a major FAK autophosphorylation site at tyrosine 397 (Tyr-397), which has been shown to regulate cell motility [12,13]. The C-terminal domain of focal adhesion kinase contains two tyrosine phosphorylation sites at Tyr-861 and Tyr-925 and four serine phosphorylation sites at Ser 722, Ser 840, Ser 843 and Ser 910 [14].

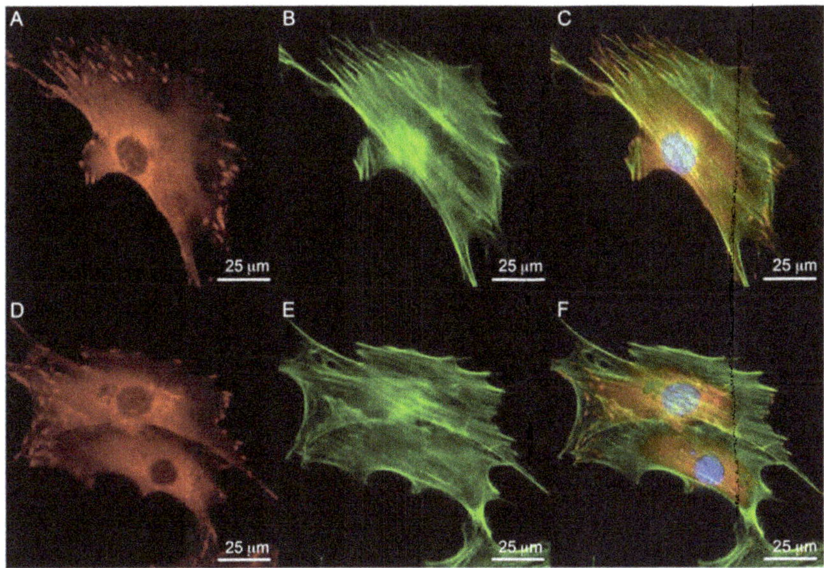

Figure 1. Focal adhesion formation and actin cytoskeleton in wild-type and FAK−/− osteoblasts. (A–C) FAK+/+ osteoblasts form focal adhesions (red) as shown by vinculin staining and display prominent actin fiber formation (green) as shown by phalloidin staining. (D–F) FAK−/− osteoblasts also exhibit actin fiber and focal adhesion formation. Panels C and F show merged images. DAPI nuclei stain in blue. Magnification = 60×. Scale bar represents 25 μm.

FAK been implicated in cellular mechanotransduction [15,16,17], including in bone cells [18]. Both bone and endothelial cells exposed to fluid flow shear stress *in vitro* exhibit increased FAK phosphorylation [18] and downstream MAPK activation [19], as compared to cells maintained in static culture. FAK phosphorylation has also been linked to NFκB activation [20] as well as calcium release via large conductance calcium channels [21]. Disruption of the FAK gene in osteoblasts *in vitro* leads to reductions in fluid flow-induced ERK phosphorylation, c-fos and Cox-2 expression, as well as prostaglandin E_2 (PGE_2) release [18], all of which are important signaling events for normal osteoblast function and bone formation [22,23]. Ablation of the FAK gene in osteoblasts and osteocytes *in vivo* slows bone regeneration and interrupts the response of bone marrow cells to anabolic mechanical stimuli in a tibial injury model [24,25]. Together, these data suggest that FAK plays an important role in osteoblast function; however, its role in mechanical adaptation of the skeleton *in vivo* is unclear. Furthermore, the precise phosphorylation sites on FAK essential to load-induced activation in bone cells have not been identified.

FAK relies on the focal adhesion associated proteins paxillin and talin to indirectly associate with integrins via their C-terminal domain binding sites [26]. Paxillin is an adaptor protein that binds vinculin and is phosphorylated by a range of growth factors, as well as by integrin activation [27]. Talin is a cytoskeletal protein that binds β integrin and activates focal adhesions [28]. Vinculin is a cytoskeletal protein that is part of the integrin-cytoskeletal protein assembly found at focal adhesions. It binds to several proteins including α-actinin, talin and paxillin, and is involved in integrin signaling [29]. Another protein that is an important mediator in integrin signaling events is proline-rich tyrosine kinase 2 (Pyk2). Pyk2 is a 116 kD cytoplasmic protein that has 45% sequence homology with FAK [30]. Overexpression of Pyk2 has been shown to result in apoptosis of fibroblast and epithelial cell lines [31], suggesting that it has an important role in mediating cell survival. Previous western blot analysis has shown increased expression of the activated versus the inactive form of Pyk2 in FAK−/− osteoblasts [32], suggesting co-dependence.

Based on previous studies, we hypothesized that FAK mediates load-induced bone formation. To address this hypothesis, we performed *in vitro* studies using clonal wild-type and FAK−/− osteoblasts and assayed PGE_2 release. Prostaglandins are released from bone cells as a result of mechanical stimulation [33] and are essential for load-induced bone formation *in vivo* [22]. We also transfected FAK−/− cells with wild-type FAK, Tyr-397, and Tyr-925 to determine importance of specific site mutations on osteoblast morphology, arrangement of cytoskeletal protein, and sensitivity to mechanical stimuli. Next, to determine whether these mechanisms are important *in vivo*, we subjected mice in which FAK was deleted in osteoblasts and osteocytes to three consecutive days of *in vivo* ulnar loading and analyzed bone formation rates and changes in bone geometry in response to axial compressive mechanical loading.

Results

FAK−/− osteoblasts exhibit reduced focal adhesion number relative to wild-type FAK osteoblasts

No differences in the actin cytoskeleton were observed (Figure 1). Vinculin expression and localization in FAK+/+ and FAK−/− osteoblasts were similar. Paxillin expression was observed in FAK+/+ and FAK−/− osteoblasts (Figure 2). The mean number of focal adhesions per cell area was significantly lower in FAK−/− osteoblasts (1.07×10^{-3}+/−0.55×10^{-3}; mean+/−SD) compared to FAK+/+ cells (2.84×10^{-3}+/−1.27×10^{-3}; mean+/−SD).

Phosphorylated Pyk2 localizes to focal adhesions in FAK−/− osteoblasts

Immunostaining for the activated form of Pyk2 (phosphorylated Tyr-402) is shown in Panels A and B of Figure 3. Panel A indicates localization of Pyk2 p-Tyr-402 to focal adhesions in FAK+/+

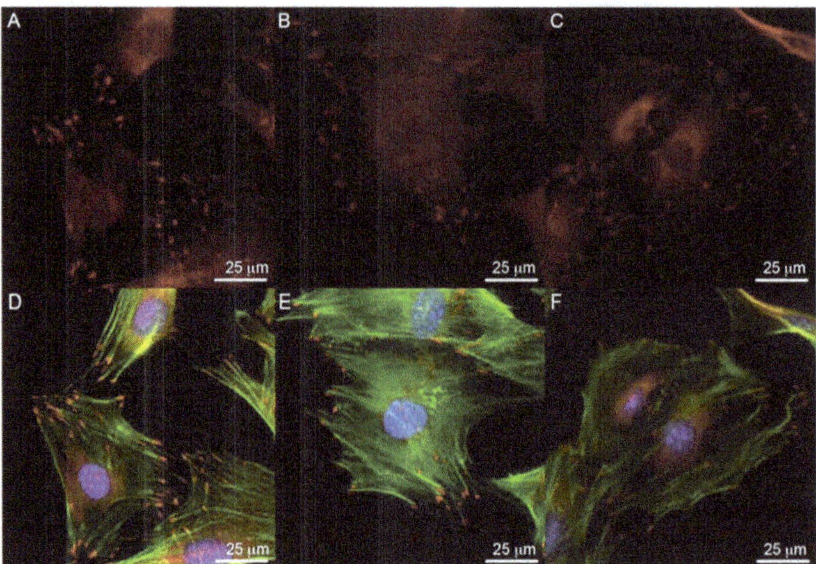

Figure 2. Paxillin expression and localization in osteoblasts. (A–C) Paxillin expression in MC3T3 osteoblasts, FAK+/+ osteoblasts and FAK−/− osteoblasts is similar. (D–F) Overlay of paxillin (red) and F-actin (green) as shown by phalloidin staining shows regions of strong paxillin expression and localization corresponding to the termini of actin fibers. FAK−/− cells exhibited fewer numbers of focal adhesions per cell area as quantified by point counting. DAPI nuclei stain in blue. Magnification = 60×. Scale bar represents 25 μm.

osteoblasts. FAK−/− osteoblasts also exhibited phosphorylated Pyk2 localized to focal adhesions, staining which appeared qualitatively more punctate but these observations were not quantified and further work is needed to explore changes in phosphorylated Pyk2 expression in the absence of FAK [24].

Absence of FAK impairs flow-induced PGE_2 release

Our results show that PGE_2 release is activated immediately following flow with a maximum 12-fold increase in PGE_2 release observed after 2 hours of flow and a 4 hour post-flow incubation (Figure 4, Panel A). FAK−/− osteoblasts exhibited only a ~5-fold increase in response to flow, a difference that was significant (n = 9–10, $p<0.05$).

Transient expression of FAK constructs partially restore flow-induced PGE_2 release in FAK−/− osteoblasts

FAK−/− osteoblasts were transiently transfected with three FAK constructs (wild-type FAK, F397 and F925) and exposed to OFF. Restoration of wild-type focal adhesion kinase by transient transfection resulted in a significantly greater fold-increase in PGE_2 release over the site-specific mutation constructs (n = 5–7, $p<0.05$) (Figure 4, Panel B). Cells transfected with site-specific mutations at Tyr-397 and Tyr-925 did not display any significant difference from the vector controls pcDNA3.1 (n = 5–7, $p>0.05$). Western blot analysis showed that FAK derived from the transiently transfected WT FAK construct was expressed at a level similar to FAK in FAK+/+ and MC3T3 cells (Figure 5).

Body weight and geometric properties of long bones in FAK−/− mice

Characterization of 16-week-old animals revealed that the average body weight of WT and FAK−/− mice was within 1.2% for males and 8.7% for females (WT male = 42.9±5.8 g; FAK−/− male = 42.4±5.3 g; WT female = 34.6±5.6 g; FAK−/− female = 31.6±5.5 g; mean±SD), a difference that was not significantly different. Baseline characterization of geometric properties of the femur showed that I_{MIN}, I_{MAX}, cortical thickness and cortical area (Ct.Ar) at midshaft, and femur length, were not significantly

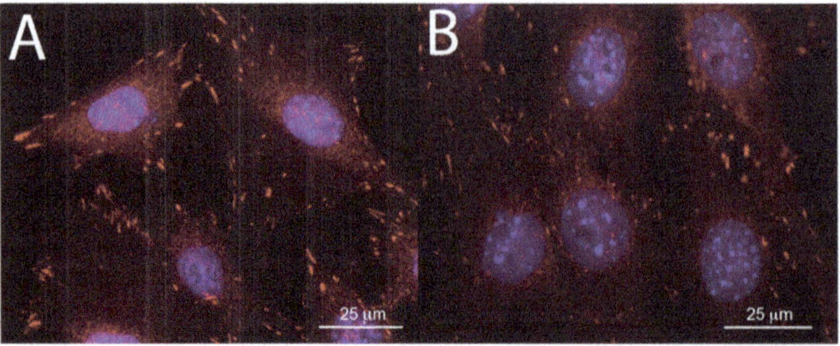

Figure 3. Expression of phosphorylated Pyk2 in FAK+/+ and FAK−/− osteoblasts. Expression and localization of phosphorylated Pyk2 at Tyr-402 (red) in FAK+/+ (A) and FAK−/− (B) osteoblasts. DAPI nuclei stain in blue. Magnification = 60×. Scale bar represents 25 μm.

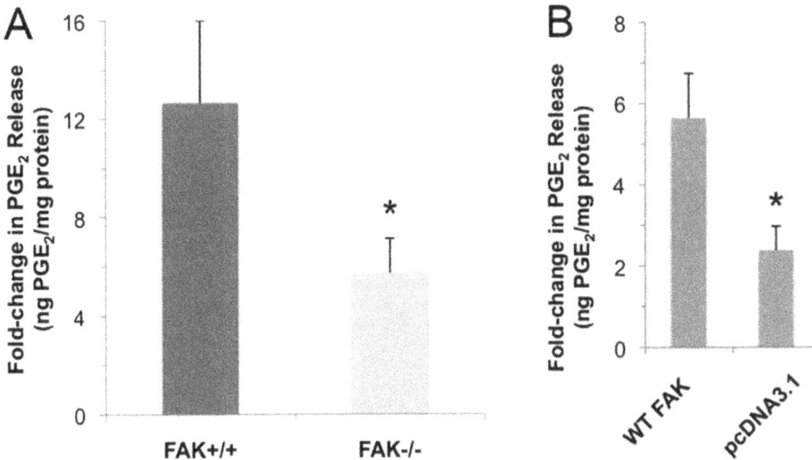

Figure 4. PGE_2 release in response to oscillatory fluid flow. (A) Fold-change in PGE_2 release in FAK+/+ and FAK−/− osteoblasts following 2 hours of oscillatory flow and a 4 hour post-flow incubation. FAK−/− osteoblasts exhibited a significantly lower fold-change in PGE_2 release in response to fluid flow compared to FAK+/+ osteoblasts. (B) Fold-change in PGE2 release following fluid flow in mutant osteoblasts transiently re-expressing wild-type focal adhesion kinase and phosphospecific site mutations. Note that differences in absolute fold-changes in PGE2 release following flow in Panel A and Panel B represent variations in parallel assays.

different between genotypes (Table 1) in male and female mice. In addition, no genotype-based differences were detected in the trabecular microarchitecture of the distal femur in male and female mice (Table 2).

Effect of conditional FAK deletion on mechanical adaptation of cortical bone

To determine whether conditional deletion of FAK had an effect on mechanical adaptation of cortical bone *in vivo*, we subjected animals to three consecutive days of ulnar loading (Figure 6), and measured fluorescently-labeled newly-formed bone *in vivo*. We estimated strain levels during loading using a load-strain dose response curve determined in *ex vivo* bones, a procedure that has been previously described by Turner and colleagues [34]. Results from the load-strain calibration procedure showed that WT and FAK−/− mice experienced similar strains at the same load level. Males experienced peak mean strains of 3250 ± 610 με (WT) and 3468 ± 495 με (FAK−/−) at 3.0N and females experienced peak mean ulnar strains of 3190 ± 610 με(WT) and 3270 ± 735 με (FAK−/−) at 2.8N. Gender did not affect bone formation parameters (ΔImax, ΔImin, rMS/BS, rMAR, rBFR/BS), and combining male and female bone formation data did not change the outcome of the analysis. Here we report male and female data separately. FAK−/− mice, both male and female, exhibited significant increases in Imax and Imin in loaded ulna (Table 3). The percent increase, however, was not significantly different between gender-matched genotypes. In both WT and FAK−/− mice, loading resulted in new bone formation on the endosteal and periosteal bone surfaces (Figure 7). The maximum difference in the mean among bone formation parameters was 16% and was not statistically significant (Table 4, Figure 8) by a t-test ($\alpha = 0.05$).

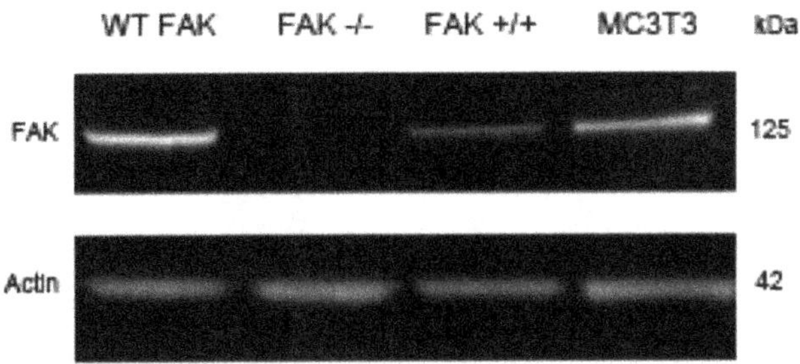

Figure 5. Western blot analysis of focal adhesion kinase expression in FAK−/− osteoblasts transiently transfected with the wild-type focal adhesion kinase (WT FAK) construct. Actin was used as a loading control. Expression in FAK−/−, FAK+/+, and MC3T3 osteoblast-like cells is shown as controls. WT FAK protein expression is similar to FAK expression in FAK+/+ and MC3T3 cells.

Discussion

FAK has been shown to be important in several cellular processes including migration [35], proliferation [36], and survival [37]. Global deletion of FAK is embryonic lethal [38], highlighting its important role in growth and development. Focal adhesions have been postulated to serve as mechanosensors in osteoblasts and osteocytes, and FAK is a key focal adhesion-associated signaling molecule implicated in mechanotransduction in bone cells. The main objective of this study was to determine the role of FAK in skeletal mechanotransduction. We hypothesized that FAK is critical in transducing mechanical forces into biochemical signals in the skeleton. We tested this hypothesis with FAK+/+ and FAK−/− osteoblast clonal lines in *in vitro* fluid flow studies to determine the precise role of FAK in osteoblast mechanotransduction. Deletion of FAK in osteoblasts *in vitro* was associated with fewer numbers of focal adhesions per cell area and reduced load-induced PGE_2 release, an effect that was reversed with the introduction of a wild-type FAK construct, suggesting that FAK can mediate an osteogenic response in osteoblasts. The observation that transient expression of constructs harboring mutations at Tyr-397 and Tyr-925 do not lead to flow-induced PGE_2 release suggests that these phosphorylation sites are involved in FAK-mediated mechanotransduction. One limitation of the present study is that mutant FAK protein expression levels following transient transfection of constructs could not be determined because anti-FAK antibodies did not recognize the mutant forms of the protein; however, transient transfection of the WT FAK

Table 1. Structural Properties of the Femur in WT and FAK−/− Adult Mice.

	Female		Male	
	WT (n = 18)	*FAK−/− (n = 32)*	*WT (n = 33)*	*FAK−/− (n = 15)*
Length, mm	16.11±0.47	16.04±0.61	16.47±0.40	16.45±0.46
I_{MAX} @ midshaft, mm^4	0.287±0.061	0.314±0.013	0.434±0.087	0.420±0.086
I_{MIN} @ midshaft, mm^4	0.166±0.037	0.164±0.045	0.239±0.060	0.219±0.038
Ct.Ar, mm^2	1.11±0.13	1.19±0.16	1.37±0.14	1.35±0.15
Ct.Th, mm^2	0.28±0.02	0.29±0.04	0.31±0.02	0.31±0.03

Mean ± SD; *n*, sample number; I_{MAX}, maximum second moment of area; I_{MIN}, minimum second moment of area; Ct.Ar, cortical area; Ct.Th, cortical thickness; $^a p<0.05$ versus gender-matched WT group.

construct into FAK−/− cells showed robust expression giving us a level of confidence that, in our hands, adequate levels of mutant protein expression are obtained.

We found that FAK cKO animals form bone with equal efficiency in response to mechanical loading compared to controls. While our *in vitro* data suggest that FAK is involved in osteoblast mechanotransduction, our *in vivo* loading data suggest that FAK is not required for load-induced bone formation in an intact system and presents the possibility of a signaling redundancy that compensates for a loss of FAK in osteoblasts and osteocytes.

Recent reports suggest an important role for FAK in reparative bone formation following skeletal injury. Using a mono-cortical tibial defect model, Kim et al. [24] showed that while progenitors were able to migrate to the site of skeletal injury and ultimately differentiate into mature osteoblasts, there was a delay in osteoblast differentiation and matrix formation in FAK−/− compared to WT animals. This difference was most evident 14 days post-surgery, but differences were lost by day 21. The authors concluded that integrin signaling via FAK was important for proper matrix deposition during healing, although deleting the FAK gene did not result in the complete abolition of matrix formation. Using a similar approach to study the role of FAK in load-enhanced reparative bone formation, Leucht et al. [25] applied a daily mechanical stimulus to a monocortical tibial implant during the healing process. Direct stimulation to bone marrow cells beneath the implant 1–3 days post-surgery and to the emerging bone regenerate 3+ days post-surgery enhanced osteogenic differentiation of bone marrow cells in WT animals during repair, but FAK−/− animals were unable to respond as robustly. They concluded that FAK inactivation blocked the ability of bone marrow cells to sense a mechanical stimulus and inhibited osteoblasts from forming matrix, suggesting an important role for FAK in mechanically enhanced bone repair.

One possible explanation for the discrepancy between our and their observations is that the ulnar loading model initiates new bone formation on the periosteal surface by activating progenitors residing in the periosteum, whereas, the tibial defect model triggers a bone healing process, which is comprised of several complex stages including inflammation, callus formation and remodeling. During the cortical repair process, a majority of the progenitor cells do not come from the periosteum but from the marrow or endosteum [39,40] whereby progenitors must migrate to the site of injury before laying down new bone. Thus, the temporal and spatial requirements for FAK may be different in reparative versus

Table 2. Trabecular Microarchitecture in the Distal Femur of Adult WT and FAK−/− Mice.

	Female		Male	
	WT (n = 18)	*FAK−/− (n = 32)*	*WT (n = 33)*	*FAK−/− (n = 15)*
BV/TV	0.031±0.016	0.048±0.018	0.072±0.031	0.078±0.030
Tb. N, 1/mm	1.61±0.36	1.65±0.57	2.27±0.60	2.30±0.48
Tb.Th, mm	0.061±0.011	0.066±0.013	0.062±0.007	0.063±0.010
Tb.Sp, mm	0.661±0.153	0.674±0191	0.472±0.120	0.449±0.140
Conn.D	7.2±3.6	10.5±2.7	25.8±17.9	27.8±23.6
SMI	2.5±0.6	2.4±0.8	2.4±0.4	2.4±0.7

Mean ± SD; *n*, sample number; BV/TV, bone volume; Tb.N, trabecular number; Tb.Th, trabecular thickness; Tb.Sp, trabecular spacing; Conn.D, connectivity density; SMI, structure model index; $^a p<0.05$ versus gender-matched WT group.

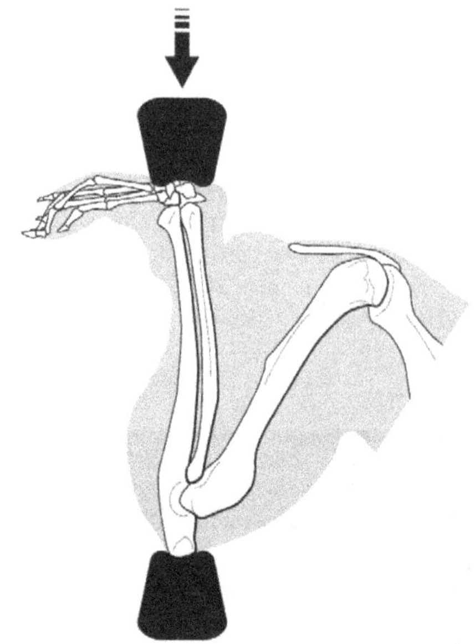

Figure 6. Rodent ulnar loading model. The right forearm in mice is subjected to cycle axial compression across the olecranon and flexed carpus while under isoflurane anesthesia. Due to the natural curvature of the ulna-radius complex in the medial direction, compressive loading creates a bending moment about the craniocaudal axis creating compressive and tensile bending strains on the medial and lateral surfaces, respectively.

Table 3. Structural Properties of the Ulna in Response to High-Load.

	Female		Male	
	WT (n = 16)	*FAK−/− (n = 16)*	*WT (n = 11)*	*FAK−/− (n = 12)*
Length, mm	13.91±0.41	13.60±0.57	14.63±0.49	14.49±0.36
I_{MAX} (initial), mm^4	0.0172±0.0063	0.0178±0.0048	0.0222±0.0046	0.0223±0.0063
I_{MAX} (final), mm^4	0.0177±0.0063^a	0.0180±0.0048^a	0.0228±0.0046^a	0.0228±0.0065^a
ΔI_{MAX}, %	2.64±2.08	1.50±0.90	2.83±2.22	2.23±1.93
I_{MIN} (initial), mm^4	0.0036±0.0006	0.0041±0.0005	0.0043±0.0010	0.0044±0.0007
I_{MIN} (final), mm^4	0.0041±0.0005^b	0.0045±0.0005^b	0.0049±0.0010^b	0.0048±0.0008^b
ΔI_{MIN}, %	12.85±8.45	9.58±3.21	14.8±8.19	10.16±6.12

Mean ± SD; *n*, sample number; I_{MAX}, maximum second moment of area; I_{MIN}, minimum second moment of area; Δ, percentage change in I_{MAX} or I_{MIN} shown in gray rows;
[a]$p<0.05$ versus initial I_{MAX} value by a paired t-test;
[b]$p<0.05$ versus gender- and genotype-matched initial I_{MIN} value by a paired t-test.

load-induced bone formation and may involve other molecular mechanosensing mechanisms.

Recent *in vitro* studies suggest a role for FAK in bone cell mechanotransduction [18,41,42]. Young et al. [18] showed that disruption of FAK signaling in osteoblasts attenuated the load-induced activation of several key osteogenic outcomes including ERK phosphorylation, c-fos, Cox-2, PGE_2 release, and osteopontin expression. Furthermore, the phenotype was rescued by re-expression of wild-type FAK. In a separate study, Santos et al. [42] reported that flow-induced activation of Wnt/β-catenin signaling in MLO-Y4 osteocytes was attenuated by the addition of FAK inhibitor-14. In addition, flow-enhanced proliferation of osteoblast-like cells was abolished with F397Y, a dominant-negative mutant of FAK [41] that blocks binding at the SH2 domain of Src-family non-receptor tyrosine kinases and Grb2 [43], both of which are important for integrin activated signaling.

We found that mechanically stimulated PGE_2 release in FAK−/− osteoblasts was impaired in comparison to FAK+/+ osteoblasts, a result similar to that reported by Young et al. [18] supporting a role for FAK in osteoblast mechanotransduction. Cells expressing FAK harboring a mutation at two major tyrosine phosphorylation sites, Tyr-397 and Tyr-925, exhibited no such release, suggesting that these sites are essential in mediating PGE_2 release following fluid flow. That is, autophosphorylation at Tyr-397 within the N-terminal domain and phosphorylation of Tyr-925 within the focal adhesion targeting C-terminal domain are important in transmitting external mechanical stimuli into osteogenic signals.

The presence of an intact cytoskeleton in the absence of focal adhesion kinase, even though the number of focal adhesions is reduced, still permits transmission of forces sensed at the points of cell-surface contact and permits other signaling molecules to compensate for the loss of FAK. This may explain the unaltered osteogenic response to *in vivo* loading observed in FAK−/− mice. Indeed, recent data suggest that Pyk2 may compensate for loss of FAK in various cell types including endothelial cells [44] and fibroblasts [45]. Others [24] have shown that phosphorylated Pyk2 was expressed more robustly in FAK−/− osteoblasts at focal

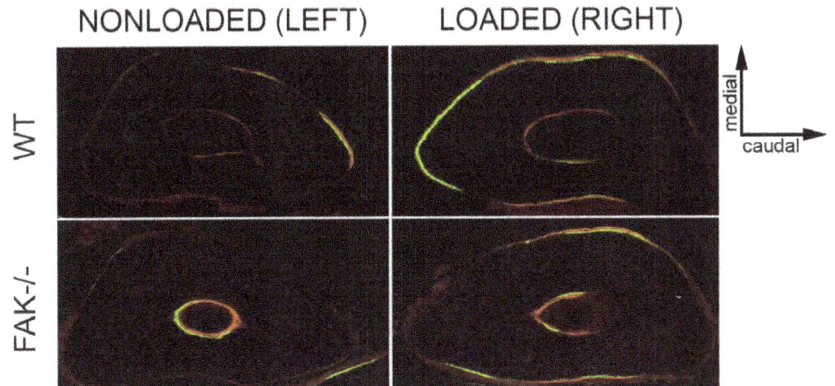

Figure 7. Transverse cross-sections at ulnar midshaft in nonloaded (left) and loaded (right) forearms in WT (top) and FAK−/− (bottom) mice given calcein (green) and alizarin (red) fluorochrome bone labels at 4 and 11 days, respectively, after the first day of loading. In response to applied mechanical loading, most new bone is formed on the medial and lateral surfaces where bending strains are highest. Note the appearance of double bone labels (green and red) on the medial and lateral surfaces of the ulna, as well as on the rostral surface, in the loaded ulna (top, right) compared to the nonloaded internal control (top, left) where very little bone formation is observed. The loaded ulna (bottom, right) in FAK−/− mice exhibit bone formation on the medial and lateral ulnar surfaces, but much less new bone formation, in terms of percent mineralizing surface, is observed relative to the nonloaded ulna (bottom, left). Sections are representative of the response observed for WT and FAK−/− mice. Magnification = 10×.

Table 4. Ulnar Bone Formation Parameters.

	Female		Male	
	WT (n = 16)	*FAK−/− (n = 16)*	*WT (n = 11)*	*FAK−/− (n = 12)*
NL-MS/BS, %	14.3±12.3	12.1±9.8	14.6±9.8	18.7±17.8
L-MS/BS, %	39.6±17.4[a]	37.9±10.7[a]	35.9±7.7[a]	42.0±14.6[a]
rMS/BS, %	25.3±19.1	25.8±12.0	21.3±9.1	23.3±15.1
NL-MAR, µm/day	0.57±0.16	0.59±0.21	0.65±0.27	0.78±0.34
L-MAR, µm/day	1.11±0.34[b]	0.94±0.22[b]	1.40±0.38[b]	0.31±0.31[b]
rMAR, µm/day	0.54±0.35	0.35±0.32	0.74±0.44	0.53±0.42
NL-BFR/BS, µm³/µm²/yr	32.23±30.43	29.0±28.5	39.4±38.3	72.8±86.2
L-BFR/BS, µm³/µm²/yr	171.3±104.5[c]	133.7±53.2[c]	179.9±56.7[c]	207.0±113.4[c]
rBFR/BS, µm³/µm²/yr	139.0±99.6	104.7±56.4	140.5±70.5	134.2±97.6

Mean ± SD; *n*, sample number; NL, nonloaded; L, loaded; r, relative values (initial-final) are shown in gray rows; MS/BS, mineralizing surface; MAR, mineral apposition rate; BFR/BS, bone formation rate;
[a]$p<0.05$ versus gender- and genotype-matched NL-MS/BS by a paired t-test.
[b]$p<0.05$ versus gender- and genotype-matched NL-MAR by a paired t-test.
[c]$p<0.05$ versus gender- and genotype-matched NL-BFR/BS by a paired t-test.

adhesions by immunofluorescence, suggesting enhanced Pyk2-focal adhesion interactions. Others have reported that Pyk2 expression levels are not altered in FAK−/− osteoblasts [18]; however, the change in localization of Pyk2 to focal adhesions may be sufficient to restore some functional activity to integrin-mediated mechanotransduction. In fact, Pyk2−/− mice exhibit increased bone formation due to disruption of osteoclast function [46] and repression of osteoblastic activity [47]. Furthermore, Turner and colleagues have shown that Pyk2 knockout mice exhibit greater load-induced bone formation rates compared to wild-type controls [48], suggesting that Pyk2 may normally repress an adaptive response to mechanical stimuli. While we did not definitively show that phosphorylated Pyk2 expression levels are altered in FAK−/− osteoblasts, expression qualitatively appeared more punctate. Additional data are needed to determine the precise role of Pyk2 in bone mechanotransduction *in vivo*.

In summary, we showed that FAK−/− osteoblasts were less responsive to mechanical stimulation *in vitro* as measured by PGE_2 release, and that Tyr-397 and Tyr-925 phosphorylation sites conferred functional activity; however, deletion of FAK in osteocytes and osteoblasts *in vivo* had no significant effect on the ability of mice to form bone in response to mechanical loading.

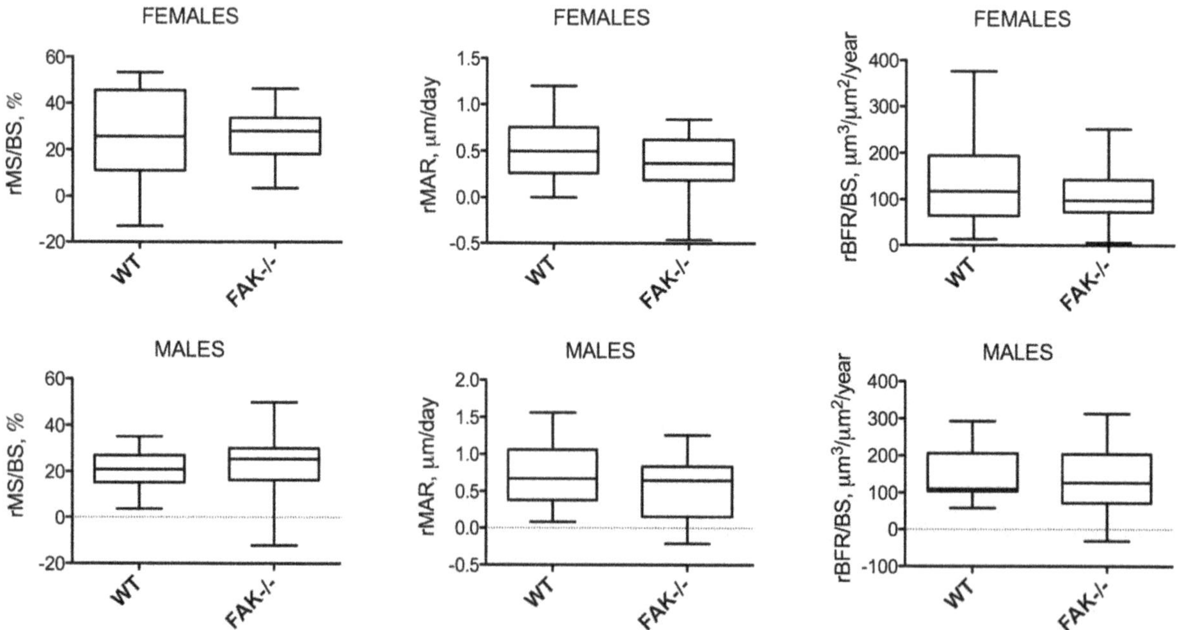

Figure 8. Relative bone formation parameters in WT and FAK−/− male and female mice. Conditional deletion of FAK did not affect relative mineralizing surface (rMS/BS), relative mineral apposition rate (rMAR) or relative bone formation rate (rBFR/BS), which is a product of rMS/BS and rMAR. Data are presented as box and whisker plots where the median, Q2, Q3 and whiskers, representing the 5% and 95% confidence intervals, are depicted.

These results challenge the current hypothesized role for FAK in bone mechanotransduction *in vivo* and suggest that alternative signaling molecules mediate integrin-specific signal transduction in mechanical adaptation of the skeleton.

Materials and Methods

Ethics statement

All work was performed in accordance with the guidelines of the American Association for the Accreditation of Laboratory Animal Care. In addition, the Palo Alto Veterans Affairs Medical Center Institutional Animal Care and Use Committee approved all procedures (IACUC No. CAT1350 CAT090501MOU, approved 03/27/12).

Bone cell culture

Primary immortalized osteoblastic clonal lines expressing native wild-type FAK (FAK$^{+/+}$ clone 1E11) and a FAK−/− mutation (FAK$^{-/-}$ clone ID8) were previously established as described in Kim et al. [24]. All cells were maintained at 37°C with 5% CO_2 in complete growth media (MEMα+ 10% FBS +1% Penicillin-Streptomycin). Cells were passaged using 0.05% trypsin (Invitrogen). Passages 7 to 9 were used in all experiments.

Transient DNA transfections

FAK−/− osteoblasts were transiently transfected with three FAK plasmids separately using Lipofectamine 2000 reagent (Invitrogen). An empty vector was used as a negative control. The FAK plasmids consisted of wild-type FAK [pcDNA3.1/Hygro(+)-WT], FAK with a site specific mutation at Tyr-397 [pcDNA3.1/Hygro(+)-F397 FAK], and FAK with a site specific mutation at phosphorylation site Tyr-925 [pcDNA3.1/Hygro(+)-F925 FAK]. FAK−/− osteoblasts were plated at 70–75% confluence onto 100 mm tissue culture dishes and grown overnight in antibiotic free media prior to transfection. The conditions for transfection were optimized by varying the ratio of plasmid DNA (µg) to the volume of Lipofectamine 2000 (µl) from 1:1 to 1:4 in Opti-MEM media (Invitrogen). The optimal transfection ratio (20 µg of plasmid DNA per 40 µl of Lipofectamine 2000 reagent) was determined by Western blot analysis for FAK protein expression. At 24 hours post-transfection, cells were used for described experiments.

Antibodies

Primary antibodies used were anti-mouse monoclonal FAK antibody (clone 4.47) (Millipore), rabbit polyclonal antibody against phosphospecific FAK Tyr-397 (Santa Cruz Biotechnology), rabbit polyclonal antibody against phosphospecific p-proline-rich tyrosine kinase 2 (Pyk2)-Tyr 402 conjugated to Alexa Fluor 488 (Invitrogen), chicken antibody against paxillin (clone 349) (BD Biosciences), monoclonal anti-vinculin (clone hVIN-1) (Sigma) and actin mouse monoclonal antibody (clone AC-40) (Abcam). Secondary antibodies used were goat anti-rabbit-HRP (Santa Cruz Biotechnology), goat anti-mouse-HRP (Santa Cruz Biotechnology), anti-mouse monoclonal FAK (clone 4.47) conjugated to Alexa Fluor 555 (Upstate), phalloidin-conjugated Alexa Fluor 488 (Invitrogen) and goat anti-mouse Alexa Fluor 568 (Invitrogen).

Western blot analysis

Expression of transiently transfected WT FAK construct was verified by Western blot. Cells were rinsed twice in cold PBS and lysed using RIPA lysis buffer (Santa Cruz Biotechnology). Cell lysates were sheared using a 21 gauge needle and centrifuged for 10 min at 16,000 rpm. The protein concentration of the resultant supernatants was quantified by bicinchoninic acid analysis (BCA) (Pierce Chemical). Protein was denatured for 10 min at 70°C, and 10–20 µg per lane were loaded into a NuPAGE 4–12% Bis-Tris polyacrylamide gel (Invitrogen) for separation and transferred to nitrocellulose for immunoblotting. Nonspecific binding sites were blocked with 5% bovine serum albumin (Sigma) in 1% Tris-buffered saline solution containing 0.1% Tween 20 (TTBS) for 2 hours at room temperature. After blocking, immunoblots were probed with FAK and actin antibodies diluted in 5% BSA/TTBS overnight at 4°C at a 1:1000 dilution and then incubated with goat anti-mouse (1:4000) and goat anti-rabbit (1:8000) antibodies conjugated to horseradish peroxidase (HRP) for one hour at room temperature. HRP was detected using Immun-Star WesternC Chemiluminescence (Bio-Rad) and quantified using an automated imager (LAS-4000, Fujifilm).

Immunofluorescence staining

To examine cellular morphology and localization of FAK, vinculin, talin, paxillin and Pyk2, MLO-Y4 osteocytes, MC3T3 osteoblasts, and wild-type FAK and FAK−/− osteoblasts were seeded onto fibronectin-coated cover slips and cultured overnight in 24-well plates. The cover slips were rinsed twice in PBS, fixed in 4% paraformaldehyde, and permeabilized in 0.1% Triton-X (Sigma). The samples were incubated in primary blocking solution containing 1% BSA in PBS (1% BSA/PBS) for 1 hour at room temperature. The cell-seeded cover slips were probed for focal adhesion kinase, vinculin, talin, or paxillin followed by the appropriate secondary antibodies (see *Antibodies*). Cells were imaged on an Olympus IX71 microscope mounted with a Hamamatsu C9100 digital camera. Images were captured and processed using MetaMorph software (Molecular Devices). The number of focal adhesions was quantified in wild-type FAK and FAK−/− osteoblasts. Focal adhesions were visualized by paxillin localization in individual cells and quantified by manual point-counting using Image J software. Individual cell area was determined by phalloidin-stained actin using a thresholding technique.

Oscillatory fluid flow (OFF)

An *in vitro* model of fluid flow in bone [49] was used to investigate the role of focal adhesion kinase in bone cell mechanotransduction. FAK$^{+/+}$ and FAK−/− osteoblasts were cultured on fibronectin-coated (10 µg/ml) glass slides at a density of approximately $2–3\times10^5$ cells/slide. Cells were incubated for 24 to 48 hours and serum starved in reduced serum media (MEMα+ 0.5% FBS +1% Penicillin-Streptomycin) overnight. At 80% confluence, cells were loaded into parallel-plate flow chambers as previously described [49]. Cells were exposed to laminar oscillatory fluid flow at a peak shear stress of 1 Pa (10 dynes/cm^2) and a frequency of 1 Hz for 5, 30 and 120 min to determine the time course of mechanically-induced PGE_2 release. The chambers were placed in the incubator at 37°C with 5% CO_2 throughout the duration of flow to maintain a constant temperature and pH. Static control samples were maintained in 100 mm tissue culture dishes at the same conditions. After flow, slides were immediately removed from the flow chambers and prepared for PGE_2 release.

Prostaglandin E_2 (PGE_2) release

Peak levels of PGE_2 release from FAK+/+ and FAK−/− osteoblasts were determined using ELISA. Immediately following OFF, slides were removed from the flow chambers, rinsed with warm PBS, placed in sterile tissue culture dishes, and covered with approximately 1 ml of fresh flow media. Following an incubation period of 4 or 24 hours at 37°C and 5% CO_2, media was collected and assayed. A PGE_2 Enzyme Immunoassay (EIA) Kit (Assay Designs) was used to measure PGE_2 concentrations in media samples per the manufacturers instructions.

Animals

The Palo Alto Veterans Affairs Medical Center Institutional Animal Care and Use Committee (IACUC) approved all experimental procedures. Global deletion of FAK results in embryonic lethality [50], therefore we deleted FAK specifically in osteoblasts and osteocytes by crossing mice with conditional floxed FAK alleles [24,51] (gift from Jill Helms, Stanford University) and transgenic mice harboring the Cre gene under the control of the 2.3-kb proximal fragment of the α1(I) collagen promoter [52] to generate experimental animals [$FAK^{flox/flox}$;Col2.3 α 1(I)-Cre^- (WT) and $FAK^{flox/flox}$;Col2.3 α 1(I)-Cre^+ (FAK−/−)] in which FAK was ablated in osteoblasts and osteocytes [51]. Offspring were on a mixed FVB/C67BL/6 background. Cre expression under the control of the 2.3-kb proximal fragment of the α1(I) collagen promoter is observed at high levels in osteoblasts and osteocytes [52] and results in effective deletion of FAK with a Cre-LoxP approach [24]. Previous studies show that Col2.3-Cre animals express Cre specifically in osteoblasts and osteocytes [52], and osteoblast/osteocyte deletion of FAK in the FAKfloxed::Col2.3-Cre offspring has been confirmed previously by *in situ* hybridization [24].

Offspring were genotyped using DNA from tail clips and primers P1(F): 5′-GAC CTT CAA CTT CTC ATT TCT CC-3′, P2(R): 5′-GAA TGC TAC AGG AAC CAA ATA AC-3′ and P3(F): 5′-GAG AAT CCA GCT TTG GCT GTT G-3′ [51] yielding a 327 bp fragment for the Cre-mediated recombined region (P1/P2), a 290 bp fragment for the WT allele (P2/P3) and a 400 bp fragment for the floxed FAK gene (P2/P3). $FAK^{flox/flox}$;Col2.3α1(I)-Cre- and $FAK^{flox/flox}$;Col2.3α1(I)-Cre+ male and female animals were used in loading experiments. Siblings were housed in groups of up to five animals at the VAPA Medical Center Veterinary Unit where they had *ad libitum* access to standard mouse chow and water. Animals were weighed at 16 weeks of age and body weight was recorded.

Micro-computed tomography (μCT)

Trabecular bone microarchitecture in the distal femur and cortical bone geometry at the femur midshaft were evaluated using high-resolution computed tomography (vivaCT40, Scanco Medical). The femur was chosen for analysis because it is a load-bearing bone and its distal region provides enough trabecular tissue for analysis of basal levels of trabecular bone in the adult skeleton. Bones were secured in a custom sample holder and scanned transverse to the long axis using a 55 kVp energy x-ray source and 2048×2048 pixel slices with a 10.5 μm isotropic voxel size. The slices were reconstructed using the manufacturer's software. From the resulting grayscale images, a region of interest (ROI) was manually outlined in each CT slice encompassing trabecular bone. For the distal femur, the ROI started at approximately 0.25 mm proximal to the distal femoral growth plate and spanned ~4 mm (400 slices) proximally. The edge of the ROI in individual slices was manually drawn at approximately 0.1 mm from the endocortical surface. The slices were evaluated at a fixed threshold to distinguish bone tissue from surrounding soft tissue. Approximately 200 transverse slices were evaluated for morphometric parameters including bone volume fraction (BV/TV, %), trabecular number (Tb.N, 1/mm), trabecular thickness (Tb.Th, mm), trabecular spacing (Tb.Sp, mm), connectivity density (Conn.D), and structure model index (SMI). SMI is a measure of the structure of cancellous bone and relates to the trabecular convexity. An ideal (flat) plate, cylinder and sphere have SMI values of 0, 3 and 4, respectively [53]. An ROI spanning ~1 mm was scanned at the femur midshaft, and approximately 50 slices were used to calculate cortical area (Ct.Ar), cortical thickness (Ct.Th), and moments of inertia I_{MIN} and I_{MAX} at the femur midshaft using Scanco software.

In situ ulnar strain analysis

Mechanical strains achieved during loading were measured as described previously [54] using 16-wk-old animals from each experimental group (n = 5 per group). Briefly, immediately following euthanasia (isoflurane to effect and cervical dislocation) the forelimbs were dissected free at the shoulder, keeping the soft tissue surrounding the forearm intact. The musculature was retracted exposing only the medial diaphysis of the ulna, and a 120 Ω single-element strain gauge (EA-06-015DJ-120, Vishay Measurements Group) was bonded to the surface with cyanoacrylate adhesive centered approximately 3.5 mm distal to the insertion point of the brachialis muscle. Previous studies showed that this was the most reliable method of positioning the gauge at the ulnar midshaft [34]. Each gauge was conditioned with a 0.8 V bridge excitation voltage and amplified with a gain of 300× using a signal conditioner (Model 2210, Vishay Measurements Group). The amplified analog strain signals were digitized using an AD-DA board (aISA-A57, Adtek-System Science, Kanagawa, Japan). For the strain calibration procedure, each forearm was axially loaded (Figure 6) using a Bose ElectroForce® 3200 mechanical testing machine at increasing peak load levels (1N, 1.5N, 2.0N, 2.5N and 3.0N). Voltage data for each of the loading waveforms were converted to strain values using a conversion factor determined by electronic shunt calibration of the measuring hardware and confirmed by calculated strains using an aluminum cantilever.

In vivo ulnar loading

Sixteen-week-old experimental male and female mice were divided into low, medium and high loading groups. Each group was subjected to axial cyclic ulnar loading while under isoflurane anesthesia (Baxter International) using the mechanical testing system described above. Due to the natural curvature of the ulna in the medial direction, loading in this manner causes bending about the craniocaudal axis creating compressive and tensile bending strains on the medial and lateral surfaces, respectively [34]. Thus, most new bone formation occurs on the medial and lateral surfaces where bending strains are highest. The applied force was controlled via load feedback using a 50 g load cell (Honeywell Sensotec). The right forearm was loaded on three consecutive days, while the left ulna served as an internal nonloaded control. Peak loads were 3.0N for males and 2.8N for females, which correspond to approximately 3500 με. All animals were given *in vivo* sequential bone labels at 7 (calcein, 30 mg/kg, IP) and 14 (alizarin, 50 mg/kg, IP) days after the first day of loading. Fluorochrome labels bind to calcium ions and are incorporated into newly forming matrix on bone surfaces. When labels are administered at different times, the amount of new bone formed between label administration times can be quantified using standard dynamic histomorphometric techniques.

At sacrifice, the right and left ulnae were harvested, fixed in 10% neutral buffered formalin for 48 h and stored in 70% ETOH at 4°C until further processing.

Histomorphometry

Right and left ulnae were dehydrated in sequential ascending concentrations of ethanol (70, 80, 90 and 100%) and embedded undecalcified in methylmethacrylate (Sigma) as described previously [55]. Three 90-μm thick sequential transverse sections were cut at the midshaft using an Isomet Precision Saw (Buehler Ltd.). The sections were ground to a final thickness of 50 μm and then mounted unstained on standard microscope slides. One section per ulna was analyzed at a magnification of 10× using a Nikon TE-2000/C1 confocal microscope (Nikon, Inc.). 'Measured' histomorphometric variables on the periosteal surface were obtained using ImageJ, and dynamic bone formation indices calculated. Variables measured included total bone perimeter (B.Pm, mm), single label perimeter (sL.Pm, mm), double label perimeter measured along the innermost label (dL.Pm, mm), and the interlabel width (Ir.L.Wi, μm), which is the distance between the first and second labels [56]. When only single labels were present on a bone section, mineral apposition rate was estimated as the minimum value observed in that particular experimental group [55]. 'Derived' or calculated variables were mineralizing surface (MS/BS = 100*[0.5*sL. Pm+dL.Pm]/B.Pm, %), mineral apposition rate (MAR = dL.Ar/dL.Pm/days between labels, μm/day) and bone formation rate (BFR/BS = MAR*[MS/BS]*3.65, $\mu m^3/\mu m^2$/year). Relative values (rMS/BS, rMAR, and rBFR/BS) for each animal were calculated by subtracting nonloaded (left) from loaded (right) values to control for individual differences between animals.

Structural properties of the ulna

Load-induced changes in cortical cross sectional geometry are represented by changes in maximum and minimum second moments of area (I_{MAX}, I_{MIN}), measures of resistance to bending about two perpendicular principal axes in the plane of the bone section. One section from the loaded (right) ulnar midshaft was imaged at a magnification of 10×. Initial and final cortical bone geometry was determined by observing bone labels administered at the beginning and end of the loading period as previously described [55]. Images of initial and final cross-sections were imported into ImageJ (Scion Corporation), and I_{MIN} (mm^4) and I_{MAX} (mm^4) were calculated for each image using a customized macro. Percent change in I_{MIN} and I_{MAX} before and after loading [$100*(I_{final}-I_{initial})/I_{initial}$] was calculated [55]. I_{MIN} and I_{MAX} were calculated directly from sections because it is only by visualizing bone labels that one can distinguish between cortical geometry both pre- and post-loading.

Data analysis

In vivo data were checked for normality and constancy of variance. The effects of gender and genotype on all outcome measures were analyzed by a two-factor ANOVA. When a significant effect of gender was detected, male and female data were analyzed separately. Estimated peak ulnar strain was calculated for each genotype using a load-strain calibration procedure. Unpaired t-tests (SPSS® Base 16.0 Statistical Software) were used to assess differences in males and females separately based on genotype in body weight, structural properties of the femur, and relative (loaded minus nonloaded) bone formation parameters in the ulna. Effects of mechanical loading were determined by comparing histomorphometric parameters and structural properties from loaded (right) and nonloaded (left) ulnae using a paired t-test. Statistical significance was assumed for $p<0.05$. Our experimental design yielded a minimum detectable difference of mean of 0.77 standard deviations with a statistical power of 80%. Data are presented as mean ± standard deviation (SD) except for relative bone formation parameters, which are presented as box-and-whisker plots showing the median and 95% confidence intervals. *In vitro* quantitative data are presented as the mean ± standard error (SE). A one-way ANOVA followed by a Bonferroni post hoc analysis (SPSS) was used to test for differences in PGE2 release between multiple groups. For two-sample comparisons, an unpaired Student's t-test was used. Statistical significance was assumed for $p<0.05$.

Acknowledgments

The authors thank Vasavi Ramachandran and Sara Temiyasathit Jones for their assistance with animal colony maintenance.

Author Contributions

Conceived and designed the experiments: ABC JTB JCC JBK CRJ. Performed the experiments: ABC JTB JCC KLL NRY EJ SK WJT SZ JBK. Analyzed the data: ABC JTB JCC JBK. Contributed reagents/materials/analysis tools: ABC JTB JCC KLL NRY EJ SK WJT SZ JBK CRJ. Wrote the paper: ABC JTB CRJ. FAK cell culture: JCC NRY EJ SK. Multiple transfection and subcloning strategies: JCC NRY EJ SK. PGE2 and total protein content assays: JCC NRY EJ SK. Flow experiments: JCC NRY EJ SK. Western blot: JCC NRY EJ SK. Imaged slides: KL.

References

1. Chen CS, Tan J, Tien J (2004) Mechanotransduction at cell-matrix and cell-cell contacts. Annu Rev Biomed Eng 6: 275–302.
2. Litzenberger JB, Tang WJ, Castillo AB, Jacobs CR (2009) Deletion of beta-1 Integrins from cortical osteocytes reduces load-induced bone formation. Cellular and Molecular Bioengineering.
3. Cary LA, Guan JL (1999) Focal adhesion kinase in integrin-mediated signaling. Front Biosci 4: D102–113.
4. Miyauchi A, Gotoh M, Kamioka H, Notoya K, Sekiya H, et al. (2006) AlphaVbeta3 integrin ligands enhance volume-sensitive calcium influx in mechanically stretched osteocytes. J Bone Miner Metab 24: 498–504.
5. Ishida T, Peterson TE, Kovach NL, Berk BC (1996) MAP kinase activation by flow in endothelial cells. Role of beta 1 integrins and tyrosine kinases. Circ Res 79: 310–316.
6. Hanks SK, Calalb MB, Harper MC, Patel SK (1992) Focal adhesion protein-tyrosine kinase phosphorylated in response to cell attachment to fibronectin. Proc Natl Acad Sci U S A 89: 8487–8491.
7. Kapur S, Baylink DJ, Lau KH (2003) Fluid flow shear stress stimulates human osteoblast proliferation and differentiation through multiple interacting and competing signal transduction pathways. Bone 32: 241–251.
8. Schaller MD, Borgman CA, Cobb BS, Vines RR, Reynolds AB, et al. (1992) pp125FAK a structurally distinctive protein-tyrosine kinase associated with focal adhesions. Proc Natl Acad Sci U S A 89: 5192–5196.
9. Hungerford JE, Compton MT, Matter ML, Hoffstrom BG, Otey CA (1996) Inhibition of pp125FAK in cultured fibroblasts results in apoptosis. J Cell Biol 135: 1383–1390.
10. Xu LH, Owens LV, Sturge GC, Yang X, Liu ET, et al. (1996) Attenuation of the expression of the focal adhesion kinase induces apoptosis in tumor cells. Cell Growth Differ 7: 413–418.
11. Wozniak MA, Modzelewska K, Kwong L, Keely PJ (2004) Focal adhesion regulation of cell behavior. Biochim Biophys Acta 1692: 103–119.
12. Sieg DJ, Hauck CR, Schlaepfer DD (1999) Required role of focal adhesion kinase (FAK) for integrin-stimulated cell migration. J Cell Sci 112 (Pt 16): 2677–2691.
13. Sieg DJ, Hauck CR, Ilic D, Klingbeil CK, Schaefer E, et al. (2000) FAK integrates growth-factor and integrin signals to promote cell migration. Nat Cell Biol 2: 249–256.
14. Ma A, Richardson A, Schaefer EM, Parsons JT (2001) Serine phosphorylation of focal adhesion kinase in interphase and mitosis: a possible role in modulating binding to p130(Cas). Mol Biol Cell 12: 1–12.
15. Lee HS, Millward-Sadler SJ, Wright MO, Nuki G, Salter DM (2000) Integrin and mechanosensitive ion channel-dependent tyrosine phosphorylation of focal adhesion proteins and beta-catenin in human articular chondrocytes after mechanical stimulation. J Bone Miner Res 15: 1501–1509.
16. Orr AW, Murphy-Ullrich JE (2004) Regulation of endothelial cell function BY FAK and PYK2. Front Biosci 9: 1254–1266.
17. Wen H, Blume PA, Sumpio BE (2009) Role of integrins and focal adhesion kinase in the orientation of dermal fibroblasts exposed to cyclic strain. Int Wound J 6: 149–158.
18. Young SR, Gerard-O'Riley R, Kim JB, Pavalko FM (2009) Focal adhesion kinase is important for fluid shear stress-induced mechanotransduction in osteoblasts. J Bone Miner Res 24: 411–424.

19. Li S, Kim M, Hu YL, Jalali S, Schlaepfer DD, et al. (1997) Fluid shear stress activation of focal adhesion kinase. Linking to mitogen-activated protein kinases. J Biol Chem 272: 30455–30462.
20. Petzold T, Orr AW, Hahn C, Jhaveri K, Parsons JT, et al. (2009) Focal adhesion kinase modulates activation of NF-{kappa}B by flow in endothelial cells. Am J Physiol Cell Physiol.
21. Rezzonico R, Cayatte C, Bourget-Ponzio I, Romey G, Belhacene N, et al. (2003) Focal adhesion kinase pp125FAK interacts with the large conductance calcium-activated hSlo potassium channel in human osteoblasts: potential role in mechanotransduction. J Bone Miner Res 18: 1863–1871.
22. Chow JW, Chambers TJ (1994) Indomethacin has distinct early and late actions on bone formation induced by mechanical stimulation. Am J Physiol 267: E287–292.
23. Lean JM, Mackay AG, Chow JW, Chambers TJ (1996) Osteocytic expression of mRNA for c-fos and IGF-I: an immediate early gene response to an osteogenic stimulus. Am J Physiol 270: E937–945.
24. Kim J, Leucht P, Luppen CA, Park YJ, Beggs HE, et al. (2007) Reconciling the roles of FAK in osteoblast differentiation, osteoclast remodeling, and bone regeneration. Bone 41: 39–51.
25. Leucht P, Kim JB, Currey JA, Brunski J, Helms JA (2007) FAK-Mediated mechanotransduction in skeletal regeneration. PLoS ONE 2: e390.
26. Mitra SK, Hanson DA, Schlaepfer DD (2005) Focal adhesion kinase: in command and control of cell motility. Nat Rev Mol Cell Biol 6: 56–68.
27. Delmas P, Nauli SM, Li X, Coste B, Osorio N, et al. (2004) Gating of the polycystin ion channel signaling complex in neurons and kidney cells. Faseb J 18: 740–742.
28. Tadokoro S, Shattil SJ, Eto K, Tai V, Liddington RC, et al. (2003) Talin binding to integrin beta tails: a final common step in integrin activation. Science 302: 103–106.
29. Clark EA, Brugge JS (1995) Integrins and signal transduction pathways: the road taken. Science 268: 233–239.
30. Sasaki H, Nagura K, Ishino M, Tobioka H, Kotani K, et al. (1995) Cloning and characterization of cell adhesion kinase beta, a novel protein-tyrosine kinase of the focal adhesion kinase subfamily. J Biol Chem 270: 21206–21219.
31. Xiong W, Parsons JT (1997) Induction of apoptosis after expression of PYK2, a tyrosine kinase structurally related to focal adhesion kinase. J Cell Biol 139: 529–539.
32. Kim JB, Leucht P, Lam K, Luppen C, Ten Berge D, et al. (2007) Bone regeneration is regulated by wnt signaling. J Bone Miner Res 22: 1913–1923.
33. Klein-Nulend J, Semeins CM, Ajubi NE, Nijweide PJ, Burger EH (1995) Pulsating fluid flow increases nitric oxide (NO) synthesis by osteocytes but not periosteal fibroblasts–correlation with prostaglandin upregulation. Biochem Biophys Res Commun 217: 640–648.
34. Robling AG, Turner CH (2002) Mechanotransduction in bone: genetic effects on mechanosensitivity in mice. Bone 31: 562–569.
35. Wang HB, Dembo M, Hanks SK, Wang Y (2001) Focal adhesion kinase is involved in mechanosensing during fibroblast migration. Proc Natl Acad Sci U S A 98: 11295–11300.
36. Pirone DM, Liu WF, Ruiz SA, Gao L, Raghavan S, et al. (2006) An inhibitory role for FAK in regulating proliferation: a link between limited adhesion and RhoA-ROCK signaling. J Cell Biol 174: 277–288.
37. Lim ST, Chen XL, Lim Y, Hanson DA, Vo TT, et al. (2008) Nuclear FAK promotes cell proliferation and survival through FERM-enhanced p53 degradation. Mol Cell 29: 9–22.
38. Ilic D, Furuta Y, Suda T, Atsumi T, Fujimoto J, et al. (1995) Focal adhesion kinase is not essential for in vitro and in vivo differentiation of ES cells. Biochem Biophys Res Commun 209: 300–309.
39. Monfoulet L, Rabier B, Chassande O, Fricain JC (2009) Drilled Hole Defects in Mouse Femur as Models of Intramembranous Cortical and Cancellous Bone Regeneration. Calcif Tissue Int.
40. Colnot C (2009) Skeletal cell fate decisions within periosteum and bone marrow during bone regeneration. J Bone Miner Res 24: 274–282.
41. Lee DY, Li YS, Chang SF, Zhou J, Ho HM, et al. (2009) Oscillatory flow-induced proliferation of osteoblast-like cells is mediated by {alpha}v{beta}3 and {beta}1 integrins through synergistic interactions of FAK and Shc with PI3K and the Akt/mTOR/p70S6K pathway. J Biol Chem.
42. Santos A, Bakker AD, Zandieh-Doulabi B, de Blieck-Hogervorst JM, Klein-Nulend J (2009) Early activation of the beta-catenin pathway in osteocytes is mediated by nitric oxide, phosphatidyl inositol-3 kinase/Akt, and focal adhesion kinase. Biochem Biophys Res Commun.
43. Schlaepfer DD, Hunter T (1996) Evidence for in vivo phosphorylation of the Grb2 SH2-domain binding site on focal adhesion kinase by Src-family protein-tyrosine kinases. Mol Cell Biol 16: 5623–5633.
44. Weis SM, Lim ST, Lutu-Fuga KM, Barnes LA, Chen XL, et al. (2008) Compensatory role for Pyk2 during angiogenesis in adult mice lacking endothelial cell FAK. J Cell Biol 181: 43–50.
45. Sieg DJ, Ilic D, Jones KC, Damsky CH, Hunter T, et al. (1998) Pyk2 and Src-family protein-tyrosine kinases compensate for the loss of FAK in fibronectin-stimulated signaling events but Pyk2 does not fully function to enhance FAK-cell migration. EMBO J 17: 5933–5947.
46. Gil-Henn H, Destaing O, Sims NA, Aoki K, Alles N, et al. (2007) Defective microtubule-dependent podosome organization in osteoclasts leads to increased bone density in Pyk2(−/−) mice. J Cell Biol 178: 1053–1064.
47. Buckbinder L, Crawford DT, Qi H, Ke HZ, Olson LM, et al. (2007) Proline-rich tyrosine kinase 2 regulates osteoprogenitor cells and bone formation, and offers an anabolic treatment approach for osteoporosis. Proc Natl Acad Sci U S A 104: 10619–10624.
48. Nguyen KT, Robling AG, Turner CH (2009) Knockout of Pyk2 improves the mechanical loading response of bone; Pittsburgh, PA.
49. Jacobs CR, Yellowley CE, Davis BR, Zhou Z, Cimbala JM, et al. (1998) Differential effect of steady versus oscillating flow on bone cells. J Biomech 31: 969–976.
50. Ilic D, Furuta Y, Kanazawa S, Takeda N, Sobue K, et al. (1995) Reduced cell motility and enhanced focal adhesion contact formation in cells from FAK-deficient mice. Nature 377: 539–544.
51. Beggs HE, Schahin-Reed D, Zang K, Goebbels S, Nave KA, et al. (2003) FAK deficiency in cells contributing to the basal lamina results in cortical abnormalities resembling congenital muscular dystrophies. Neuron 40: 501–514.
52. Dacquin R, Starbuck M, Schinke T, Karsenty G (2002) Mouse alpha1(I)-collagen promoter is the best known promoter to drive efficient Cre recombinase expression in osteoblast. Dev Dyn 224: 245–251.
53. Hildebrand T, Rüegsegger P (1997) Quantification of Bone Microarchitecture with the Structure Model Index. Computer methods in biomechanics and biomedical engineering 1: 15–23.
54. Robling A, Li J, Shultz KL, Beamer W, Turner C (2003) Evidence for a skeletal mechanosensitivity gene on mouse chromosome 4. The FASEB Journal 17: 324–326.
55. Castillo AB, Alam I, Tanaka SM, Levenda J, Li J, et al. (2006) Low-amplitude, broad-frequency vibration effects on cortical bone formation in mice. Bone 39: 1087–1096.
56. Parfitt AM, Drezner MK, Glorieux FH, Kanis JA, Malluche H, et al. (1987) Bone histomorphometry: standardization of nomenclature, symbols, and units. Report of the ASBMR Histomorphometry Nomenclature Committee. J Bone Miner Res 2: 595–610.

Activation of Fms-Like Tyrosine Kinase 3 Signaling Enhances Survivin Expression in a Mouse Model of Rheumatoid Arthritis

Sofia E. M. Andersson*, Mattias N. D. Svensson, Malin C. Erlandsson, Mats Dehlin, Karin M. E. Andersson, Maria I. Bokarewa

Department of Rheumatology and Inflammation Research, Sahlgrenska University Hospital, University of Göteborg, Göteborg, Sweden

Abstract

Survivin is known as an inhibitor of apoptosis and a positive regulator of cell division. We have recently identified survivin as a predictor of joint destruction in patients with rheumatoid arthritis (RA). Flt3 ligand (Flt3L) is expressed in the inflamed joints and has adjuvant properties in arthritis. Studies on 90 RA patients (median age 60.5 years [range, 24–87], disease duration 10.5 years [range, 0–35]) show a strong positive association between the levels of survivin and Flt3L in blood. Here, we present experimental evidence connecting survivin and Flt3L signaling. Treatment of BALB/c mice with Flt3L led to an increase of survivin in the bone marrow and in splenic dendritic cells. Flt3L changed the profile of survivin splice variants, increasing transcription of the short survivin40 in the bone marrow. Treatment with an Flt3 inhibitor reduced total survivin expression in bone marrow and in the dendritic cell population in spleen. Inhibition of survivin transcription in mice, by shRNA lentiviral constructs, reduced the gene expression of Flt3L. We conclude that expression of survivin is a downstream event of Flt3 signaling, which serves as an essential mechanism supporting survival of leukocytes during their differentiation, and maturation of dendritic cells, in RA.

Editor: Serge Nataf, University of Lyon, France

Funding: This work was funded by grants from the Medical Society of Göteborg, the Swedish Association against Rheumatism, the King Gustaf V:s 80-year Foundation, the Commission of European Union (HEALTH-F2-2010-261460), the Swedish Research Council, IngaBritt and Arne Lundberg Foundation, Professor Nanna Swartz Foundation, Torsten Söderberg Foundation, AME Wolff Foundation, Rune and Ulla Amlövs Trust, the Swedish Research Agency for Innovation Systems (VINNOVA), the Swedish Foundation for Strategic Research, the Pharmacist Hedberg's Foundation, Magnus Bergwall Foundation, the University of Göteborg, the Family Thölen and Kristlers Foundation, the Regional agreement on medical training and clinical research between the Western Götaland county council and the University of Göteborg (LUA/ALF). The funders had no role in study design, data collection and analysis, decision to publish, or preparation of the manuscript.

Competing Interests: The authors have declared that no competing interests exist.

* E-mail: sofia.andersson@rheuma.gu.se

Introduction

Survivin is an intracellular protein and a member of the inhibitor of apoptosis proteins (IAPs), with many functions in cytoprotection, cell division and cellular adaptation. It is encoded by the *BIRC5* gene on the human chromosome 17q25, into a 142 amino acid, 16.5 kDa protein but can be extensively alternatively spliced into several variants and form homodimers and heterodimers with two different splice variants, or an IAP-IAP complex by pairing with X-linked IAP (XIAP) [1,2]. Transcription of survivin is negatively regulated by p53 [3] and positively regulated by STAT3 [4] and TCF-4 [5].

Similar to human protein, full-length murine survivin (survivin140) contains a single BIR-domain, which is critical for its anti-apoptotic function [6], and a carboxy-terminal coiled-coil domain that links its function to the cell cycle [7]. Murine survivin121 contains a BIR-domain that makes it able to inhibit caspase activity but lacks the coiled-coil structure. Additionally, there is a splice variant that predicts a 40 aa residue protein (survivin40), which lacks both the BIR- and a coiled-coil regions. The differential expression of these forms of survivin is believed to affect the balance between cell proliferation and programmed cell death [8].

Survivin has only limited expression in adult tissues, but is overexpressed in tumors and is therefore regarded as a cancer gene. Survivin is expressed in a cell-cycle dependent manner with a peak at G2/M. Together with Aurora B, borealin and INCENP, survivin forms the chromosomal passenger complex, which is recruited to chromosomes by the phosphorylation by histones which is recognized by the BIR domain of survivin. In anaphase, the chromosomal passenger complex relocalizes to form the mitotic spindle and stimulate cytokinesis. The requirement of survivin during fetal development has been demonstrated by lethality of knockout embryos [1].

Survivin is also expressed independently of cell cycle progression and is linked to the inhibition of apoptosis [3]. The pool of survivin with apoptotic inhibiting properties seems to be localized to the mitochondria [1,9], and is released into the cytoplasm in response to death stimuli. Survivin inhibits apoptosis in complex with hepatitis B X interacting protein [10] or XIAP, perhaps by separating Smac/Diablo from XIAP, thus enabling caspase degradation [1]. There is an emerging role for survivin in normal adult CD34+ hematopoetic stem cells [11,12] and in the development, maturation and survival of immune cells, for example in T cells [13–16] and neutrophils [17]. It is upregulated in response to stimulation with hematopoetic cytokines and growth factors [18–20].

Expression of survivin in malignancies is associated with unfavorable outcome [21,22] and resistance to cytotoxic treatment [23–25]. In the context of rheumatoid arthritis (RA), extracellular survivin is a marker of poor prognosis. A prospective study on 651 patients at the early stage of RA with the mean disease duration of 6 month showed that high serum levels of survivin were predictive for severe cause of RA, characterized by persistent joint inflammation and progressive joint destructions [26]. The proportion of survivin-positive patients may vary from 20–30% in the group of established and treated RA patients [27] to 60% in the population of early RA patients [26]. Successful anti-rheumatic treatment may reduce serum levels of survivin, while survivin-positive patients accumulate among the patients who do not respond to anti-rheumatic treatment [26–28]. A growing number of publications [26,27,29–31] support the idea that survivin has a role in progression of RA. We have previously shown that survivin has a key function in the regulation of invasive properties of fibroblasts in the inflamed rheumatic joint, and that intracellular survivin is essential for urokinase expression and for the up-regulation of urokinase receptor [32]. Also, serum survivin modifies surface pattern of leukocyte adhesion molecules [33].

Fms-like tyrosine kinase 3 (Flt3) is a receptor tyrosine kinase class III, a class that also includes c-KIT, PDGFRα/β and c-FMS receptors. It is expressed on hematopoietic stem cells and promotes differentiation, maturation and survival of lymphoid progenitors in the bone marrow [34]. Flt3 is essential for the development of antigen presenting cells, such as B cells and dendritic cells (DC) [35–37]. Mutations in the Flt3 receptor, leading to its constant activation, are frequently found in acute myeloid leukemia (AML) [38]. It has been shown that bone marrow cells expressing Flt3 with internal tandem duplication mutations which keeps Flt3 signaling constantly active, have an increased survivin expression [39,40] and this is associated with development of resistance to Flt3 inhibition [39].

Flt3 ligand (Flt3L) is expressed by many cell types, and is present in a soluble intracellular form, and in a membrane bound form [41]. Flt3L has recently been outlined within a panel of preclinical biomarkers of predictive value for the development of RA [42]. We have recently shown that Flt3L is elevated in RA patients and that Flt3L has adjuvant properties when injected into the joint, facilitating development of arthritis in experimental settings [43]. Blockade of Flt3 signaling using a synthetic Flt3 inhibitor alleviates signs of synovitis and cartilage destruction in antigen-induced model of arthritis [44].

Since expression of the Flt3 receptor and survivin in adults is present in hematopoietic stem cells, we address the question whether Flt3L signaling could actually be linked to survivin in rheumatoid arthritis. We further tested the pathological significance of this relation using in vivo treatment with Flt3L and evaluated the possibility of targeting this pathway with an Flt3 inhibitor and lentiviral shRNA knockdown of survivin.

Results

Higher Levels of Flt3 Ligand in Survivin Positive Rheumatoid Arthritis Patients

Survivin levels in the blood of 104 healthy controls (male n = 16, female n = 88, mean age 52.4 years [range 18–67]) were measured by ELISA. The evaluation of the results showed a non-Gaussian distribution of survivin levels in the studied group. The 95% confidence interval was calculated which indicated that the levels of survivin above 450 pg/ml was present in less than 5% of healthy individuals. Thus, the patients with serum or synovial fluid levels of survivin above 450 pg/ml represented the survivin-positive group (n = 29) and the remaining were survivin-negative (n = 61, Table 1). In the present material, 32% of the RA patients were survivin-positive. This is in agreement with our previous reports [27]. As expected, survivin-positive RA patients were significantly more often RF-positive (p = 0.0006) and a majority of the survivin positive patients had erosive joint disease (p = 0.003). The comparison between the groups revealed significantly higher levels of Flt3L in the blood of the survivin-positive RA patients compared to survivin-negative (pg/ml: 110 [range 30–3320] vs 70 [range 10–230], p = 0.003, Fig. 1A). This was also the case for synovial fluid (pg/ml: 200 [range 40–2000] vs 150 [range 30–930], p = 0.055), although not statistically significant (Fig. 1A). There was no significant difference in the levels of acute-phase reactants (e.g., C-reactive protein, serum amyloid A protein levels, IL-6 levels) between the survivin-positive and survivin-negative groups (Table 1).

Survivin Expression is Upregulated in Mouse Bone Marrow Following Treatment with Flt3 Ligand

To elucidate a causative relation behind the observed association between survivin and Flt3L levels in RA patients, arthritic mice were challenged with Flt3L. Two independent experiments were performed containing 15 Flt3L-treated mice and 19 PBS-treated controls. After 14 days of Flt3L treatment, survivin levels in bone marrow cell lysates were increased compared to the PBS treated group (pg/ml: 472.5±193.4 vs 286.5±48.9, $p = 0.01$, Fig. 1B). At day 28, the number of survivin+ cells in bone marrow of Flt3L treated mice was higher compared to PBS treated controls (28.1±6.3% vs 21.9±4.3%, $p = 0.02$, Fig. 1B). Additionally, Flt3L-treated mice tended to have somewhat higher survivin concentration per cell, measured as the intensity of intracellular staining (gMFI: 336±54 vs 288±29, n.s.). The intensity of survivin staining was higher in the Flt3+ cells compared to the Flt3− cell population ($p = 0.003$). Flt3L treatment tended to upregulate survivin expression in both Flt3+ and Flt3− cell populations (Fig. 1C).

Despite the similar size of survivin+ population in bone marrow and spleen, survivin gene expression in spleen was 4 times lower compared to bone marrow (p = 0.002, Fig. 2A, PBS). Flt3L treatment of arthritic mice did not affect total survivin levels in the spleen, since the percentage of survivin+ spleen cells was similar in the Flt3L treated group and the control group (20.3±5.3% vs. 19.5±6.3%). High intensity of survivin expression was attributed to the $MHCII^{+}CD11c^{hi}$ dendritic cell population in the spleen (Fig. 1D). Flt3L treatment increased the proportion of survivin+ cells within the $MHCII^{+}CD11c^{hi}$ population (73.9±6.2% vs 66.0±4.2%, p = 0.005, Fig. 1E). When cultured *in vitro*, splenocytes of Flt3L-treated mice (n = 7) secreted significantly higher levels of survivin compared to splenocytes of PBS-treated controls (n = 7) (pg/ml: 32.6±7.7 vs 24.3±6.2, p = 0.04), but Flt3L treatment did not increase serum levels of survivin (pg/ml: 1772±2503 vs 1190±1335).

Flt3L Changes the Profile of Survivin Splice Variants in Bone Marrow

Gene expression analysis showed an increase in the overall transcription of *survivin* in the bone marrow of Flt3L-treated mice ($n = 6$) compared to PBS treated controls ($n = 6$) (Fig. 2A). This increase was not seen in spleen. Moreover, *survivin* gene expression

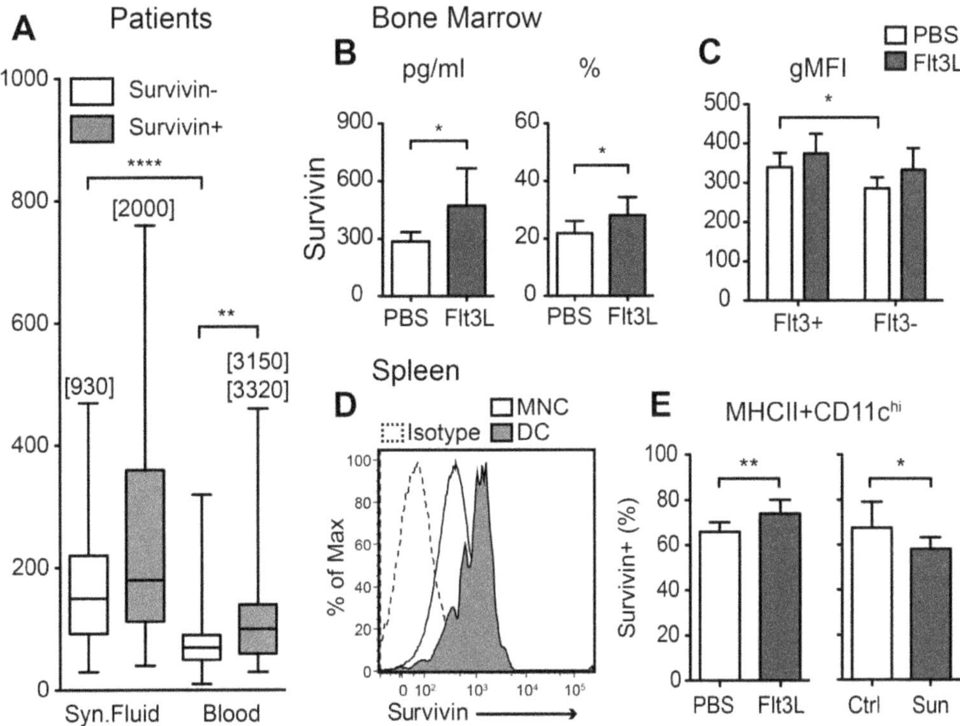

Figure 1. Treatment with Flt3 ligand increases expression of surviving. (A) Levels of Flt3L in blood and synovial fluid of patients with rheumatoid arthritis. Stratification of patients was done into the groups of survivin+ (serum or synovial fluid levels above 450 pg/ml, n = 29) and compared to survivin- (serum and synovial fluid levels below 450 pg/ml, n = 61). (B) Survivin levels in bone marrow from Flt3L or PBS treated mice measured by sandwich ELISA (left panel; Flt3L, n = 8; PBS, n = 8), and the percentage of the survivin positive bone marrow cells measured by flow cytometry (right panel; Flt3L, n = 7; PBS, n = 11). (C) Flt3L treatment increased the intensity of survivin (expressed as gMFI) in the Flt3+ and Flt3- cell populations. (D) Flow cytometry histogram showing survivin staining in spleen MHCII+CD11c^{hi} dendritic cells (dark) compared to total spleen mononuclear cells (open) and isotype control staining (dashed). (E) Percentage of survivin positive cells in the MHCII^{+}CD11c^{hi} dendritic cell population in the spleen after treatment with Flt3L (n = 7) or Flt3-inhibitor sunitinib (Sun) (n = 10) compared to control groups (n = 10 and 11 respectively). Comparison between the groups was done by the Mann-Whitney statistics. (*), p<0.05; (**), p<0.01; (***), p<0.001.

in spleen was lower compared to the expression in the bone marrow (p = 0.002, Fig. 2A). Further analysis of different splice variants of survivin (Fig. 2C) was done on spleen and bone marrow samples. Flt3L treatment increased transcription of the short *survivin40* variant in bone marrow, while no increase in the transcription of the full-length variant *survivin140* could be detected (Fig. 2D). Since it was hard to design specific primers for the *survivin121* transcript, a primer pair localized in the exon 1 and exon 2 was used. These primers were able to detect *survivin140* and *survivin121* transcripts, but not *survivin40* transcript. The transcription of *survivin140* and *survivin121* variants was similar in Flt3L treated and in PBS treated mice. Western blot showed the dominating expression of survivin140 in spleen and survivin140 and survivin121 in bone marrow samples (Fig. 2B).

Survivin Expression in the Bone Marrow is Dependent on Flt3 Receptor Activity

We hypothesized that blockade of Flt3 receptor would affect survivin production in the bone marrow. Survivin was measured in arthritic mice treated with the Flt3 inhibitor SU11248 (sunitinib) in 3 independent experiments containing totally 24 sunitinib-treated mice and 25 control mice treated with citric acid. On day 28, a reduction of total survivin levels was observed in bone marrow lysates of sunitinib treated mice compared to the citric acid treated controls (pg/ml: 1796±388 vs. 2590±1107, p = 0.049, Fig. 3A). Sunitinib significantly reduced the number of survivin+ cells in mouse bone marrow (46.8±4.2% vs 59.3±6.8%, p = 0.0007), and the intensity of intracellular survivin staining (p = 0.002, Fig. 3C). This reduction of survivin expression could be seen mainly on Flt3− cells (p = 0.003, Fig. 3B).

To assess whether sunitinib suppressed the expression of survivin in secondary lymphoid organs, we analyzed survivin levels in the spleen. The total survivin levels in the spleen were not reduced following sunitinib treatment (Fig. 3C), however a significant reduction of survivin expression in the MHCII^{+}CD11c^{hi} dendritic cell population was identified (gMFI: 2684±607 vs 2179±207, p = 0.02). The number of survivin+ dendritic cells was also reduced with sunitinib treatment (58.1±5.3 vs 67.6±11.5%, p = 0.05, Fig. 1E). In spleen, Flt3 inhibition resulted in a reduction of CD11c+ cell population (p = 0.02, Table 2). The latter observation was in consistence with our previous findings on the inhibitory effect of sunitinib on the development of dendritic cells [44].

Survivin shRNA Reduces Flt3 Ligand Expression in the Spleen

Finally, we studied if Flt3/Flt3L system was changed by survivin inhibition. BALB/c mice received lentiviral constructs, containing a sequence coding for shRNA targeting survivin gene transcripts (n = 8), or the same lentiviral construct containing a non-targeting shRNA sequence (n = 9), by a single intra-articular injection. On day 28, the efficacy of survivin inhibition was confirmed on the

Table 1. Clinical characteristics of patients with rheumatoid arthritis.

	Survivin+ $n=29$	Survivin− $n=61$	p-value*
Gender, f/m (n)	22/7	45/16	n.s.
Age, years	60 [24–84]	61 [28–84]	n.s.
Rheumatoid factor + (n, %)	25 (86%)	31 (41%)	0.0006
Disease duration, years	8 [1–33]	9 [1–35]	n.s.
Erosions (n, %)	25 (86%)	35 (57%)	0.003
Treated with DMARDs** (n, %)	22 (76%)	35 (57%)	n.s.
Methotrexate (n, %)	19 (66%)	26 (43%)	n.s.
Other (n, %)	3 (10%)	9 (15%)	n.s.
Non-treated (n, %)	7 (24%)	26 (43%)	n.s.
CRP, mg/L	29 [5–230]	28 [5–170]	n.s.
SAA, mg/L	100 [22–600]	42 [22–600]	n.s.
IL-6, pg/ml (SF)	1.68 [0.03–4.52]	1.81 [0.05–2.69]	n.s.
WBC count, $\times 10^9$/L			
blood	8.0 [3.6–16.8]	8.2 [5.5–14.2]	n.s.
synovial fluid	15.2 [0.1–43.8]	10.4 [0.7–33.2]	n.s.
Survivin, ng/ml			
blood	2.5 [0.45–160]	0 [0–0.38]	<0.0001
synovial fluid	1.81 [0.53–40]	0 [0–0.37]	<0.0001

Data presented as median [range].
*p-values are referred to a comparison between the groups of Survivin+ and survivin- patients, calculated using Mann-Whitney U test or Chi-Square test for categorial data.
**DMARDs, disease modifiying anti-rheumatic drugs SAA, Serum Amyloid A protein. SF, synovial fluid. CRP, C-reactive protein. n.s = not significant.

transcription level by qPCR and on the protein level by flow cytometry. shRNA successfully reduced the total population of survivin+ cells by 35% (17.1±5.2 vs 26.4±3.4, $p=0.002$), and the intensity of survivin expression in the spleen (gMFI: 582±95 vs 789±61, p<0.0001, Fig. 4A). The gene transcription of survivin in spleen tissue and bone marrow was not significantly changed

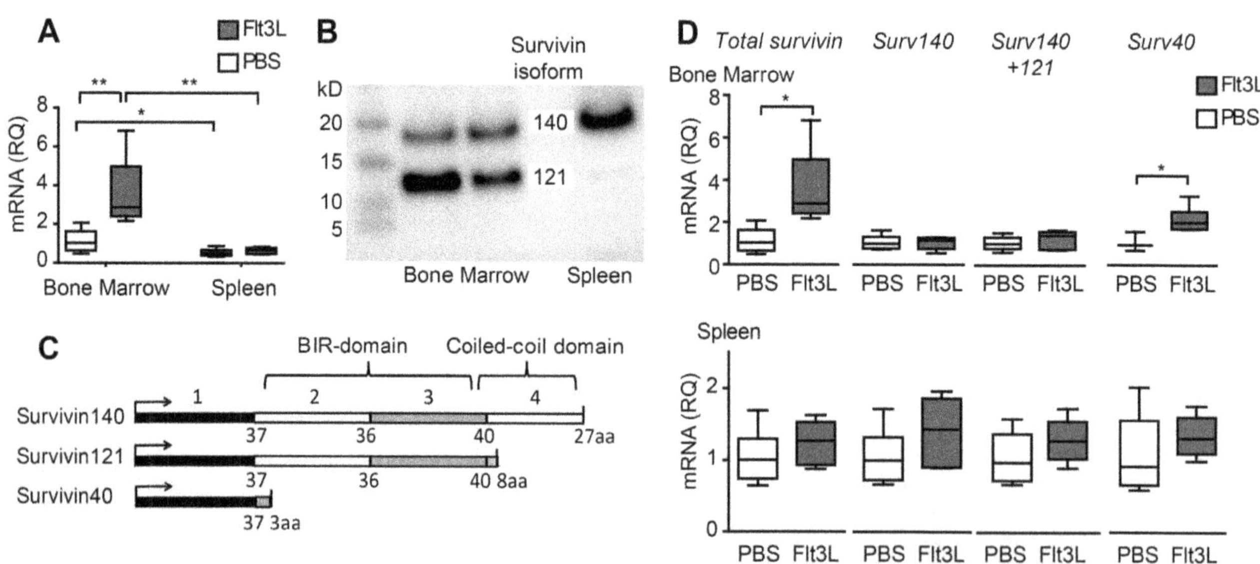

Figure 2. The effect of Flt3L-treatment of BALB/c mice on the expression profile of the survivin splice variants. Mice treated with Flt3L (n = 6) or PBS (n = 6) for 14 days. (A) Total survivin gene expression in bone marrow and spleen, RQ = relative quantity, all values are related to bone marrow from PBS-treated mice. (B) Western blot showing survivin protein isoforms survivin140 and survivin121 in cell lysates from bone marrow and spleen. (C) A schematic overview of the three splice variants of survivin in mice. (D) Gene expression of the different survivin transcripts in bone marrow and spleen, RQ = relative quantity, Flt3L-treated related to PBS-treated for each assay. Data shown as median, whiskers = min to max, (*) p<0.05, (**) p<0.01.

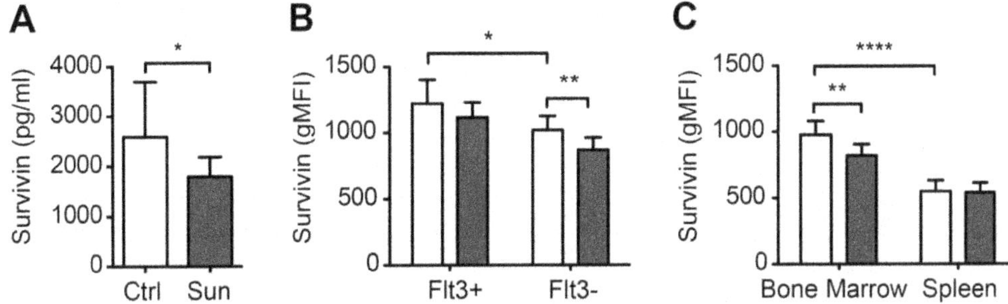

Figure 3. Survivin levels in bone marrow and spleen of BALB/c AIA mice after Flt3 inhibition in vivo. Survivin levels in bone marrow and spleen of mice treated with Flt3 inhibitor sunitinib (Sun, 40 mg/kg/d, n = 10, grey bars) compared to control mice treated with citric acid (Ctrl, *n* = 10, open bars). (A) Survivin levels in bone marrow lysates, measured by sandwich ELISA. (B) The intensity of survivin (expressed as gMFI) in bone marrow Flt3+ and Flt3- cells, and (C) in total bone marrow and spleen. This experiment was repeated with similar results. Comparison between the groups was done by the Mann-Whitney statistics. (*), $p<0.05$; (**), $p<0.01$; (***), $p<0.001$.

(Fig. 4A and data not shown). Inhibition of survivin led to a reduction in Flt3L transcription in the spleen (0.85±0.12 vs 1.01±0.12, $p = 0.04$, Fig. 4B), and to a reduction of survivin+ $MHCII^+CD11c^{hi}$ dendritic cells (40.8±9.1 vs 52.5±3.4, $p = 0.006$, Fig. 4C).

Discussion

High levels of survivin and Flt3L in blood and synovial fluid of patients with rheumatoid arthritis are implied in the pathogenesis of joint inflammation [26,27,43]. Additionally, a tight clinical association observed between these parameters with respect to joint destruction and effect of anti-rheumatic treatment [28] prompted us to study common biological processes linking high expression of survivin and Flt3L in RA patients. The analysis of a cohort of RA patients with the established joint disease showed a clear association of high Flt3L levels with high levels of survivin in blood. Neither Flt3L nor survivin was a consequence of inflammation, measured by CRP, WBC count, serum amyloid A protein and IL6. Due to the cross-sectional nature of the study, one can see a clear difference in the frequency of radiologic erosions, which is a sign of severe disease, in the survivin positive group compared to the survivin negative group. The survivin-positive group contains higher proportion of patients treated with immunosuppressive anti-rheumatic drugs compared to the survivin-negative group. High levels of survivin characterize patients with therapy resistant cause of RA, suggesting that many patients responding to anti-rheumatic treatment convert from survivin-positive to survivin-negative. The results from the patient material show an association between Flt3L and survivin in RA, suggesting the existence of a mutual mechanism regulating levels of these proteins. Similarity of the groups with respect to disease duration, age, levels of C-reactive protein and white blood cell count further support this argument.

Our clinical observations were further extended in the experimental setting, where the requirement of Flt3/Flt3L signaling for expression of survivin *in vivo* was assessed. Survivin levels were increased following treatment with recombinant Flt3L and they were decreased with Flt3 receptor blockade. This proves that survivin production in the bone marrow is dependent on Flt3 signaling and makes Flt3L a major trigger of survivin transcription and expression in leukocytes. Interestingly, we showed the existence of a negative regulation loop where the low expression of survivin in spleen (induced by shRNA) resulted in the low levels of Flt3L in spleen. In the joints of RA patients, the elevated levels of Flt3L could originate from immune cells or fibroblast-like stromal cells in the synovium, by an inflammation caused shedding of the membrane bound form [45] or as a response to lack of antigen presenting cells. It is for example known that the human syndrome of dendritic cell, monocyte, B and NK lymphoid deficiency is associated with elevated levels of Flt3L in humans [37] and the same is true in mice following Flt3 inhibition [44,46].

Flt3/Flt3L signaling is important for the maturation of hematopoietic cells [34]. Here, we show that Flt3L induces survivin production in the Flt3+ progenitors in bone marrow, and in dendritic $MHCII^+CD11c^{hi}$ cells in spleen. Survivin is increased after Flt3L treatment also in the Flt3− population in the bone marrow, suggesting that survivin is induced in Flt3 positive hematopoietic progenitors and remains upregulated after internalization of activated Flt3. Thus, survivin expression induced by Flt3L is associated with differentiation of cells rather than cell proliferation. Our findings are in agreement with previous reports on the induction of survivin production in CD34+ stem cells [20] prior to their differentiation.

Spleen is a maturation site for the peripheral dendritic cells and the process has recently been shown to be dependent on Flt3 expression [47,48]. In our study, a reduction of the intracellular pool of survivin by inhibition of Flt3 led to a pronounced reduction of CD11c+ population of dendritic cells in the spleen. The obvious effect of Flt3L treatment/Flt3 inhibition on survivin levels in the $MHCII^+CD11c^{hi}$ population in the spleen further supports a strong relationship between the induction of survivin and DC development. We have previously shown that inhibition of Flt3 receptor reduces the DC population in spleen [44]. In RA patients, we have seen that high levels of extracellular survivin are

Table 2. Percentage of major leukocyte populations in bone marrow and spleen of sunitinib treated mice.

	Bone Marrow			Spleen		
	Control	Sunitinib	P value	Control	Sunitinib	P value
CD3+ (%)	8.7±0.8	7.3±0.7	0.001	30.2±1.5	31.8±4.7	n.s.
B220+ (%)	26.2±4.6	22.0±4.0	0.04	56.0±7.1	54.0±5.7	n.s.
CD11b+ (%)	49.0±4.3	59.5±6.7	0.002	4.2±0.9	3.9±1.2	n.s.
Gr-1 (%)	47.0±4.3	55.1±6.2	0.007	12.9±1.2	13.4±1.4	n.s.
CD11c+ (%)	2.9±0.3	3.1±0.7	n.s.	4.1±1.5	2.8±0.7	0.02

1–3 pooled experiments, 9–19 mice, n.s = not significant.

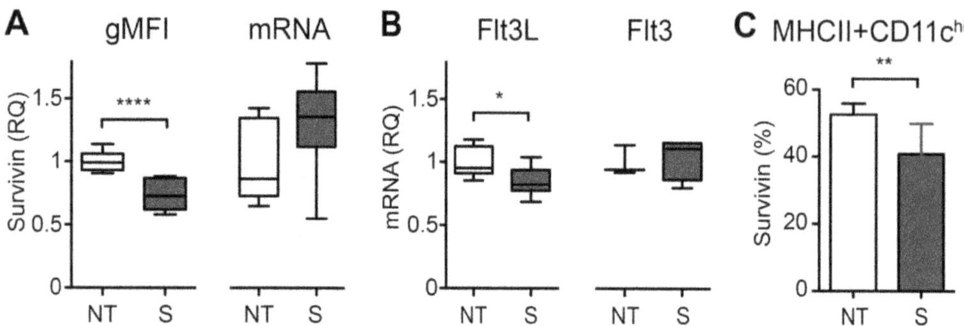

Figure 4. *In vivo* downregulation of survivin using shRNA in BALB/c mice. Lentiviral particles containing a sequence coding for shRNA targeting survivin gene (S, n = 8) were injected intra-articular. The control group received lentiviral particles containing non-targeting shRNA (NT, n = 9). (A) Levels of survivin protein (survivin gMFI analyzed using flow cytometry) and survivin mRNA (RT-qPCR analysis of survivin gene expression) in the spleen (NT, n = 9; S, n = 8). (B) *Flt3L* (NT, n = 7; S, n = 7) and *Flt3* (NT, n = 3; S, n = 4) gene expression in spleen tissue. (C) Percentage of survivin positive MHCII$^+$CD11c^{hi} dendritic cells in the spleen analyzed using flow cytometry (NT, n = 9; S, n = 8). Comparison between the groups was done by the Mann-Whitney statistics. (*), $p<0.05$; (**), $p<0.01$; (***), $p<0.001$.

associated with an increased number of circulating CD11c+ survivin expressing cells in blood [33]. Our present results suggest that modulation of survivin levels is an essential mechanism regulating homeostasis of peripheral dendritic cells.

Interestingly, studies on the Flt3L-induced expressions of different survivin-transcripts revealed an effect on the short *survivin40*-transcript in bone marrow. This variant lacks both the BIR-domain, essential for the interaction with caspases and for the anti-apoptotic effects of survivin [6], as well as the coiled coil-domain required for the formation of chromosomal passenger complex [7]. As survivin40 retains the N-terminal domain, it has been believed to bind other survivin variants [8], and to modulate their function by preventing homodimerization and facilitating interaction through the BIR- and coiled-coil domains. However, we could not detect survivin40 on protein level with western blot, as this has been shown earlier by another group [8] and might either indicate that this transcript is not translated or that the antibodies used are not able to detect the survivin40. The increase in survivin protein after Flt3L treatment can either be a result of an increased survivin40-expression or of a decrease in survivin140- or survivin121- turnover. In spleen, high survivin expression is seen within the MHCII$^+$CD11c^{hi} population. This population represents a small part of the total amount of spleen cells and verification of survivin changes requires cell sorting prior to the RNA analyses.

In conclusion, our findings indicate that expression of survivin is a downstream event of Flt3L signaling, which serves as an essential mechanism supporting survival of hematopoietic cells during their differentiation and maturation of antigen presenting cells in bone marrow and spleen during arthritis.

Materials and Methods

Ethics Statement

The study involving human participants (S441-01) was approved by the Ethics Committee of Sahlgrenska University Hospital. All studies were conducted in compliance with the Declaration of Helsinki, and all patients gave written informed consent to participate in the study. All animal experiments (Protocol Numbers: 176-2008, 328-2008) were approved by the Ethical Committee on Animal Experiments in Gothenburg.

Patients

Synovial fluid and serum samples were obtained from 90 patients with RA attending the Rheumatology Clinic at Sahlgrenska University Hospital, Göteborg, Sweden, for acute joint effusion. All the patients met the diagnostic criteria for RA suggested by the American College of Rheumatology (ACR) [49]. The presence of bone erosions, defined as the loss of cortical definition at the joint, was recorded in proximal interphalangeal, metacarpophalangeal, carpus, wrist and metatarsophalangeal joints using recent radiographs of hands and feet. The presence of one erosion was sufficient to fulfill the requirement of an erosive disease. The presence of rheumatoid factor of any of the immunoglobulin isotypes was considered positive. Clinical characteristics of the patients are presented in Table 1. Blood from 104 healthy blood donors (male n = 16, female n = 88, mean age 52,4 years [range 18–67]) was used to calculate normal levels of survivin.

Collection and Preparation of Samples

Synovial fluid was obtained by arthrocentesis, aseptically aspirated and transmitted into sodium citrate (0.129 mol/l; pH 7.4) containing tubes. In most cases synovial fluid was obtained from knee joints. Synovial fluid samples were aliquoted and frozen in −70°C immediately after joint injections. Blood samples were centrifuged at 1000 rpm and serum was aliquoted and stored at -70°C.

Laboratory Measures of Disease Activity

Serum levels of C-reactive protein (CRP) were measured by standard nephelometry, with established normal range 0–5 mg/ml. Serum amyloid A protein (SAA) levels were detected by an ELISA (Biosource, Camarillo, CA). White blood cell (WBC) counts in blood and synovial fluid samples were obtained with a microcell counter F300 (Sysmex, Toa, Japan). Levels of IL-6 were measured as described previously [43], and rheumatoid factor (RF) were measured using standard laboratory techniques at Sahlgrenska University Hospital, Göteborg, Sweden.

Antigen Induced Arthritis using Methylated Bovine Serum Albumin (mBSA)

Female Balb/c mice were purchased from the Charles River Laboratory (Germany) and housed at the animal facility at the Department of Rheumatology & Inflammation Research, under

Table 3. Primers for real time PCR.

Target	Forward primer		Reverse primer	
Survivin140	TGGACAGACAGAGAGCCAAG	Exon 3	CTGACGGGTAGTCTTTGCAG	Exon4
Survivin121	GTCAAGAAGCAGATGGAAG	Exon 3	TCAGTCCTTATTCTCAATCAT	Retained part of intron3
Survivin40	CCTCAAGAACTACCGCATCG	Exon 1	TATGCTCCTCTTCGCTCTGG	Exon 1/3
Total survivin	AGATCTGGCAGCTGTACCTCA	Exon 1	AGTTCTTGAAGGTGGCGATG	Exon 1
Survivin140+ Survivin121	TCGCCACCTTCAAGAACTG	Exon 1	ATCAGGCTCGTTCTCGGTAG	Exon 2

standard conditions of temperature and light, and fed laboratory chow and water ad libitum. Mice (10 weeks old) were immunized with subcutaneous injection of mBSA (200 µg/mouse, Sigma-Aldrich) dissolved in PBS and mixed with IFA (Sigma-Aldrich) at day 0, followed by booster with mBSA (100 µg/mouse) at the tail root at day 7. Arthritis was induced by a single intra-articular injection of mBSA (30 µg/mouse) in PBS given at day 21. Mice were sacrificed on day 10 or 28. Samples of serum, bone marrow and spleen were collected for further analysis.

In Vivo Treatment with Flt3 Ligand and Flt3 Inhibitor

Arthritic mice were treated with a daily intraperitoneal injection of recombinant Flt3L, in the dose of 1.5µg/mouse, starting 4 days prior to first immunization. Flt3L was purchased from Creative BioMart (Shirley, NY) or purified from Sp2.0 hybridoma transfected with Flt3L gene [43]. Control mice were treated with PBS injection or a control cell line supernatant purified with the same procedure. Flt3 receptor was inhibited using sunitinib (SU11248, Pfizer). Treatment was given by gavage (day 7–28, 40 mg/kg mouse), and the control group was treated with the same volume of citrate buffer as previously described [44]. Specificity of sunitinib for Flt3 inhibition in our model has been previously shown [44].

Knockdown of Survivin using Lentiviral Vector

Lentiviral construct, encoding short hairpin (sh)RNA targeting survivin with the sequence CCGGCAAAGACTACCCGT-CAGTCAACTCGAGTTGACTGACGGGTAGTCTTTGTT-TTTG (TRCN0000054616, Sigma-Aldrich), were selected after *in vitro* evaluation. Lentiviral particles were given by a single intra-articular injection at immunization day 0 (10^7 transduction particles/knee, n = 8). The control group received the same amount of lentiviral particles with non-targeting scrambled sequence (n = 9). Downregulation of survivin was confirmed in bone marrow and spleen.

Cell Preparation and Cell Culture

Bone marrow cells from femur and tibia were flushed with PBS. Single cell suspensions from spleens were prepared by mechanically disruption of tissues through a 70 µm cell strainer. Erythrocytes were lysed in NH_4Cl solution (0.83%, pH 7.29). Leukocyte pellet was resuspended in Iscoves complete medium (10% FBS, 4 mM L-glutamine, 50 µM β-mercaptoethanol, 50 µg/ml gentamycin sulphate) or FACS buffer (PBS, 10% FBS, 0.09% NaN3, 0.5 mM EDTA). Freshly prepared mouse spleen cells were plated on 96-well plate at 2×10^5 cells/well in Iscoves complete medium. Supernatants were collected after 48 hours. Cell lysates were prepared by freezing the cells in −20°C overnight in 6 M urea.

Determination of Survivin and Flt3 Ligand Levels

Survivin and Flt3L protein levels in plasma, synovial fluid, supernatant and lysates were determined by ELISA (DYC647E, DY308, DY427, R&D Systems). Plasma and synovial fluid samples were tested in parallel ELISA plates, in dilution 1:10, lysates 1:3 and supernatant 1:2 in PBS-BSA. The obtained absorbance values were compared to serial dilution of the recombinant proteins and presented as pg/mL. For intracellular staining of survivin, cells were permeabilized with Cytofix/Cytoperm™ Fixation/Permeabilization Solution Kit (BD Pharmingen™) and stained with anti-Survivin antibody (IC6472P, clone 91630, R&D Systems) or with isotype-matched IgG (IC002P, clone 11711, R&D systems).

Flow Cytometry

2×10^6 cells were plated on a 96-well plate, washed with FACS buffer and pelleted (4 min, 1200 rpm, 4°C). Cells were pre-incubated with Fc-block (BD Biosciences) for 30 minutes at 4°C and stained at 4°C for surface markers. Flt3 expression was detected using a biotinylated anti-mouse CD135 antibody (A2F10, Biolegend) followed by a Streptavidin-APC incubation (BD Biosciences). Then the following antibodies against surface markers were used; CD3-APC-eFluor® 780 (17A2), MHC-II-eFluor® 450 (M5/114.15.2), (eBioscience), Gr-1-PerCp (RB6-8C5), CD11b-PerCp (M1/70) (Biolegend), B220-FITC (RA3-6B2), CD11b-V450 (M1/70), CD11c-APC (HL3), B220-V500 (RA3-6B2) (BD Biosciences). Following staining, cells were washed, resuspended in FACS buffer, and collected in FACS-Canto II equipped with FACSDiva software (BD Biosciences). Data were analyzed using the FlowJo software (Tree Star Inc., Ashland, OR). The gating of the cells was based on the isotype control values as well as fluorochrome minus one (FMO) settings when needed. Data is shown as percentage or geometric mean fluorescence intensity (gMFI), calculated in FlowJo and compared to data acquired on the same run.

Protein Preparation and Western Blotting

Total protein was prepared from cells and tissue by homogenization and sonication in the presence of protease inhibitors (Complete Mini, Roche Diagnostics GmbH, Mannheim, Germany). Protein concentrations were measured using the BCA Protein Assay kit (Pierce, Rockford, IL) according to the manufacturer's protocol. Proteins were separated on SDS-PAGE 4–12% Bis-Tris gels (NuPAGE, Invitrogen), and transferred to PVDF membranes (NuPAGE, Invitrogen). Membranes were blocked with 5% non-fat milk and incubated with rabbit-anti-survivin antibodies (840471, R&D systems) at 4°C over night. Detection was performed with peroxidase conjugated anti-rabbit secondary antibody (NA934VS, GE Healthcare) and ECL Prime™ Western Blotting Reagents (GE Healthcare). Chemiluminescent signals were visualized by the Chemidoc equipment and Quantity-One software (BioRad Laboratories).

Gene Expression Analysis

Total RNA from spleen tissue and bone marrow cells was extracted using the RNeasy Mini Kit (Qiagen, Valencia, CA) according to the manufacturer's instructions. Concentration and quality of the RNA was evaluated with NanoDrop spectrophotometer (Thermo Scientific, USA) and Experion (BioRad Laboratories). 400 ng RNA was used for cDNA synthesis using RT^2 First Strand Kit (SABiosciences, Qiagen). Real-time amplification was performed with RT^2 SYBR® Green qPCR Mastermix (SABioscences, Qiagen) using a ViiA^{TM} 7 Real-Time PCR System (Applied Biosystems) according to the manufacturer's instructions. A negative control (no template) reaction was also performed for each primer pair tested. A melting curve for each PCR was performed between 60 and 95°C to ensure that only a single product had been amplified. For *Flt3* and *Flt3L* PCR Assays from SABiosciences (Qiagen) were used (sequences available upon request). Primers used for quantification of *survivin* expression were designed using Primer3 [50], uniqueness checked using the In silico PCR feature of the UCSC Genome Browser, and NetPrimer (PremierBiosoft) was used to check for secondary structures. Primers were ordered from Sigma-Aldrich, and are noted in table 3. Expression levels of the genes were normalized to the two reference genes, *Gapdh* and *Ppia* (TATAA, Sweden, sequences available upon request). Primer concentration used was 0.5 µM. The results were expressed as the fold change compared with the expression level in the control cells with the ddCq-method.

Statistical Analysis

Patient data was expressed as mean (±SD) and analyzed with GraphPad Prism, version 5.0 for Mac (GraphPad, San Diego, CA). The patient material was stratified by the level of survivin, and the difference between the groups regarding Flt3L levels, age, rheumatoid factor, disease duration, presence of erosions, CRP, and WBC count in blood and synovial fluid, was calculated using the Mann-Whitney test or Chi-Square test for categorical data. Experimental data was also analyzed using GraphPad Prism, expressed as mean with SD and significance regarding differences between groups was calculated using the Mann-Whitney test. The two-tailed tests were used and for the statistical evaluation of the results p values <0.05 was considered significant.

Author Contributions

Conceived and designed the experiments: SEMA MNDS MCE MD MIB. Performed the experiments: SEMA MNDS MCE MD KMEA MIB. Analyzed the data: SA KMEA MIB. Contributed reagents/materials/analysis tools: MIB. Wrote the paper: SEMA MNDS KMEA.

References

1. Altieri DC (2010) Survivin and IAP proteins in cell-death mechanisms. Biochem J 430: 199–205.
2. Noton EA, Colnaghi R, Tate S, Starck C, Carvalho A, et al. (2006) Molecular analysis of survivin isoforms: evidence that alternatively spliced variants do not play a role in mitosis. J Biol Chem 281: 1286–1295.
3. Xia F, Altieri DC (2006) Mitosis-independent survivin gene expression in vivo and regulation by p53. Cancer Res 66: 3392–3395.
4. Aoki Y, Feldman GM, Tosato G (2003) Inhibition of STAT3 signaling induces apoptosis and decreases survivin expression in primary effusion lymphoma. Blood 101: 1535–1542.
5. Kim PJ, Plescia J, Clevers H, Fearon ER, Altieri DC (2003) Survivin and molecular pathogenesis of colorectal cancer. Lancet 362: 205–209.
6. Takahashi R, Deveraux Q, Tamm I, Welsh K, Assa-Munt N, et al. (1998) A single BIR domain of XIAP sufficient for inhibiting caspases. J Biol Chem 273: 7787–7790.
7. Jeyaprakash AA, Klein UR, Lindner D, Ebert J, Nigg EA, et al. (2007) Structure of a Survivin-Borealin-INCENP core complex reveals how chromosomal passengers travel together. Cell 131: 271–285.
8. Conway EM, Pollefeyt S, Cornelissen J, DeBaere I, Steiner-Mosonyi M, et al. (2000) Three differentially expressed survivin cDNA variants encode proteins with distinct antiapoptotic functions. Blood 95: 1435–1442.
9. Kang BH, Xia F, Pop R, Dohi T, Socolovsky M, et al. (2011) Developmental Control of Apoptosis by the Immunophilin Aryl Hydrocarbon Receptor-interacting Protein (AIP) Involves Mitochondrial Import of the Survivin Protein. J Biol Chem 286: 16758–16767.
10. Marusawa H, Matsuzawa S, Welsh K, Zou H, Armstrong R, et al. (2003) HBXIP functions as a cofactor of survivin in apoptosis suppression. EMBO J 22: 2729–2740.
11. Leung CG, Xu Y, Mularski B, Liu H, Gurbuxani S, et al. (2007) Requirements for survivin in terminal differentiation of erythroid cells and maintenance of hematopoietic stem and progenitor cells. J Exp Med 204: 1603–1611.
12. Li F, Cheng Q, Ling X, Stablewski A, Tang L, et al. (2010) Generation of a novel transgenic mouse model for bioluminescent monitoring of survivin gene activity in vivo at various pathophysiological processes: survivin expression overlaps with stem cell markers. Am J Pathol 176: 1629–1638.
13. Xing Z, Conway EM, Kang C, Winoto A (2004) Essential role of survivin, an inhibitor of apoptosis protein, in T cell development, maturation, and homeostasis. J Exp Med 199: 69–80.
14. Okada H, Bakal C, Shahinian A, Elia A, Wakeham A, et al. (2004) Survivin loss in thymocytes triggers p53-mediated growth arrest and p53-independent cell death. J Exp Med 199: 399–410.
15. Song J, So T, Cheng M, Tang X, Croft M (2005) Sustained survivin expression from OX40 costimulatory signals drives T cell clonal expansion. Immunity 22: 621–631.
16. Kornacker M, Verneris MR, Kornacker B, Scheffold C, Negrin RS (2001) Survivin expression correlates with apoptosis resistance after lymphocyte activation and is found preferentially in memory T cells. Immunol Lett 76: 169–173.
17. Altznauer F, Martinelli S, Yousefi S, Thurig C, Schmid I, et al. (2004) Inflammation-associated cell cycle-independent block of apoptosis by survivin in terminally differentiated neutrophils. J Exp Med 199: 1343–1354.
18. Fukuda S, Pelus LM (2001) Regulation of the inhibitor-of-apoptosis family member survivin in normal cord blood and bone marrow CD34(+) cells by hematopoietic growth factors: implication of survivin expression in normal hematopoiesis. Blood 98: 2091–2100.
19. Carter BZ, Milella M, Altieri DC, Andreeff M (2001) Cytokine-regulated expression of survivin in myeloid leukemia. Blood 97: 2784–2790.
20. Gu L, Chiang KY, Zhu N, Findley HW, Zhou M (2007) Contribution of STAT3 to the activation of survivin by GM-CSF in CD34+ cell lines. Exp Hematol 35: 957–966.
21. Williams NS, Gaynor RB, Scoggin S, Verma U, Gokaslan T, et al. (2003) Identification and validation of genes involved in the pathogenesis of colorectal cancer using cDNA microarrays and RNA interference. Clin Cancer Res 9: 931–946.
22. Kuttler F, Valnet-Rabier MB, Angonin R, Ferrand C, Deconinck E, et al. (2002) Relationship between expression of genes involved in cell cycle control and apoptosis in diffuse large B cell lymphoma: a preferential survivin-cyclin B link. Leukemia 16: 726–735.
23. Morgillo F, Woo JK, Kim ES, Hong WK, Lee HY (2006) Heterodimerization of insulin-like growth factor receptor/epidermal growth factor receptor and induction of survivin expression counteract the antitumor action of erlotinib. Cancer Res 66: 10100–10111.
24. Tran J, Master Z, Yu JL, Rak J, Dumont DJ, et al. (2002) A role for survivin in chemoresistance of endothelial cells mediated by VEGF. Proc Natl Acad Sci U S A 99: 4349–4354.
25. Petrarca CR, Brunetto AT, Duval V, Brondani A, Carvalho GP, et al. (2011) Survivin as a predictive biomarker of complete pathologic response to neoadjuvant chemotherapy in patients with stage II and stage III breast cancer. Clin Breast Cancer 11: 129–134.
26. Svensson B, Hafstrom I, Forslind K, Albertsson K, Tarkowski A, et al. (2010) Increased expression of proto-oncogene survivin predicts Joint destruction and persistent disease activity in early rheumatoid arthritis. Ann Med 42: 45–54.
27. Bokarewa M, Lindblad S, Bokarew D, Tarkowski A (2005) Balance between survivin, a key member of the apoptosis inhibitor family, and its specific antibodies determines erosivity in rheumatoid arthritis. Arthritis Res Ther 7: R349–358.
28. Isgren A, Forslind K, Erlandsson M, Axelsson C, Andersson S, et al. (2012) High survivin levels predict poor clinical response to infliximab treatment in patients with rheumatoid arthritis. Semin Arthritis Rheum 41: 652–657.
29. Ahn JK, Oh JM, Lee J, Bae EK, Ahn KS, et al. (2010) Increased extracellular survivin in the synovial fluid of rheumatoid arthritis patients: fibroblast-like synoviocytes as a potential source of extracellular survivin. Inflammation 33: 381–388.
30. Dharmapatni AA, Smith MD, Findlay DM, Holding CA, Evdokiou A, et al. (2009) Elevated expression of caspase-3 inhibitors, survivin and xIAP correlates

with low levels of apoptosis in active rheumatoid synovium. Arthritis Res Ther 11: R13.

31. Smith MD, Weedon H, Papangelis V, Walker J, Roberts-Thomson PJ, et al. (2010) Apoptosis in the rheumatoid arthritis synovial membrane: modulation by disease-modifying anti-rheumatic drug treatment. Rheumatology (Oxford) 49: 862–875.
32. Baran M, Mollers LN, Andersson S, Jonsson IM, Ekwall AK, et al. (2009) Survivin is an essential mediator of arthritis interacting with urokinase signalling. J Cell Mol Med 13: 3797–3808.
33. Mera S, Magnusson M, Tarkowski A, Bokarewa M (2008) Extracellular survivin up-regulates adhesion molecules on the surface of leukocytes changing their reactivity pattern. J Leukoc Biol 83: 149–155.
34. Boyer SW, Schroeder AV, Smith-Berdan S, Forsberg EC (2011) All hematopoietic cells develop from hematopoietic stem cells through Flk2/Flt3-positive progenitor cells. Cell Stem Cell 9: 64–73.
35. McKenna HJ, Stocking KL, Miller RE, Brasel K, De Smedt T, et al. (2000) Mice lacking flt3 ligand have deficient hematopoiesis affecting hematopoietic progenitor cells, dendritic cells, and natural killer cells. Blood 95: 3489–3497.
36. Mackarehtschian K, Hardin JD, Moore KA, Boast S, Goff SP, et al. (1995) Targeted disruption of the flk2/flt3 gene leads to deficiencies in primitive hematopoietic progenitors. Immunity 3: 147–161.
37. Bigley V, Haniffa M, Doulatov S, Wang XN, Dickinson R, et al. (2011) The human syndrome of dendritic cell, monocyte, B and NK lymphoid deficiency. J Exp Med 208: 227–234.
38. Small D (2006) FLT3 mutations: biology and treatment. Hematology Am Soc Hematol Educ Program: 178–184.
39. Zhou J, Bi C, Janakakumara JV, Liu SC, Chng WJ, et al. (2009) Enhanced activation of STAT pathways and overexpression of survivin confer resistance to FLT3 inhibitors and could be therapeutic targets in AML. Blood 113: 4052–4062.
40. Fukuda S, Singh P, Moh A, Abe M, Conway EM, et al. (2009) Survivin mediates aberrant hematopoietic progenitor cell proliferation and acute leukemia in mice induced by internal tandem duplication of Flt3. Blood 114: 394–403.
41. Chklovskaia E, Nissen C, Landmann L, Rahner C, Pfister O, et al. (2001) Cell-surface trafficking and release of flt3 ligand from T lymphocytes is induced by common cytokine receptor gamma-chain signaling and inhibited by cyclosporin A. Blood 97: 1027–1034.
42. Deane KD, O'Donnell CI, Hueber W, Majka DS, Lazar AA, et al. (2010) The number of elevated cytokines and chemokines in preclinical seropositive rheumatoid arthritis predicts time to diagnosis in an age-dependent manner. Arthritis Rheum 62: 3161–3172.
43. Dehlin M, Bokarewa M, Rottapel R, Foster SJ, Magnusson M, et al. (2008) Intra-articular fms-like tyrosine kinase 3 ligand expression is a driving force in induction and progression of arthritis. PLoS One 3: e3633.
44. Dehlin M, Andersson S, Erlandsson M, Brisslert M, Bokarewa M (2011) Inhibition of fms-like tyrosine kinase 3 alleviates experimental arthritis by reducing formation of dendritic cells and antigen presentation. J Leukoc Biol 90: 811–817.
45. Horiuchi K, Morioka H, Takaishi H, Akiyama H, Blobel CP, et al. (2009) Ectodomain shedding of FLT3 ligand is mediated by TNF-alpha converting enzyme. J Immunol 182: 7408–7414.
46. Tussiwand R, Onai N, Mazzucchelli L, Manz MG (2005) Inhibition of natural type I IFN-producing and dendritic cell development by a small molecule receptor tyrosine kinase inhibitor with Flt3 affinity. J Immunol 175: 3674–3680.
47. Karsunky H, Merad M, Cozzio A, Weissman IL, Manz MG (2003) Flt3 ligand regulates dendritic cell development from Flt3+ lymphoid and myeloid-committed progenitors to Flt3+ dendritic cells in vivo. J Exp Med 198: 305–313.
48. Schmid MA, Kingston D, Boddupalli S, Manz MG (2010) Instructive cytokine signals in dendritic cell lineage commitment. Immunol Rev 234: 32–44.
49. Arnett FC, Edworthy SM, Bloch DA, McShane DJ, Fries JF, et al. (1988) The American Rheumatism Association 1987 revised criteria for the classification of rheumatoid arthritis. Arthritis Rheum 31: 315–324.
50. Rozen S, Skaletsky H (2000) Primer3 on the WWW for general users and for biologist programmers. Methods Mol Biol 132: 365–386.

4

Porous Surface Modified Bioactive Bone Cement for Enhanced Bone Bonding

Qiang He[1,⁹], Huiling Chen[2,⁹], Li Huang[3], Jingjing Dong[1], Dagang Guo[4], Mengmeng Mao[4], Liang Kong[5], Yang Li[1], Zixiang Wu[1]*, Wei Lei[1]*

1 Institute of Orthopaedics, Xijing Hospital, Fourth Military Medical University, Xi'an, Shaanxi, People's Republic of China, **2** Department of Health Service, School of Public Health and Military Preventive, Fourth Military Medical University, Xi'an, Shaanxi, People's Republic of China, **3** Department of General Dentistry, School of Stomatology, Fourth Military Medical University, Xi'an, Shaanxi, People's Republic of China, **4** State Key Laboratory for Mechanical Behavior of Materials, School of Materials Science and Engineering, Xi'an Jiaotong University, Xi'an, Shaanxi, People's Republic of China, **5** Department of Oral and Maxillofacial Surgery, School of Stomatology, Fourth Military Medical University, Xi'an, Shaanxi, People's Republic of China

Abstract

Background: Polymethylmethacrylate bone cement cannot provide an adhesive chemical bonding to form a stable cement-bone interface. Bioactive bone cements show bone bonding ability, but their clinical application is limited because bone resorption is observed after implantation. Porous polymethylmethacrylate can be achieved with the addition of carboxymethylcellulose, alginate and gelatin microparticles to promote bone ingrowth, but the mechanical properties are too low to be used in orthopedic applications. Bone ingrowth into cement could decrease the possibility of bone resorption and promote the formation of a stable interface. However, scarce literature is reported on bioactive bone cements that allow bone ingrowth. In this paper, we reported a porous surface modified bioactive bone cement with desired mechanical properties, which could allow for bone ingrowth.

Materials and Methods: The porous surface modified bioactive bone cement was evaluated to determine its handling characteristics, mechanical properties and behavior in a simulated body fluid. The in vitro cellular responses of the samples were also investigated in terms of cell attachment, proliferation, and osteoblastic differentiation. Furthermore, bone ingrowth was examined in a rabbit femoral condyle defect model by using micro-CT imaging and histological analysis. The strength of the implant–bone interface was also investigated by push-out tests.

Results: The modified bone cement with a low content of bioactive fillers resulted in proper handling characteristics and adequate mechanical properties, but slightly affected its bioactivity. Moreover, the degree of attachment, proliferation and osteogenic differentiation of preosteoblast cells was also increased. The results of the push-out test revealed that higher interfacial bonding strength was achieved with the modified bone cement because of the formation of the apatite layer and the osseointegration after implantation in the bony defect.

Conclusions: Our findings suggested a new bioactive bone cement for prosthetic fixation in total joint replacement.

Editor: Nuno M. Neves, University of Minho, Portugal

Funding: This work was supported by the Research Fund for the National Natural Science Foundation of China (No.31170913/C1002). The funders had no role in study design, data collection and analysis, decision to publish, or preparation of the manuscript.

Competing Interests: The authors have declared that no competing interests exist.

* E-mail: fmmuleiwei@gmail.com (WL); wuzixiang@fmmu.edu.cn (ZW)

⁹ These authors contributed equally to this work.

Introduction

Tight fixation between polymethylmethacrylate (PMMA) bone cement and bone is of great importance for a successful outcome of total joint replacement. The fixation strength of PMMA cement to bone is primarily dependent on mechanical interlocking [1,2]. To achieve interlock, the bone surface must be rough and irregular. Although a good fixation of PMMA cement can be achieved by interlocking into pores of implants and bone [3], a fibrous tissue layer always intervenes between cement and bone [4,5]. The layer is known as the weak-link zone and can lead to loosening of the prosthesis [6].

Several strategies are employed to improve PMMA based cement-bone interactions. One of the strategies attempted is to develop bioactive bone cements by incorporation of all sorts of bioceramics into PMMA bone cement. Various bioceramics have been studied, including bone, glass, and calcium phosphate compounds, such as hydroxyapatite and tricalcium phosphates [7–10]. The bioactive bone cements can bond directly to the bone, but the pre-clinical results are far from satisfactory. The addition of excess amounts of ceramic power to the PMMA cement adversely affects the mechanical and handling properties [11–12]. Moreover, bone resorption is observed after implantation in the bioactive bone cement group, which will gradually compromise fixation. This is because weakness of the calcium phosphorous layer formed on the surface of the bioactive bone cement results in particles of wear debris and stimulates bone resorption [13]. Another strategy is to provide porosity in PMMA bone cement with the addition of carboxymethylcellulose (CMC) [14], alginate [15] and gelatin microparticles (GMPs) [16]. The porous PMMA can promote ingrowth of soft and hard tissue into the material, thereby creating more interlocking and the anchorage of the PMMA. However, the mechanical properties of the porous PMMA are too low to be used in orthopedic applications. Previous studies revealed that bone ingrowth into bone cement could decrease the possibility of bone resorption and promote the formation of a stable interface [17]. Therefore, bone ingrowth into bioactive bone cement is of importance in developing adequate initial fixation. Recently, Lye KW et al proposed a porous PMMA cement incorporated with β-TCP particles, but the addition of β-TCP did not convey any advantage in terms of increase in bone formation and ingrowth due to the way the β-TCP particles were included into the PMMA matrix [18]. Scarce literature is reported on bioactive bone cements that allow bone ingrowth.

The objective of this study was to prepare a bioactive bone cement with desired mechanical properties, which could allow for bone ingrowth. The bioactive bone cement consisted of low content of bioactive glass as bioactive fillers, chitosan particles as porogen, and polymethylmethacrylate as the matrix. Chitosan is a safe ingredient that is biodegradable and environmentally biocompatible. The porous surface structure obtained by the degradation of the chitosan particles will promote bone ingrowth and improve the interfacial bonding strength. In addition, with the low content of bioactive fillers, proper handling characteristics, adequate mechanical properties and direct bone contact can be achieved. In the present study, the porous surface modified bioactive bone cement was evaluated to determine its handling characteristics, mechanical properties and behavior in a simulated body fluid (SBF). The in vitro cellular responses of the samples were also investigated in terms of cell attachment, proliferation, and osteoblastic differentiation. Furthermore, bone ingrowth was examined in a rabbit femoral condyle defect model by using micro-CT imaging and histological analysis. The strength of the implant-bone interface was also investigated by push-out tests.

Table 1. Compositions of the bone cements prepared.[a]

	PSB bone cement	PMMA bone cement
Solid component		
PMMA	48.5	98.5
Glass	40.0	0
CS	10.0	0
BPO	1.5	1.5
Liquid component		
MMA	99.0	99.0
DMPT	1.0	1.0

[a]by weight ratio (wt%) of solid component and liquid component, respectively.

Table 2. Values of curing parameters of different cements (n = 6).

Cement	Dough time(min)	Setting time(min)
PSB bone cement	3.8±0.4	12.7±0.3*
PMMA bone cement	3.0±0.2	8.6±0.3

*, $P<0.05$ compared to PMMA bone cement.

Materials and Methods

1. Preparation of the Porous Surface Modified Bioactive Bone Cement

The raw materials used for the preparation and composition of the bone cement are listed in Table 1. Two types of cements, the porous surface modified bioactive bone cement (designated as PSB bone cement) and PMMA bone cement, were prepared. The PMMA bone cement was used as a control material. The bioactive glass (glass) was glass 45S5 particles, which were pulverized from NovaBone® product (LLC, Alachua, USA). This glass has a composition of 45 wt% SiO_2, 24.5 wt% CaO, 24.5 wt% Na_2O and 6 wt% P_2O_5. Chitosan (CS) was purchased from Biochemical Medicine Plant of Qingdao (Qingdao, China) and obtained by the method described in a previous study [19]. The average molecular weight of CS particles was 2000–3000 g/mol, and the extent of deacetylation was approximately 85%. The microstructures of the CS and glass particle were examined by scanning electron microscopy (SEM, Hitachi S-2400, Japan). Pure PMMA powder was obtained from Industrias Quirúrgicas de Levante (Asturias, Spain). Methyl methacrylate (MMA, Acros Organics, Fisher Scientific, UK) was used as received. Benzoyl peroxide (BPO, Fluka, Sigma–Aldrich, UK) initiator and N,N-dimethyl-p-toluidine (DMPT, Fluka) activator were used as received for the polymerization reaction. The solid component consisted of PMMA beads, glass particles, CS particles, and BPO as the initiator. The liquid component consisted of MMA monomer and DMOH as activator of reduced toxicity. The paste was prepared by mixing the powder with the liquid using a solid: liquid mass ratio of 2:1 under ambient conditions at room temperature.

2. Characterisation of the PSB Bone Cement

Sample of the PSB bone cement was gently washed with distilled water three times to remove the polymer on the surface and dried in a fume hood overnight. Then the sample surface was examined with scanning electron microscopy (SEM, Hitachi S-2400, Japan).

3. Curing Parameters

In order to compare curing parameters of the PSB bone cement with those of the PMMA bone cement, dough time and setting time were measured. Dough time and setting time were determined according to International Standard Specification (ISO 5833) [20]. Dough time is defined as the time at which the cement mass no longer adheres to a surgically gloved finger. The setting time of cement sample was measured using a vicat needle (SS-S-403, Shinohara Manufacturing Co., Ltd., Tochigi, Japan). The cement paste was mixed for 3 min and cast into a cylindrical mold made of polytetrafluoroethylene (inner diameter = 6 mm, inner depth = 6 mm). The vicat needle with cross-sectional area of 1 mm^2 was gently placed on the surface of the molded cement for

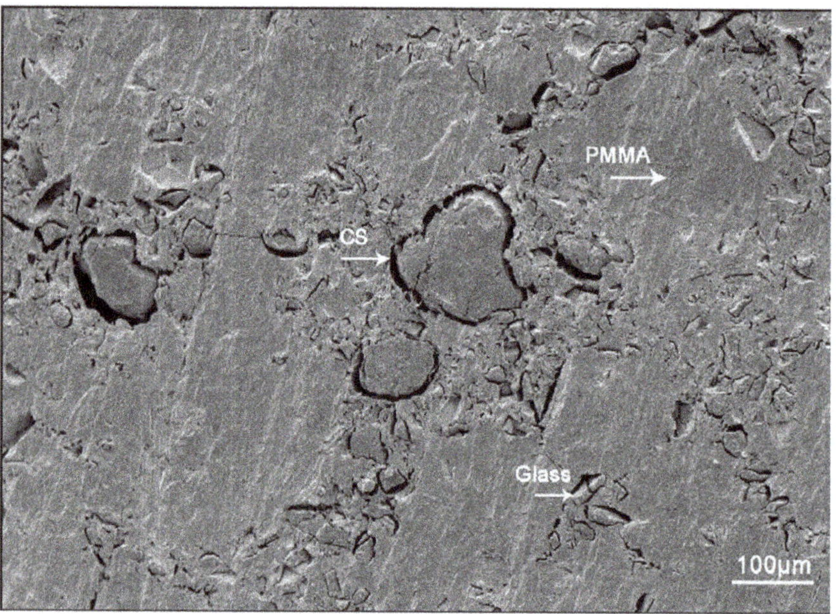

Figure 1. SEM images of the PSB bone cement fresh prepared. The glass and CS particles were uniformly distributed in the polymeric matrix for dry cement samples.

time intervals of 30 s. The time required for the needle trace to disappear after placing the vicat needle on the surface was measured under ambient conditions of temperature = 21–22°C and humidity = 26–28%. The setting time was defined as the point when the vicat needle no longer gave a trace in the cement surface [21].

4. Compressive Strength and Degradation Testing

For the compressive strength test, cylindrical samples of cured cement were prepared with diameters of 6 mm and lengths of 12 mm [22]. Then samples were immersed in 15 ml phosphate buffered saline (PBS) at 37°C and kept for 4 weeks. Every 2 days, the immersion solution was renewed. Six samples were taken out and dried for measurements at 1, 2, and 4 weeks, respectively. The

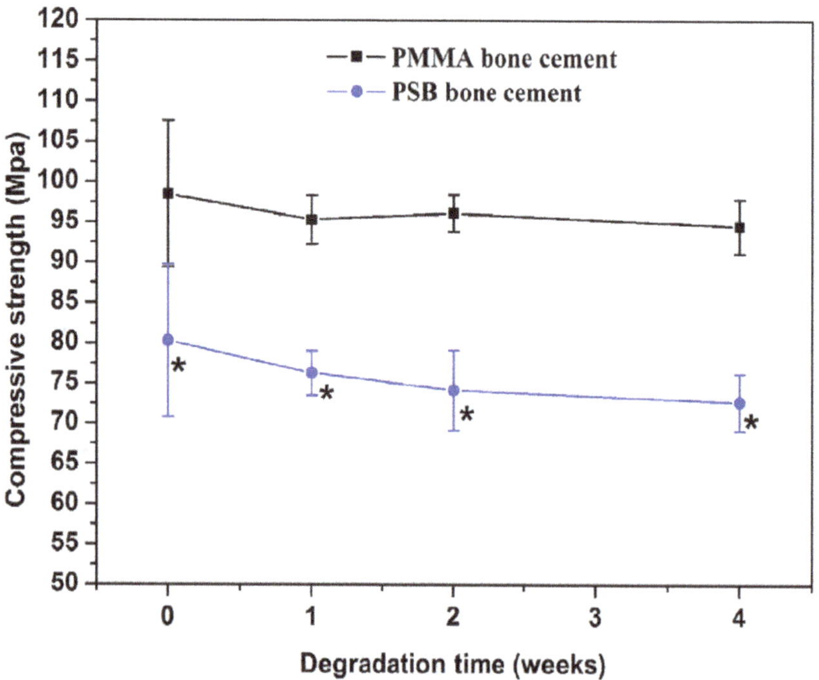

Figure 2. The degradation of mechanical properties of the PMMA and PSB bone cement. A significantly lower compressive strength ($P<0.05$) was observed for the PSB bone cement compared to the PMMA bone cement at each degradation time.

compressive load was applied at a loading rate of 0.01 mm/s using an MTS materials testing system (MTS 858 Bionix machine, MTS System Inc., Minneapolis, MN). The compressive strength was calculated from the compressive load and geometric area of the samples.

5. Behavior of the Sample in SBF

The PSB bone cement was molded into rectangular shapes of 5 mm×5 mm×5 mm. Then the prepared specimens were soaked in 10 ml of SBF at 37°C. The SBF solution was prepared by dissolving NaCl, $NaHCO_3$, KCl, $K_2PO_4{\bullet}3H_2O$, $MgCl_2{\bullet}6H_2O$, 1.0 M HCl, $CaCl_2$, Na_2SO_4 and $(HOCH_2)_3CNH_2$ in ultrapure water [23]. After 7 days, the specimens were removed from the solution, and gently washed with distilled water. Surface changes on the specimens were characterized by scanning electron microscopy (SEM, Hitachi S-2400, Japan) and an energy dispersive spectrometer (EDS, Falcon, USA).

6. *In vitro* Cellular Response

6.1 Cell culture. MC3T3-E1 subclone 4 mouse preosteoblast cells (American Type Culture Collection) were grown in culturing medium consisting of a-MEM (Hyclone, USA) containing 100 units per ml penicillin and 100 µg per ml streptomycin and supplemented with 10 vol. % fetal bovine serum (Hyclone, USA) at 37°C with 5% CO_2. Osteogenic medium was prepared by adding 10 mM b-glycerophosphate (Sigma–Aldrich, UK) and 50 mg/ml ascorbic acid (Sigma–Aldrich, UK) into culturing medium for the alkaline phosphatase (ALP) test.

6.2 Cell attachment, proliferation and differentiation. Disk samples of bone cement with dimensions of 10 mm in diameter and 1 mm in thickness were prepared, briefly submersed in 70% ethyl alcohol and allowed to dry under sterile conditions for all experiments. Tissue culture polystyrene (TCPS) plates were used as a positive control. The pre-incubated cell lines were placed on disk samples at densities of 5×10^4, 2×10^4 and 1.5×10^4 cells/cm^2 for the cell attachment, proliferation and differentiation tests. The time for MC3T3-E1 cell attachment on TCPS is usually 4 hours [24]. At 3 hours of adhesion the MC3T3-E1 cells had not yet completely adhered to the substrate and the difference of cell attachment could be found. Then attached cells were fixed using 3.7% formaldehyde solution, permeabilized with 0.2% Triton X-100 and stained using Rhodamine-phalloidin (Invitrogen, USA) and DAPI (Sigma–Aldrich, UK) for photographing using an Olympus FV1000 confocal microscope (Japan). The cell number attached on substrates was determined using MTS (methoxyphenyl tetrazolium salt) assay at this time. Normalized cell adhesion was calculated using the following equation: Normalized cell adhesion (%) = OD of test sample/OD of TCPS. The sample area for cell proliferation was only 0.785 cm^2. The MC3T3-E1 cells will be in contact with each other and stop proliferation if the cells are incubated in culturing medium for over 7 days. Therefore, the MTS assay was used to evaluate cell numbers at 1, 4, 7 days. Cell differentiation from pre-osteoblasts to osteoblasts was determined as ALP activity. The enzyme ALP has been used as an indicator of osteoblastic activity for many years. The MC3T3-E1 cell is a clonal pre-osteoblastic cell line derived from newborn mouse calvaria [25]. The cells must be differentiated in osteogenic medium for over 7 days before a dramatic increase in the ALP activity can be measured. After culturing for 7 and 14 days in osteogenic medium, the ALP activity of cells on disk samples was measured using p-nitrophenyl phosphate (pNPP) (Sigma–Aldrich, UK) as described in a recent paper [26]. PNPP was converted into p-nitrophenol (pNP) in the presence of ALP at a rate that was proportional to the ALP activity. The production of pNP was determined using the absorbance that was measured at 405 nm wavelength using a micro-reader. The ALP activities were normalized to the total protein content.

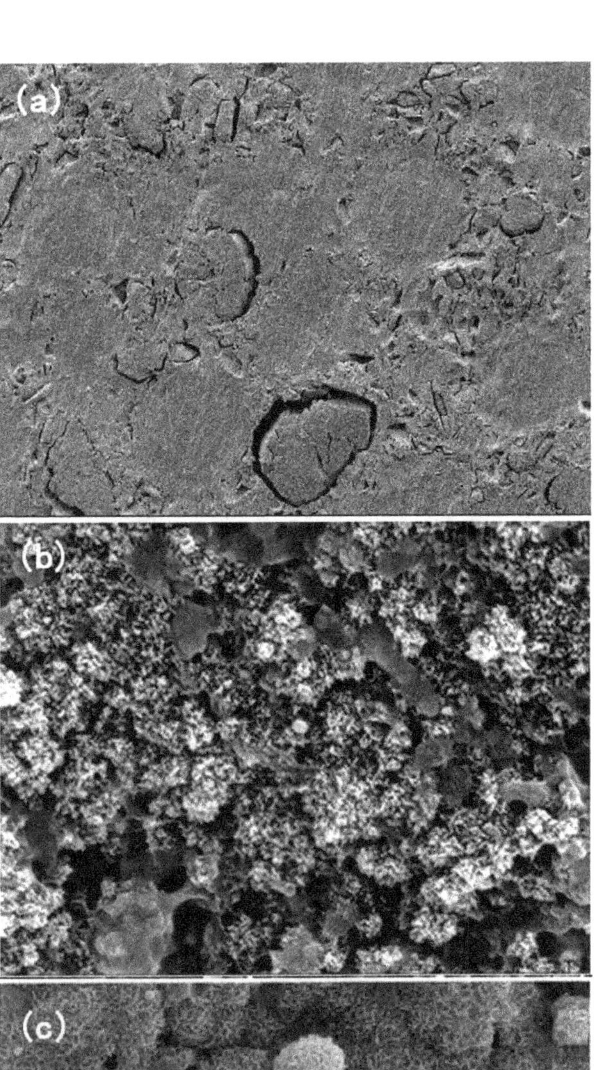

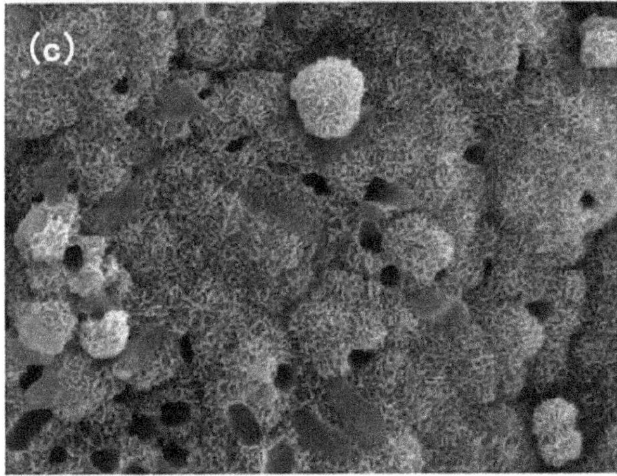

Figure 3. SEM photographs of the surface of PSB bone cement before and after soaking in SBF for different periods. (a) Samples before soaked in SBF. (b) Samples after soaking in SBF for 3 days. (c) Samples after soaking in SBF for 7 days. After 3 days, the surface changed considerably (as compared to the non-immersed specimens), but no deposits were visible even at high magnifications. Apatite crystals of needle-like morphology were observed on the surface of the cement sample soaked in SBF for 7 days.

(a)

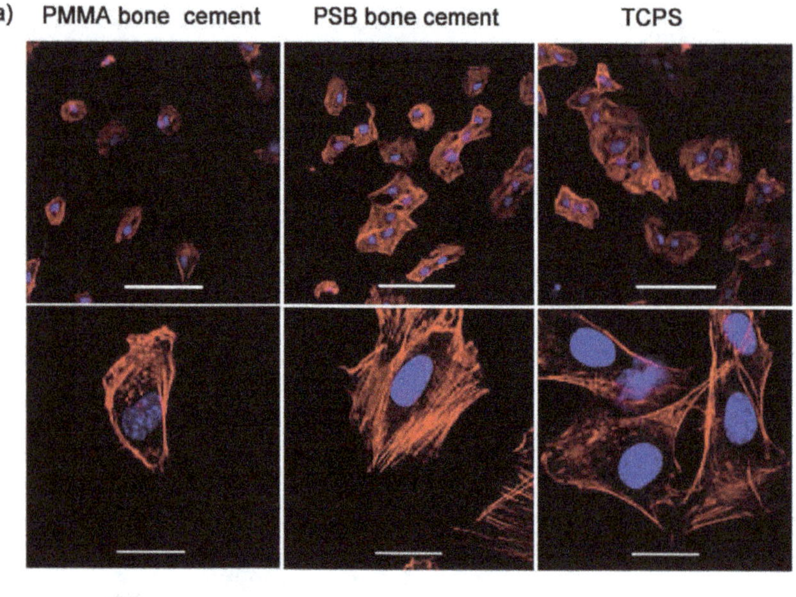
PMMA bone cement
PSB bone cement
TCPS

(b)

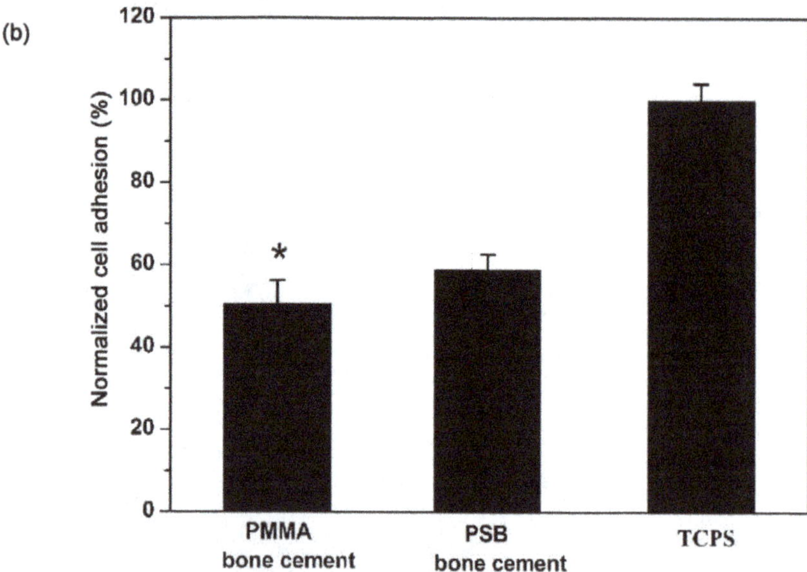
Normalized cell adhesion (%)
120
100
80
60
40
20
0
*
PMMA
bone cement
PSB
bone cement
TCPS

(c)

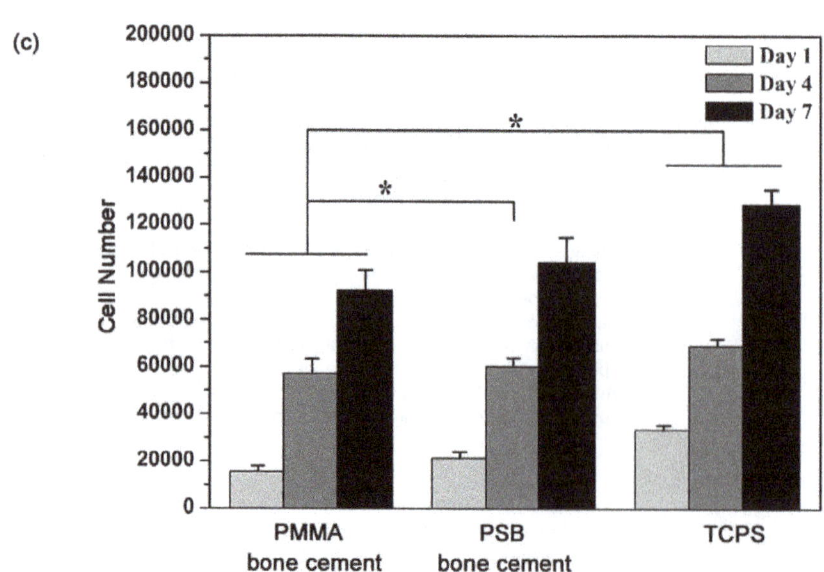
Cell Number
200000
180000
160000
140000
120000
100000
80000
60000
40000
20000
0
Day 1
Day 4
Day 7
*
*
PMMA
bone cement
PSB
bone cement
TCPS

Figure 4. Cell adhesion and proliferation on disks of different bone cements. (a) Confocal images of F-actin and nuclei stained MC3T3-E1 cells cultured for 3 h on cement surfaces. Scale bar represents 100µm (top row) and 20 µm (bottom row). (b) Normalized cell adhesion 3 h post-seeding on the PMMA and PSB bone cement compared to cell-seeded TCPS as positive (+) control. Data are shown as mean ± standard deviation (n = 3).*, $p<0.05$ compared to TCPS and the PSB bone cement. (c) The number of MC3T3-E1 cells 1, 4, 7 days post-seeding on disks of the PMMA and PSB bone cement compared to cell-seeded TCPS as positive (+) control. Data are shown as mean ± standard deviation (n = 3).*, $P<0.05$ between two marked samples.

7. *In vivo* Test

For the *in vivo* animal tests, 44 adult female New Zealand white rabbits 5 months of age weighing between 3.5 and 4 kg were used. This study was carried out in strict accordance with the recommendations in the Guide for the Care and Use of Laboratory Animals of the National Institutes of Health. The animal protocol was approved by the Animal Care and Use Committee at Fourth Military Medical University (Permit Number: 08–269). A combination of ketamine hydrochloride (50 mg/kg, IM) and fentanile (0.17 mg/kg, IM) was used as the general anesthesia and 2% lidocaine with 1:100000 epinephrine was injected as the local anesthesia. Hardened cylindrical specimens (10 mm in length and 6 mm in diameter) of the cement were prepared. The specimens were implanted into each medial femoral condyle. After surgery, the wounds were sutured with vicryl and penicillin (240,000 UI) was injected into the rabbits for 3 days. After 6 and 12 weeks, the rabbits were sacrificed with an overdose of sodium pentobarbital. For the micro-CT and histological analysis, harvested medial femoral condyles were fixed in a 10% neutral formaldehyde solution. Then the rabbit femur with hardened cement was imaged with three-dimensional microfocus computed tomography (micro-CT, eXplore Locus SP, GE, USA), at a voltage of 80 kVp and an electric current of 80 mA. The voxel size after reconstruction was 62.5 µm×62.5 µm×62.5 µm. To evaluate the *in vivo* resorption of the implanted materials, the residual material volume fraction (RMVF) was calculated as the ratio between the volume of residual material and the total volume of the materials. The porosity was quantified from the micro-CT data and calculated using the formula: $\Phi = V_V/V_T$, where V_V is the volume of void-space and V_T is the total volume of material [27]. Based on the micro-CT results, the amount of bone ingrowth into the cement was quantified as the bone volume (BV) within the defined VOI (volume of interest) in each defect site. After the micro-CT scanning, the samples were embedded in methacrylate resin [28]. A total of 5 µm sections were obtained with a microtome (Microm-HM 350S, Thermo Fisher Scientific, USA). The sections were stained with Van Gieson's Stain and examined with a light microscope (Nikon Microphot FXA). To investigate the strength of the implant–bone interface, push-out tests were conducted on a biomechanical test apparatus (SHIMADZU EHF-F01, Shimadzu Co., Kyoto, Japan). The test was performed following the procedure described in a previous report [29]. The maximum push-out force was determined and used to indicate the quality of the attachment to bone tissue.

8. Statistical Analysis

All statistical processing was completed using SPSS 16.0 (SPSS, Chicago, IL). A student's t-test was used to analyze data between two groups. Differences between three groups were tested by a one-way analysis of variance (ANOVA) and differences between two groups were then compared using a Bonferroni post-hoc test.

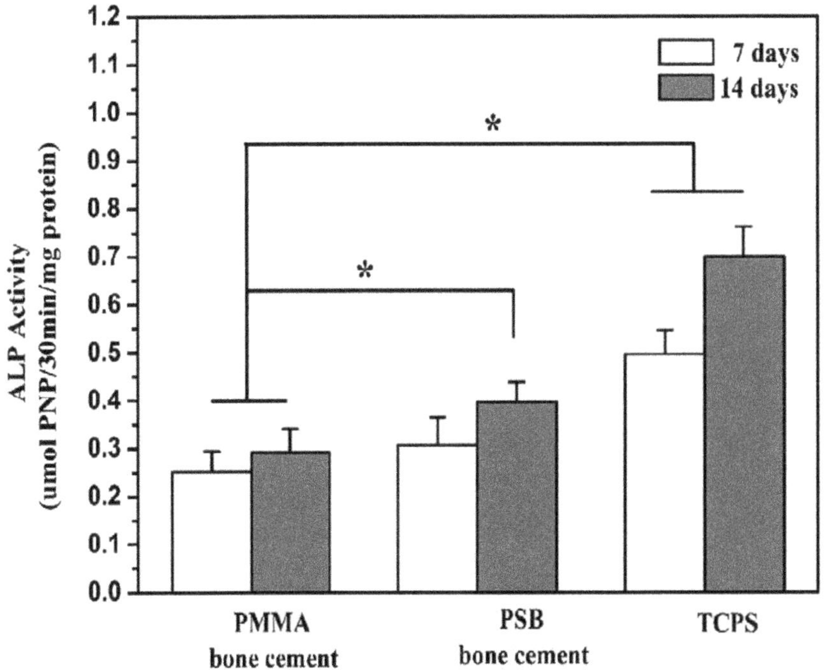

Figure 5. Cell differentiation on disks of different bone cements. ALP activities of MC3T3-E1 cells cultured on disks of the PMMA and PSB bone cement for 7 and 14 days, compared to cell-seeded TCPS as positive (+) control. Data are shown as mean ± standard deviation (n = 3).*, $P<0.05$ between two marked samples.

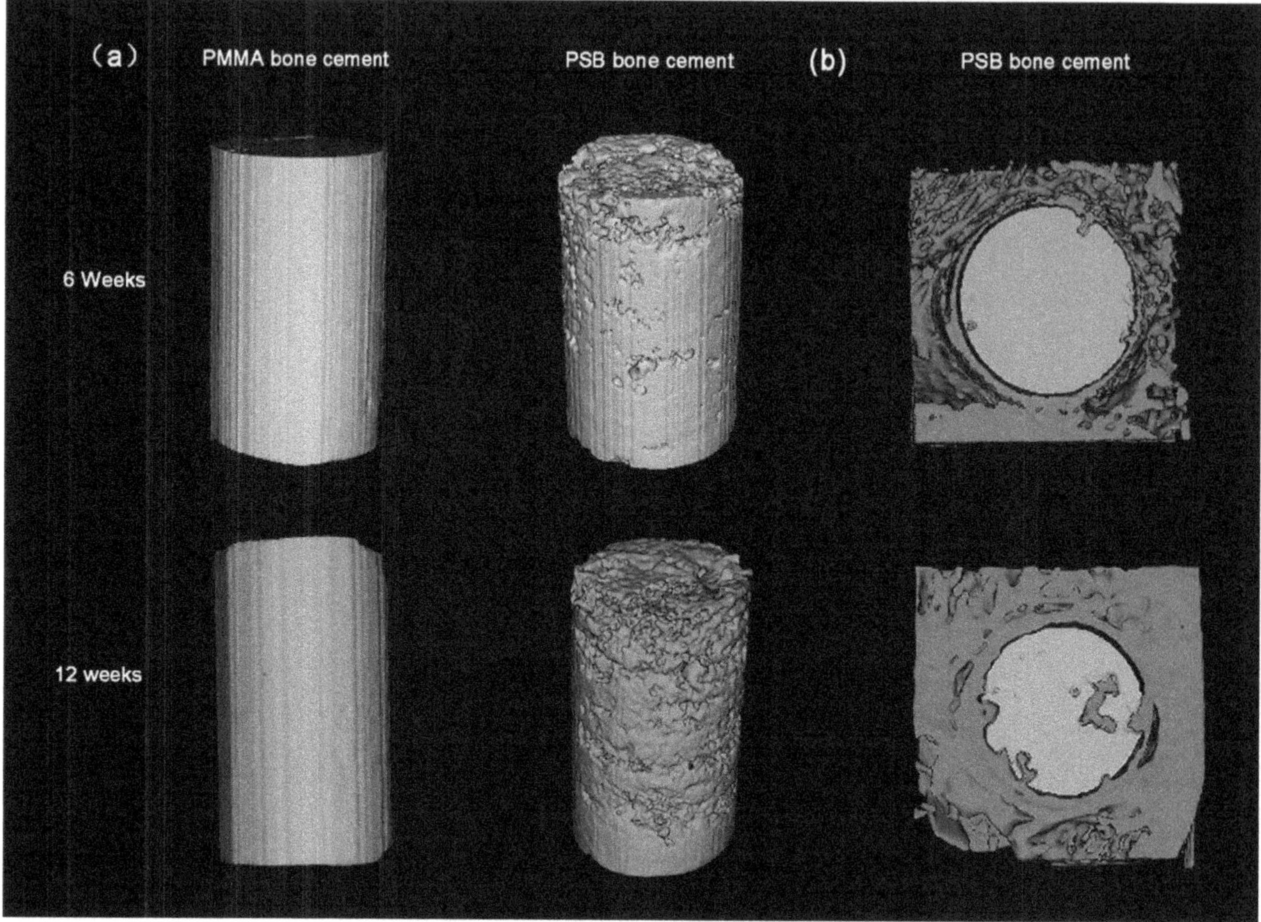

Figure 6. Tridimensional reconstruction using micro-CT analysis. (a) Residual material of the PMMA and PSB bone cement and (b) cross section images of rabbit femur after implantation for different periods.

P values less than 0.05 were considered statistically significant. All errors are given as standard deviations.

Results

1. Formulation and Setting Time of Cements Used

The CS particles displayed irregular shapes with the average diameter of about 200 μm. The glass particles consisted of numerous fine grains. The average diameter of the particles was about 40 μm. Table 2 shows the values of dough time and setting time of the cements used. The setting time of the PSB bone cement was longer than that of the PMMA bone cement ($p<0.05$). There was a small difference between the dough times of the PSB bone cement and those values of the PMMA bone cement.

2. Surface Morphologies of the PSB Bone Cement

SEM images of the PSB bone cement are shown in Fig. 1. The glass and CS particles were uniformly distributed in the polymeric matrix for dry cement samples. The space around the particles was present as the particles were not firmly integrated into PMMA matrix. However, the particles did not separate out. It's already known that space around particles can increase the contact area between materials and body, thus accelerating the degradation rate of particles and promoting the formation of macropores [30].

3. Mechanical and Degradation Properties

Fig. 2 shows the compressive strength of the PSB and PMMA bone cement before and after degradation. It can be seen that the PSB bone cement had a lower initial compressive strength than the PMMA bone cement ($p<0.05$). Initially, the PSB bone cement had 80.31 Mpa in strength, which is in the range of that of bone (80–200 MPa). After 28 days degradation, the strength of the PSB bone cement decreased to 72.71 Mpa, which still meets the criterion (>70 MPa) listed in ISO 5833. In contrast, there was no significant decrease in the value of the PMMA bone cement after 28 days degradation.

4. Assessment of *in vitro* Bioactivity

The *in vitro* bioactivity of the PSB bone cement was investigated by soaking the samples in SBF. Fig. 3 shows SEM photographs of the surface of the cements before and after soaking in SBF for different periods. After 3 days, the surface changed considerably (as compared to the non-immersed specimens), but no deposits were visible even at high magnifications. Apatite crystals of needle-like morphology were observed on the surface of the cement sample soaked in SBF for 7 days. The EDS spectra of cement samples after immersion in SBF showed that silicon peaks almost disappeared and Ca and P peaks increased. The other elements (plus Cl from the solution) were also present in residual amounts on the surface.

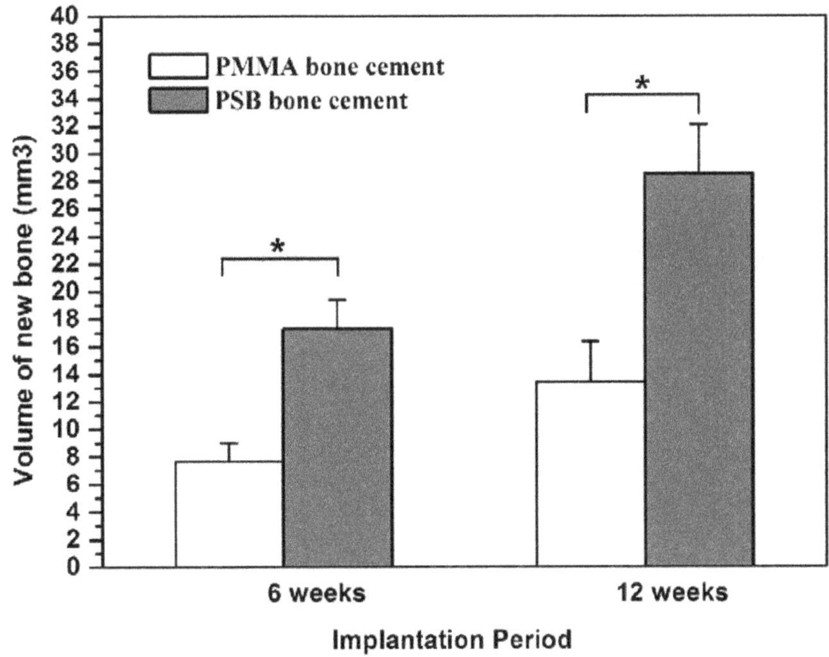

Figure 7. Quantitative analysis of new bone formation from micro-CT images. Data are shown as mean ± standard deviation (n = 5).*, $P<0.05$ between two marked samples.

5. Cell Attachment

Fig. 4a shows cytoskeletal and adhesion structures of MC3T3-E1 cultured for 3 h on disks of different bone cements. A significant difference in cytoskeleton organization was observed. The PMMA bone cement showed that F-actin in the seeded cells was disorganized while cells assumed a more or less spherical morphology. The PSB bone cement showed that cells developed well-organized F-actin bundles at their peripheries. The cell numbers attached on the disks of the PMMA bone cement at 3 h post-seeding were lower than those of the PSB bone cement (Fig. 4b) ($p<0.05$), suggesting that the PSB bone cement had better cell adhesion.

6. Cell Proliferation

MC3T3-E1 cell proliferation on bone cement disks was evaluated using MTS at different time points, as shown in Fig. 4c. It is evident that cell numbers increased continuously with the culture time, which indicates that all bone cements have good biocompatibility. The number of viable cells on the PSB bone cement was greater than that on the PMMA bone cement after 4 days culture ($p<0.05$), which suggests that the PSB bone cement was more beneficial for cell proliferation than the PMMA bone cement.

7. Cell Differentiation

Degree of differentiation of the MC3T3-E1 cells that were cultured in an osteogenic medium for 7 and 14 days on bone cements are shown in Fig. 5. The ALP activities of cells on the PSB bone cement were higher than those of cells on the PMMA bone cement after 14 days culture ($p<0.05$), suggesting that the glass particles in the PSB bone cement modulates preosteoblast cell differentiation.

8. Micro-CT Analysis

As shown in Fig. 6a, the 3D reconstruction images of residual material of the PMMA and PSB bone cement after implantation for 6 and 12 weeks were used to evaluate the *in vivo* resorption of the implanted cements. The areas and the volumes of the PSB bone cement can be seen to decrease with an increase of the implantation times. The dissolution of CS particles can result in macropore formation after 6 weeks of degradation. The pore size became greater when the bioglass particles close to the macropores degraded with time. It is clear to see that a porous surface construct was obtained after 12 weeks implantation. Furthermore, the porosity does not appear to be uniform. Obvious pore formation was found at the outer side of implant because the subcutaneous muscle layers generally contain large amounts of vascular tissues, which will accelerate the degradation process. However, no obvious pore formation was observed at the inner side of implant. Conversely, PMMA bone cement showed few observable changes even after 12 weeks of degradation. With increasing the implantation time from 6 to 12 weeks, the porosity of the PSB bone cement increased from 8.59±2.54% to 13.95±3.11%. In contrast, after 12 weeks of degradation, porosity was only 1.57±1.05% for the PMMA bone cement. Assessment of bone ingrowth into the implanted cements was also performed with micro-CT scanning (Fig. 6b). At 6 weeks, a small amount of newly formed bone was observed surrounding the PSB bone cement. And more extensive bone formations were observed throughout the cross-section of the bone cement at week 12 after implantation. Whereas only a few newly formed bones in the PMMA bone cement group appeared at the native bone margins and the defect periphery 12 weeks after implantation. The volume of new bone within the defect was calculated to evaluate the bone ingrowth more precisely (Fig. 7). The results indicated that the PSB bone cement contained a higher bone volume than the PMMA bone cement at both 6 and 12 weeks ($p<0.05$). The RMVF of the PSB bone cement decreased with the increase of the implantation time from 6 to 12 weeks, the RMVF decreased from 91.41±2.54% to 86.05±3.11%. Conversely, the RMVF of the PMMA bone cement remained 98.44±1.05% after 12 weeks

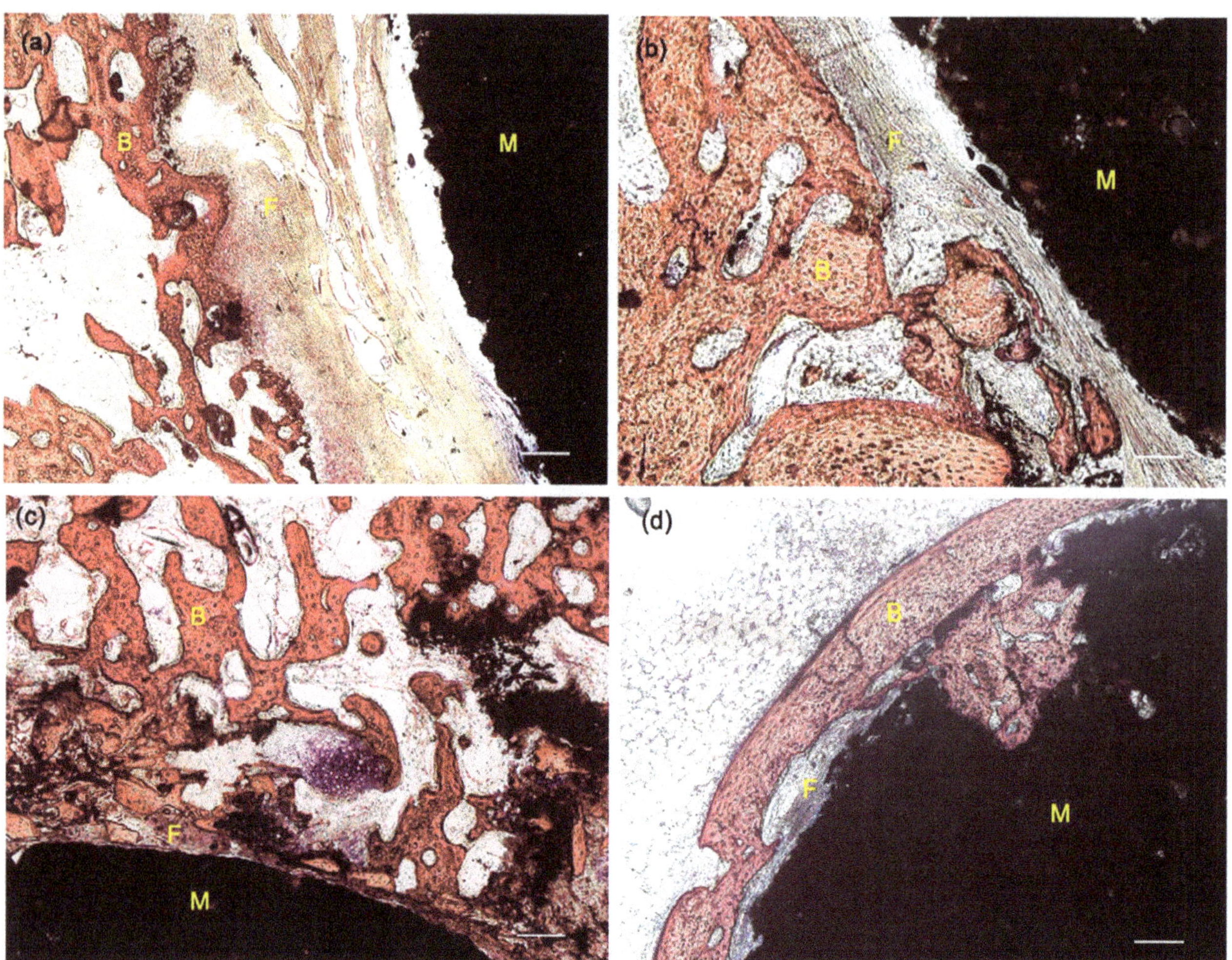

Figure 8. Histological morphologies of the interface between bone tissue and cement. (a, b) The PMMA and (c, d) PSB bone cement after implantation for 6 and 12 weeks, respectively. M: materials, B: bone, F: fibrous tissue, Arrow: bone ingrowth into macropores formed by the degradation of bone cement, bars = 100 μm.

implantation, which suggests the degradation rate of the PSB bone cement was much higher than that of the PMMA bone cement.

9. Histological Analysis

Bone-cement contact was confirmed using histological analysis at 6 and 12 weeks (Fig. 8). At 6 weeks after implantation, a dense fibrous layer was observed at the interface of the PMMA bone cement (Fig. 8a). On the other hand, direct contact with bone cement was observed at 6 weeks after implantation in the PSB bone cement. However, a thin fibrous layer was seen on those surface areas of the bone cement where PMMA was present (Fig. 8c). With the increase of the implantation period to 12 weeks, a thin fibrous layer was still observed at the interface of the PMMA bone cement, preventing bone contact (Fig. 8b). In contrast, for the PSB bone cement, obvious bone ingrowth into macropores formed by the degradation of bone cement occurred at 12 weeks after implantation (Fig. 8d).

10. Biomechanics

The strength of the implant–bone interface was examined using the push-out test after 6 and 12 weeks implantation (Fig. 9). It was obvious that the PSB bone cement had a higher value of push-out load than the PMMA bone cement at each implantation period. At week 12 after implantation, the push-out load of the PSB bone cement reached 1.89 Mpa, which was 4.7-fold higher than that of the PMMA bone cement.

Discussion

Since the current PMMA bone cement used in total joint replacement is far from optimal, the bonding strength between bone and cement still needs to be enhanced. Many studies have been steadily conducted to improve the bonding strength at the interface. An early trial using Ceravital® particles reported tight bonding between the newly formed osseous tissue and the glass ceramic particles at the interface, but obtaining a bioactive composite cement with high mechanical properties was not achieved [31]. In this study, chitosan particles were chosen as porogen for the following reason: The addition of chitosan particles does not significantly reduce the mechanical property of the PMMA cement because no "macroscopic" weak links were present in the cement [32]. Therefore, the adequate mechanical property was achieved. Although the reduction in the compressive strength from 80 to 72 Mpa was observed after immersion in PBS for 4 weeks (Fig. 2), the value of strength still meets mechanical

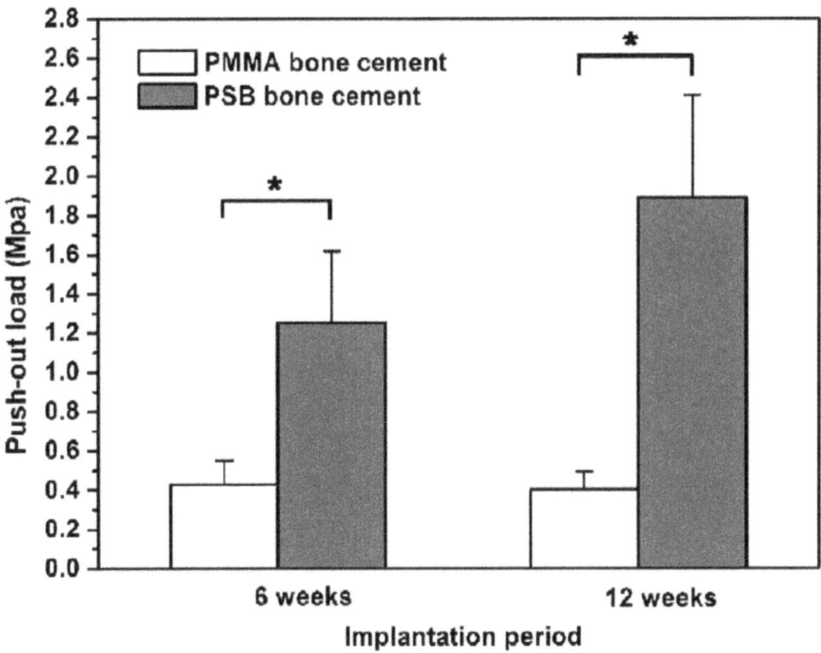

Figure 9. Results of push-out strength after implantation in rabbit femur. Data are shown as mean ± standard deviation (n = 6).*, $P<0.05$ between two marked samples.

properties required by ISO 5833. Moreover, the mechanical properties would be enhanced by bone ingrowth under *in vivo* conditions.

One of the most important properties of cement is its setting time. The optimal time required is between 10 and 15 min [33]. If the setting time is too long, the surgeon must wait until he/she can close the wound [34]. Tsukeoka et al developed a bioactive PMMA cement through modification with gmethacryloxypropyltrimethoxysilane and calcium acetate, but the bone cement had a setting time of 18 min [29], which was beyond the range of clinical demands. In this study the PSB bone cement had a setting time of 12.7 min, which met clinical demands from a biological point of view.

We found the bioactivity was affected slightly by the low content of bioactive fillers. The results of SEM and EDS revealed that the formation of an apatite layer on the cement surface was confirmed until 7 days after soaking in SBF. Correspondingly, a histological examination also showed a thin fibrous layer on those surface areas of the bone cement where PMMA was present at week 12 after implantation (Fig. 8). This may be because of the low content of additives, which probably leaves less area of the bioactive fillers to react with the surrounding body fluid.

The *in vivo* degradation studies revealed that the formation of the porous surface structure was confirmed by the micro-CT analysis after implantation of the PSB bone cement in the rabbit femur defect. The *in vivo* resorption occurs with the increase of the implantation times. The residual material volume fraction of the PSB bone cement decreased to 86.05±3.11% at 12 weeks after implantation. The micro-CT results showed that the macropores seem to be formed by the degradation of the biodegradable CS particles, which was also observed in the histological images. Previous studies have shown that the pore size required for successful ingrowth of bone cells in orthopedics is at least 150 μm [35–38]. In the study, the average size of the macropores is about 200 μm, which is favorable for new bone ingrowth.

The findings of the present study suggest that the PSB bone cement resulted in a higher binding strength than the PMMA bone cement (Fig. 9). The results might be caused by the formation of the apatite layer and the osseointegration after implantation in the bony defect. The *in vitro* bioactivity using SBF clearly showed that the PSB bone cement had the ability to form apatite in the body environment. The apatite formation and release of calcium and phosphate ions were probably attributed to the increased degree of attachment, proliferation, and osteogenic differentiation of preosteoblast cells *in vitro*. A similar response was observed for osteoblast cells grown on PMMA/HA, where the proliferation of the cells on the composite was higher compared to PMMA after 8 days in the culture [39]. The formation of the apatite layer induced osteoconduction of the PSB bone cement through the surface reaction with surrounding body fluids *in vivo*. The micro-CT and histological analysis revealed that the newly formed bone was present around the PSB bone cement and direct bone apposition to the PSB bone cement was observed. In contrast, a dense soft tissue layer was seen at the interface of the PMMA bone cement. Quantitative analysis also showed that the volume of new bone in the PSB bone cement was remarkably higher than that in the PMMA bone cement (Fig. 7). The PSB bone cement stimulated more new bone formation than the PMMA bone cement on their surface during the implantation periods. More importantly, we observed obvious bone ingrowth into the PSB bone cement after implantation. The results indicated that the PSB bone cement possesses osseointegration properties, which is considered to be vital to firmly anchor the implant in place [40].

The results of the present study indicate that higher bonding strengths between bone and implant can be achieved with a porous surface modified bioactive bone cement. The low content of bioactive fillers resulted in proper handling characteristics and adequate mechanical properties, but slightly affected its bioactivity. The degree of attachment, proliferation and osteogenic differentiation of preosteoblast cells was also increased. Histological observation and micro-CT images showed that the modified bone cement exhibited osteoconductive properties and induced bone ingrowth into the porous surface structure. Our findings suggested a new bioactive bone cement for prosthetic fixation in total joint replacement. Further studies will attempt to investigate whether bone ingrowth into the bioactive bone cement will decrease the possibility of bone resorption in canine total hip arthroplasty.

Acknowledgments

We thank for assistance and advices on laboratory technology support by Dai Cheng-Long, Department of Chemical and Biomolecular Engineering, The Ohio State University, Columbus, USA.

Author Contributions

Conceived and designed the experiments: WL ZW. Performed the experiments: QH HC LH JD MM. Analyzed the data: QH LK YL. Contributed reagents/materials/analysis tools: QH DG MM. Wrote the paper: QH HC. Obtained permission for use of cell line: JD.

References

1. Friedman RJ, Black J, Galante JO, Jacobs JJ, Skinner HB (1993) Current concepts in orthopaedic biomaterials and implant fixation. J Bone Joint Surg 75: 1086–109.
2. Lewis G (1997) Properties of acrylic bone cement: state of the art review. J Biomed Mater Res (APPL Biomater) 38: 155–88.
3. Martens M, Ducheyne P, De Meester P, Mulier JC (1980) Skeletal fixation of implants by bone ingrowth into surface pores. Arch Orthop Trauma Surg 97: 111–6.
4. Freeman MA, Bradley GW, Revell PA (1982) Observations upon the interface between bone and polymethylmethacrylate cement. J Bone Joint Surg Br 64: 489–93.
5. Jasty M, Maloney WJ, Bragdon CR, Haire T, Harris WH (1990) Histomorphological studies of the long-term skeletal responses to well fixed cemented femoral components. J Bone Joint Surg Am 72: 1220–9.
6. Ohashi KL, Dauskardt RH (2000) Effects of fatigue loading and PMMA precoating on the adhesion and subcritical debonding of prosthetic–PMMA interfaces. J Biomed Mater Res 51: 172–83.
7. Knabe C, Driessens FC, Planell JA, Gildenhaar R, Berger G, et al (2000) Evaluation of calcium phosphates and experimental calcium phosphate bone cements using osteogenic cultures. Journal of Biomedical Materials Research 52: 498–508.
8. Yuan H, Yang Z, De Bruij JD, De Groot K, Zhang X (2001) Material dependent bone induction by calcium phosphate ceramics: a 2.5-year study in dogs. Biomaterials 22: 2617–23.
9. Fini M, Giavaresi G, Aldini NN, Torricelli P, Botter R, et al (2002) A bone substitute composed of polymethylmethacrylate and alpha-tricalcium phosphate: results in terms of osteoblast function and bone tissue formation. Biomaterials 23: 4523–31.
10. HeikkiläJT, Aho AJ, Kangasniemi I, Yli-Urpo A (1996) Polymethylmethacrylate composites: disturbed bone formation at the surface of bioactive glass and hydroxyapatite. Biomaterials 17: 1755–60.
11. Shinzato S, Nakamura T, Kokubo T, Kitamura Y (2001) A new bioactive bone cement: effect of glass bead filler content on mechanical and biological properties. J Biomed Mater Res 54: 491–500.
12. Ralf S, Per A (1999) Attachment of PMMA cement to bone: force measurements in rats. Biomaterials 21: 2137–46.
13. Fujita H, Ido K, Matsuda Y, Iida H, Oka M, et al (2000) Evaluation of bioactive bone cement in canine total hip arthroplasty. J Biomed Mater Res 49: 273–88.
14. Gettleman L, Nathanson D (1980) Confirmation of bone ingrowth into porous PMMA materials. J Dent Res 59: 139.
15. Qi X, Ye J, Wang Y (2009) Alginate/poly (lactic-co-glycolic acid)/calcium phosphate cement scaffold with oriented pore structure for bone tissue engineering. J Biomed Mater Res A 89: 980–7.
16. Shi M, Kretlow JD, Spicer PP, Tabata Y, Demian N, et al (2011) Antibiotic-releasing porous polymethylmethacrylate/gelatin/antibiotic constructs for craniofacial tissue engineering. J Control Release 152: 196–205.
17. Bauer TW, Schils J (1999) The pathology of total joint arthroplasty. II. Mechanisms of implant failure. Skeletal Radiol 28: 483–97.
18. Lye KW, Tideman H, Wolke JC, Merkx MA, Chin FK, et al (2011) Biocompatibility and bone formation with porous modified PMMA in normal and irradiated mandibular tissue. Clin Oral Implants Res 8: 1–10.
19. Tunney MM, Brady AJ, Buchanan F, Newe C, Dunne NJ (2008) Incorporation of chitosan in acrylic bone cement: effect on antibiotic release, bacterial biofilm formation and mechanical properties. J Mater Sci Mater Med 19: 1609–15.
20. (1992) International Standard ISO 5833 Implants for surgery-acrylic resins cements.
21. Kawashita M, Kawamura K, Li Z (2010) PMMA-based bone cements containing magnetite particles for the hyperthermia of cancer. Acta Biomater 6: 3187–92.
22. Guo D, Xu K, Zhao X, Han Y (2005) Development of a strontium-containing hydroxyapatite bone cement. Biomaterials 26: 4073–83.
23. Kokubo T, Takadama H (2006) How useful is SBF in predicting in vivo bone bioactivity? Biomaterials 27: 2907–15.
24. Bernards MT, Qin C, Ratner BD, Jiang S (2008) Adhesion of MC3T3-E1 cells to bone sialoprotein and bone osteopontin specifically bound to collagen I. J Biomed Mater Res A 86: 779–87.
25. Jeong JC, Lee JW, Yoon CH, Kim HM, Kim CH (2004) Drynariae Rhizoma promotes osteoblast differentiation and mineralization in MC3T3-E1 cells through regulation of bone morphogenetic protein-2, alkaline phosphatase, type I collagen and collagenase-1. Toxicol In Vitro 18: 829–34.
26. Horii A, Wang X, Gelain F, Zhang SG (2007) Biological designer self-assembling peptide nanofiber scaffolds significantly enhance osteoblast proliferation, differentiation and 3-D migration. PLoS One 2: e190.
27. Guldberg RE, Duvall CL, Peister A, Oest ME, Lin AS, et al (2008) 3D imaging of tissue integration with porous biomaterials. Biomaterials 29: 3757–61.
28. Wang W, Itoh S, Tanaka Y, Nagai A, Yamashita K (2009) Comparison of enhancement of bone ingrowth into hydroxyapatite ceramics with highly and poorly interconnected pores by electrical polarization. Acta Biomaterialia 5: 3132–40.
29. Tsukeoka T, Suzuki M, Ohtsuki C, Sugino A, Tsuneizumi Y, et al (2006) Mechanical and histological evaluation of a PMMA-based bone cement modified with gmethacryloxypropyltrimethoxysilane and calcium acetate. Biomaterials 27: 3897–903.
30. Ramakrishnan N, Sivakumar K (1990) An expression for contact area between particles in a powder compact in terms of the porosity. Bulletin of Materials Science 13: 217–225.
31. Hennig W, Blencke BA, BrÖmer H, Deutscher KK, Gross A, et al (1979) Investigations with bioactivated polymethylmethacrylate. J Biomed Mater Res 13: 89–99.
32. Shi Z, Neoh KG, Kang ET, Wang W (2006) Antibacterial and mechanical properties of bone cement impregnated with chitosan nanoparticles. Biomaterials 27: 2440–9.
33. Ginebra MP, Fernández E, Boltong MG, Bermúdez O, Planell JA, et al (1994) Compliance of an apatitic calcium phosphate cement with the short-term clinical requirements in bone surgery, orthopaedics and dentistry. Clin Mater 17: 99–104.
34. Abd Samad H, Jaafar M, Othman R, Kawashita M, Abdul Razak NH (2011) New bioactive glass-ceramic: Synthesis and application in PMMA bone cement composites Journal Bio-Medical Materials and Engineering. Biomed Mater Eng 21: 247–58.
35. Markus DS, Philip PR, Jan S, Christina T, Sonja S, et al (2011) Electrospun PLLA nanofiber scaffolds and their use in combination with BMP-2 for reconstruction of bone defects. PLoS One 6: e25462.
36. Kim SB, Kim YJ, Yoon TL, Park SA, Cho IH, et al (2004) The characteristics of a hydroxyapatite–chitosan–PMMA bone cement. Biomaterials 25: 5715–23.
37. Itoh S, Nakamura S, Nakamura M, Shinomiya K, Yamashita K (2006) Enhanced bone ingrowth into hydroxyapatite with interconnected pores by electrical polarization. Biomaterials 27: 5572–9.
38. Ito Y, Tanaka N, Fujimoto Y, Yasunaga Y, Ishida O, et al (2004) Bone formation using novel interconnected porous calcium hydroxyapatite ceramic hybridized with cultured marrow stromal stem cells derived from Green rat. J Biomed Mater Res 69: 454–61.
39. Moursi AM, Winnard AV, Winnard PL, Lannutti JJ, Seghi RR (2002) Enhanced osteoblast response to a polymethylmethacrylate-hydroxyapatite composite. Biomaterials 23: 133–44.
40. Hennessy KM, Clem WC, Phipps MC, Sawyer AA, Shaikh FM, et al (2008) The effect of RGD peptides on osseointegration of hydroxyapatite. Biomaterials 29: 3075–83.

5

Of Mice, Men and Elephants: The Relation between Articular Cartilage Thickness and Body Mass

Jos Malda[1,2,3]*, Janny C. de Grauw[3], Kim E. M. Benders[1], Marja J. L. Kik[4], Chris H. A. van de Lest[3,5], Laura B. Creemers[1], Wouter J. A. Dhert[1,3], P. René van Weeren[3]

1 Department of Orthopaedics, University Medical Center Utrecht, Utrecht, The Netherlands, **2** Institute of Health and Biomedical Innovation, Queensland University of Technology, Kelvin Grove, Queensland, Australia, **3** Department of Equine Sciences, Faculty of Veterinary Medicine, Utrecht University, Utrecht, The Netherlands, **4** Department of Pathobiology, Faculty of Veterinary Medicine, Utrecht University, Utrecht, The Netherlands, **5** Department of Biochemistry and Cell Biology, Faculty of Veterinary Medicine, Utrecht University, Utrecht, The Netherlands

Abstract

Mammalian articular cartilage serves diverse functions, including shock absorption, force transmission and enabling low-friction joint motion. These challenging requirements are met by the tissue's thickness combined with its highly specific extracellular matrix, consisting of a glycosaminoglycan-interspersed collagen fiber network that provides a unique combination of resilience and high compressive and shear resistance. It is unknown how this critical tissue deals with the challenges posed by increases in body mass. For this study, osteochondral cores were harvested post-mortem from the central sites of both medial and lateral femoral condyles of 58 different mammalian species ranging from 25 g (mouse) to 4000 kg (African elephant). Joint size and cartilage thickness were measured and biochemical composition (glycosaminoclycan, collagen and DNA content) and collagen cross-links densities were analyzed. Here, we show that cartilage thickness at the femoral condyle in the mammalian species investigated varies between 90 µm and 3000 µm and bears a negative allometric relationship to body mass, unlike the isometric scaling of the skeleton. Cellular density (as determined by DNA content) decreases with increasing body mass, but gross biochemical composition is remarkably constant. This however need not affect life-long performance of the tissue in heavier mammals, due to relatively constant static compressive stresses, the zonal organization of the tissue and additional compensation by joint congruence, posture and activity pattern of larger mammals. These findings provide insight in the scaling of articular cartilage thickness with body weight, as well as in cartilage biochemical composition and cellularity across mammalian species. They underscore the need for the use of appropriate *in vivo* models in translational research aiming at human applications.

Editor: Joseph P. R. O. Orgel, Illinois Institute of Technology, United States Of America

Funding: JM is supported by the Dutch Arthritis Foundation (www.reumafonds.nl). KB is supported by an Alexandre Suerman Fellowship (www.umcutrecht.nl). The funders had no role in study design, data collection and analysis, decision to publish, or preparation of the manuscript.

Competing Interests: The authors have declared that no competing interests exist.

* E-mail: j.malda@umcutrecht.nl

Introduction

Articular cartilage is a heavily challenged tissue, as its main functions (shock absorption, force transmission and enabling low-friction movement of joints) require a combination of both great resilience and high compressive and shear resistance [1]. These demands are difficult to reconcile, but the tissue succeeds in doing so by the specific characteristics of its extracellular matrix (ECM) that consists of a glycosaminoglycan-interspersed collagen fiber network [2]. As articular cartilage is aneural, avascular and of low cellularity, its ECM is of relatively homogeneous composition. The downside, however, is that this constitution is thought to be the underlying cause of the very limited regenerative capacity of the tissue [3].

There is a huge difference in adult body mass amongst the currently living mammalian species. A mouse may weigh as little as 25 grams, whereas an African elephant easily reaches 4 tons, which represents 150,000-fold increase in body mass. The cube square law [4] stipulates that with increasing volume of a body, total mass increases with the third power of unit length, while the cross-sections of the supporting structures only increase with the second power, thus resulting in a linear increase in potential load (force per unit area) on these structures. The mammalian skeleton (y) generally scales proportionally [5] (isometrically; $y = bx^a$; $a = 0.33$) with body mass (x), and to compensate for the relatively higher loading of specific supporting structures, bone mass increases at certain sites[5,6,7,8] and thus scales with positive allometry ($a > 0.33$). However, the basic biological requirement for bone is to provide rigidity, which is more straightforward than the specific demands cartilage has to meet. Thus far, little is known about how articular cartilage deals with the challenges posed by increases in body mass [9]. The biochemical composition of the cartilage varies significantly over different topographical locations of the joint surface [10,11,12], and glycosaminoglycan (GAG) content appears to be dependent on local tissue loading [10,13,14]. While some significant differences in cartilage biochemical composition have been demonstrated between species [15], it is not known to what extent a similar mechanism would be necessary and may indeed exist to accommodate for the much larger differences in loading generated by the size differences between species.

Increases in thickness are likely to be limited by the avascular nature of cartilage. Previous studies in small groups of mammals, however, demonstrated that cartilage thickness does increase with increasing body mass [16,17,18]. Simon [16] found that cartilage thickness in 5 species of quadrupeds (mouse, rat, dog sheep, and cow) generally increased with body mass although marked variations were noted. Interestingly, Simon did not observe a consistent relationship between tissue thickness and the estimated compressive stress on the joint [16]. Stockwell [17] also showed that overall articular cartilage thickness is proportional to body mass in 8 mammalian species (mouse, rat, cat, rabbit, dog, sheep, man, and cow), although human cartilage was found to be relatively thicker. While these studies are helpful, they unfortunately comprised only a few species, were not fully conclusive, and failed to find evidence of a mechanism that may compensate for the more than proportional increase in potential loading that follows from the cube-square law.

We investigated the thickness and composition of the articular cartilage at the femoral condyle in 58 mammalian species with a wide variation in body mass. The hypotheses to be tested were that, (1) due to diffusional constraints [19,20], cartilage thickness, unlike the dimensions of bones, cannot scale isometrically with increasing body mass and hence will be relatively thinner in larger animals; (2) a high cellularity of the articular cartilage could only be sustained in mammals with a low body mass; and (3) dramatic changes in extracellular matrix composition would not be required in view of the previously reported similar static compressive stresses in the articular cartilage of various species [16]. The results indeed show that cartilage thickness scales with negative allometry with body mass and that collagen and glycosaminoglycan content remain relatively constant over a wide body mass range.

Materials and Methods

Tissue harvest

Osteochondral cores were harvested post-mortem from the central sites of both the medial and lateral femoral condyles of different-sized mammals sent in for autopsy at the Department of Pathobiology, Faculty of Veterinary Medicine, Utrecht University, The Netherlands. Prior to harvest, animal species, age and body mass were recorded and macroscopic photographs of the joints were taken. Joints demonstrating macroscopic signs of cartilage degeneration, a microscopic Mankin score above 7 (see histology) or originating from skeletally immature animals were excluded. Human tissue samples were obtained from the Department of Pathology, University Medical Center Utrecht, The Netherlands, with approval of the local ethics committee and in line with the Dutch code of conduct "Proper Secondary Use of Human Tissue" as installed by the Federation of Biomedical Scientific Societies. In total, tissue was harvested (121 samples for histological and 84 for biochemical analysis) from mammals belonging to 58 different species (Table 1).

Histology

Osteochondral tissue samples for histology were decalcified using Luthra solution (3.2% 11 M HCl, 10% formic acid in distilled water), dehydrated, cleared in xylene, embedded in paraffin and cut to yield 5 µm sections. Sections were either stained with hematoxylin and eosin for image analysis or with hematoxylin, fast green and safranin-O for measurement of cartilage thickness from the surface down to the chondro-osseous junction and for osteoarthritic grading using the Mankin score [21]. Digital images were analyzed using cellF software (Olympus, USA). The average thickness of the articular cartilage of each sample was determined by averaging 4 measurements per image at different locations.

Glycosaminoglycan and DNA content

Cartilage samples for biochemical analyses were digested overnight at 60°C in 20 µL papain solution (0.01 M cysteine, 250 µg/ml papain, 0.2 M NaH_2PO_4 and 0.01 M $EDTA.2H_2O$) per mg cartilage tissue. Glycosaminoglycan (GAG) content of the digests was determined spectrophotometrically after reaction with dimethylmethylene blue reagent (DMMB, Sigma-Aldrich, USA) [22]. DNA content was determined using the Picogreen DNA assay [23] (Invitrogen, P7589) in accordance with the manufacturer's instructions.

Collagen content

Hydroxyproline content (as a measure of collagen content) and collagen cross-links were analyzed by HPLC-MS/MS using multiple reaction monitoring (MRM) as previously described [24]. Briefly, aliquots of digested cartilage samples were hydrolyzed (110°C, 18–20h) in 6 M HCl. Homo-arginine was added to the hydrolyzed samples as an internal standard. Samples were vacuum-dried and dissolved in 30% methanol containing 0.2% heptafluor buteric acid (HFBA). After centrifugation at 13,000 *g* for 10 min, the supernatants were analyzed with HPLC-MS/MS, using an API3000 mass-spectrometer (Applied Biosystems/MDS Sciex, Foster City, CA) at a source temperature of 300°C and a spray voltage of 4.5 kV. Amino acids were separated on a Synergi MAX-RP 80A (250×3 mm, 4 µm) column (Phenomenex Inc., Torrance, CA) at a flow rate of 400 µL/min, using a gradient from 0.2% HFBA in MilliQwater (Millipore, Billerica, MA) to 100% methanol (Biosolve, Valkenswaard, The Netherlands).

Statistics

Statistical comparison of the medial and lateral cartilage thicknesses was conducted using a paired one-sample Student's t-test on the ratios. For correlations between body mass and cartilage thickness, a regression analysis using a power curve fit was performed. Statistical comparison of the obtained power coefficient with the theoretical coefficient of 0.33 (isometric scaling) was performed using a one-sample T-test. Significance of both tests was assumed at $p<0.05$.

Results

The total width of the lateral and medial condyles was analyzed (Figure 1) as a measure of joint size in the 58 different species of mammals evaluated (Table 1). We found an increase in total condyle size with body mass that scaled according to an isometric relation ($a = 0.337$, Figure 1), in line with previous observations on the scaling of the mammalian skeleton. Histological analysis revealed a relatively higher bone density of the subchondral bone in larger species in our study (Figure 2).

Within the cartilage tissue of all species, a decreased intensity of safranin O staining was observed within the superficial layers compared to the deeper layers, indicative of lower glycosaminoglycan content in the upper tissue regions (Figure 2).

We found that the thickness of the calcified plus non-calcified cartilage layer on the summits of the lateral and medial femoral condyles varied widely between species (Figure 3), ranging from about 90 µm in the mouse to 2,000 µm in humans and approximately 3,000 µm in the Asian elephant (Figure 3, Table 2). Moreover, cartilage thickness was (on average per species) significantly greater at the medial than at the lateral condyle (15%, $p = 0.004$).

Table 1. Number of animals per species included in this study.

	Species	*Average body mass (kg)*	*Histology (n)*	*Biochemistry (n)*
1	Mouse (*Mus Musculus*)	0.025	5	
2	Pygmy marmoset (*Callithrix pygmaea*)	0.13	1	
3	Common marmoset (*Callithrix jacchus*)	0.3	1	1
4	Rat (*Rattus sp.*)	0.3	5	4
5	Cotton-top or Pinché tamarin (*Saguinus oedipus*)	0.34	1	1
6	Eurasian Red squirrel (*Sciurus vulgaris*)	0.4		1
7	Cape Ground squirrel (*Xerus inauris*)	0.65		1
8	Guinea pig (*Cavia porcellus*)	0.78	3	3
9	Potto (*Perodicticus potto*)	0.99	1	1
10	Ferret (*Mustela putorius furo*)	1.3	1	2
11	White-faced saki (*Pithecia pithecia*)	2	1	1
12	Ring-tailed lemur (*Lemur catta*)	2.2	1	2
13	Opossum (*Didelphis sp.*)	2.4	1	1
14	Oriental small-clawed otter (*Aonyx cinerea*)	2.81		1
15	Hare (*Lepus sp.*)	3.1	2	4
16	Rabbit (*Oryctolagus cuniculus*)	3.7	6	7
17	South American coati (*Nasua Nasua*)	5.1	2	1
18	European otter (*Lutra lutra*)	6.5	1	1
19	Linnaeus's two-toed sloth (*Choloepus didactylus*)	6.5	1	1
20	Black Mangabey (*Lophocebus albigena*)	7	1	1
21	Vervet monkey (*Chlorocebus pygerythrus*)	7.7	2	1
22	Southern or Chilean Pudú (*Pudu puda*)	7.8	2	2
23	Woolly Monkey (*Lagothrix lagotricha*)	8.4	1	1
24	Barbary macaque (*Macaca sylvanus*)	8.5	2	2
25	Badger (*Meles meles*)	10	2	2
26	Dikdik (*Madoqua kirkii*)	10	1	
27	Beagle dog (*Canis sp.*)	12	4	2
28	Tammar wallaby (*Macropus eugenii*)	12.5	2	1
29	Hamadryas baboon (*Papio hamadryas*)	15.8	3	3
30	Indian crested porcupine (*Hystrix indica*)	16	1	1
31	Thomson's gazelle (*Eudorcas thomsoni*)	18	4	1
32	Roe deer (*Capreolus capreolus*)	19.2	5	2
33	Capybara (*Hydrochoerus hydrochaeris*)	22	1	1
34	Dutch milk goat (*Capri hircus*)	25	1	
35	West African dwarf goat (*Capri sp.*)	29	1	1
36	Cheetah (*Acinonyx jubatus*)	39.5	4	1
37	Impala (*Aepyceros melampus*)	41	2	2
38	Red Kangaroo (*Macropus rufus*)	52.5	2	1
39	Human (*Homo Sapiens*)	68.3	10	2
40	Fallow deer (*Dama dama*)	70	1	1
41	Gorilla (*Troglodytes gorilla*)	74		1
42	Siberian tiger (*Panthera tigris*)	80	1	1
43	Reindeer (*Rangifer tarandus*)	125	1	
44	Lion (*Panthera leo*))	148	1	
45	Horse (mini-shetland) (*Equus sp.*)	150	1	
46	Kudu (*Tragelaphus strepsiceros*)	150	1	
47	Llama (*Lama Glama*)	160	1	
48	Polar bear (*Ursus Maritimus*)	175	1	1
49	South American tapir (*Tapirus terrestris*)	250	1	1

Table 1. Cont.

	Species	Average body mass (kg)	Histology (n)	Biochemistry (n)
50	European moose (*Alces alces alces*)	343	1	1
51	Watoessi (*Bos Taurus Taurus watussi*)	350	1	
52	Dairy cow (*Bovinae*)	450	2	
53	Giraffe (*Giraffa camelopardalis*)	555	3	1
54	Horse (*Equus ferus caballus*)	557	15	13
55	Banteng (*Bos javanicus*)	600	1	1
56	White rhinoceros (*Ceratotherium simum*)	1550	2	2
57	Asian elephant (*Elaphus maximus*)	3350	2	1
58	African Elephant (*Loxodonta africanus*)	4000	1	
	Total		**121**	**84**

There was a direct relationship between cartilage thickness and body mass, but our data reveal that cartilage thickness increased less than would be expected based on isometric scaling of the skeleton (as illustrated in Figure 1), and consequently bore a negative allometric relationship to body mass over the range 25 g (mouse) – 4,000 kg (African elephant) for both the lateral ($a = 0.262$; $R^2 = 0.80$, $p < 0.001$) and medial ($a = 0.280$; $R^2 = 0.79$, $p < 0.001$) condyles (Figure 3). The obtained power coefficients (a) were significantly different from the theoretical coefficient of 0.33 for both lateral ($p < 0.001$) and medial ($p = 0.01$) sites.

The average overall GAG content across species (lateral: 47±14 µg per mg, medial: 49±15 µg per mg cartilage) appeared not to be related to body mass (Figure 4A). In addition, hydroxyproline content, as a measure of collagen content, (lateral: 350±154 nmol hydroxyproline per mg, medial: 419±180 nmol hydroxyproline per mg) was also independent of body mass across different species (Figure 4B). In contrast, an inverse relationship between DNA content and body mass was observed (lateral: $R^2 = 0.50$ and medial: $R^2 = 0.51$) (Figure 4C), resulting in a rapid decrease in DNA content with increasing body mass, particularly in the 25 g–10 kg range.

Since structural features of the collagen network might also influence the mechanical properties of the tissue, collagen cross-links were analyzed as well. However, no significant correlation between lysyl-pyridinoline (LP) or hydroxylsyl-pyridinoline (HP) cross-link density and body mass was found (Figure 5).

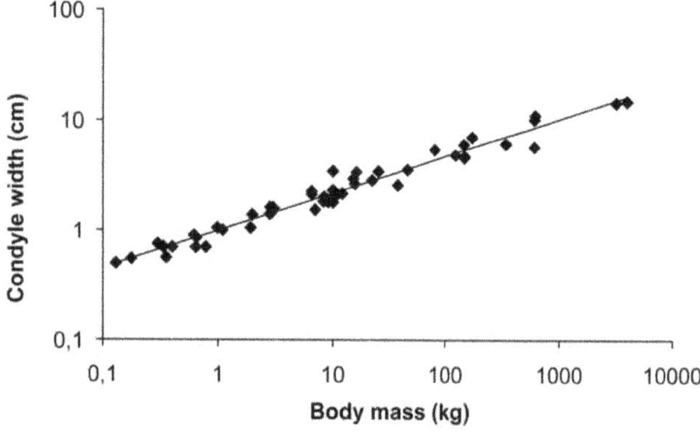

Figure 1. Scaling of the knee joint. The total average width of the articulating lateral and medial condyles per species follows an isometric relationship with body mass ($a = 0.337$, $R^2 = 0.96$), illustrating the isometric scaling of the entire skeleton. Image shows the lateral and medial condyles of a cheetah.

Discussion

The present study shows for the first time that cartilage thickness at the femoral condyle bears a negative allometric relationship body mass, unlike the size of the mammalian skeleton that generally scales proportionally (isometrically) with body mass [5,6,7,8]. In addition, we show that cellular density (as determined by DNA content) decreases with increasing body mass particularly in the lower end of the mass spectrum, but that gross biochemical composition is remarkably constant over a wide range of mammalian body mass.

The condylar cartilage thicknesses reported here are in line with the outcomes of earlier studies investigating cartilage thicknesses in small groups of animals of different species [16,17,18]. Moreover, the average greater thickness of the medial compared to the lateral condyle is also in line with previous reports on a number of different species including the horse [25], cow [26], sheep [27] and rabbit [28]. Cartilage thickness scaled according to a negative allometric relationship with body mass; *i.e.*, based on the thickness observed in small mammals and assuming proportional scaling, one would have expected a considerably greater tissue thickness (approximately 4,500–6,000 µm) than the actual observed value (3,000 µm) for the African elephant. This lower-than-expected increase in tissue thickness may be related to diffusional constraints, as adult articular cartilage lacks vascularization [20,29]. Interestingly, recent research on fossilized material of the largest land creatures that ever lived, the dinosaurs, revealed traces of vascularization to potentially sustain the substantially thicker articular cartilage [30]. In contrast to our findings, previous investigations [16,17,26] have suggested a positive allometric relationship between articular cartilage thickness and body mass. These studies were however performed on only a small number (5–8) of mammalian species of less than 300 kg, analyzed the maximum cartilage thickness in the joint and included skeletally immature animals [16,17,26]. These factors likely explain the overestimation of cartilage thickness in the larger species in these studies.

Besides variation in thickness, the mechanical characteristics of articular cartilage are determined by the interplay of its three main biochemical constituents: collagen, proteoglycans and water. Although some species differences in biochemical composition of the articular cartilage have previously been demonstrated[15], we

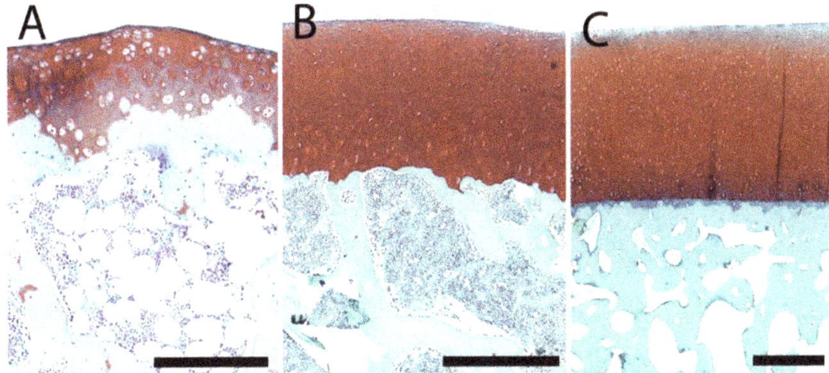

Figure 2. Safranin-O staining (stains GAGs red) of osteochondral tissue of the (A) rat, (B) barbary macaque and (C) white rhinoceros. Scale bars indicate (A) 200 μm, (B) 400 μm, and (C) 1000 μm.

found that gross biochemical composition is remarkably constant. It should be noted however that the DMMB assay [22] we employed is a rather crude technique for GAG quantitation that for example does not discriminate between keratan sulphate and chondrotin sulphate [31]. The ratio of these components in the cartilage may significantly affect the overall fixed charge density [31], which in turn will affect the mechanical characteristics of the tissue [32]. Nevertheless, our results indicate a certain immutability of cartilage ECM with respect to gross composition, as both collagen content and the abundance of pyridinoline cross-links that heavily influence mechanical properties, were likewise found to be relatively stable over a wide range of mammalian body mass.

Cartilage DNA content, as a measure of cellular density, decreases with increasing body mass. This observation is consistent with the finding that cell density in thinner cartilages is considerably higher [17], although in the current study potential species-specific differences in DNA content per cell were not taken into account. The relatively high DNA content in mouse and rat cartilage is not a specific feature of rodent cartilage, as the cartilage of the Capybara (the largest extant rodent in the world), showed considerably lower DNA content, which is in the range of other similarly-sized mammals. The high DNA content of the thinner cartilages could also be related to the high cell content in the superficial zone of the tissue [17,25,33,34], which likely contributes relatively more to total tissue thickness in thin cartilage than in thicker cartilage. Regardless, the relatively high DNA content in the lighter species is indicative of a higher cellularity of thinner cartilage (as supported by histological evaluation of tissue cell density). This may impact (positively) on the regenerative capacity of cartilage in these smaller animals and underscores the need for the use of appropriate *in vivo* models [35,36], which approximate the human situation, when evaluating experimental approaches for cartilage repair.

An increase in mammalian body mass will require adaptations of the musculoskeletal system to accommodate for higher loading. Alterations in tissue dimensions and/or composition constitute a logical response to such changes. Indeed, articular cartilage biochemical composition (and with it biomechanical characteristics) have been shown to be both location and age dependent [37,38,39], which may explain the higher variation of the biochemical data in comparison to the joint sized in our study.

When gross ECM composition is remarkably stable over a large range of species and body mass, differences may exist at a more detailed (structural / molecular) level. These may explain previously reported interspecies differences in mechanical properties [32]. Although cartilage is a relatively homogeneous tissue, distinct zones, each with their own specific compressive properties, biochemical composition and structural organization, can be

Table 2. Cartilage thickness at the lateral en femoral condyles of selected species.

Species	(n)	Thickness Lateral ±SD (μm)	Thickness Medial ±SD (μm)
Mouse (Mus Musculus)	5	99±32	87±13
Rat (Rattus sp.)	5	213±29	235±46
Rabbit (Oryctolagus cuniculus)	6	455±119	470±139
Vervet monkey (Chlorocebus pygerythrus)	2	540±142	707±48
Beagle dog (Canis sp.)	4	476±146	849±184
Hamadryas baboon (Papio hamadryas)	3	805±85	1087±145
Cheetah (Acinonyx jubatus)	4	919±152	999±297
Human (Homo Sapiens)	10	2014±512	2050±780
Horse (Equus ferus caballus)	15	1283±205	2309±726
White rhinoceros (Ceratotherium simum)	2	2119*	2502±192
Asian elephant (Elaphus maximus)	2	2413±101	3021±335

* = only one sample was available.

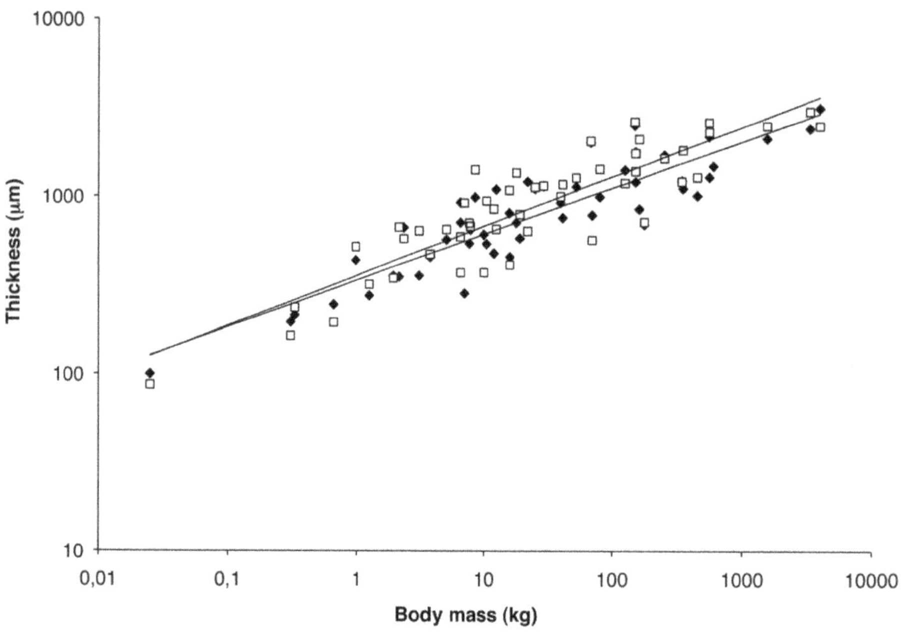

Figure 3. Average mammalian articular cartilage thickness per species at the center of lateral (black diamonds) and medial (open squares) condyles varies allometrically with body mass ($a=0.262$ and $a=0.280$, respectively).

distinguished from the articular surface down to the cartilage-bone interface. For example, the superficial zone is known to exhibit larger strain [40] and to have lower GAG content [25] compared to deeper zones (in line with our histological safranin O stainings). Moreover, the superficial zone contains a number of specific extracellular matrix components, including lubricin (proteoglycan-4) [41] and clusterin [42] that are not found in the deeper zones. In addition, the chondroitin sulphate sulphation motifs and the ratio of chondroitin sulphate to keratan sulphate also vary with depth [31,43]. Collagen content is relatively stable throughout the depth of the tissue [25], but collagen fibril orientation is notably depth-dependent [44]. These depth-dependent differences clearly have implications for the overall mechanical characteristics of tissue with a specific thickness and may hence contribute to the adaptation to higher loads. Consequently, the potential variation in depth-dependent biochemical properties of the cartilage over a range of species and body masses warrants further investigation.

The limited increase in thickness of cartilage and its biochemical constancy are probably largely compensated for, as supported by the fact that static compressive stresses in the joint cartilage among various species are within one order of magnitude and are unrelated to cartilage thickness [16]. Moreover, compression of the tissue is radially confined and shear forces are further resisted by bonding with the subchondral bone and periarticular structures. This, together with the increase in joint surface area in the larger species and accompanying changes in joint alignment, posture and activity pattern (which are related to body mass [9]), might be sufficient to compensate for the additional loading. However, whether the less-than-proportional increase of articular cartilage thickness in larger mammals contributes to a greater susceptibility to degenerative joint disorders in these animals remains unclear and could be an interesting area of future investigation.

Conclusion

Articular cartilage thickness scales according to negative allometry, and, as a result, cartilage is relatively thinner in larger animals. This is potentially due to diffusional constraints, as is illustrated by the presence of high cell densities only in thin cartilages. However, gross biochemical composition is remarkably constant over a wide range of body mass, which, together with the

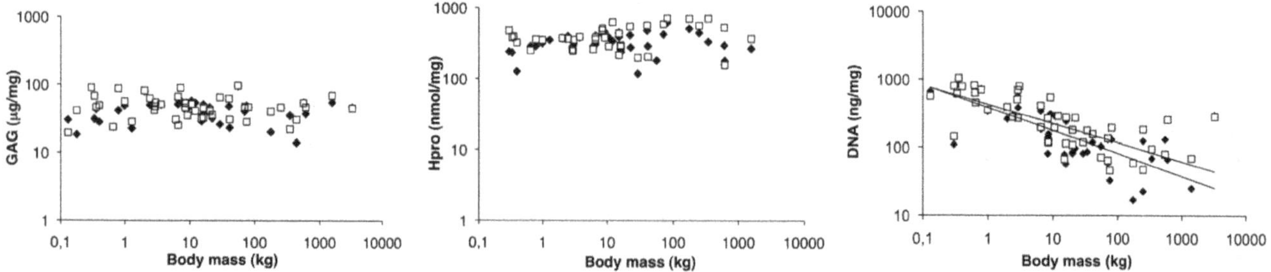

Figure 4. Average (A) glycosaminoglycan (GAG) and (B) hydroxyproline (Hpro) content of the articular cartilage per species is independent of body mass, whilst an inverse relation was observed for (C) DNA at the lateral (black diamonds, $a=-0.327$) and medial (open squares, $a=-0.282$) condyles.

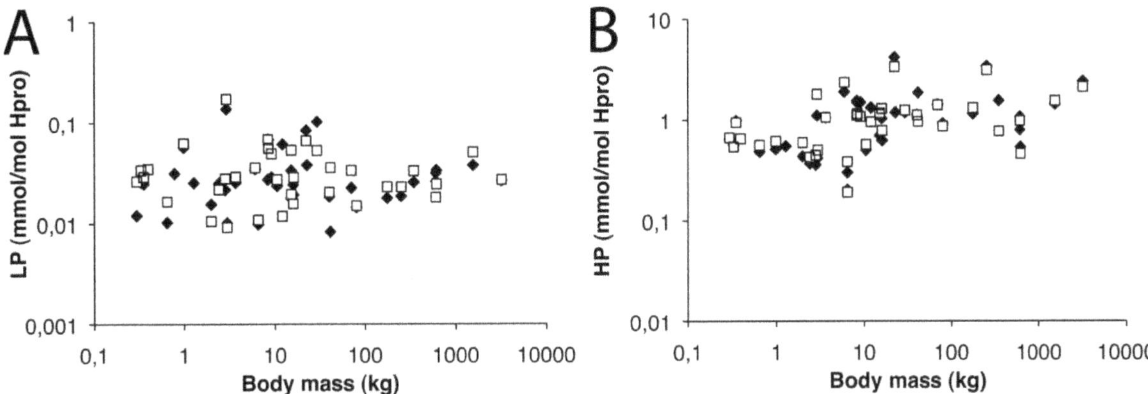

Figure 5. Average collagen cross-link content as a function of body mass. (A) Lysyl-pyridinoline (LP) and (B) hydroxylsyl-pyridinoline (HP) cross-links are independent of body mass at the lateral (black diamonds) and medial (open squares) condyles.

negative allometric scaling of thickness, theoretically leads to a decrease in biomechanical resistance with increasing body weight. However, an isometric increase in thickness may not be required for life-long performance, in light of relatively constant static compressive stresses on the tissue perhaps facilitated by additional compensatory factors like congruence, posture and activity pattern of the animal.

Acknowledgments

The authors thank R. Wagensveld, L. van den Boom, J. van Amerongen, P. Bürgisser, W. Schuurman and J.M. Blom of Utrecht University for their assistance with tissue harvest and P. Levett of Queensland University of Technology for proofreading the manuscript.

Author Contributions

Conceived and designed the experiments: JM JdG KB MK CvdL LC WD PRvW. Performed the experiments: JM JdG KB CvdL. Analyzed the data: JM JdG KB MK CvdL PRvW. Contributed reagents/materials/analysis tools: JM MK WD PRvW. Wrote the paper: JM JdG KB MK CvdL LC WD PRvW.

References

1. Grodzinsky AJ, Levenston ME, Jin M, Frank EH (2000) Cartilage tissue remodeling in response to mechanical forces. Annu Rev Biomed Eng 2: 691–713.
2. Buckwalter J, Mankin H (1997) Articular Cartilage. Part I: Tissue Design and Chondrocyte-Matrix Interactions. J Bone Joint Surg Am 79: 600–611.
3. Steinert AF, Ghivizzani SC, Rethwilm A, Tuan RS, Evans CH, et al. (2007) Major biological obstacles for persistent cell-based regeneration of articular cartilage. Arthritis Res Ther 9: 213.
4. Galilei Linceo G (1683) Discorzsi e demostrazioni matematiche, intorno à duo nuoue scienze. Leiden: Elsevier.
5. Schmidt-Nielsen K (1984) Scaling; Why is animals size so important? Cambridge: University of Cambridge.
6. Christiansen P (2002) Mass allometry of the appendicular skeleton in terrestrial mammals. Journal of Morphology 251: 195–209.
7. Doube M, Klosowski MM, Wiktorowicz-Conroy AM, Hutchinson JR, Shefelbine SJ (2011) Trabecular bone scales allometrically in mammals and birds. Proc Biol Sci.
8. Reynolds WW (1977) Skeleton weight allometry in aquatic and terrestrial vertebrates. Hydrobiology 56: 35–37.
9. Biewener AA (2005) Biomechanical consequences of scaling. Journal of Experimental Biology 208: 1665–1676.
10. Brama PA, Tekoppele JM, Bank RA, Karssenberg D, Barneveld A, et al. (2000) Topographical mapping of biochemical properties of articular cartilage in the equine fetlock joint. Equine Vet J 32: 19–26.
11. Rogers BA, Murphy CL, Cannon SR, Briggs TW (2006) Topographical variation in glycosaminoglycan content in human articular cartilage. J Bone Joint Surg Br 88: 1670–1674.
12. Esquisatto MA, Pimentel ER, Gomes L (1997) Extracellular matrix composition of different regions of the knee joint cartilage in cattle. Ann Anat 179: 433–437.
13. Kiviranta I, Jurvelin J, Tammi M, Saamanen AM, Helminen HJ (1987) Weight bearing controls glycosaminoglycan concentration and articular cartilage thickness in the knee joints of young beagle dogs. Arthritis Rheum 30: 801–809.
14. Kempson GE, Muir H, Swanson SA, Freeman MA (1970) Correlations between stiffness and the chemical constituents of cartilage on the human femoral head. Biochim Biophys Acta 215: 70–77.
15. Buckwalter JA, Pedrini-Mille A, Dobrowolski AM, Olmstead M, Grood E (1989) Differences in articular cartilage matrices of humans monkeys and rabbits. Trans Orthop Res Soc 14: 155.
16. Simon WH (1970) Scale effects in animal joints. I. Articular cartilage thickness and compressive stress. Arthritis Rheum 13: 244–256.
17. Stockwell RA (1971) The interrelationship of cell density and cartilage thickness in mammalian articular cartilage. J Anat 109: 411–421.
18. Frisbie DD, Cross MW, McIlwraith CW (2006) A comparative study of articular cartilage thickness in the stifle of animal species used in human pre-clinical studies compared to articular cartilage thickness in the human knee. Vet Comp Orthop Traumatol 19: 142–146.
19. Brighton C, Heppenstall R (1971) Oxygen tension in zones of the epiphyseal plate, the metaphysis and diaphysis. An in vitro and in vivo study in rats and rabbits. J Bone Joint Surg Am 53: 719–728.
20. Malda J, Rouwkema J, Martens DE, Le Comte EP, Kooy FK, et al. (2004) Oxygen gradients in tissue-engineered Pegt/Pbt cartilaginous constructs: Measurement and modeling. Biotechnol Bioeng 86: 9–18.
21. Mankin HJ, Dorfman H, Lippiello L, Zarins A (1971) Biochemical and metabolic abnormalities in articular cartilage from osteo-arthritic human hips. II. Correlation of morphology with biochemical and metabolic data. J Bone Joint Surg Am 53: 523–537.
22. Farndale R, Buttle D, Barrett A (1986) Improved quantitation and discrimination of sulphated glycosaminoglycans by use of dimethylmethylene blue. Biochim Biophys Acta 883: 173–177.
23. McGowan KB, Kurtis MS, Lottman LM, Watson D, Sah RL (2002) Biochemical quantification of DNA in human articular and septal cartilage using PicoGreen and Hoechst 33258. Osteoarthritis Cartilage 10: 580–587.
24. Souza MV, van Weeren PR, van Schie HT, van de Lest CH (2010) Regional differences in biochemical, biomechanical and histomorphological characteristics of the equine suspensory ligament. Equine Vet J 42: 611–620.
25. Malda J, Benders KE, Klein TJ, de Grauw JC, Kik MJ, et al. (2012) Comparative study of depth-dependent characteristics of equine and human osteochondral tissue from the medial and lateral femoral condyles. Osteoarthritis Cartilage 20: 1147–1151.
26. McLure SW, Fisher J, Conaghan PG, Williams S (2012) Regional cartilage properties of three quadruped tibiofemoral joints used in musculoskeletal research studies. Proceedings of the Institution of Mechanical Engineers, Part H 226: 652–656.
27. Armstrong SJ, Read RA, Price R (1995) Topographical variation within the articular cartilage and subchondral bone of the normal ovine knee joint: a histological approach. Osteoarthritis Cartilage 3: 25–33.
28. Rasanen T, Messner K (1996) Regional variations of indentation stiffness and thickness of normal rabbit knee articular cartilage. J Biomed Mater Res 31: 519–524.

29. Silver IA (1975) Measurement of pH and ionic composition of pericellular sites. Philos Trans R Soc Lond B Biol Sci 271: 261–272.
30. Holliday CM, Ridgely RC, Sedlmayr JC, Witmer LM (2010) Cartilaginous Epiphyses in Extant Archosaurs and Their Implications for Reconstructing Limb Function in Dinosaurs. PLoS One 5.
31. Han E, Chen SS, Klisch SM, Sah RL (2011) Contribution of proteoglycan osmotic swelling pressure to the compressive properties of articular cartilage. Biophys J 101: 916–924.
32. Athanasiou KA, Rosenwasser MP, Buckwalter JA, Malinin TI, Mow VC (1991) Interspecies comparisons of in situ intrinsic mechanical properties of distal femoral cartilage. J Orthop Res 9: 330–340.
33. Hunziker EB, Quinn TM, Hauselmann HJ (2002) Quantitative structural organization of normal adult human articular cartilage. Osteoarthritis Cartilage 10: 564–572.
34. Schuurman W, Gawlitta D, Klein TJ, ten Hoope W, van Rijen MH, et al. (2009) Zonal chondrocyte subpopulations reacquire zone-specific characteristics during in vitro redifferentiation. Am J Sports Med 37 Suppl 1: 97S-104S.
35. McIlwraith CW, Fortier LA, Frisbie D, Nixon AJ (2011) Equine Models of Articular Cartilage Repair. Cartilage 2: 317–326.
36. Chu CR, Szczodry M, Bruno S (2010) Animal models for cartilage regeneration and repair. Tissue Eng Part B Rev 16: 105–115.
37. Brama PA, Holopainen J, van Weeren PR, Firth EC, Helminen HJ, et al. (2009) Influence of exercise and joint topography on depth-related spatial distribution of proteoglycan and collagen content in immature equine articular cartilage. Equine Vet J 41: 557–563.
38. Brama PAJ, TeKoppele JM, Bank RA, van Weeren PR, Barneveld A (1999) Influence of site and age on biochemical characteristics of the collagen network of equine articular cartilage. American Journal of Veterinary Research 60: 341–345.
39. Brommer H, Brama PA, Laasanen MS, Helminen HJ, van Weeren PR, et al. (2005) Functional adaptation of articular cartilage from birth to maturity under the influence of loading: a biomechanical analysis. Equine Vet J 37: 148–154.
40. Schinagl RM, Ting MK, Price JH, Sah RL (1996) Video microscopy to quantitate the inhomogeneous equilibrium strain within articular cartilage during confined compression. Ann Biomed Eng 24: 500–512.
41. Schumacher BL, Block JA, Schmid TM, Aydelotte MB, Kuettner KE (1994) A novel proteoglycan synthesized and secreted by chondrocytes of the superficial zone of articular cartilage. Arch Biochem Biophys 311: 144–152.
42. Malda J, ten Hoope W, Schuurman W, van Osch GJ, van Weeren PR, et al. (2010) Localization of the potential zonal marker clusterin in native cartilage and in tissue-engineered constructs. Tissue Eng Part A 16: 897–904.
43. Hayes AJ, Hall A, Brown L, Tubo R, Caterson B (2007) Macromolecular organization and in vitro growth characteristics of scaffold-free neocartilage grafts. Journal of Histochemistry and Cytochemistry 55: 853–866.
44. Benninghoff A (1925) Form und Bau der Gelenkknorpel in Ihren Beziehungen zur Funktion. Z Zellforsch 2: 783–862.

6

Predicting Cortical Bone Strength from DXA and Dental Cone-Beam CT

Jui-Ting Hsu[1], Ying-Ju Chen[2], Ming-Tzu Tsai[3], Howard Haw-Chang Lan[4,5], Fu-Chou Cheng[2], Michael Y. C. Chen[1], Shun-Ping Wang[6]*

1 School of Dentistry, College of Medicine, China Medical University, Taichung, Taiwan, **2** Stem Cell Center, Department of Medical Research, Taichung Veterans General Hospital, Taichung, Taiwan, **3** Department of Biomedical Engineering, Hungkuang University, Taichung, Taiwan, **4** Department of Radiology, Taichung Veterans General Hospital, Taichung, Taiwan, **5** School of Radiological Technology, Central Taiwan University of Science and Technology, Taichung, Taiwan, **6** Department of Orthopaedics, Taichung Veterans General Hospital, Taichung, Taiwan

Abstract

Objective: This study compared the capabilities of dual-energy X-ray absorptiometry (DXA) and dental cone-beam computed tomography (CBCT) for predicting the cortical bone strength of rat femurs and tibias.

Materials and Methods: Specimens of femurs and tibias obtained from 14 rats were first scanned with DXA to obtain the areal bone mineral density (BMD) of the midshaft cortical portion of the bones. The bones were then scanned using dental CBCT to measure the volumetric cortical bone mineral density (vCtBMD) and the cross-sectional moment of inertia (CSMI) for calculating the bone strength index (BSI). A three-point bending test was conducted to measure the fracture load of each femur and tibia. Bivariate linear Pearson analysis was used to calculate the correlation coefficients (*r* values) among the CBCT measurements, DXA measurements, and three-point bending parameters.

Results: The correlation coefficients for the associations of the fracture load with areal BMD (measured using DXA), vCtBMD (measured using CBCT), CSMI (measured using CBCT), and BSI were 0.585 ($p = 0.028$) and 0.532 ($p = 0.050$) (for the femur and tibia, respectively), 0.638 ($p = 0.014$) and 0.762 ($p = 0.002$), 0.778 ($p = 0.001$) and 0.792 ($p < 0.001$), and 0.822 ($p < 0.001$) and 0.842 ($p < 0.001$), respectively.

Conclusions: CBCT was found to be superior to DXA for predicting cortical bone fracture loads in rat femurs and tibias. The BSI, which is a combined index of densitometric and geometric parameters, was especially useful. Further clinical studies are needed to validate the predictive value of BSI obtained from CBCT and should include testing on human cadaver specimens.

Editor: Yi-Hsiang Hsu, Harvard Medical School, United States of America

Funding: This research was supported by China Medical University, Taiwan (Grant number: CMU99-COL-43). The funders had no role in study design, data collection and analysis, decision to publish, or preparation of the manuscript.

Competing Interests: The authors have declared that no competing interests exist.

* E-mail: richard@ms32.url.com.tw

Introduction

The ability to measure bone strength using noninvasive methods is important for evaluating fracture risk according to the severity of osteoporosis [1,2], as well as to the early-stage stabilization of artificial implants after implantation in bone (e.g., dental or orthopedic implants) [3,4]. Dual-energy X-ray absorptiometry (DXA) is one of the methods commonly used in the clinical field of orthopedics for evaluating bone mineral content (BMC) and bone mineral density (BMD) [5]. The areal BMD (in g/cm^2) measured through DXA is calculated by dividing the obtained BMC (in g) by the projected bone area (in cm^2) [6–8]. Bone quality cannot be determined simply using BMD since, in addition to the intrinsic mechanical quality of the bone, geometric characteristics (size, shape, and macroarchitecture) are important attributes influencing the strength of particular bones [9]. For example, BMD obtained using DXA represents two-dimensional (2D) bone-density information that does not provide data regarding the structural stiffness characteristics, which are related to the bone's shape [6,10].

Numerous researchers have recently used microcomputed tomography (micro-CT) to measure bone geometry and strength [11–13]. Micro-CT also provides three-dimensional (3D) images of bone architecture and various parameters that influence the strength of trabecular bone (e.g., trabecular bone volume, trabecular number, trabecular separation, trabecular thickness, and structure model index). However, because of the limited scan range, micro-CT is mostly used for the bones of small animals (rats or mice) or extracted human bones [12,14,15], and is applied more in laboratory-based research than in the clinical field of orthopedics. In clinical orthopedic practice, quantitative computed tomography (QCT) [5,16,17] or peripheral quantitative computed tomography (pQCT) [6,9,10,18–20] are commonly used to assist in determining the bone BMD. In addition to measuring BMD, pQCT can obtain the 3D geometric parameters of bones. Ferretti and colleagues [7,9] proposed predicting bone bending strength by using pQCT to measure several bone parameters, including the bone strength index (BSI), cross-sectional moment of inertia (CSMI), and volumetric cortical bone mineral density (vCtBMD). Siu et al. [6] and Moisio et al. [10] suggested that bone strength can be predicted more accurately using pQCT than DXA.

In addition to QCT and pQCT, which are commonly used in orthopedics, in recent years dental computed tomography (CT)—also known as dental cone-beam CT (CBCT)—has been used in the dental field. The resolution of CBCT (typically 75–400 μm) is better than that of traditional CT. Nomura et al. [21] found a linear correlation between the voxel values of CBCT and the contents of hydroxyapatite (HA) rod samples, and some researchers have used CBCT to examine the alveolar bone density of patients to serve as references in presurgical evaluations for dental implants [22–24]. Furthermore, the dosage required for CBCT is much less than that for traditional CT [25–28], making CBCT an appropriate method for postsurgical follow-up assessments of changes in bone quality [29,30].

While several studies have evaluated the feasibility of pQCT and DXA for measuring bone strength, few have examined the utility of dental CBCT in assessing cortical bone strength. Most studies have focused on CBCT as a tool for evaluating alveolar bone density before performing dental implantation. Therefore, the present study compared the abilities of DXA and CBCT to predict cortical bone strength in rat femurs and tibias. The hypothesis tested was that the capabilities of CBCT in elucidating and judging BMD and bone shape would make CBCT a better predictor of cortical bone strength than is DXA.

Materials and Methods

Specimen Preparation

Fourteen femurs and 14 tibias were collected from 14 healthy male Sprague-Dawley rats [age = 4 months of age, weight = 335 ± 10 g (mean ± standard deviation)]. The femurs and tibias of each rat were harvested within 5 min after death. The bone specimens were wrapped with gauze soaked in saline and stored in a −20°C freezer. The study procedures were carried out in strict accordance with the recommendations in the Guide for the Care and Use of Laboratory Animals of the National Institutes of Health. Animal Research Ethics approval was obtained from the Research Ethics Committee of the Taichung Veterans General Hospital (Permit Number: La-101955). All surgery was performed under sodium pentobarbital anesthesia, and all efforts were made to minimize suffering.

DXA and Dental CBCT Measurements

The BMDs of the femur and tibia were measured at the midshaft region using the small-laboratory-animal scan mode of the Lunar Prodigy Advanced System (GE, Madison, WI, USA) (Figure 1). The midshaft regions of the femur and tibia were defined as shown in Figure 1. The BMD was calculated from the BMC of the measured area. The measurement values were calculated automatically using Encore 2007 small-animal software (version 11.20.068, GE, Madison, WI, USA). The DXA machine was calibrated according to the manufacturer's instructions.

A dental CBCT device (AZ 3000, Asahi Roentgen, Japan) was used to obtain the CBCT images of each femur and tibia (Figure 1). The scanning parameters were set at 85 kV, 3 mA, and a voxel resolution of 155 μm. When performing the CBCT scans for all bone specimens, two phantoms with predetermined HA concentrations [0.25 and 0.75 g/cm^3 HA BMD phantoms obtained from Skyscan (Skyscan, Aartselaar, Belgium)] were constructed in order to calculate the vCtBMD of the bones. The obtained CBCT images were loaded into professional medical imaging software (Mimics, Materialise, Leuven, Belgium) to calculate the vCtBMD values (in g/cm^3) of the midshaft portions of the femurs and tibias (Figure 2). Five images of the midshaft portion of each femur and tibia were then imported into ImageJ 1.45 s (Rasband, W.S., ImageJ, US National Institutes of Health, Bethesda, Maryland, USA) [31] to measure the CSMI (in mm^4) of the femurs and tibias and for finally calculating the BSI (= vCtBMD × CSMI) [9].

Three-Point Bending Test

After removing their soft tissues, each femur or tibia was placed on a specially designed loading apparatus on a material testing system (JSV-H1000, Japan Instrumentation System, Nara, Japan), as shown in Figure 2. Loads were applied at distances of 40% and 45% of the total femoral and tibial lengths from the anatomic inferior side. The two supporting locations were separated by 20 mm (Figure 2). A static preload of 1 N was applied to fix the bone specimens between the contacts. The loading speed of the crosshead was set to 20 mm/min using the displacement control mode. The force-vs-displacement data were acquired and recorded at a sampling rate of 40 points/second until the bone specimen was fractured. The strength (fracture load) was determined as the highest point of the obtained curve.

Statistical Analysis

The mean, standard deviation, and coefficient of variation (CV) were calculated for all measurements. The Shapiro-Wilk test was used to determine if the measurements conformed to a normal distribution. The paired-sample t-test was used to compare differences between the measurements and the results of the CBCT, DXA, and three-point bending test between the femurs and tibias from the same rat. A bivariate linear Pearson analysis was used to calculate the corresponding correlation coefficients (r values). All statistical analyses of the data were performed using OriginPro software (Version 8, OriginLab, Northampton, MA, USA). The level of the statistical significance was set at $P<0.05$.

Results

Densitometric, geometric, and mechanical test results

The measured densitometric, geometric, and mechanical parameters of the rat femurs and tibias are summarized in Table 1. All of the experimental data were normally distributed ($p<0.05$). The CV was largest for the BSI (32.75% and 35.11% for femurs and tibias, respectively) and smallest for the vCtBMD (6.74% and 8.06%). The densitometric parameters (BMD measured by DXA and vCtBMD measured by CBCT), geometric parameter (CSMI measured by CBCT), combined densitometric and geometric parameters (BSI, = CSMI × vCtBMD), and fracture load were all significantly higher for the femurs than for the tibias ($P<0.001$).

Correlations between radiologic measurements and mechanical test results

The correlation coefficients for the associations of the fracture loads with the areal BMD (measured using DXA), vCtBMD (measured using CBCT), CSMI (measured using CBCT), and BSI (combined densitometric and geometric parameters) were 0.585 ($p = 0.028$) and 0.532 ($p = 0.050$) (for the femur and tibia, respectively; Figure 3), 0.638 ($p = 0.014$) and 0.762 ($p = 0.002$) (Figure 4), 0.778 ($p = 0.001$) and 0.792 ($p<0.001$) (Figure 5), and 0.822 ($p<0.001$) and 0.842 ($p<0.001$) (Figure 6), respectively. The strong associations meant that the following linear expressions

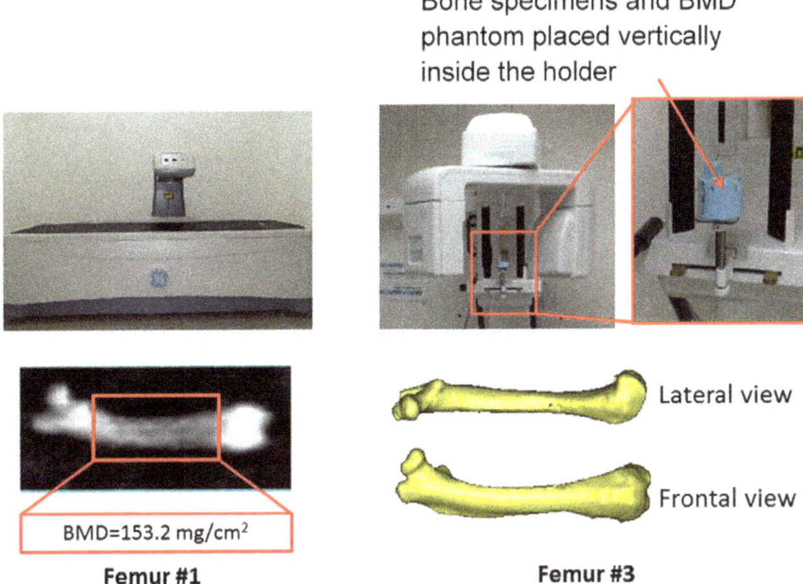

Figure 1. Radiologic measurements of bone specimens: DXA (left) and CBCT (right).

accurately describe the fracture load for the bone specimens: Fracture $load_{Femur} = 0.0029\ BSI_{Femur} + 80.562$ and Fracture $load_{Tibia} = 0.0088\ BSI_{Tibia} + 65.123$.

Discussion

It would be very helpful if noninvasive methods could be used to accurately measure the BMD in order to predict bone strength. DXA has been the most common method, but it only provides 2D information regarding bone density and hence is of limited use in determining the strength of an actual bone structure. Previous studies have shown that compared to DXA, pQCT provides more information about the geometric parameters of bones, and is superior for predicting bone strength [6,10]. Dental CBCT has recently become a popular method for evaluating alveolar bone density prior to dental implantation [22–24]. Researchers have recognized the ability of CBCT to predict BMD [21], although no

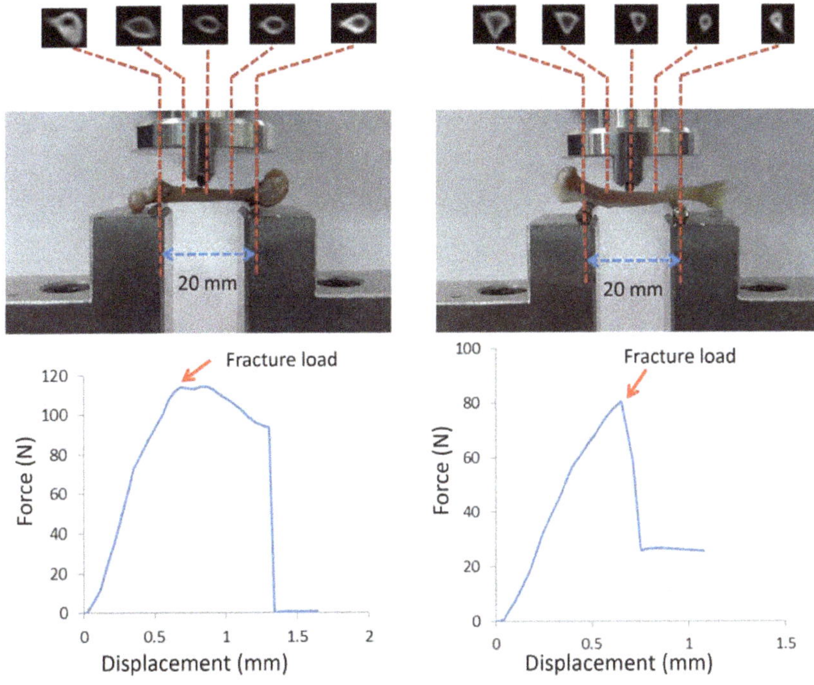

Figure 2. Five CBCT cross-sectional scans, the sites of the DXA scanning measurements, and the three-point bending test: femur (left) and tibia (right). (The force-vs-displacement curves were recorded using the three-point bending test for femur #6 and tibia #10.)

Table 1. Experimentally measured densitometric and geometric parameters of the femurs and tibias obtained from DXA and CBCT. The fracture loads based on the three-point bending test are also listed.

	Parameter	Unit	Femur (N = 14)		Tibia (N = 14)		P values
			Mean±SD	CV(%)	Mean±SD	CV(%)	
DXA	BMD	mg/cm^2	133.69±13.69	10.23	103.29±10.34	10.00	<0.0001
CBCT	vCtBMD	mg/cm^3	1264.48±85.21	6.74	936.50±75.44	8.06	<0.0001
	CSMI	mm^4	8.58±2.55	29.68	3.98±1.17	29.36	<0.0001
	BSI		10937.58±3582.43	32.75	3775.20±1325.60	35.11	<0.0001
MT	Fracture load	N	111.26±12.63	11.25	98.51±13.93	14.14	0.006

SD = standard deviation; CV = coefficient of variation (SD/mean × 100%); DXA = dual-energy X-ray absorptiometry (DXA); CBCT = cone beam computed tomography; MT = mechanical test (three-point bending test); BMD = bone mineral density; vCtBMD = volumetric cortical bone mineral density; CSMI = cross-sectional moment of inertia; BSI = bone strength index.

studies have predicted the strength of long bones using dental CBCT. The present study is the first to evaluate the bone strength of cortical bones using dental CBCT, and the obtained results indicate that CBCT is superior to DXA for predicting cortical bone fracture loads.

Bone strength is commonly used in evaluations of the risk of bone fractures. Both the material (or densitometric) parameters (i.e., the intrinsic mechanical quality of the bone) and the geometric parameters of the bone shape (i.e., the size, shape, and macroarchitecture) affect bone strength. Therefore, the 2D areal BMD (measured using DXA) cannot be used to accurately determine the bone strength [9]. The correlation coefficient between the areal BMD of rat femurs as measured using DXA and fracture loading was found to be 0.585 ($p = 0.028$). This represents a moderate correlation, slightly weaker than that obtained by Siu et al. [6] ($r = 0.612$) for the correlation between fracture load and areal BMD (measured using DXA) for the femurs of 23 goats. These different findings can be attributed to the sample variance of the two studies. The variances among the rats included in the present study (age = 4 months, weight = 335±10 g) were small, leading to a narrower distribution of the BMD for the femurs with a CV of 10.23%, which was smaller than the value of 15.0% found by Siu et al. (age = 4–6 years, weight = 26–30 kg).

The measurements of the geometric parameters of bones obtained using noninvasive methods could be useful when evaluating bone strength. Although micro-CT provides several parameters for trabecular and cortical bones, it is not commonly used in clinical settings because it can only be applied to small specimens. Siu et al. [6] and Moisio et al. [10] studied goat femurs, goat humeri, and beagle femurs, and found that the BSI of the midshaft cortical bone portions of long bones measured using pQCT yielded better predictions of the bone fracture load than did the areal BMD obtained using DXA. These findings imply that pQCT not only measures densitometric parameters (volumetric BMD) of bones but also—with the addition of the geometric parameters (i.e., CSMI) of bones—can more accurately predict bone strength.

Dental CBCT is characterized by lower cost, smaller spatial

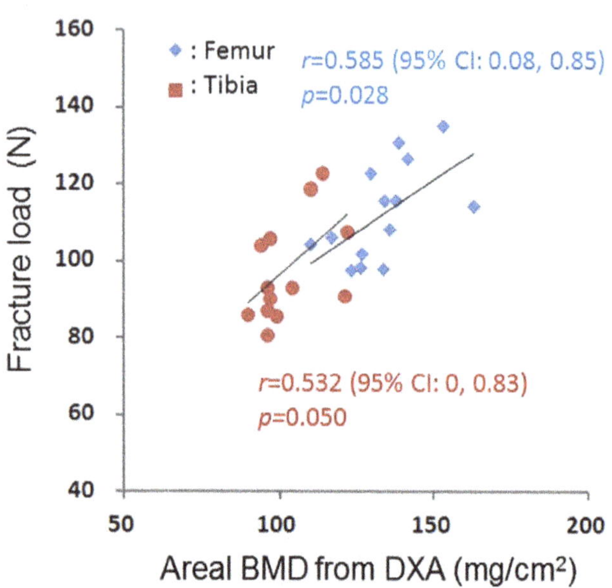

Figure 3. Correlation between fracture load (measured using a three-point bending test) and areal BMD (measured using DXA).

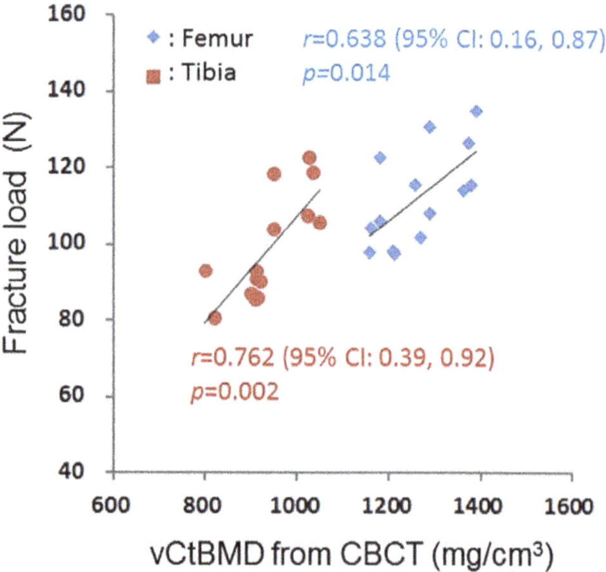

Figure 4. Correlation between fracture load (measured using a three-point bending test) and vCtBMD (measured using CBCT).

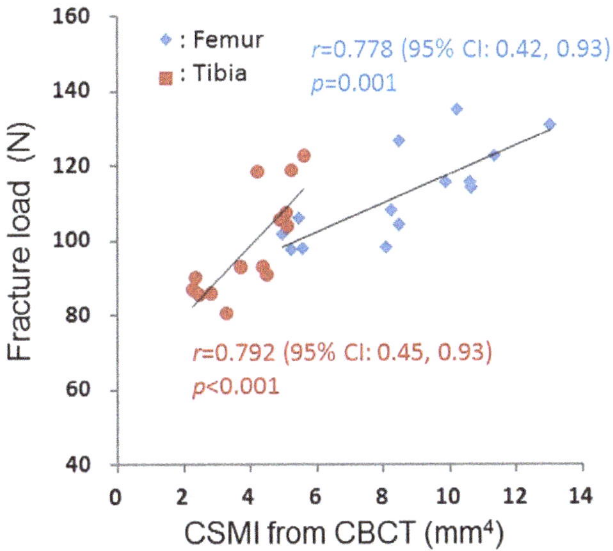

Figure 5. Correlation between fracture load (measured using a three-point bending test) and CSMI (measured using CBCT).

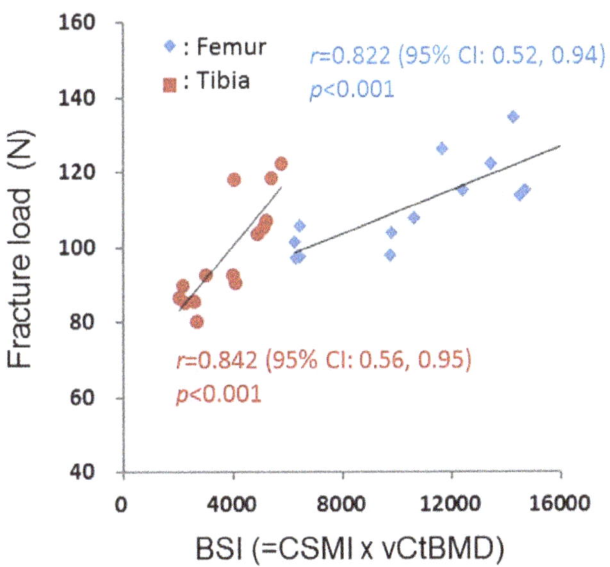

Figure 6. Correlation between fracture load (measured using a three-point bending test) and BSI (=CSMI×vCtBMD).

volume, and lower radiological dosages relative to traditional CT, which has made CBCT popular in clinical dental diagnosis and treatment services. CBCT can be used to determine the shape of bones precisely [32,33] due to its ability to differentiate among bone tissues. In addition, its higher spatial resolution means that it should be possible to use it to measure the CSMI of rat femurs and tibias accurately, such as those used in this study. In addition to the ability of CBCT to precisely measure geometric shapes, recent studies have examined its effectiveness in determining the bone BMD. Nackaerts et al. [34] showed that the intensity values in CBCT were not reliable because they are influenced by the actual device used and the sample positioning. However, most CBCT models use a flat panel detector (FPD) instead of image intensifier (I.I) type [21]. The FPD is quiet, has a wider dynamic range than I.I., and provides improved image quality [35]. In addition, Nomura et al. [36] demonstrated that there was strong correlation between the voxel values and concentrations of iodine solutions, but that the variance of the voxel values was larger than the CT number from multiplied CT. Nomura et al. [21] have recently indicated that CBCT might be able to determine BMC from the voxel values of dental CBCT. Therefore, the present study used dental CBCT to measure the vCtBMD of rat bones.

Animal bones are typically used in biomechanical studies since human cadaveric bones are difficult to obtain. Although the results of studies that use bones from large animals with similar bone structures to humans, such as dogs and goats, are more appreciated, many studies have used rat femurs or tibias in such tests [9,19,37,38]. In addition, although the three-point bending test does not measure the pure bending moment, since this type of measurement includes the shear stress, it is used for measuring bone strength [6,9,10,18,19,37,39,40] more often than are compression, torsion, and tension tests. Furthermore, the groups in this study were larger (comprising 14 samples/group) than the recommended minimum of 11 samples proposed by Leppanen et al. [41] when applying the three-point bending test to evaluate the bone fracture load.

The fracture load was slightly higher for the femurs (111.26±12.63 N) than for the tibias (98.51±13.93 N). This contrasts with Jamsa et al. [18] finding that the fracture load was slightly higher for mouse tibias (21.1±6.4 N) than for mouse femurs (19.9±4.3 N) when using a three-point bending test, which may reflect differences in the bone structure between rats and mice. We further analyzed the findings of studies that used rat femurs. The measured femur fracture load was 111.26±12.63 N in our study, while it was 162.22±17.06 N, 163±26.1 N (for a daily intake of 2000 ppm Mg), and 340±60 N (estimated from figures) in the studies of Jiang et al. [19], Stendig-Lindberg et al. [39], and Iwamoto [42], respectively. In addition to factors such as the type, age, and weight of the rats possibly leading to significantly different results, the span distance between the two ends in the three-point bending test is a primary factor influencing the measured fracture load. In the present study the span distance was set to 20 mm, which was wider than that used in previous experiments and therefore yielded a lower fracture load. However, the rat femur vCtBMD densitometric parameter was slightly smaller in this study (1264.48±85.21 mg/cm^3) than those obtained by Leppanen et al. [40] (1431±334 mg/cm^3) and Jiang et al. [19] (1334.15±11.97 mg/cm^3), while the femur CSMI geometric parameter obtained in this study (8.58±2.55 mm^4) was slightly larger than that obtained by Leppanen et al. (7.85±2.29 mm^4).

Our experimental results show that the correlation coefficients of the obtained BSI (=CSMI×vCtBMD) with the femur and tibia fracture loads were 0.822 and 0.842, respectively. These values are lower than that of 0.94 obtained by Ferretti et al. [9] for between the fracture load and the BSI of rat femurs measured using pQCT. This could be mainly attributable to Ferretti et al. [9] using both rats that had normal bone quality and those that were treated with dexamethasone or aluminum hydroxide, which is likely to have resulted in a larger variation in the cortical BMD values of the specimens. However, Siu et al. [6] found (using pQCT) a correlation coefficient of only 0.334 between BSI_{CSMI} and the fracture load of goat femurs whose quality was similar to that of the normal bone in the present study. Nevertheless, using $BSI_{cross\text{-}sectional\ area}$ as an indicator to predict the fracture load of femurs increased the correlation coefficient to 0.697. In addition, Moisio et al. [10] also used pQCT to measure beagle femurs, and found that the adjusted r^2 between the BSI and the fracture load was 0.877. Both the CBCT used in the present study and the pQCT used in previous studies to measure the combined densitometric and geometric parameters of bones, such as BSI (= vCtBMD×CSMI or vCtBMD×cross-sectional area), yield better predictions of bone strength than the areal BMD that is measured using DXA. These results show that, in addition to pQCT, CBCT is an appropriate method for evaluating the strength of cortical bone (quantified as the fracture load).

The limitations of this study should be considered. First, because of the difficulty of obtaining human cadaveric bones, rat bones were used in this preliminary study. Although the results of this study are based on a rat model, the described experimental procedure could be applied to human bones when they become available. Second, only 14 femurs and tibias were used in this study. Although this is more than the 11 samples proposed by Leppanen et al. [41] when applying the bending test to evaluate the bone fracture load, more samples may be needed to better quantify the association between fracture load and measured parameters. Third, this study used dental CBCT to evaluate only the cortical bone strength, and so future studies should explore the ability of CBCT to predict the strength of trabecular bone. Fourth, the bone strength is affected not only by densitometric (density) and geometric (CSMI) parameters, but also by other factors such as inhomogeneity (in the bone density distribution), anisotropy, and the strain rate.

Conclusions

Based on the results obtained from rat bones *in vitro*, the vCtBMD, CSMI, and BSI obtained using dental CBCT all provided superior predictions of cortical bone bending fracture loads than did areal BMD measured using DXA. Furthermore, strong correlations were found between the BSI (= vCtBMD×CSMI) and the fracture loads ($r = 0.822$ and 0.842 for femurs and tibias, respectively). Subject to the limitations of the sample size and the experimental setup, dental CBCT is a noninvasive method that requires low radiological dosages to predict bone strength, and might constitute a suitable alternative to pQCT, especially when frequent radiological examinations must be conducted within a short time period.

Acknowledgments

The authors thank Dr. Yu-Fen Li from the Institute of Biostatistics, China Medical University for her assistance with the statistical analyses.

Author Contributions

Conceived and designed the experiments: JTH MTT MYCC SPW. Performed the experiments: JTH YJC FCC SPW. Analyzed the data: JTH YJC MTT FCC. Contributed reagents/materials/analysis tools: JTH YJC MYCC SPW. Wrote the paper: JTH MTT SPW.

References

1. Cawthon PM, Ewing SK, Mackey DC, Fink HA, Cummings SR, et al. (2012) Change in hip bone mineral density and risk of subsequent fractures in older men. J Bone Miner Res doi: 10.1002/jbmr.1671.
2. Scibora LM, Ikramuddin S, Buchwald H, Petit MA (2012) Examining the Link Between Bariatric Surgery, Bone Loss, and Osteoporosis: a Review of Bone Density Studies. Obes Surg: 1–14.
3. Hsu JT, Lai KA, Chen Q, Zobitz ME, Huang HL, et al. (2006) The relation between micromotion and screw fixation in acetabular cup. Comput Methods Programs Biomed 84: 34–41.
4. Huang HL, Tu MG, Fuh LJ, Chen YC, Wu CL, et al. (2010) Effects of elasticity and structure of trabecular bone on the primary stability of dental implants. J Med Biol Eng 30: 85–89.
5. Link TM (2012) Osteoporosis Imaging: state of the art and advanced imaging. Radiology 263: 3–17.
6. Siu WS, Qin L, Leung KS (2003) pQCT bone strength index may serve as a better predictor than bone mineral density for long bone breaking strength. J Bone Miner Metab 21: 316–322.
7. Ferretti J (1995) Perspectives of pQCT technology associated to biomechanical studies in skeletal research employing rat models. Bone 17: S353–S364.
8. Genant HK, Engelke K, Fuerst T, Glüer CC, Grampp S, et al. (1996) Noninvasive assessment of bone mineral and structure: state of the art. J Bone Miner Res 11: 707–730.
9. Ferretti JL, Capozza RF, Zanchetta JR (1996) Mechanical validation of a tomographic (pQCT) index for noninvasive estimation of rat femur bending strength. Bone 18: 97–102.
10. Moisio K, Podolskaya G, Barnhart B, Berzins A, Sumner D (2003) pQCT provides better prediction of canine femur breaking load than does DXA. J Musculoskelet Neuronal Interact 3: 240–245.
11. Bagi CM, Hanson N, Andresen C, Pero R, Lariviere R, et al. (2006) The use of micro-CT to evaluate cortical bone geometry and strength in nude rats: correlation with mechanical testing, pQCT and DXA. Bone 38: 136–144.
12. Dumas A, Brigitte M, Moreau M, Chrétien F, Baslé M, et al. (2009) Bone mass and microarchitecture of irradiated and bone marrow-transplanted mice: influences of the donor strain. Osteoporos Int 20: 435–443.
13. Ravoori M, Czaplinska AJ, Sikes C, Han L, Johnson EM, et al. (2010) Quantification of mineralized bone response to prostate cancer by noninvasive in vivo microCT and non-destructive ex vivo microCT and DXA in a mouse model. PLoS One 5: e9854.
14. Huang HL, Hsu JT, Chen MYC, Liu C, Chang CH, et al. (2012) Microcomputed tomography analysis of particular autogenous bone graft in sinus augmentation at 5 months: differences on bone mineral density and 3D trabecular structure. Clin Oral Investig: 1–8.
15. Fei J, Peyrin F, Malaval L, Vico L, Lafage-Proust MH (2010) Imaging and quantitative assessment of long bone vascularization in the adult rat using microcomputed tomography. Anat Rec (Hoboken) 293: 215–224.
16. Chen WP, Hsu JT, Chang CH (2003) Determination of Young's modulus of cortical bone directly from computed tomography: a rabbit model. J Chin Inst Eng 26: 737–745.
17. Huang HL, Tsai MT, Lin DJ, Chien CS, Hsu JT (2010) A new method to evaluate the elastic modulus of cortical bone by using a combined computed tomography and finite element approach. Comput Biol Med 40: 464–468.
18. Jämsä T, Jalovaara P, Peng Z, Väänänen HK, Tuukkanen J (1998) Comparison of three-point bending test and peripheral quantitative computed tomography analysis in the evaluation of the strength of mouse femur and tibia. Bone 23: 155–161.
19. Jiang GZ, Matsumoto H, Hori M, Gunji A, Hakozaki K, et al. (2008) Correlation among geometric, densitometric, and mechanical properties in mandible and femur of osteoporotic rats. J Bone Miner Metab 26: 130–137.
20. Bensamoun SF, Hawse JR, Subramaniam M, Ilharreborde B, Bassillais A, et al. (2006) TGFbeta inducible early gene-1 knockout mice display defects in bone strength and microarchitecture. Bone 39: 1244–1251.
21. Nomura Y, Watanabe H, Shirotsu K, Honda E, Sumi Y, et al. (2012) Stability of voxel values from cone-beam computed tomography for dental use in evaluating bone mineral content. Clin Oral Implants Res doi: 10.1111/j.1600-0501.2012.02420.x.
22. Isoda K, Ayukawa Y, Tsukiyama Y, Sogo M, Matsushita Y, et al. (2012) Relationship between the bone density estimated by cone-beam computed tomography and the primary stability of dental implants. Clin Oral Implants Res 23: 832–836.
23. Benavides E, Rios HF, Ganz SD, An CH, Resnik R, et al. (2012) Use of cone beam computed tomography in implant dentistry: the international congress of oral implantologists consensus report. Implant Dent 21: 78–86.
24. Song YD, Jun SH, Kwon JJ (2009) Correlation between bone quality evaluated by cone-beam computerized tomography and implant primary stability. Int J Oral Maxillofac Implants 24: 59.
25. Fanning B (2011) CBCT–the justification process, audit and review of the recent literature. J Ir Dent Assoc 57: 256.
26. Koong B (2010) Cone beam imaging: is this the ultimate imaging modality? Clin Oral Implants Res 21: 1201–1208.
27. Gray CF (2010) Practice-based cone-beam computed tomography: a review. Prim Dent Care 17: 161–167.
28. Nada RM, Maal TJ, Breuning KH, Berge SJ, Mostafa YA, et al. (2011) Accuracy and reproducibility of voxel based superimposition of cone beam computed tomography models on the anterior cranial base and the zygomatic arches. PLoS One 6: e16520.
29. Chang HW, Huang HL, Yu JH, Hsu JT, Li YF, et al. (2012) Effects of orthodontic tooth movement on alveolar bone density. Clin Oral Investig 16: 679–688.
30. Hsu JT, Chang HW, Huang HL, Yu JH, Li YF, et al. (2011) Bone density changes around teeth during orthodontic treatment. Clin Oral Investig 15: 511–519.
31. Doube M, Klosowski MM, Arganda-Carreras I, Cordelieres FP, Dougherty RP, et al. (2010) BoneJ: Free and extensible bone image analysis in ImageJ. Bone 47: 1076–1079.
32. Marmulla R, Wörtche R, Mühling J, Hassfeld S (2005) Geometric accuracy of the NewTom 9000 cone beam CT. Dentomaxillofac Radiol 34: 28–31.

33. Bissonnette JP, Moseley D, White E, Sharpe M, Purdie T, et al. (2008) Quality assurance for the geometric accuracy of cone-beam CT guidance in radiation therapy. Int J Radiat Oncol Biol Phys 71: S57–S61.
34. Nackaerts O, Maes F, Yan H, Couto Souza P, Pauwels R, et al. (2011) Analysis of intensity variability in multislice and cone beam computed tomography. Clin Oral Implants Res 22: 873–879.
35. Baba R, Ueda K, Okabe M (2004) Using a flat-panel detector in high resolution cone beam CT for dental imaging. Dentomaxillofac Radiol 33: 285–290.
36. Nomura Y, Watanabe H, Honda E, Kurabayashi T (2010) Reliability of voxel values from cone-beam computed tomography for dental use in evaluating bone mineral density. Clin Oral Implants Res 21: 558–562.
37. Ke H, Shen V, Qi H, Crawford D, Wu D, et al. (1998) Prostaglandin E2 increases bone strength in intact rats and in ovariectomized rats with established osteopenia. Bone 23: 249–255.
38. Yamano S, Berley JA, Kuo WP, Gallucci GO, Weber HP, et al. (2010) Effects of nicotine on gene expression and osseointegration in rats. Clin Oral Implants Res 21: 1353–1359.
39. Stendig-Lindberg G, Koeller W, Bauer A, Rob PM (2004) Prolonged magnesium deficiency causes osteoporosis in the rat. J Am Coll Nutr 23: 704S–711S.
40. Leppanen O, Sievanen H, Jokihaara J, Pajamaki I, Jarvinen TL (2006) Three-point bending of rat femur in the mediolateral direction: introduction and validation of a novel biomechanical testing protocol. J Bone Miner Res 21: 1231–1237.
41. Leppänen OV, Sievänen H, Järvinen TLN (2008) Biomechanical testing in experimental bone interventions—May the power be with you. J Biomech 41: 1623–1631.
42. Iwamoto J, Seki A, Takeda T, Sato Y, Yamada H (2005) Effects of risedronate on femoral bone mineral density and bone strength in sciatic neurectomized young rats. J Bone Miner Metab 23: 456–462.

7

Influence of Architecture of β-Tricalcium Phosphate Scaffolds on Biological Performance in Repairing Segmental Bone Defects

Ya-Fei Feng[1]☯, Lin Wang[1]☯, Xiang Li[2]☯, Zhen-Sheng Ma[1], Yang Zhang[1], Zhi-Yong Zhang[3,4]*, Wei Lei[1]*

1 Department of Orthopedics, Xijing Hospital, The Fourth Military Medical University, Xi'an, China, **2** School of Mechanical Engineering, Shanghai Jiao Tong University, State Key Laboratory of Mechanical System and Vibration, Shanghai, China, **3** Department of Plastic and Reconstructive Surgery, Shanghai 9th People's Hospital, Shanghai Key Laboratory of Tissue Engineering, School of Medicine, Shanghai Jiao Tong University, Shanghai, China, **4** National Tissue Engineering Center of China, Shanghai, China

Abstract

Background: Although three-dimensional (3D) β-tricalcium phosphate (β-TCP) scaffolds serve as promising bone graft substitutes for the segmental bone defect treatment, no consensus has been achieved regarding their optimal 3D architecture.

Methods: In this study, we has systematically compared four types of β-TCP bone graft substitutes with different 3D architectures, including two types of porous scaffolds, one type of tubular scaffolds and one type of solid scaffolds, for their efficacy in treating segmental bone defect in a rabbit model.

Results: Our study has demonstrated that when compared to the traditional porous and solid scaffolds, tubular scaffolds promoted significantly higher amount of new bone formation in the defect regions as shown by X-ray, micro CT examinations and histological analysis, restored much greater mechanical properties of the damaged bone evidenced by the biomechanical testing, and eventually achieved the complete union of segmental defect. Moreover, the implantation of tubular scaffolds enhanced the neo-vascularization at the defect region with higher bone metabolic activities than others, as indicated by the bone scintigraphy assay.

Conclusions: This study has further the current knowledge regarding the profound influence of overall 3D architecture of β-TCP scaffolds on their in vivo defect healing performance and illuminated the promising potential use of tubular scaffolds as effective bone graft substitute in treating large segmental bone defects.

Editor: Abhay Pandit, National University of Ireland, Ireland

Funding: This work was supported by the Research Fund for the National Natural Science Foundation of China (No.31170913/C1002) to Wei Lei and National Natural Science Foundation of China (No.81101353) and Xijing Zhutui Project (SJZT10Z09) to Zhi-Yong Zhang. The funders had no role in study design, data collection and analysis, decision to publish, or preparation of the manuscript.

Competing Interests: The authors have declared that no competing interests exist.

* E-mail: leiwei@fmmu.edu.cn (WL); mr.zhiyong@gmail.com (ZYZ)

☯ These authors contributed equally to this work.

Introduction

Treatment of large segmental bone defects caused by severe trauma, non-union fractures or tumor resection remains as a major clinical challenge. Nowadays, the usual strategy for large bone defect treatment involves the use of autologous or allogeneic bone grafts, with more than 500,000 bone grafting procedures conducted annually in the United States alone, making bone tissue the second largest transplanted tissue in the world [1]. The autologous bone grafts, which are considered to be the gold standard [2], require two seperate surgical operations associated with various complications such as wound dehiscence, vessel injuries, hematoma and infections [3,4,5]. The use of allografts can avoid the secondary surgery, nevertherless, is harrased by the concerns of disease transmission and decreased donor tissue sources [6]. The development of three-dimensional (3D) synthetic scaffold as bone graft substitutes has become the promising attempt to overcome these limitations and eventually addressed the ever-increasing clinical need for large bone defect treatment [4,7,8]. A suitable 3D scaffold for bone defect treatment should be able to fullfil the following criteria: (1) provide the initial mechanical support to protect the defect area from the collapse of surrounding tissue; (2) be able to prevent the invasion of fibrous tissue; (3) possess favorable osteoconductivity to promote bone tissue ingrowth; (4) allow sufficient vascularization within the constructs to promote the new bone regeneration [9].

In order to fabricate a favorable 3D scaffold as bone graft substitute to promote bone defect healing, various types of materials with different chemical properties were carefully investigated, including metal, polymeric material, ceramic material and so on. Bioactive ceramic materials such as β-tricalcium phosphate (β-TCP) have been demonstrated as attractive material candidates for 3D scaffold fabrication, because of their chemical similarity to the inorganic phase of natural bone, favorable biocompatibility, osteoconductivity and bioresorbable properties [10,11,12,13]. Besides the chemical properties of material for fabrication, the physical characteristics, especially the 3D architecture of the constructs have been proven to be another determinant for developing a suitable bone graft substitute, which influenced in vivo performance of 3D constructs profoundly [14]. However, there has been still no consensus regarding the optimal architecture of 3D scaffolds as bone substitutes for bone regeneration and vascularization. Porous architecture has been widely used for the fabrication of 3D scaffold, because it is similar to the nature structure of bone tissue, allowing certain degree of bone tissue infiltration and vascularization without compromising the mechanical property [15,16]. The detailed architecture characteristics of porous scaffolds such as porosity and pore size have been intensively investigated for their influence on the in vivo bone tissue ingrowth and vascularization [17,18]. But the use of porous scaffolds as bone substitutes for large segmental bone defect treatment is usually hindered by the limited bone ingrowth, especially in the center region of grafts [19]. On the other hand, tubular design has been proposed in several studies as well, in order to mimic the tubular structure of long bone, with potential efficacy to facilitate bone tissue infiltration and vascularization [20,21]. However, how the tubular scaffolds compared to porous ones as bone graft substitutes in terms of their osteoconductivity (bone tissue ingrowth) and vascularization during the defect treatment still remains elusive. Therefore, in current study, we conducted a head-to-head comparison of β-TCP scaffolds with different porous architecture as well as tubular architecture for their in vivo performance. Firstly, we precisely designed and fabricated four types of β-TCP constructs with different architectures, then implanted them into a rabbit radius defect model for 12 weeks and evaluated the influence of their architecture on the infiltration of fibrous tissue, bone tissue ingrowth, vascularization and in vivo mechanical properties.

Materials and Methods

Fabrication and Characterization of β-TCP Scaffolds

Commercial β-TCP powder was obtained from Edward Keller (Shanghai, China). The β-TCP scaffolds were manufactured as described previously [11]. In brief, large β-TCP cylinders were designed with computer-aided design (CAD) software. The epoxy molds were made by stereolithography (SL), one of the solid freeform fabrication (SFF) techniques. Prepared β-TCP suspension was cast into the molds and sintered at 1100°C, so that the epoxy mold with interconnected beams can be removed by pyrolysis to create the channel space in the scaffolds. Four types of cylindrical β-TCP scaffolds were fabricated with the diameter of 4 mm and the height of 16 mm. The morphology and 3D structure of the scaffolds were characterized by micro-computerized tomography (micro-CT) (eXplore Locus SP, GE Healthcare, Canada). The β-TCP scaffolds were individually double packed and steam sterilized at 121°C for 20 min before implantation.

Animal Study

Animals ethics and experiment design. All animal experiments were performed in strict accordance with protocols approved by the Institutional Animal Care Committee of Xijing Hospital. Forty New Zealand rabbits (Male, 6 months age, 3.5–3.75 kg) were randomly divided into six experimental groups: (Group A-D) β-TCP scaffold group (n = 8 in each group), in which defects were implanted with four types of β-TCP scaffolds respectively according to a randomized complete block design; (Group E) autologous bone control group (n = 4), in which defects were implanted with autologous radius; and (Group F) control untreated group (n = 4), in which defects were left untreated to validate that the defects created here are critical sized defect. In order to analyze the biological performance of β-TCP scaffolds for large bone defect treatment, X-ray, gross view, fluorochrome marker, micro-computer tomography (micro-CT), biomechanical testing, histology and emission computed tomography (ECT) analysis were carried out in the present study (Fig. 1).

Surgical procedure. General anesthesia was performed on rabbits before the surgery using an intramuscular injection of a mixture of Ketamine and Xylazine. Limbs were shaved, skin was disinfected with iodine solution and a longitudinal incision was made to expose the radius, and a 16-mm segmental bone defect was created with a miniature oscillating saw [22]. The cylindrical β-TCP scaffolds or autologous bone grafts were then press-fitted into the radius defect (Fig. 1B). The subcutaneous tissue and skin were closed in layers using degradable sutures. The surgical site was finally covered with an adhesive bandage. Each rabbit was administered 400,000 U of penicillin intraoperatively and on the first postoperative day to prevent infection. At the predetermined time point, the animals were anaesthetized and sacrificed by intracardiac overdose of sodium pentobarbital. The middle radius were immediately dissected and prepared for testing.

Radiographic imaging and gross view. At 12 weeks post-surgery, under the anesthesia, the defect region of rabbits was subject to the radiographic imaging (distance: 1 mm; X-ray source: 46 Kv, 50 mA; exposure time: 0.14 s) to assess the healing of bone defect. The status of bone repair and growth of callus were studied in samples taken out through the original incision after the animals were sacrificed.

Fluorochrome labeling. Sequential fluorochrome markers were administered 2 weeks and 3 days before the animals were sacrificed. Tetracycline (30 mg/kg, Sigma, USA) was administered using intramuscular injection. After the animals were sacrificed at 12 weeks post-surgery, the implants were retrieved for fluorescence analysis.

Micro-CT analysis. Specimens containing the scaffold construct and some surrounding tissue were harvested (n = 8 in Group A-D) and fixed in 10% neutral buffered formalin, placed in the sample holder and scanned under the micro CT (eXplore Locus SP, GE Healthcare, Canada). About 1600 projections of 1024^2 pixels were acquired for each tomogram. The X-ray source voltage was set at 80 kV and beam current at 200 mA using filtered Bremsstrahlung radiation. The scanning angular rotation was 180°, and the angular increment was 0.40°. To minimize beam hardening artifacts a 1 mm aluminum X-ray beam filter was used to attenuate soft X-rays at the source. The projections were reconstructed using a modified parallel Feldkamp algorithm, and segmented into binary images (8-bit BMP images). For determination of the 3D micro-architectural properties within the bone regeneration area, specimens were evaluated using 3D analysis software (Microview, GE Healthcare, Canada). The percentage of bone volume out of total volume (BV/TV) and degradation rate were calculated using the threshold of 2000 for bone tissue and 3000 for scaffold.

Biomechanical testing. Immediately after the animals were sacrificed, the mechanical properties of the implants (n = 4 in Group A–D) were evaluated with the use of a destructive compression test. Cubes of 8mm×4mm×4mm from each specimen were sawed and tested under wet conditions at room temperature. The compressive load was applied at cross-head speed of 1 mm/min using the material testing machine (AGS-10kN, Shimadzu Co., Kyoto, Japan) until fracture occurred. From the load-displacement curve, the compressive strength was

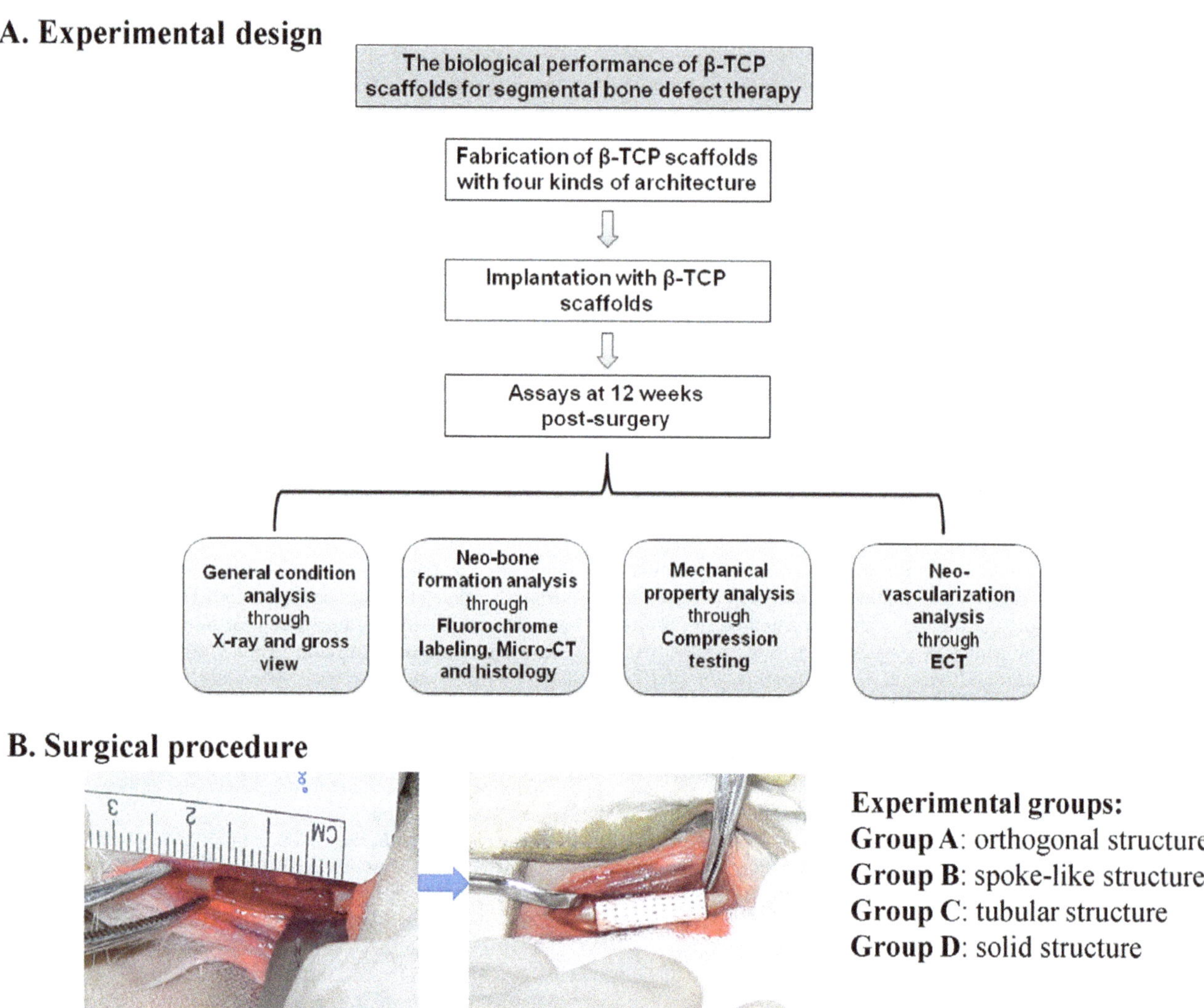

Figure 1. Experimental design and surgical procedure. (**A**) The experimental design of the whole study. (**B**) A 16 mm-long segmental defect was created on the radius of each rabbit and implanted with four types of β-TCP scaffolds with different architectures.

calculated from compressive load and geometric area of the specimens. The compression test of the β-TCP scaffold was also done before implanted.

Histology analysis. Specimens from bone defect sites (n = 4 in Group A–D) were fixed in 10% formalin solution for 7 days. All implants were dehydrated in a graded ethanol series (70–100%) and transferred into a methylmethacrylate (MMA) solution that polymerized at 37°C within 1 week. Three slices of histology section (about 50 μm in thickness) were conducted longitudinally alone the long axis of tibia at the central region using the modified interlocked diamond saw (Leica Microtome, Wetzlar, Germany). Histological sections remained unstained first and were subjected to the fluorescence analysis using epifluorescence microscopy. Then they were stained with 1.2% trinitrophenol and 1% acid fuchsin (Van Gieson staining) for light microscopy analysis. The qualitative analysis of bone formation and fluorochrome markers were performed using a light/fluorescence microscope (Leica LA Microsystems, Bensheim, Germany). Prior to histomorphometry analysis, bone and material were pseudocoloured respectively using Adobe Photoshop 6.0 and then measured using an image analysis system (Image-Pro Plus software, Media Cybernetics, Silver Spring, USA). Bone formation was quantified from the pixels that represented bone tissue, while the total area was defined as the implanted bone site (4 mm × 16 mm). The rate of new bone formation was presented as the percentage of bone area in total implant area [(bone area/total area) × 100%]. In addition, the bone mineralization apposition rate (MAR, vertical spacing between two fluorochrome markers/injection interval) was analyzed from the images of fluorochrome labeling.

ECT analysis. ECT was performed at 2, 4, 8 and 12 weeks after surgery. ^{99m}Tc-methylene- diphosphonate (MDP) was injected through the ear vein at a dose of 5 MBq/kg. ECT images were acquired (140 Kev maximum) 4 h after injection, and delayed images were obtained (512×512 acquisition matrix). During the dynamic imaging, manually drawn rectangular regions of interest (ROIs) (1cm × 1cm, 40 pixels) were established on the implanted bone sites. The uptake ratio of ^{99m}Tc-MDP (T/NT) between the implant site and the contralateral radius was determined for quantitative analysis.

Statistical analysis. The results were expressed as the means ± SD. Statistical analysis was performed using one way ANOVA followed by a SNK-q test for multiple comparisons. Values of p<0.05 were considered to be statistically significant.

Results

Characterization of β-TCP Scaffolds

Four types of cylindrical β-TCP scaffolds with different architectures were manufactured and characterized by micro-CT respectively (Fig. 2). Two types of porous scaffolds were fabricated to mimic the structures of human trabecular bone: the orthogonal structure scaffold (Group A, Fig. 2) had the porosity of around 42% and the pore size of about 500 μm; the spoke-like structure scaffold (Group B, Fig. 2) had the porosity of around 40% and pore size of about 500 μm. The third type of scaffold was tubular shaped (Group C, Fig. 2) with inner diameter of 2 mm, mimicking the tubular structure of long bone. The forth type of scaffold was solid cylindrical (Group D, Fig. 2) as a control.

X-rays Examinations and Gross Observation

[TIGHTER All rabbits exhibited normal diets and movements after surgery, without any surgical complications and sign of infection. X-ray images were taken to evaluate the position of the scaffolds and the development of bone regeneration within the defects (Fig. 3, the upper row). At 12 weeks postoperatively, the newly formed bone tissue infiltrated and integrated well with the scaffold constructs in Group A–C, which was similar to the complete integration found between implanted autologous bone graft and surrounding bone tissue in Group E. Whereas, Group D showed limited osteointegration between the solid scaffold and the surrounding bone tissue, as evidenced by the clear boundary line observed (Fig. 3, red arrow) between the implants and bone tissue. Group F led to the non-union healing of the bone defect, validating that the segmental bone defect created in this study was the critical-sized bone defect.

In agreement with the radiographic analysis, the gross images of the radius repaired with the implantation of porous and tubular β-TCP constructs (Group A–C) and autologous bone graft (Group E) showed well integration of implants with the surrounding tissue (Fig. 3, the lower row). In Group D, the radius, which was implanted with solid β-TCP constructs, achieved partial bony union and limited bone defects healing. In Group F, the defects were filled with fibrous-like tissue and the medullary cavities were blocked.

Fluorochrome Labeling

Fluorescent labeling was detected in the regenerated bone in all specimens. Bone remodeling was validated by interrupted bone

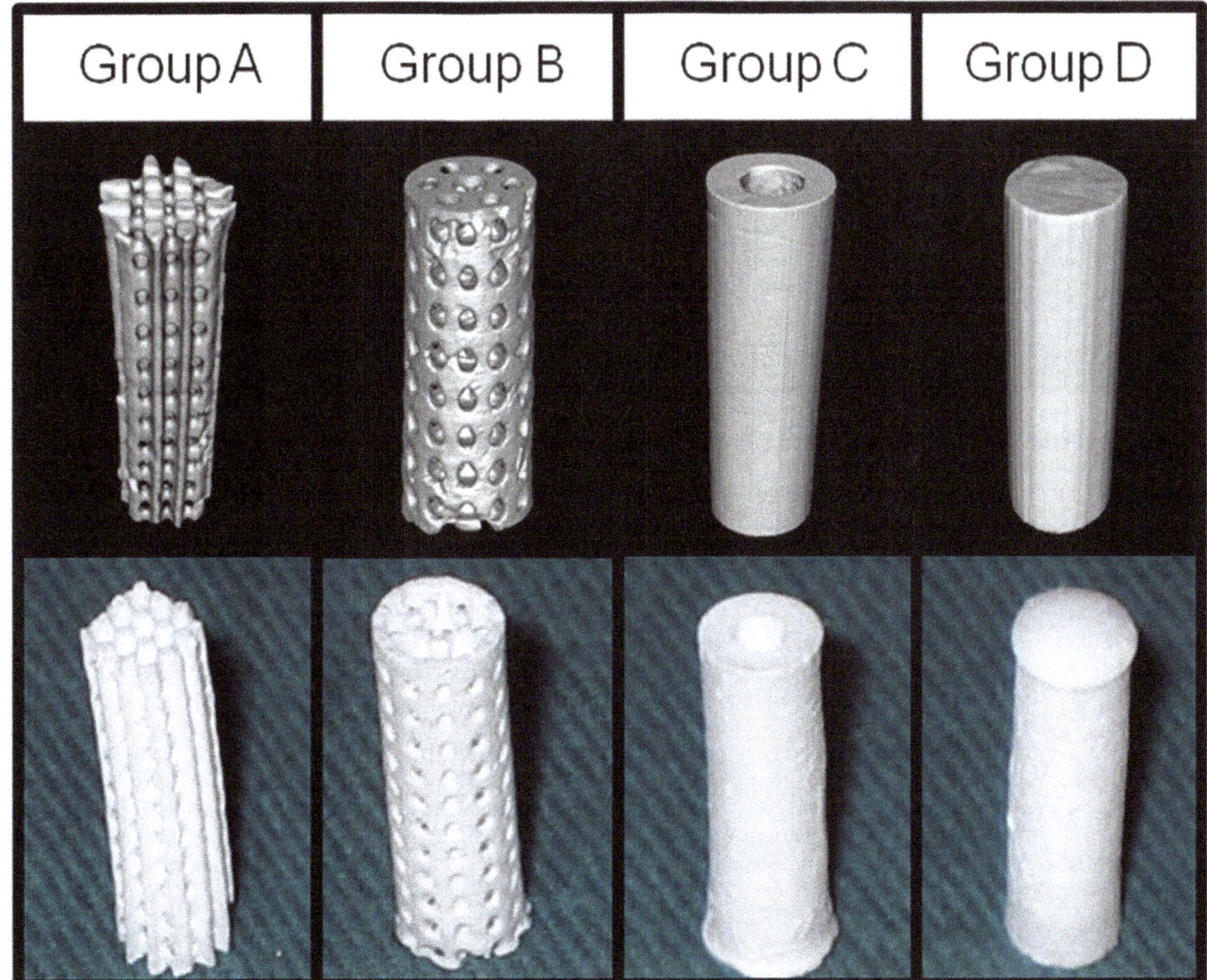

Figure 2. Characterization of β-TCP scaffolds. Micro-CT 3D image (upper row) and gross view (lower row) showed the general constructions of the four types of scaffolds. Two porous scaffolds (Group A and B) with porosity of around 40% and pore size of 500 μm, the tubular scaffolds (Group C) with inner diameter of 2 mm and the solid scaffolds (Group D) were manufactured and used in this study.

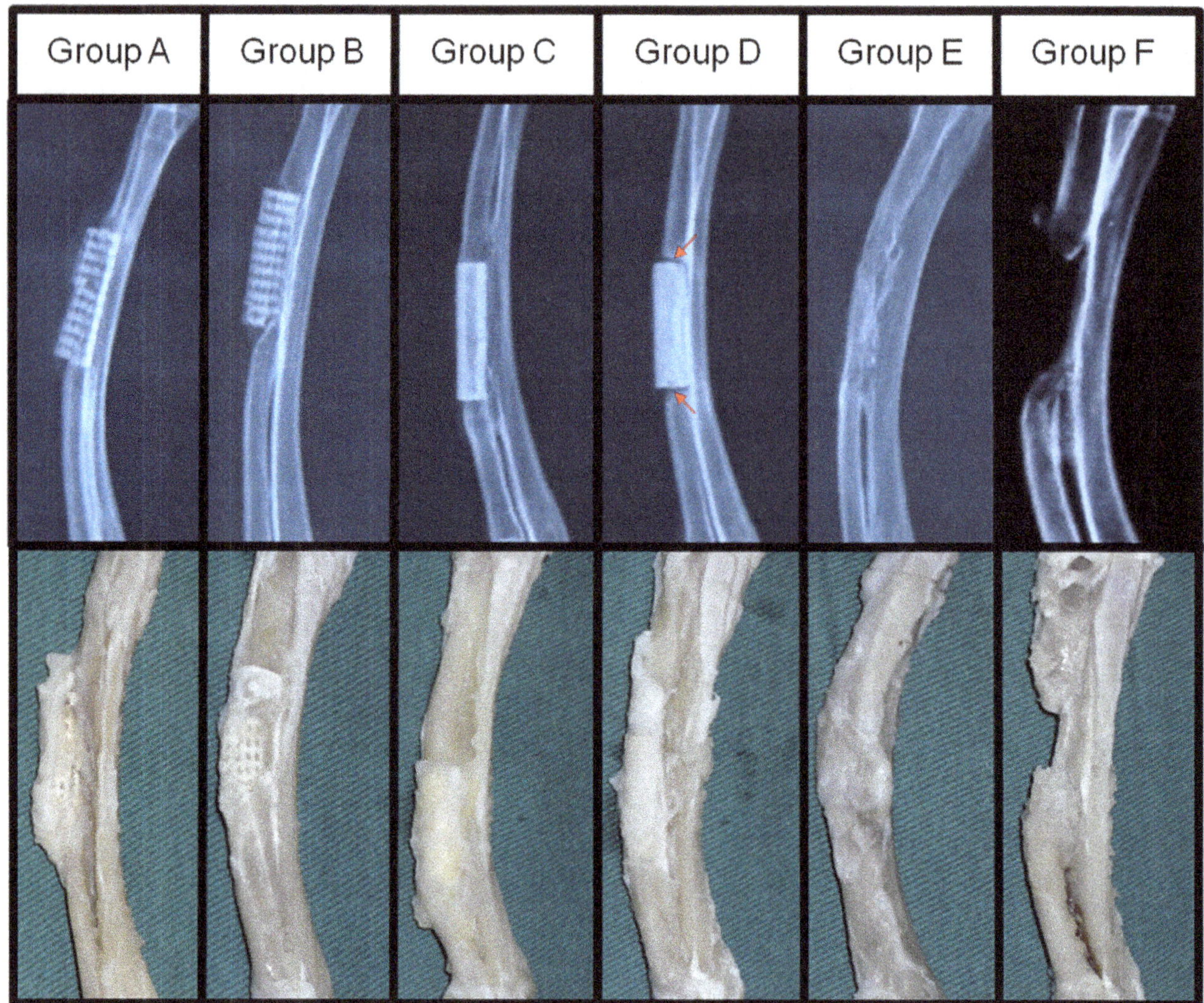

Figure 3. X-ray and gross examinations of the radius with different treatment at 12 weeks post-surgery. X-ray examination (upper row) showed evident ingrowth of new bone tissue into the porous (Group A and B) and tubular (Group C) scaffolds. Tubular scaffolds showed better graft/bone integration than porous ones, which was comparable to the implantation of autologous bone graft (Group E). The solid scaffolds (Group D) showed the poorest osteointegration as evidenced by clear boundary line (red arrow) between the scaffold and bone tissue. Non-union healing of the bone defect in Group F (no treatment) validated that the segmental defect used in this study was the critical sized bone defect. Gross view of the radius (lower row) showed treatment with porous or tubular scaffolds and autologous bone graft exerted better bony union than solid scaffolds.

labeling and new bone deposition. The bone labeling was detected in the pores of both porous scaffolds (Group A–B) and tubular scaffolds (Group C), while only limited amount of new bone formed around the solid scaffolds (Group D) (Fig. 4A). It was noted that most of the newly formed bone was observed on the peripheral area rather than the center area of porous scaffolds. The quantitative analysis of fluorochrome markers (Fig. 4B) showed that the bone MAR of porous scaffolds (Group A and B) was slightly higher than that of tubular and solid scaffolds (Group C and D) but without statistically significant difference ($p>0.05$), indicating a similar growth rate of bone tissue in these four kinds of scaffolds.

Micro-CT Evaluation

Bone tissue regeneration within the scaffold was evaluated by micro-CT at 12 weeks post-surgery (Fig. 5). In Group D, limited amount of bone has formed in the defects postoperatively, while in Group A, B and C, significant amount of bone formation was observed with better healing of the defect. Bony callus has formed in the interspaces between the implants and the bone tissue, and newly formed bone had tight contact with the scaffolds and infiltrated into the pore region of implants. However, in Group A and B, the ingrowth of newly formed bone tissue only limited to the peripheral region of the porous scaffolds, with little bone regeneration amount in the center of scaffold (Fig. 5A, red arrows). On the contrary, the tubular scaffolds had better bone ingrowth within the center tube, which was fully filled with new bone tissue. The ratio of bone volume/total volume (%BV/TV) in Group C (56.8±2.5%) was about 1.5-fold of Group A (37.0±3.0%) or Group B (34.8±3.0%) and 10-fold of Group D (5.9±0.9%) at 12 weeks post-surgery (n = 8 in each group, all $p<0.05$), indicating better osteogenesis of tubular scaffolds than porous or solid scaffolds (Fig. 5B, threshold of 2000 for bone tissue and 3000 for scaffold).

In addition, by comparing the micro CT images of the scaffolds before and after implantation, we observed considerable scaffold

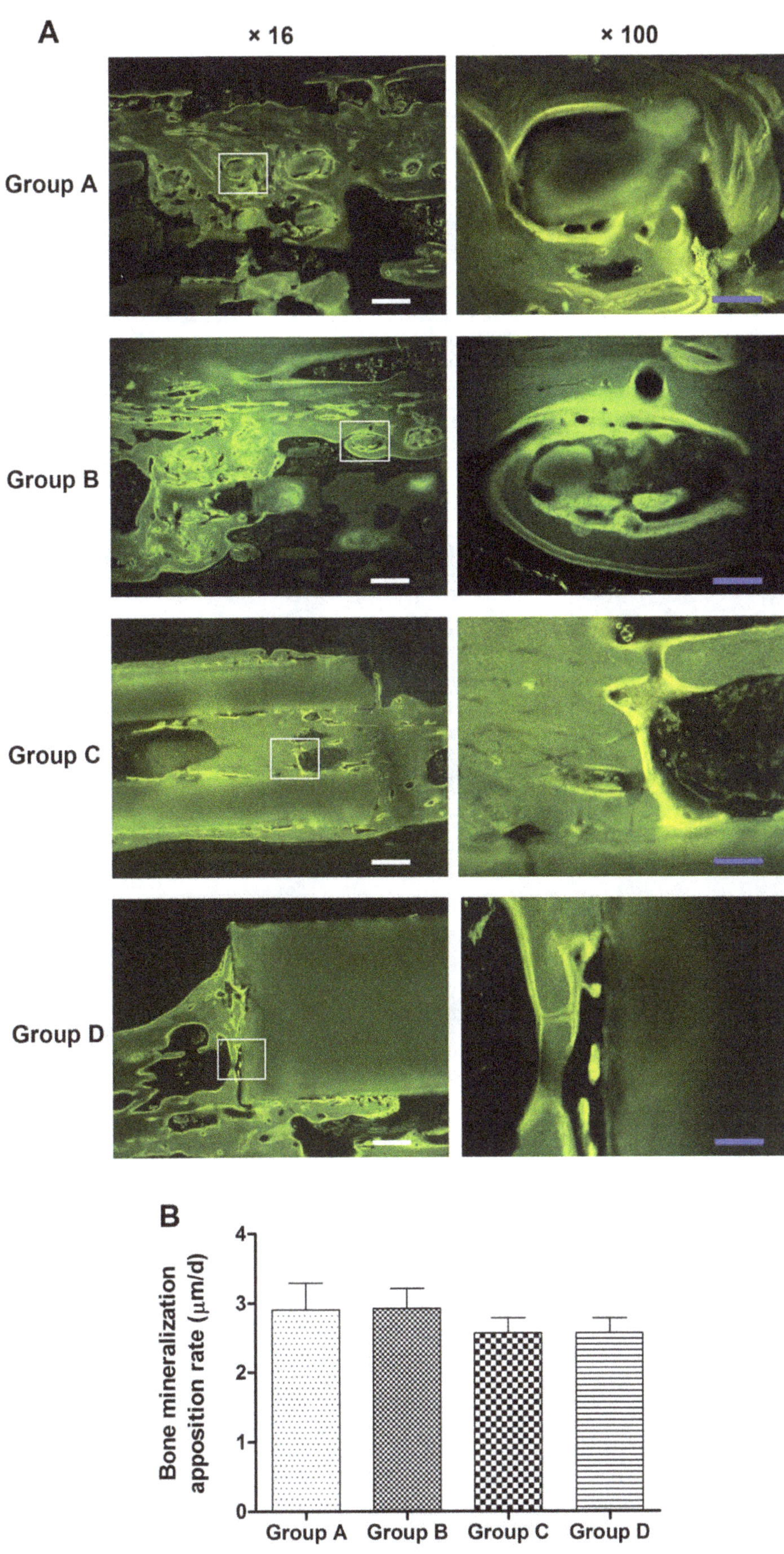
A
× 16
× 100
Group A
Group B
Group C
Group D
B
Bone mineralization apposition rate (μm/d)
4
3
2
1
0
Group A
Group B
Group C
Group D

Figure 4. Fluorochrome labeling of bone regeneration at 12 weeks post-surgery. (**A**) The fluorescent labeling images indicated that more new bone growth into the porous (Group A–B) and tubular scaffolds (Group C), while very limited bone tissue formed around the solid scaffolds (Group D). (**B**) Quantitative analysis showed there were no significant differences in the bone mineralization apposition rate ($p>0.05$), indicating similar bone growth rate in these four kinds of scaffolds. Scale bar: 50 μm (white), 10 μm (blue).

degradation occurring in vivo (Fig. 5C). At 12 weeks, the biodegradation percentages (%) of two porous scaffolds in Group A and B were 54.8±2.7% and 58.3±2.2%, both of which were remarkably faster than that of tubular scaffolds in Group C (29.0±2.8%, $p<0.05$), while Group D showed the least amount of degradation (15.9±1.8%) (Fig. 5D). The results in Fig.5 indicated that the biodegradation rate of porous scaffolds exerted a more rapid replacement than the degree of osteogenesis within the scaffolds, whereas the tubular scaffolds were resorbed at a rate corresponding to the new bone deposition.

Biomechanical Testing

In order to evaluate the mechanical properties of the scaffolds and the integration of the new bone tissue within scaffolds, we carried out compression tests on the native and implanted scaffolds 12 weeks post transplantation. The solid shaped scaffolds (Group D) showed the highest compression strength of native scaffolds but achieved the lowest strength of harvested scaffolds after 12 weeks implantation, indicating little bone formation and osteointegration with scaffolds (Fig.6). Tubular scaffolds (Group C) demonstrated significantly higher compression strength for both native (8.10±0.44 MPa) and implanted scaffolds (49.89±2.62 MPa) compared to porous ones of Group A (3.24±0.48 MPa for native and 37.12±2.13 MPa for implanted scaffolds, both $p<0.05$) or

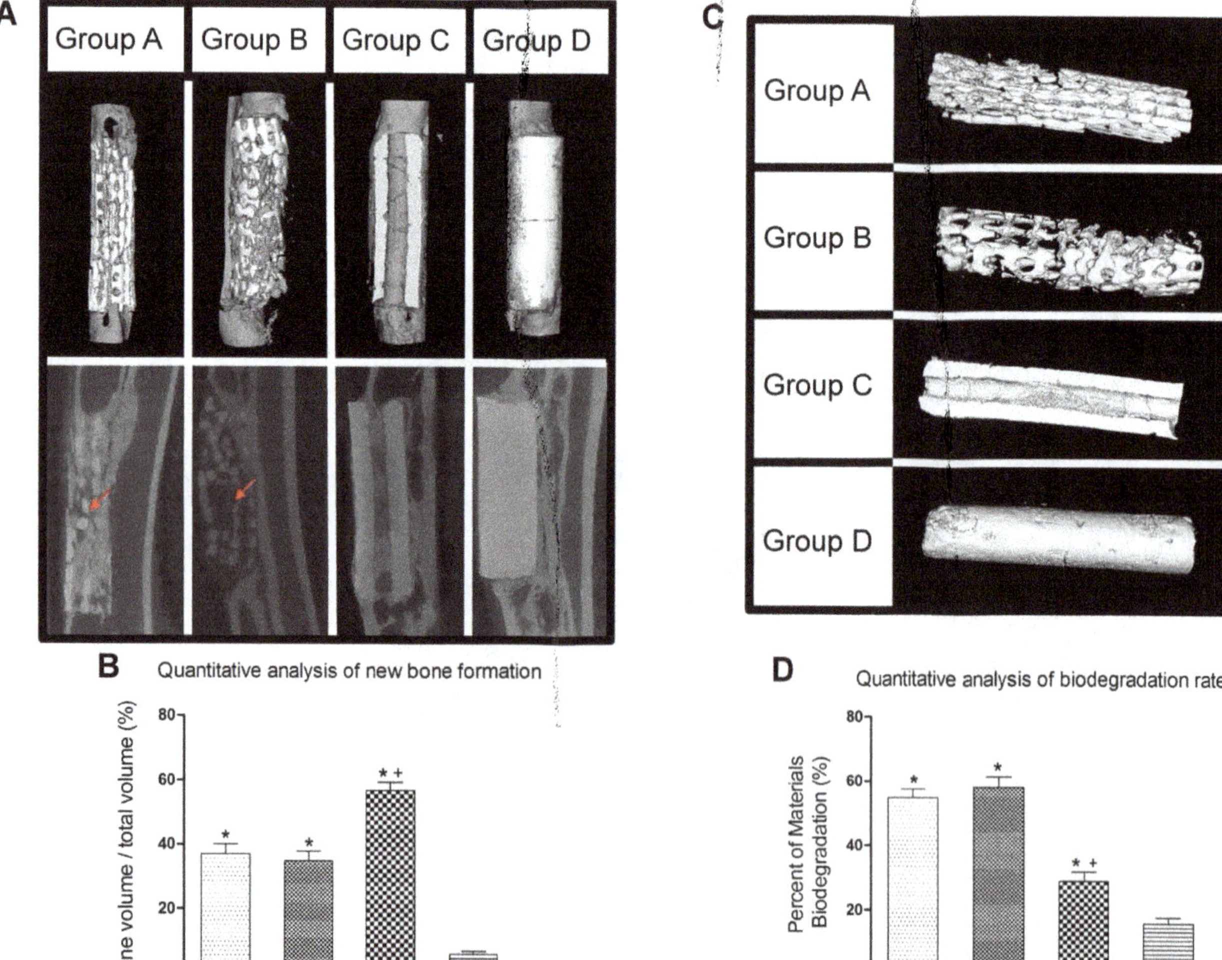

Figure 5. Micro-CT analysis of new bone formation and biodegradation rate of scaffolds at 12 weeks post-surgery. (**A**) Micro-CT images showed more bone ingrowth within the tubular scaffolds (Group C) than porous ones (Group A and B), especially in the center of grafts (red arrow). Little new bone generated in solid scaffolds (Group D). (**B**) The ratio of bone volume/total volume (%BV/TV) in Group C was higher than that of Group A, B and D. (**C**) Micro CT images indicated that porous scaffolds experienced faster degradation rate with ruptured overall structure, while tubular scaffolds maintained intact for its overall structure. (**D**) Quantitative analysis confirmed lower biodegradation rate in tubular scaffolds (Group C) than porous scaffolds (Group A and B) (*$p<0.05$ *vs.* Group D, $^{+}p<0.05$ *vs.* Group A and B).

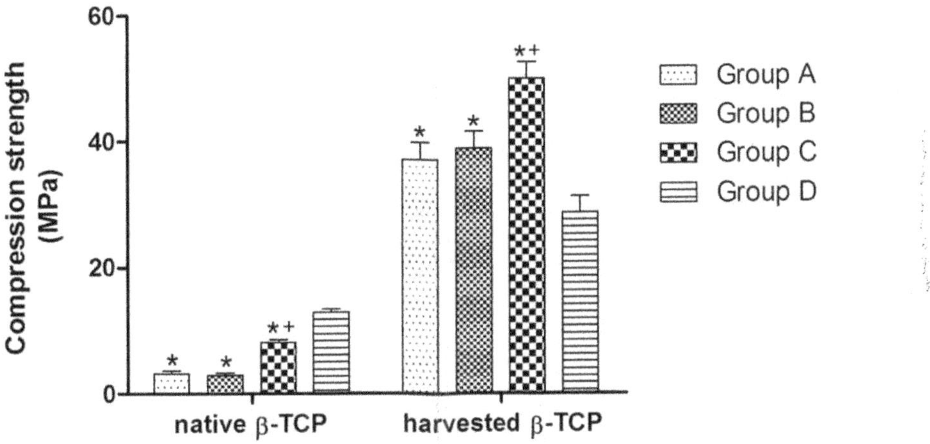

Figure 6. Compression testing of the scaffolds and radius defect. The results of compression testing showed that tubular scaffolds (Group C) demonstrated improved mechanical properties with higher compression strength in vivo than porous ones (Group A and B), indicating better bone formation and integration with the tubular scaffolds; the native solid scaffolds (Group D) showed the highest compression strength, but the lowest in vivo data after implantation (* $p<0.05$ *vs.* Group D, $^{+}p<0.05$ *vs.* Group A and B).

Group B (2.93±0.38 MPa for native and 38.79±2.70 MPa for implanted scaffolds, both $p<0.05$), indicating better mechanical property and improved osteointegration capability of the tubular bone grafts.

Histological Analysis

To evaluate the tissue response to the implanted scaffolds and the defect healing progress, we performed histological analysis on the tissue/biomaterial interface and the area of the implant. As shown in Fig. 7, there was little bone tissue in Group D, and the defects around the scaffolds were filled with fibrous tissue. The implants in Group A–C showed significantly better new bone formation, with bone trabecular structure found at 12 weeks compared to Group D. However, Group A and B experienced limited ingrowth of bone tissue, which only formed in peripheral regions of the scaffold, with the central region of the scaffold occupied by fibrous tissue (Fig. 7, red arrow). On the contrary, Group C achieved much better bone formation and bone infiltration, with central tube fully filled with newly formed bone tissue at week 12 after surgery. Furthermore, bone marrow cavity achieved recanalization in the central tube of Group C (Fig. 7, blue arrow). The percentage of new bone formation (bone area/total area) in Group C (55.9±2.9%) was significantly higher than that of Group A (33.2±2.3%), B (31.8±2.0%) and D (7.6±1.3%) (n = 8 in each group, all $p<0.05$), indicating better bone ingrowth in tubular scaffolds than other ones (Fig. 8).

ECT Examination

Bone scintigraphy with radioactive tracers has been widely used in the imaging of vascularization and metabolic activity of bone tissue. In this study, ECT was conducted at 2, 4, 8 and 12 weeks after surgery to analyze the vascularization of the TCP scaffolds. Four hours after injection of 99mTc-MDP, about half of the tracer was deposited in the bone and delayed images were obtained (Fig. 9A). The uptake ratio of ^{99m}Tc-MDP (T/NT) in the defect region tended to increase with time after the surgery throughout the whole study in each group, while the rate of increase became gradually steady after 4 weeks post-surgery. The solid scaffolds (Group D) had the lowest uptake ratio which changed slightly after implantation, indicating limited infiltration of capillary vessels. Group A, B and C displayed comparable 99mTc-MDP uptake ratio (T/NT) at 2 weeks, while tubular scaffolds (Group C) had a higher degree of blood flow perfusion from 4 weeks post-surgery than that of porous scaffolds (Group A and B) (Fig. 9B). At 12 weeks post-surgery, the T/NT value of tubular scaffolds reached to peak at 4.00±0.30, which was 1.5-fold higher than that of porous ones (2.77±0.32 in Group A and 2.87±0.32 in Group B, both $p<0.05$).

Discussion

Porous scaffolds as bone graft substitutes have been widely investigated for segmental bone defect treatment [23,24], while their in vivo application could be harassed by the limited bone ingrowth and poor vascularization in the central region of the bone grafts when implanted in the large bone defect, especially the segmental bone defect [25,26,27]. The current advance in manufacturing technology facilitates the accurate control of 3D scaffold structure parameters and makes the optimization of internal structure possible [17,28]. However, most of these studies concentrate on changing internal structural properties instead of adjusting overall architecture. In the present study, we investigated the use of tubular architecture scaffolds which mimicked the overall shape of long bone and systematically compared to porous scaffolds with different internal structures. Our results demonstrated that compared to porous scaffolds, the tubular scaffolds were more favorable for segmental bone defect treatment, demonstrating higher degree of bone tissue ingrowth and vascularization, as well as better biomechanical properties both in vitro and in vivo.

Scaffolds that mimic natural bone structures could be used as a favorable bone graft substitutes for cell and bone ingrowth when implanted, with reported efficacy in promoting in vivo osteogenesis and integration with surrounding bone tissue [29,30,31]. Porous scaffolds with interconnected pores have been widely investigated for bone defect treatment, since it can imitate the structure of cancellous bone and provide an open and connected porous framework for cellular migration, extracellular matrix production, new bone formation and the neo-vascularization from adjacent bone tissue [32,33]. It is well known that the pore size is one of the most critical architecture factors, which impose profound influence on the progression of osteogenesis [14,34],

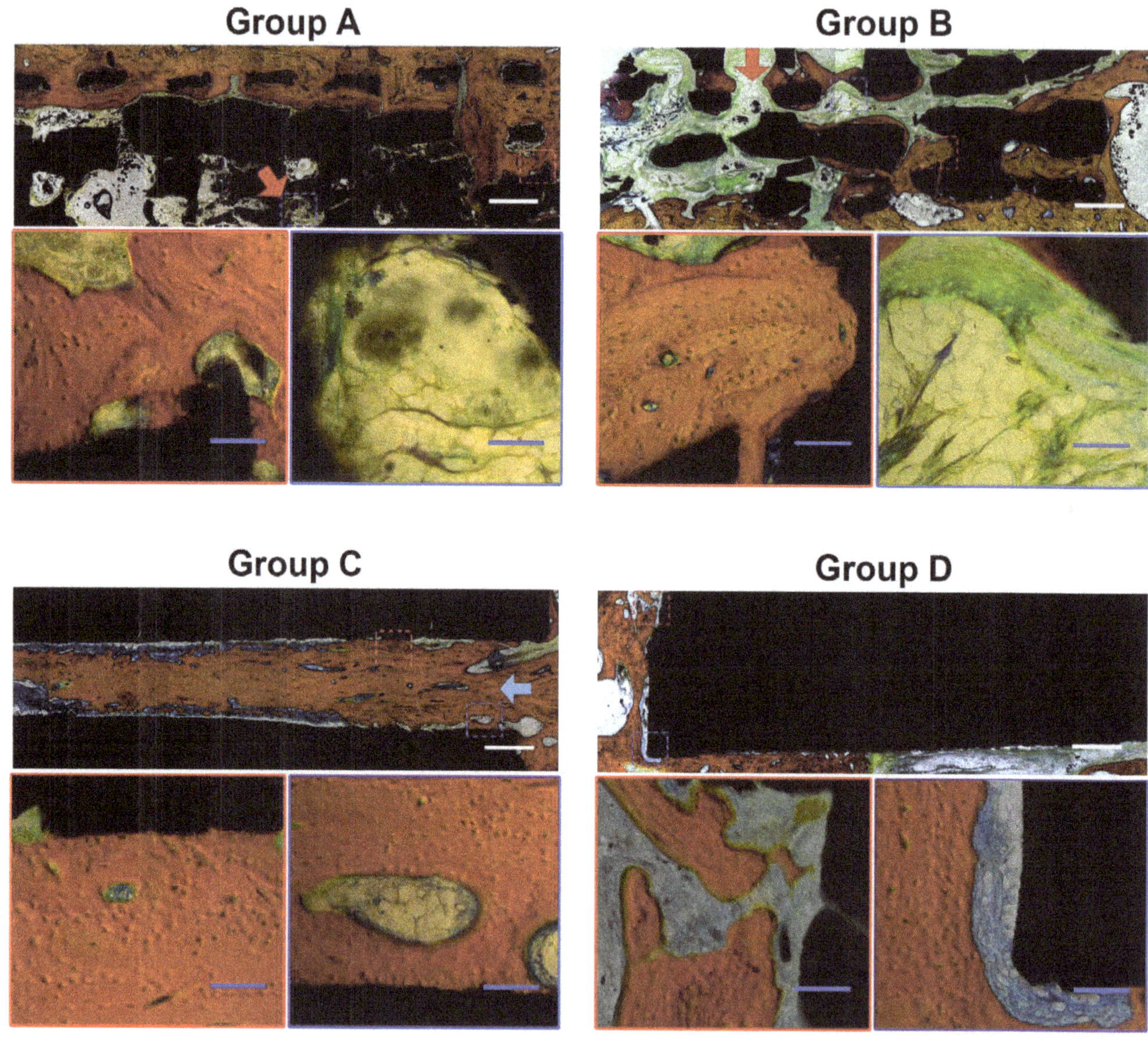

Figure 7. Histological analysis of new bone formation at 12 weeks post-surgery. Van Gieson staining showed more bone formed in tubular scaffolds (Group C) than porous (Group A and B) and solid (Group D) ones, especially in the center of grafts (blue arrow). The center region of porous scaffold was occupied by soft tissue with poor osteogenesis (red arrow). The tissue stained in red color was the newly formed bone with visible cell nuclei. The tissue stained in yellow/green/blue color was fibrous tissue. Scale bar: 1 mm (white), 100 μm (blue).

with the studies showing that 300–900 μm pore size is suitable for BTE application [35]. Porous scaffolds have been proved to be an effective bone substitute in the treatment of cavity defect which is surrounded predominantly by bone tissue [27,36]. However, when porous scaffolds were implanted in certain defect region which is surrounded by soft tissue predominantly, such as the segmental defect, the fibrous tissue may easily outgrow the bone tissue and occupy the space for new bone formation, thus compromising the bone regeneration efficacy. In our previous study, we have observed that the implantation of porous scaffolds led to the non-union treatment of femoral segmental defect in a rat model with massive fibrous tissue invasion [25]. Zhou et al reported that only a small amount of new bone and blood vessel were formed within the porous β-TCP scaffolds, which contributed to poor biomechanical strength and failed in repairing large segmental bone defect [26]. Although 500 μm of pore size for porous scaffold was suggested in Kujala et al's study, demonstrating a significantly less degree of fibrosis than the scaffold with smaller pore (260 μm), in our study, the implantation of 500 μm porous scaffold still led to the rapid infiltration of peri-implant fibrous tissue at early stage, which grew faster than bone tissue, as demonstrated by micro CT analysis (Fig. 5) and histology assay (Fig. 7). Besides precluding the new bone formation by occupying the defect space, the fibrous tissue influx can also generated a thick tissue layer around the surface of grafts, adversely affecting the sufficient blood perfusion, which may further jeopardize the bone regeneration process [37,38].

When compared to porous scaffolds, tubular scaffolds demonstrated to be better bone graft substitute design in treating the segmental defect, achieving considerably better quantity and quality of new bone formation. Generally, it is more challenging to repair the segmental bone defect than a cavity bone defect, due to

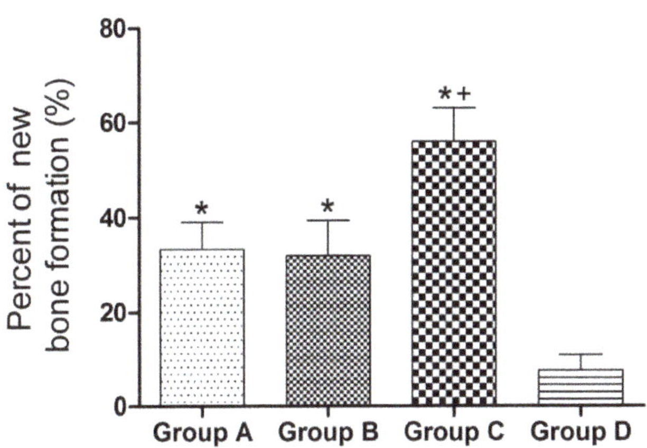

Figure 8. Histomorphology analysis of new bone formation. Quantitative analysis showed the percentage of new bone formation in Group C was significantly higher than that of Group A, B and D at 12 weeks post-surgery (*$p<0.05$ *vs.* Group D, $^{+}p<0.05$ *vs.* Group A and B).

poor bone formation environment of segmental defect, which is surrounded predominantly by soft tissue. To prevent the rapid invasion of surrounding soft tissue and protect the defect space for subsequent bone tissue ingrowth has become the key for successful defect healing [1,39]. Unlike porous scaffolds allowing the tissue ingrowth from all the interfaces with surrounding tissues, tubular scaffolds can selectively permit the ingrowth of surrounding tissue only from the tubular openings. When implanted into the segmental defect, the openings of tubular scaffolds are in tight contact with bone tissue; while the other interfaces contacting soft tissue is non-permeable for tissue infiltration, hence preventing the invasion of soft tissue effectively, as demonstrated by histological analysis (Fig. 7). With the well-protected space and favorable chemical surface of osteo-conductive TCP material, osteogenic cells could migrate from adjacent bone tissue, proliferate along inner wall of tubular scaffolds and deposit new bone tissue into the core region of grafts; in this way, implantation of tubular scaffolds have helped to achieve the complete union of segmental bone defect, evidenced by the X-ray examination, micro-CT analysis and histology assay (Fig. 3,5 and 7).

Moreover, tubular scaffolds facilitated higher volume of vascularization within the grafts than porous ones, as indicated by the radionuclide bone imaging. Radionuclide bone imaging is a

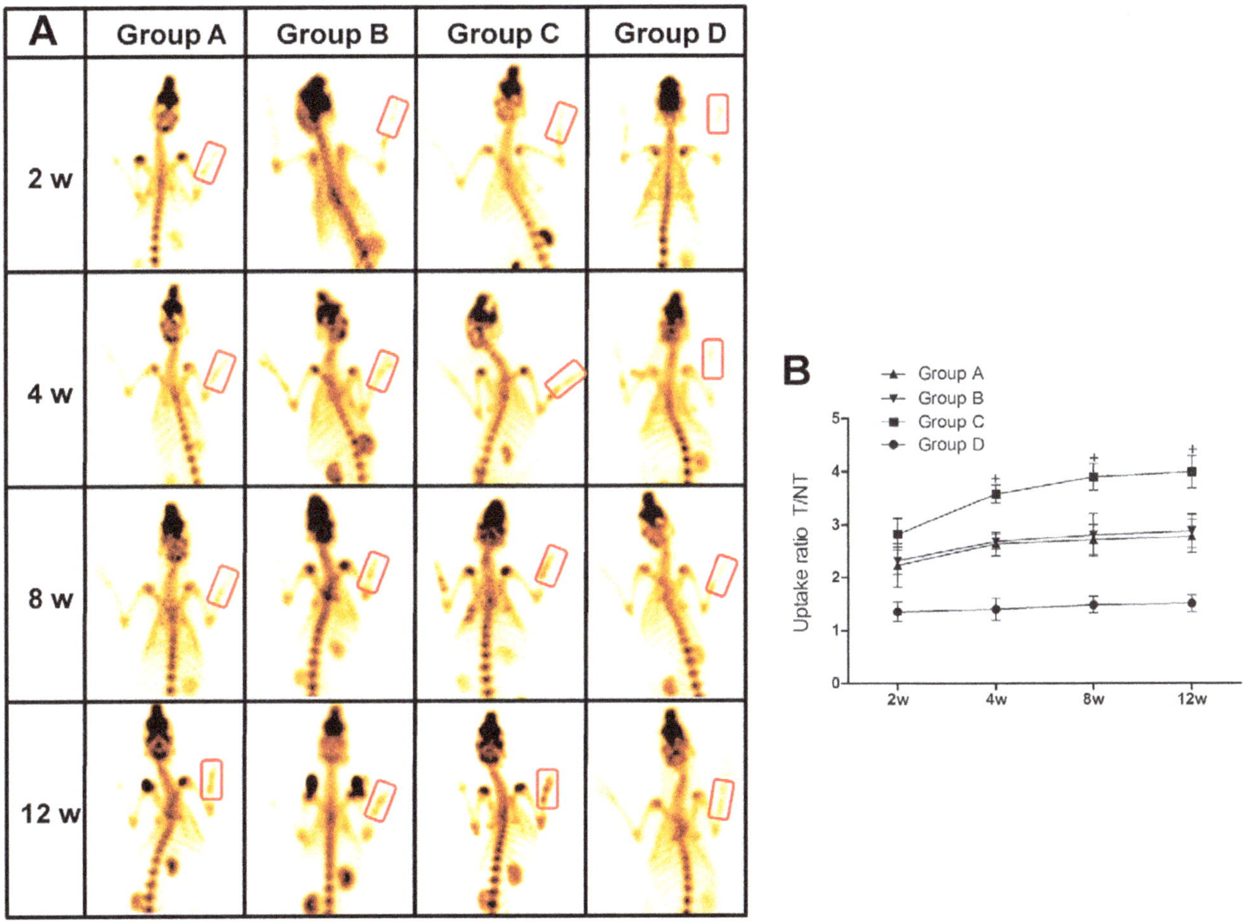

Figure 9. ECT analysis of vascularization at 2, 4, 8 and 12 weeks post-surgery. (**A**) ECT images of rabbits showed that despite of no difference among the four groups at 2 weeks post-surgery, higher counts were observed in tubular scaffolds (Group C) than other groups (Group A, B and D) since week 4 post-surgery, suggesting enhanced vascularization and metabolic activities. (**B**) Quantitative measurement of the uptake ratio (T/NT) further confirmed better vascularization and higher metabolic activities of tubular scaffolds than others since week 4 post-surgery ($^{+}p<0.05$ *vs.* Group A, B and D).

well-established clinical examination technique to assess the abnormalities of bone tissue [26,40,41]. The uptake of the radiopharmaceutical depends both on an adequate delivery system and on a living network of osteocytes [42]. ^{99m}Tc-MDP, the most commonly used tracers in clinical bone research, will be accumulated mainly into the bone tissue after injection, especially in the highly vascularized region and the accumulation dosage is closely correlated to the degree of vascularization. The capacity and accuracy of ECT to evaluate the vascularization has been validated by a number of other methods such as magnetic resonance imaging (MRI) [43], digital subtraction angiography (DSA) [44] and histology [26,45]. The ECT examination showed a significantly higher uptake of 99mTc-MDP in the defect region with the implantation of tubular scaffolds throughout the whole study (Fig. 8). Although scaffolds with porous structure are thought to favor vascular ingrowth from surrounding tissue, they allow the ingrowth of fibrous tissue as well, which may adversely affect the subsequent vascularization especially in the centre space of the implants [46]. Furthermore, it has been acknowledged that the persistent peri-implant inflammation could inhibit the process of vascularization [47,48]. As the porous scaffolds with the open structure were inevitably exposed to the surrounding environment, the sustained inflammatory reaction accompanied with traumatic condition of segmental bone defect may possibly influence the vascularization of porous scaffolds more easily than that of tubular scaffolds which provided a relatively enclosed environment to block the prolonged inflammatory reaction. This hypothesis could partially explain the finding in our study that although being similar at the first 2 weeks, the vascularization became more pronounced in tubular scaffolds than in the porous ones since 4 weeks. The histological analysis and molecular pathways examination for the specific underlying mechanism of better angiogenesis in tubular scaffolds will be conducted in our further studies.

Despite of its osteoconductive properties, the in vivo application of β-TCP is generally fraught with the problem of rapid degradation after the implantation [49,50]. Because of its higher surface/volume ratio, β-TCP scaffold with porous structure could experience faster in vivo degradation than tubular structure, as evidenced by micro CT analysis in our study (Fig.5). This rapid degradation of porous β-TCP scaffolds could result in the early disintegration of overall structure, eliminating the space for the bone tissue formation, and the TCP degradation debris may block the porous channel for the ingrowth of vessel and bone tissues [51,52]. On the contrary, tubular scaffolds could maintain the integrity of scaffold structure in a longer period of time for the ingrowth of the vessels and bone tissue. In addition, tubular scaffolds possessed better inherent mechanical property as shown by the in vitro compression testing (Fig.6). When implanted in vivo, it can restore significantly higher mechanical strength of the damaged bone than porous scaffolds, which could be explained by its slower degradation profile, better preservation of its structure integrity and more bone tissue ingrowth, thus demonstrating its promising potential in the load-bearing application.

Conclusions

In this study, we have systematically compared the efficacy of tubular scaffolds with porous scaffolds for segmental bone defect treatment, and demonstrated that compared with the traditional porous structure, scaffolds with tubular structure can promote much better defect healing with significantly higher amount of bone tissue formation and neo-vascularization, greater in vivo biomechanical strength and eventually achieving the complete union of segmental defect. These findings have provided a further knowledge about the influence of scaffold architecture on their in vivo defect healing performance and illuminated the great potential to use tubular scaffolds as effective bone graft substitutes in the segmental defect treatment.

Acknowledgments

We thank Professor Jun Wang and Professor Rong Lv for providing helpful advice of the micro-CT and histology.

Author Contributions

Conceived and designed the experiments: YFF LW XL ZYZ WL. Performed the experiments: YFF LW XL YZ. Analyzed the data: YFF LW. Contributed reagents/materials/analysis tools: YZ ZSM. Wrote the paper: YFF LW ZYZ. Revised the manuscript: WL.

References

1. Greenwald AS, Boden SD, Goldberg VM, Khan Y, Laurencin CT, et al. (2001) Bone-graft substitutes: facts, fictions, and applications. J Bone Joint Surg Am 83-A Suppl 2 Pt 2: 98–103.
2. Damien CJ, Parsons JR (1991) Bone graft and bone graft substitutes: a review of current technology and applications. J ApplBiomater 2: 187–208.
3. Bucholz RW (2002) Nonallograft osteoconductive bone graft substitutes. Clin Orthop Relat Res: 44–52.
4. De LWG Jr, Einhorn TA, Koval K, McKee M, Smith W, et al. (2007) Bone grafts and bone graft substitutes in orthopaedic trauma surgery. A critical analysis. J Bone Joint SurgAm 89: 649–658.
5. Van der Stok J, Van Lieshout EM, El-Massoudi Y, Van Kralingen GH, Patka P (2011) Bone substitutes in the Netherlands - a systematic literature review. Acta biomaterialia 7: 739–750.
6. Prolo DJ, Rodrigo JJ (1985) Contemporary bone graft physiology and surgery. ClinOrthopRelat Res: 322–342.
7. Lohfeld S, Cahill S, Barron V, McHugh P, Durselen L, et al. (2012) Fabrication, mechanical and in vivo performance of polycaprolactone/tricalcium phosphate composite scaffolds. Acta biomaterialia.
8. Schofer MD, Roessler PP, Schaefer J, Theisen C, Schlimme S, et al. (2011) Electrospun PLLA nanofiber scaffolds and their use in combination with BMP-2 for reconstruction of bone defects. PLoS One 6: e25462.
9. Laschke MW, Strohe A, Scheuer C, Eglin D, Verrier S, et al. (2009) In vivo biocompatibility and vascularization of biodegradable porous polyurethane scaffolds for tissue engineering. Acta biomaterialia 5: 1991–2001.
10. Hench LL, Polak JM (2002) Third-generation biomedical materials. Science 295: 1014–1017.
11. Wang L, Hu YY, Wang Z, Li X, Li DC, et al. (2009) Flow perfusion culture of human fetal bone cells in large beta-tricalcium phosphate scaffold with controlled architecture. J BiomedMaterRes A 91: 102–113.
12. Yu HD, Zhang ZY, Win KY, Chan J, Teoh SH, et al. (2010) Bioinspired fabrication of 3D hierarchical porous nanomicrostructures of calcium carbonate for bone regeneration. Chem Commun (Camb) 46: 6578–6580.
13. Zhong W, Sumita Y, Ohba S, Kawasaki T, Nagai K, et al. (2012) In Vivo Comparison of the Bone Regeneration Capability of Human Bone Marrow Concentrates vs. Platelet-Rich Plasma. PLoS One 7: e40833.
14. Karageorgiou V, Kaplan D (2005) Porosity of 3D biomaterial scaffolds and osteogenesis. Biomaterials 26: 5474–5491.
15. Li JP, Habibovic P, van den Doel M, Wilson CE, de Wijn JR, et al. (2007) Bone ingrowth in porous titanium implants produced by 3D fiber deposition. Biomaterials 28: 2810–2820.
16. Nishikawa M, Myoui A, Ohgushi H, Ikeuchi M, Tamai N, et al. (2004) Bone tissue engineering using novel interconnected porous hydroxyapatite ceramics combined with marrow mesenchymal cells: quantitative and three-dimensional image analysis. Cell Transplant 13: 367–376.
17. Mastrogiacomo M, Scaglione S, Martinetti R, Dolcini L, Beltrame F, et al. (2006) Role of scaffold internal structure on in vivo bone formation in macroporous calcium phosphate bioceramics. Biomaterials 27: 3230–3237.
18. Simon JL, Roy TD, Parsons JR, Rekow ED, Thompson VP, et al. (2003) Engineered cellular response to scaffold architecture in a rabbit trephine defect. Journal of biomedical materials research Part A 66: 275–282.
19. Das A, Botchwey E (2011) Evaluation of Angiogenesis and Osteogenesis. Tissue engineering Part B, Reviews.

20. Gerard C, Doillon CJ (2010) Facilitating tissue infiltration and angiogenesis in a tubular collagen scaffold. Journal of biomedical materials research Part A 93: 615–624.
21. Kokemueller H, Spalthoff S, Nolff M, Tavassol F, Essig H, et al. (2010) Prefabrication of vascularized bioartificial bone grafts in vivo for segmental mandibular reconstruction: experimental pilot study in sheep and first clinical application. Int J Oral Maxillofac Surg 39: 379–387.
22. Geiger F, Bertram H, Berger I, Lorenz H, Wall O, et al. (2005) Vascular endothelial growth factor gene-activated matrix (VEGF165-GAM) enhances osteogenesis and angiogenesis in large segmental bone defects. Journal of bone and mineral research : the official journal of the American Society for Bone and Mineral Research 20: 2028–2035.
23. Cao L, Liu X, Liu S, Jiang Y, Zhang X, et al. (2012) Experimental repair of segmental bone defects in rabbits by angiopoietin-1 gene transfected MSCs seeded on porous beta-TCP scaffolds. J Biomed Mater Res B Appl Biomater 100: 1229–1236.
24. Henslee AM, Spicer PP, Yoon DM, Nair MB, Meretoja VV, et al. (2011) Biodegradable composite scaffolds incorporating an intramedullary rod and delivering bone morphogenetic protein-2 for stabilization and bone regeneration in segmental long bone defects. Acta biomaterialia 7: 3627–3637.
25. Zhang ZY, Teoh SH, Chong MS, Lee ES, Tan LG, et al. (2010) Neo-vascularization and bone formation mediated by fetal mesenchymal stem cell tissue-engineered bone grafts in critical-size femoral defects. Biomaterials 31: 608–620.
26. Zhou J, Lin H, Fang T, Li X, Dai W, et al. (2010) The repair of large segmental bone defects in the rabbit with vascularized tissue engineered bone. Biomaterials 31: 1171–1179.
27. Zhou M, Peng X, Mao C, Xu F, Hu M, et al. (2010) Primate mandibular reconstruction with prefabricated, vascularized tissue-engineered bone flaps and recombinant human bone morphogenetic protein-2 implanted in situ. Biomaterials 31: 4935–4943.
28. Roldan JC, Detsch R, Schaefer S, Chang E, Kelantan M, et al. (2010) Bone formation and degradation of a highly porous biphasic calcium phosphate ceramic in presence of BMP-7, VEGF and mesenchymal stem cells in an ectopic mouse model. Journal of cranio-maxillo-facial surgery : official publication of the European Association for Cranio-Maxillo-Facial Surgery 38: 423–430.
29. Calori GM, Mazza E, Colombo M, Ripamonti C (2011) The use of bone-graft substitutes in large bone defects: any specific needs? Injury 42 Suppl 2: S56–63.
30. Son JS, Kim SG, Oh JS, Appleford M, Oh S, et al. (2011) Hydroxyapatite/polylactide biphasic combination scaffold loaded with dexamethasone for bone regeneration. Journal of biomedical materials research Part A 99: 638–647.
31. Taboas JM, Maddox RD, Krebsbach PH, Hollister SJ (2003) Indirect solid free form fabrication of local and global porous, biomimetic and composite 3D polymer-ceramic scaffolds. Biomaterials 24: 181–194.
32. Habibovic P, de Groot K (2007) Osteoinductive biomaterials–properties and relevance in bone repair. J Tissue Eng RegenMed 1: 25–32.
33. Habibovic P, Kruyt MC, Juhl MV, Clyens S, Martinetti R, et al. (2008) Comparative in vivo study of six hydroxyapatite-based bone graft substitutes. J OrthopRes 26: 1363–1370.
34. Bai F, Wang Z, Lu J, Liu J, Chen G, et al. (2010) The correlation between the internal structure and vascularization of controllable porous bioceramic materials in vivo: a quantitative study. Tissue engineering Part A 16: 3791–3803.
35. Kuboki Y, Jin Q, Takita H (2001) Geometry of carriers controlling phenotypic expression in BMP-induced osteogenesis and chondrogenesis. J Bone Joint Surg Am 83-A Suppl 1: S105–115.
36. Wang L, Fan H, Zhang ZY, Lou AJ, Pei GX, et al. (2010) Osteogenesis and angiogenesis of tissue-engineered bone constructed by prevascularized beta-tricalcium phosphate scaffold and mesenchymal stem cells. Biomaterials 31: 9452–9461.
37. Keselowsky BG, Bridges AW, Burns KL, Tate CC, Babensee JE, et al. (2007) Role of plasma fibronectin in the foreign body response to biomaterials. Biomaterials 28: 3626–3631.
38. Kneser U, Polykandriotis E, Ohnolz J, Heidner K, Grabinger L, et al. (2006) Engineering of vascularized transplantable bone tissues: induction of axial vascularization in an osteoconductive matrix using an arteriovenous loop. Tissue Eng 12: 1721–1731.
39. Zhang ZY, Teoh SH, Hui JH, Fisk NM, Choolani M, et al. (2012) The potential of human fetal mesenchymal stem cells for off-the-shelf bone tissue engineering application. Biomaterials 33: 2656–2672.
40. Love C, Din AS, Tomas MB, Kalapparambath TP, Palestro CJ (2003) Radionuclide bone imaging: an illustrative review. Radiographics 23: 341–358.
41. Zhang ZY, Huang AW, Fan JJ, Wei K, Jin D, et al. (2012) The potential use of allogeneic platelet rich plasma for large bone defect treatment–Immunogenicity and defect healing efficacy. Cell Transplant.
42. Schimming R, Juengling FD, Lauer G, Schmelzeisen R (2000) Evaluation of microvascular bone graft reconstruction of the head and neck with 3-D 99mTc-DPD SPECT scans. Oral Surg Oral Med Oral Pathol Oral Radiol Endod 90: 679–685.
43. Jamell GA, Hollsten DA, Hawes MJ, Griffin DJ, Klingensmith WC, et al. (1996) Magnetic resonance imaging versus bone scan for assessment of vascularization of the hydroxyapatite orbital implant. Ophthal Plast Reconstr Surg 12: 127–130.
44. Wang M, Sun YQ, Zhou H, Ye Z, Sun XH (2009) [Imaging evaluation of the contribution of the deep circumflex iliac arterial vascularized iliac bone grafting to the reconstruction of blood supply of the femoral head]. Zhongguo Gu Shang 22: 609–611.
45. Ogunsalu CO, Rohrer M, Persad H, Archibald A, Watkins J, et al. (2008) Single photon emission computerized tomography and histological evaluation in the validation of a new technique for closure of oro-antral communication: an experimental study in pigs. West Indian Med J 57: 166–172.
46. Yu H, VandeVord PJ, Mao L, Matthew HW, Wooley PH, et al. (2009) Improved tissue-engineered bone regeneration by endothelial cell mediated vascularization. Biomaterials 30: 508–517.
47. Rucker M, Laschke MW, Junker D, Carvalho C, Schramm A, et al. (2006) Angiogenic and inflammatory response to biodegradable scaffolds in dorsal skinfold chambers of mice. Biomaterials 27: 5027–5038.
48. Sung HJ, Meredith C, Johnson C, Galis ZS (2004) The effect of scaffold degradation rate on three-dimensional cell growth and angiogenesis. Biomaterials 25: 5735–5742.
49. Ghanaati S, Barbeck M, Orth C, Willershausen I, Thimm BW, et al. (2010) Influence of beta-tricalcium phosphate granule size and morphology on tissue reaction in vivo. Acta biomaterialia 6: 4476–4487.
50. Kamitakahara M, Ohtsuki C, Miyazaki T (2008) Review paper: behavior of ceramic biomaterials derived from tricalcium phosphate in physiological condition. J Biomater Appl 23: 197–212.
51. Detsch R, Mayr H, Ziegler G (2008) Formation of osteoclast-like cells on HA and TCP ceramics. Acta biomaterialia 4: 139–148.
52. Lu J, Descamps M, Dejou J, Koubi G, Hardouin P, et al. (2002) The biodegradation mechanism of calcium phosphate biomaterials in bone. J Biomed Mater Res 63: 408–412.

8

Osteopontin Level in Synovial Fluid Is Associated with the Severity of Joint Pain and Cartilage Degradation after Anterior Cruciate Ligament Rupture

Mika Yamaga[1], Kunikazu Tsuji[2]*, Kazumasa Miyatake[1], Jun Yamada[1], Kahaer Abula[1], Young-Jin Ju[1], Ichiro Sekiya[3], Takeshi Muneta[1,2]

1 Department of Joint Surgery and Sports Medicine, Tokyo Medical and Dental University, Tokyo, Japan, **2** International Research Center for Molecular Science in Tooth and Bone Diseases (Global Center of Excellence Program), Tokyo Medical and Dental University, Tokyo, Japan, **3** Department of Cartilage Regeneration, Tokyo Medical and Dental University, Tokyo, Japan

Abstract

Objective: To explore the molecular function of Osteopontin (OPN) in the pathogenesis of human OA, we compared the expression levels of OPN in synovial fluid with clinical parameters such as arthroscopic observation of cartilage damage and joint pain after joint injury.

Methods: Synovial fluid was obtained from patients who underwent anterior cruciate ligament (ACL) reconstruction surgery from 2009 through 2011 in our university hospital. The amounts of intact OPN (OPN Full) and it's N-terminal fragment (OPN N-half) in synovial fluid from each patient were quantified by ELISA and compared with clinical parameters such as severity of articular cartilage damage (TMDU cartilage score) and severity of joint pain (Visual Analogue Scale and Lysholm score).

Results: Within a month after ACL rupture, both OPN Full and N-half levels in patient synovial fluid were positively correlated with the severity of joint pain. In contrast, patients with ACL injuries greater than one month ago felt less pain if they had higher amounts of OPN N-half in synovial fluid. OPN Full levels were positively correlated with articular cartilage damage in lateral tibial plateau.

Conclusion: Our data suggest that OPN Full and N-half have distinct functions in articular cartilage homeostasis and in human joint pain.

Editor: Joel Joseph Gagnier, University of Michigan, United States of America

Funding: This study was supported by the Japan Society for the Promotion of Science (22570135 to K.T.; 22600002 to Y-J. J.), by the Global Center of Excellence (GCOE) Program; the International Research Center for Molecular Science in Tooth and Bone Diseases (to K.T. and T.M.), and by the Realization of Regenerative Medicine from Japanese Government (to I.S.). The funders had no role in study design, data collection and analysis, decision to publish, or preparation of the manuscript.

Competing Interests: The authors have declared that no competing interests exist.

* E-mail: ktsuji.gcoe@tmd.ac.jp

Introduction

Osteoarthritis (OA) is a group of diseases and mechanical abnormalities involving degradation of articular cartilage and subchondral bone. Clinical manifestations of OA may include joint pain, tenderness, stiffness, creaking, locking of joints, and local inflammation [1]. It was reported that OA affects 27 million people in the U.S. in 2005 and it is estimated that 80% of the U.S. population will have radiographic evidence of OA by age 65 [1]. These statistics strongly indicate that both prevention of cartilage loss and promotion of cartilage repair in the recovery of joint function are important issues to address [2].

Currently, the major therapeutic strategy for OA is based on conservative treatments, such as muscle exercise with medications, to relieve joint inflammation and pain [3]. However, these treatments are not always satisfactory because they are not powerful enough to inhibit OA progression nor can they promote cartilage repair. To overcome these problems and to develop a new radical treatment for OA, many efforts have been concentrated to understand the molecular pathogenesis of OA. One approach to understand the molecular pathogenesis of OA may be the identification and characterization of the genes involved in joint development and homeostasis. Studies have identified gene sets with altered expression levels in the joint during the progression of OA and RA. These genes include MMP-13 [4–7], OPN [8,9], ECRG4 [10], hYKL40 [11], and hYKL39 [12]. In this study, we focused on analyzing the molecular function of OPN in the pathogenesis of human OA.

OPN is an O-glycosylated phosphoprotein produced by a variety of tissues and cells including osteoblasts, chondrocytes, synoviocytes, and T cells [13]. It was identified as a major non-collagenous bone matrix protein as well as an inflammatory cytokine [13–16]. Previous studies reported that OPN is susceptible to proteolytic fragmentation extracellularly to form different sized protein fragments [17–20]. Full length OPN (OPN Full) is shown to increase in OA synovial fluid and articular cartilage

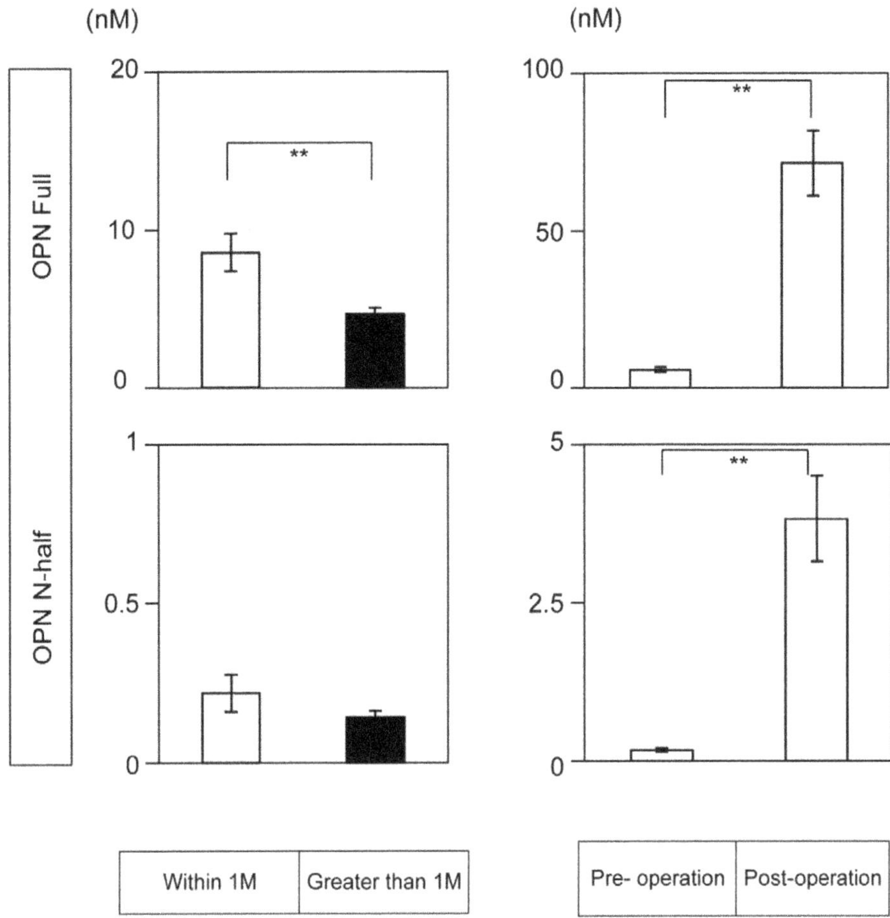

Figure 1. Kinetics of OPN Full and N-half in synovial fluid after joint injury. (Left panels) Time course changes of OPN Full (upper panel) and OPN N-half (lower panel) protein levels in synovial fluid after ACL rupture. Open bar: within 1 month after rupture n = 14, Closed bar: greater than 1 month after rupture n = 68. (Right panels) OPN Full (upper panel) and OPN N-half (lower panel) protein levels in synovial fluid collected from pre (n = 23) and post (n = 93) ACL reconstruction surgery. Data are indicated mean+/− SEM. **; $p<0.01$.

while its N-terminal fragment, OPN N-half, a proteolytic fragment produced by thrombin, is increased in the proinflammatory situation such as rheumatoid arthritis (RA) [8,9,21,22].

Since OPN contains cryptic binding sequences for several different receptors, fragmented OPN proteins are considered to have different functions in distinct pathological conditions [23–25]. It is shown that OPN Full interacts with integrin alpha-v βeta-3 through the GRGDS motif and activates various molecules involved in MAPK and NFkB signaling pathways [23,26]. It also binds to CD44, and is considered to be involved in the process of inflammation, immune response, and bone metabolism [13,27]. C-terminal sequence of OPN N-half contains SVVYGLR motif, which is reported as a cryptic alpha-1 or alpha-4 integrin binding sequence that is exposed by thrombin in an inflammatory situation. The level of OPN N-half is reported to significantly increase in the synovial fluid from rheumatoid arthritis (RA) patients in comparison with that of OA patients [21,22]. Despite of these previous studies, physiological roles of OPN Full and OPN N-half in joint maintenance have not studied in detail.

Studies utilizing OPN knockout mice have reported that aging-associated and instability-induced OA were accelerated in the absence of OPN [28]. In contrast, Yumoto et al reported that inflammation-induced articular cartilage degradation was significantly inhibited in the absence of OPN [29]. These data strongly suggest that OPN has complex roles in joint homeostasis and in the pathogenesis of arthritis by modulating multiple targets of cells in the joint. However, these studies have not elucidated distinct roles of OPN Full and N-half as both proteins were eliminated in these mice.

Since OPN is considered as a proinflammatory cytokine, we hypothesized that OPN levels in the synovial fluid were correlated with joint inflammation and pain. In this study, to examine our hypothesis and to further explore the distinct roles of OPN Full and N-half in joint homeostasis, we analyzed OPN Full and N-half levels in synovial fluid after joint injury and performed correlation analyses with various clinical parameters. Here we report that OPN Full and OPN N-half levels are associated with the severity of joint pain and articular cartilage damage in humans. We consider the two most important subjects in OA research to be the elucidation of the mechanism of joint pain and the mechanism of articular cartilage degradation in humans, both of which are quite difficult to answer using animal models.

Methods

Human Tissue Samples

This study was approved by the Ethics Committee of Tokyo Medical and Dental University. All patients included in this

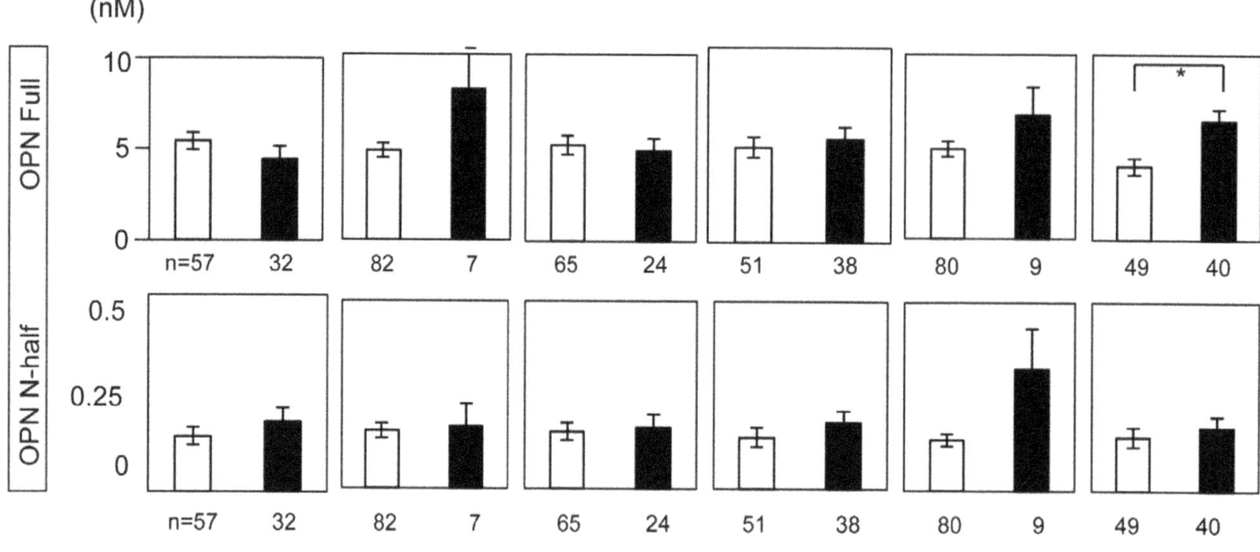

Arthroscopic observation of articular cartilage damage					
Patellofemoral joint		Femorotibial joint			
Patella	Femoral trochlear	Medial		Lateral	
		Femoral condyle	Tibial plateau	Femoral condyle	Tibial plateau

Figure 2. OPN Full levels in synovial fluid are positively correlated with joint damage in lateral tibial plateau. Severity of articular cartilage damage was scored according to the protocol described by Asano et al [32] with minor modification (Table S1). Open bar; intact articular cartilage (score = 1) Closed bar; damaged articular cartilage (score = 2~6). Number of samples is indicated below each column. Data are indicated mean+/− SEM. *; p<0.05.

study gave their full written, informed consent for participation prior to the operative procedure. For minors/children, we obtained informed written consent from their parents or guardians. In this study, we regarded ACL reconstruction patients as a high risk OA group as it was reported that more than 30% of ACL reconstruction patients develop radiographic OA on an average of 7.8 years after surgery, with most patients having no evidence of OA at the time of rupture [30,31]. One hundred and twenty-two (Male: 81, Female: 41) patients aged 14–48 (average 25) years (M: 15–47, F: 14–48), who underwent ACL reconstruction surgery in our university hospital from January 2009 through December 2011, were enrolled in the study. Duration of ACL injury until reconstruction surgery of patients was 2 weeks to 20 years (average 12.9 months). Exclusion criteria included the history of severe meniscus tear. Synovial fluid was aspirated from the knee joint just before ACL reconstruction surgery and 4 days post-surgery. All surgical procedures were performed by expert joint surgeons in our department. Aspirated synovial fluid was centrifuged to remove debris and stored immediately at −80°C.

Quantification of OPN Full and N-half in Synovial Fluid

Since OPN is shown to process by thrombin in an inflammatory environment [21,22], we quantified both intact OPN protein (OPN Full) and the thrombin-processed form (OPN N-half) in this study. Protein levels of OPN Full and N-half in synovial fluid were quantified independently using an ELISA kit according to the manufacturer's protocol (IBL Co. Ltd. Tokyo Japan). In some experiments, we divided the subjects into 2 groups, within 1 month and greater than 1 month, because our preliminary data indicated that the volume of synovial fluid quickly increased after the joint injury and usually returned to the basal level after 1 month (data not shown).

Arthroscopic Observation of Articular Cartilage Damage (TMDU Score)

The severity of articular cartilage damage was scored during ACL reconstruction surgery according to the classification protocol described by Asano et al with modification [32]. Details are shown in Table S1. These scores were determined mainly by the two skilled operators during the surgery by mutual consent.

Visual Analogue Scale (VAS) and Lysholm Score

VAS was collected in the examination room before consultation (one day before ACL reconstruction surgery). Lysholm scores were collected by expert joint surgeons in our university hospital during consultation. Details are shown in Table S2 and S3.

Statistical Analysis

All the analyses were performed by a double-blind method. Mann-Whitney's U-test or Kruskal–Wallis test followed by Steel–Dwass multiple comparison tests were employed to analyze the differences between groups. Pearson's correlation coefficient test was employed for correlation analyses. Values of $P<0.05$ were considered significant.

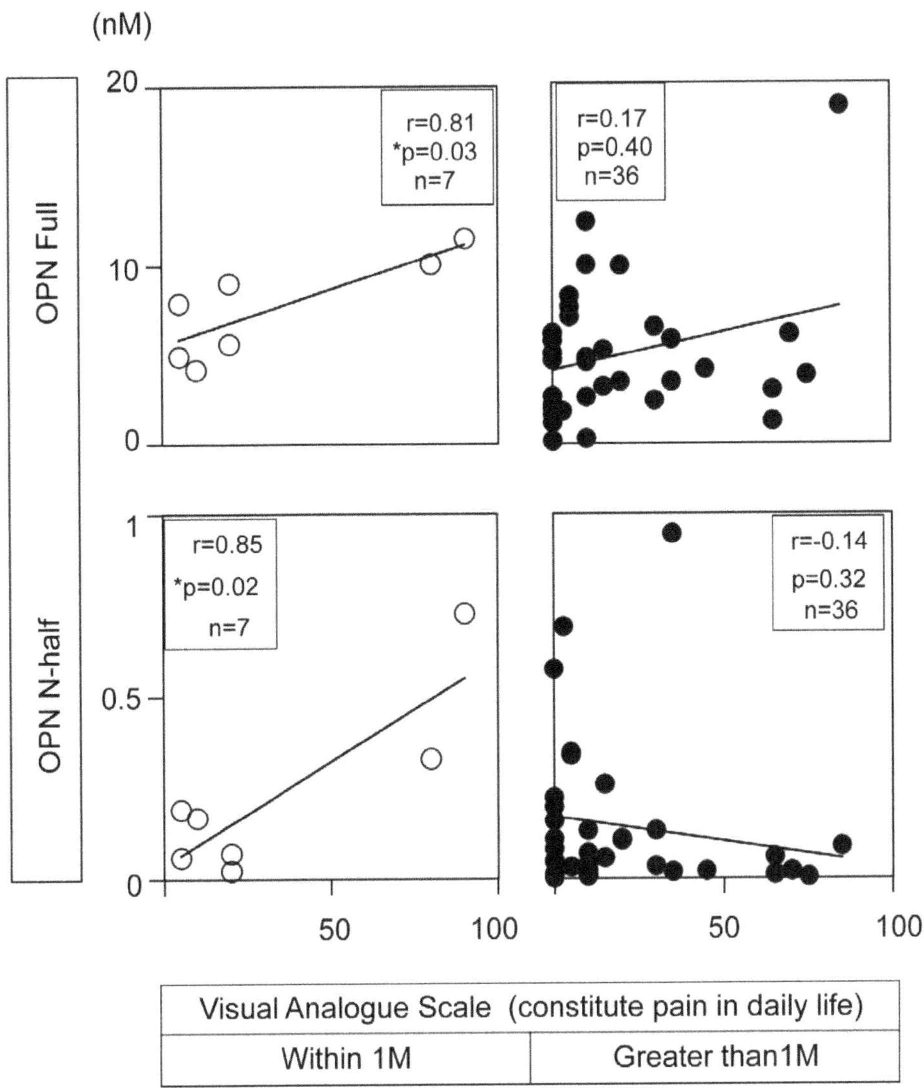

Figure 3. OPN Full and N-half levels in synovial fluid are positively correlated with the severity of joint pain within a month after ACL rupture. VAS indicating constitutive pain in a daily life (see Table S2) was collected in the examination room before consultation. Open circle; VAS from patients within 1 month after ACL rupture. Closed circle; VAS from patients who ruptured ACL greater than 1 month ago. Number of samples, correlation coefficient, and p value are indicated in each figure.

Results

Kinetics of OPN Levels in Synovial Fluid after Joint Injury

As shown in Fig. 1, OPN Full levels were significantly decreased with time after ACL rupture. In contrast, OPN N-half levels remained low and did not alter significantly between the two time periods after ACL rupture (left panels). Since it is reported that OPN gene expression is upregulated in response to injury and inflammation in various organs including bone [33,34], we analyzed OPN protein levels at pre- and 4 days post-operation. Both OPN Full and N-half levels surged by almost 10-fold at 4 days post ACL reconstruction (right panels). The base line level of OPN Full was almost 10-fold of that of OPN N-half.

Synovial Fluid OPN Levels are Positively Correlated with the Severity of Articular Cartilage Damage in Lateral Tibial Plateau

Matsui et al reported that the development of aging-associated and instability-induced osteoarthritis was accelerated in OPN deficient mice [28]. To examine if synovial fluid OPN levels were correlated with the severity of articular cartilage damage after ACL rupture in humans, we compared OPN Full and N-half levels in synovial fluid with the arthroscopic observation of cartilage damage in patellofemoral and femorotibial joints. As shown in Fig. 2, we found that synovial fluid OPN Full levels were positively correlated with the damage of articular cartilage in lateral tibial plateau in the femorotibial joint. In contrast, we did not observe any correlation between OPN N-half levels and articular cartilage damage.

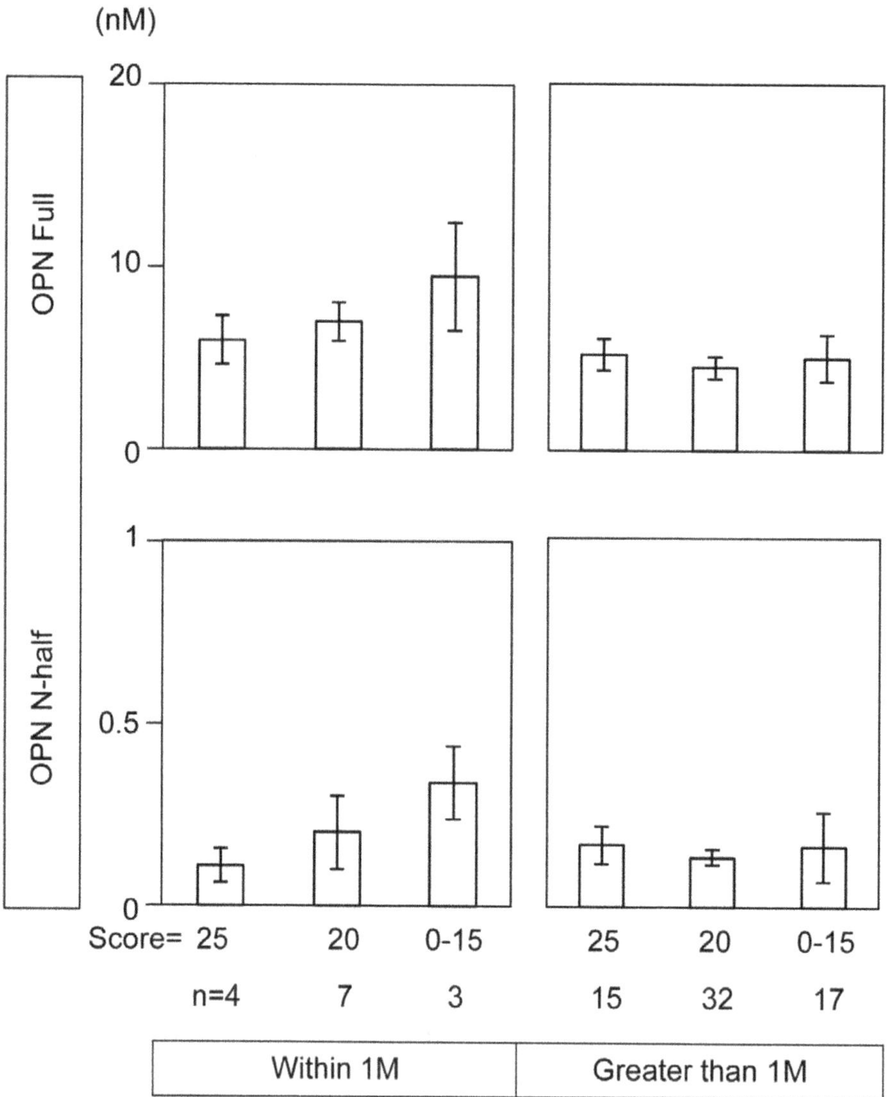

Figure 4. Correlation of OPN Full and N-half levels in synovial fluid with Lysholm scores. Lysholm scores (see Table S3) were collected in an examination room by expert joint surgeons in our university hospital. The basis of the classification of Lysholm score was 25:feel no pain at any time, 20:feel not so severe or tolerable pain even after severe exertion, 0–15:feel severe or intolerable pain sometimes in a daily life. Numbers of samples are indicated below each figure.

Synovial Fluid OPN Levels and the Severity of Joint Pain

Fig. 3 shows the correlation of synovial fluid OPN levels with constitutive pain in daily life. As shown in this figure, both OPN full and N-half levels were positively correlated with the severity of constitutive joint pain in patients suffering from ACL rupture within 1 month. These correlations were statistically significant (left panels). In contrast, we did not observe any correlation in the patients suffering from ACL rupture greater than 1 month post-injury (right panels). Interestingly, we observed a negative relationship between OPN N-half levels and VAS at this stage. These results seemed to be reproducible since we observe similar tendency between OPN levels in synovial fluid and Lysholm scores (Fig. 4). To further analyze the correlation between the severity of joint pain and synovial fluid OPN levels in patients following the acute inflammation stage, we evaluated the correlation between daily activities and joint pain in patients whose ACL injury had surpassed one month. We compared VAS of patients when they rest on a bed (first column), wake up (second column), walk (third column), and play sports (forth column) with OPN levels (Fig. 5). In parallel with the results in Fig. 3 right panels, we did not observe any correlation between OPN Full levels and VAS (Fig. 5 upper panels) at this stage. Interestingly, OPN N-half levels tended to negatively correlate with VAS at this stage, which was statistically significant when they played sports ($p = 0.03$, Fig. 5 lower 4th column).

Since local inflammation is considered to be a major contributor for joint pain, we next examined if synovial fluid OPN levels are correlated with the severity of systemic and local inflammation. As shown in Fig. 6, we did not observe any correlation between OPN levels in synovial fluid and serum C-reactive peptide (CRP) levels, a marker for systemic inflammation (Fig. 6 left and middle panels). However, we observed significant positive correlation between OPN Full levels and the volume of synovial fluid (Fig. 6 right upper panel). Since synovial fluid volume usually increases during joint inflammation, our results suggest that OPN Full levels may

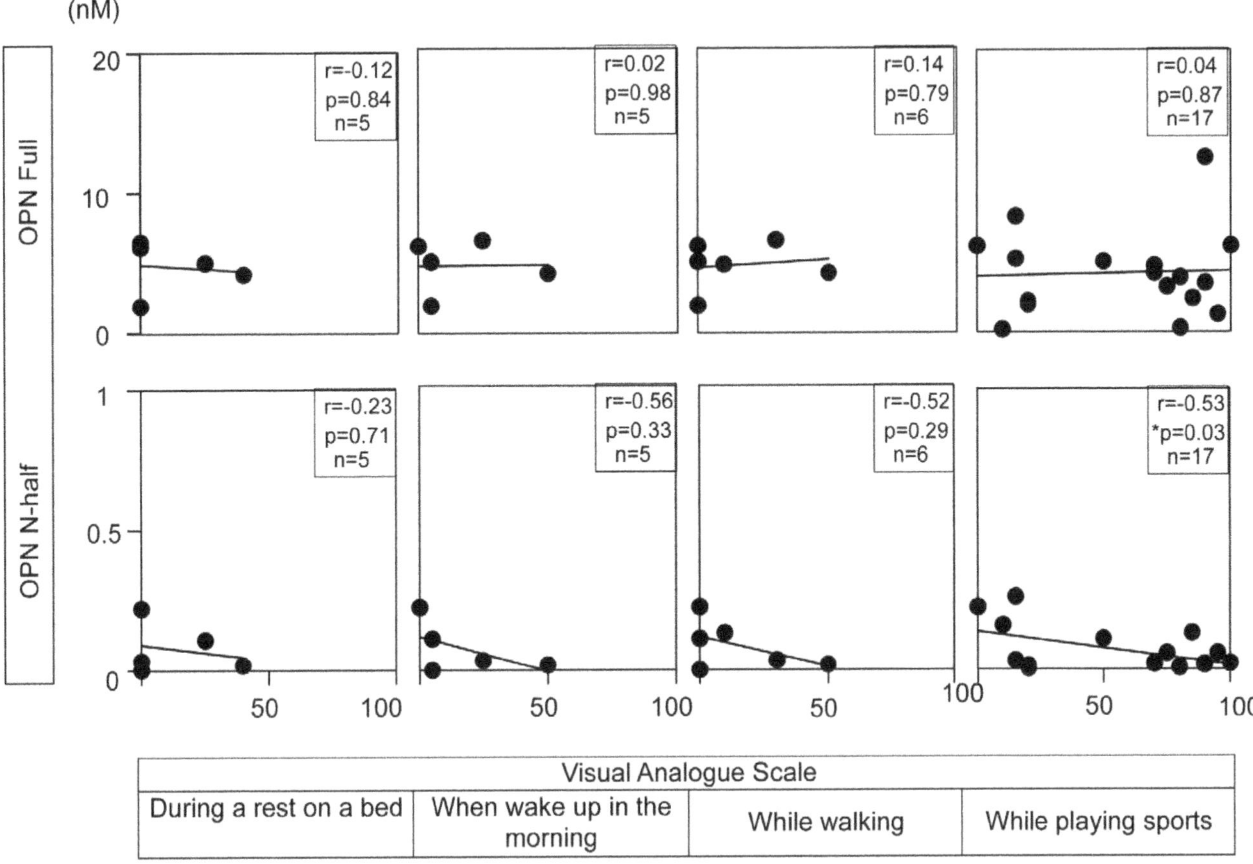

Figure 5. OPN N-half levels in synovial fluid are negatively correlated with the severity of joint pain in patients who ruptured ACL greater than 1 month ago. VAS was collected from patients who ruptured ACL more than 1 month ago using a questionnaire described in Table S2 in an examination room at our university hospital. Number of samples, correlation coefficient, and p value are indicated in each figure.

associate with joint inflammation [35]. In contrast, OPN N-half levels seemed to negatively correlate with joint inflammation (Fig. 6 right lower panel).

Discussion

OPN is a phosphorylated acidic glycoprotein with diverse functions including cell adhesion, chemoattraction, immunomodulation, and cell differentiation [13,17]. OPN is considered to be involved in the pathogenesis of human OA since its expression level is enhanced with OA progression [22]. Previous in vitro and knockout mice experiments indicated that OPN is influential in articular cartilage metabolism in both physiological and pathological conditions [28,29], however the role of OPN in the pathogenesis of human OA was still unclear. To explore the pathophysiological roles of OPN in human OA, we compared OPN expression levels in synovial fluid with various clinical conditions such as arthroscopic observation of articular cartilage and joint pain. In this manuscript we report that OPN levels were correlated with the severity of articular cartilage damage in lateral tibial plateau and joint pain. This is the first report showing that OPN is involved in joint pain in human OA.

In the present study we demonstrated that kinetics of OPN Full and N-half levels were different in synovial fluid. Both OPN Full and N-half levels surged almost 10-fold by 4 days after ACL reconstruction surgery. This result is comparable with previous reports indicating that OPN is an early response gene against various stress signals [36,37]. We observed that levels of OPN full in synovial fluid were significantly higher within 1 month than greater than 1 month after ACL rupture. In contrast, OPN N-half levels remained low and did not alter significantly between the two time periods after ACL rupture (Fig. 1 left panels). Since we could not detect OPN mRNA expression in the synovial membranes obtained from patients with ruptured ACL by RT-PCR analyses (data not shown), we expect that OPN gene expression is immediately upregulated at the point of joint injury and quickly shut down during the healing process. Posttranslational OPN processing by thrombin to produce OPN N-half may occur and quench very quickly in synovial fluid after joint injury.

With regard to the correlation of OPN levels and articular cartilage damage, we found that OPN Full levels are positively correlated with the severity of articular cartilage damage in lateral tibial plateau (Fig. 2). Lateral tibial plateau is the region where bone bruise is most frequently observed by X-ray and MRI (magnetic resonance imaging) after ACL injury [38]. This suggests that OPN Full may accelerate inflammation-induced cartilage degradation. Fig. 6 indirectly supports this idea that OPN Full levels are positively correlated with the amount of synovial fluid, which is usually positively correlated with the severity of joint inflammation [35]. OPN knockout mice experiments also support this idea since OPN knockout mice were resistant in inflammation-induced articular cartilage degradation [29]. In contrast, we did not observe any correlation between OPN N-half levels and articular cartilage damage. One reason for that may be due to the

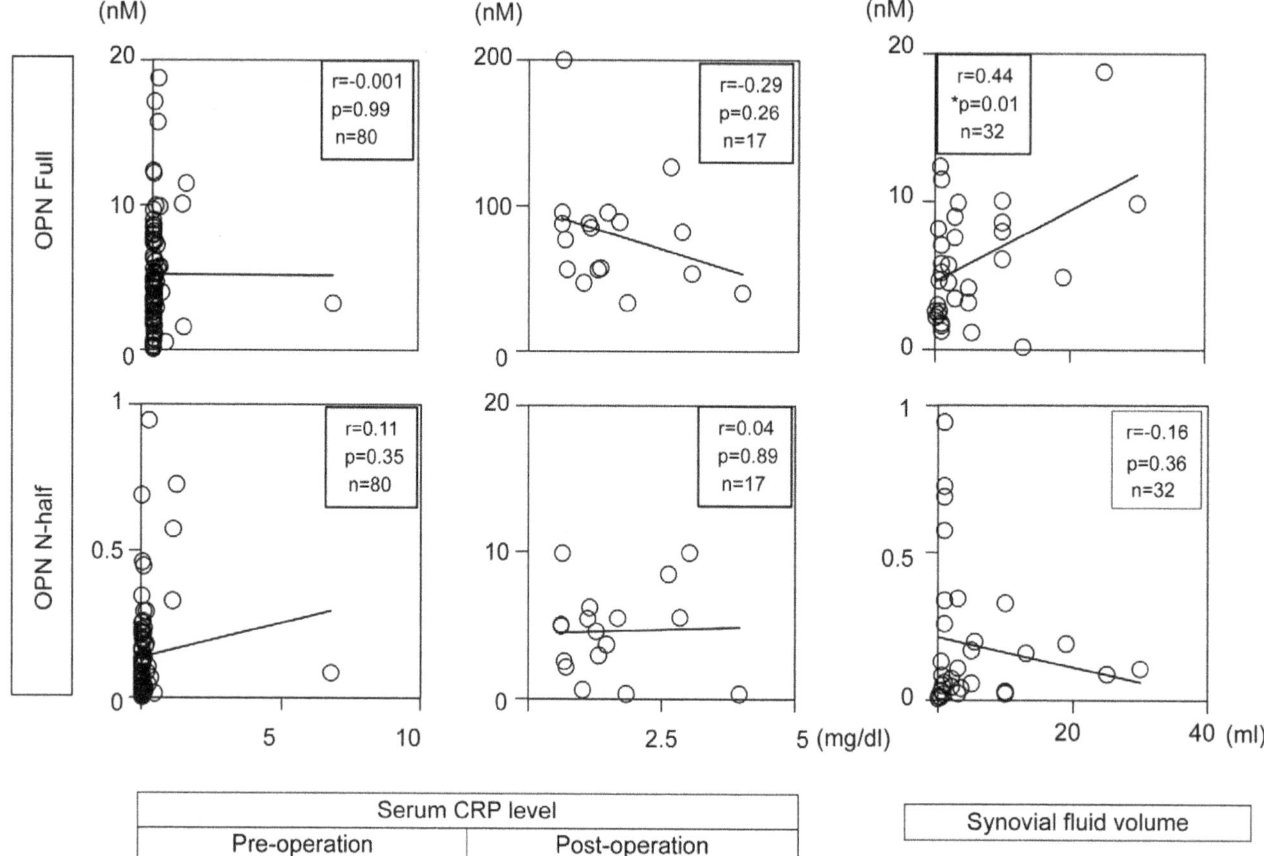

Figure 6. OPN Full and N-half levels in synovial fluid are independent from systemic inflammatory status but associate with joint inflammation. (Left and Middle panels) Blood samples were collected pre- and post-operation (at day 4) and serum CRP levels were quantified at the clinical laboratory of our university hospital. (Right panels) Synovial fluid was collected just before operation in a surgery room. Number of samples, correlation coefficient, and p value are indicated in each figure.

kinetics of OPN N-half in synovial fluid after joint injury. We showed that OPN N-half levels quickly quenched after joint damage while cartilage damage usually progresses by the month. The other possible reason for that may be due to the differences of receptor usage between OPN Full and N-half. Further studies are required to elucidate the functional differences between OPN Full and N-half on cartilage metabolism.

The most interesting finding of this study was the correlation of OPN levels with the severity of joint pain. We observed that OPN Full and N-half levels are positively correlated with the severity of joint pain in patients who suffered from ACL rupture within 1 month. Since OPN functions as a proinflammatory cytokine and regulates PTGS2 and iNOS expression [9,27], we speculate that OPN may mediate the expression of pain inducers, such as prostaglandin E2 and nitric oxide, at the acute inflammatory stage after ACL rupture. In contrast, we observed a negative correlation between OPN N-half levels and joint pain in patients whose ACL rupture surpassed one month, when the acute inflammation has already quenched. Although we do not know yet the functional differences between OPN Full and N-half, these data suggest that OPN N-half may have an inhibitory function against OPN Full. To evaluate this hypothesis, we examined the effect of OPN N-half on the regulation of PTGS2 mRNA that was induced by OPN Full in chondrogenic ATDC5 cells. However, our preliminary data indicated a subtle effect of OPN N-half on PTGS2 expression (data not shown). Since OPN is also reported as an intrinsic inhibitor of inflammation in cartilage [9], further molecular analyses of OPN Full and N-half are necessary to elucidate the specific roles of these proteins in joint pain.

In summary, we found that OPN levels were correlated with the severity of articular cartilage damage in lateral tibial plateau and joint pain. These results suggest that OPN may be an important target to relieve OA patients from severe joint pain and cartilage degradation.

Supporting Information

Table S1 Classification of arthroscopic observation of articular cartilage damage. Severity of articular cartilage damage was scored according to the protocol described by Asano et al [32] with minor modification as shown in the table.

Table S2 Visual Analogue Scale (VAS) for pain. VAS was collected using a questionnaire described in the table.

Table S3 Lysholm score for pain. Lysholm scores were collected in an examination room by expert joint surgeons in our university hospital. Classification of each score was described in the table.

Author Contributions

Conceived and designed the experiments: KT TM IS YJJ. Performed the experiments: MY KT KM JY KA. Analyzed the data: MY KT TM. Contributed reagents/materials/analysis tools: MY KT TM. Wrote the paper: KT MY TM.

References

1. (CDC) CfDCaP (2009) Prevalence and most common causes of disability among adults–United States, 2005. MMWR Morb Mortal Wkly Rep 58: 421–426.
2. Muraki S, Akune T, Oka H, En-yo Y, Yoshida M, et al. (2010) Association of radiographic and symptomatic knee osteoarthritis with health-related quality of life in a population-based cohort study in Japan: the ROAD study. Osteoarthritis Cartilage 18: 1227–1234.
3. Kon E, Filardo G, Drobnic M, Madry H, Jelic M, et al. (2011) Non-surgical management of early knee osteoarthritis. Knee Surg Sports Traumatol Arthrosc.
4. Mitchell PG, Magna HA, Reeves LM, Lopresti-Morrow LL, Yocum SA, et al. (1996) Cloning, expression, and type II collagenolytic activity of matrix metalloproteinase-13 from human osteoarthritic cartilage. J Clin Invest 97: 761–768.
5. Reboul P, Pelletier JP, Tardif G, Cloutier JM, Martel-Pelletier J (1996) The new collagenase, collagenase-3, is expressed and synthesized by human chondrocytes but not by synoviocytes. A role in osteoarthritis. J Clin Invest 97: 2011–2019.
6. Knäuper V, Will H, López-Otin C, Smith B, Atkinson SJ, et al. (1996) Cellular mechanisms for human procollagenase-3 (MMP-13) activation. Evidence that MT1-MMP (MMP-14) and gelatinase a (MMP-2) are able to generate active enzyme. J Biol Chem 271: 17124–17131.
7. Nagase H, Kashiwagi M (2003) Aggrecanases and cartilage matrix degradation. Arthritis Res Ther 5: 94–103.
8. Pullig O, Weseloh G, Gauer S, Swoboda B (2000) Osteopontin is expressed by adult human osteoarthritic chondrocytes: protein and mRNA analysis of normal and osteoarthritic cartilage. Matrix Biol 19: 245–255.
9. Attur MG, Dave MN, Stuchin S, Kowalski AJ, Steiner G, et al. (2001) Osteopontin: an intrinsic inhibitor of inflammation in cartilage. Arthritis Rheum 44: 578–584.
10. Huh YH, Ryu JH, Shin S, Lee DU, Yang S, et al. (2009) Esophageal cancer related gene 4 (ECRG4) is a marker of articular chondrocyte differentiation and cartilage destruction. Gene 448: 7–15.
11. Johansen JS, Hvolris J, Hansen M, Backer V, Lorenzen I, et al. (1996) Serum YKL-40 levels in healthy children and adults. Comparison with serum and synovial fluid levels of YKL-40 in patients with osteoarthritis or trauma of the knee joint. Br J Rheumatol 35: 553–559.
12. Steck E, Breit S, Breusch SJ, Axt M, Richter W (2002) Enhanced expression of the human chitinase 3-like 2 gene (YKL-39) but not chitinase 3-like 1 gene (YKL-40) in osteoarthritic cartilage. Biochem Biophys Res Commun 299: 109–115.
13. Wang KX, Denhardt DT (2008) Osteopontin: role in immune regulation and stress responses. Cytokine Growth Factor Rev 19: 333–345.
14. Franzén A, Heinegård D (1985) Isolation and characterization of two sialoproteins present only in bone calcified matrix. Biochem J 232: 715–724.
15. Patarca R, Freeman GJ, Singh RP, Wei FY, Durfee T, et al. (1989) Structural and functional studies of the early T lymphocyte activation 1 (Eta-1) gene. Definition of a novel T cell-dependent response associated with genetic resistance to bacterial infection. J Exp Med 170: 145–161.
16. Patarca R, Saavedra RA, Cantor H (1993) Molecular and cellular basis of genetic resistance to bacterial infection: the role of the early T-lymphocyte activation-1/osteopontin gene. Crit Rev Immunol 13: 225–246.
17. Bayless KJ, Davis GE (2001) Identification of dual alpha 4beta1 integrin binding sites within a 38 amino acid domain in the N-terminal thrombin fragment of human osteopontin. J Biol Chem 276: 13483–13489.
18. Yokosaki Y, Matsuura N, Sasaki T, Murakami I, Schneider H, et al. (1999) The integrin alpha(9)beta(1) binds to a novel recognition sequence (SVVYGLR) in the thrombin-cleaved amino-terminal fragment of osteopontin. J Biol Chem 274: 36328–36334.
19. Gao YA, Agnihotri R, Vary CP, Liaw L (2004) Expression and characterization of recombinant osteopontin peptides representing matrix metalloproteinase proteolytic fragments. Matrix Biol 23: 457–466.
20. Maeda K, Takahashi K, Takahashi F, Tamura N, Maeda M, et al. (2001) Distinct roles of osteopontin fragments in the development of the pulmonary involvement in sarcoidosis. Lung 179: 279–291.
21. Hasegawa M, Nakoshi Y, Iino T, Sudo A, Segawa T, et al. (2009) Thrombin-cleaved osteopontin in synovial fluid of subjects with rheumatoid arthritis. J Rheumatol 36: 240–245.
22. Hasegawa M, Segawa T, Maeda M, Yoshida T, Sudo A (2011) Thrombin-cleaved osteopontin levels in synovial fluid correlate with disease severity of knee osteoarthritis. J Rheumatol 38: 129–134.
23. Rodan GA (1995) Osteopontin overview. Ann N Y Acad Sci 760: 1–5.
24. Senger DR, Ledbetter SR, Claffey KP, Papadopoulos-Sergiou A, Peruzzi CA, et al. (1996) Stimulation of endothelial cell migration by vascular permeability factor/vascular endothelial growth factor through cooperative mechanisms involving the alphavbeta3 integrin, osteopontin, and thrombin. Am J Pathol 149: 293–305.
25. Agnihotri R, Crawford HC, Haro H, Matrisian LM, Havrda MC, et al. (2001) Osteopontin, a novel substrate for matrix metalloproteinase-3 (stromelysin-1) and matrix metalloproteinase-7 (matrilysin). J Biol Chem 276: 28261–28267.
26. Jain S, Chakraborty G, Kundu GC (2006) The crucial role of cyclooxygenase-2 in osteopontin-induced protein kinase C alpha/c-Src/IkappaB kinase alpha/beta-dependent prostate tumor progression and angiogenesis. Cancer Res 66: 6638–6648.
27. O'Regan A, Berman JS (2000) Osteopontin: a key cytokine in cell-mediated and granulomatous inflammation. Int J Exp Pathol 81: 373–390.
28. Matsui Y, Iwasaki N, Kon S, Takahashi D, Morimoto J, et al. (2009) Accelerated development of aging-associated and instability-induced osteoarthritis in osteopontin-deficient mice. Arthritis Rheum 60: 2362–2371.
29. Yumoto K, Ishijima M, Rittling SR, Tsuji K, Tsuchiya Y, et al. (2002) Osteopontin deficiency protects joints against destruction in anti-type II collagen antibody-induced arthritis in mice. Proc Natl Acad Sci U S A 99: 4556–4561.
30. Louboutin H, Debarge R, Richou J, Selmi TA, Donell ST, et al. (2009) Osteoarthritis in patients with anterior cruciate ligament rupture: a review of risk factors. Knee 16: 239–244.
31. Li RT, Lorenz S, Xu Y, Harner CD, Fu FH, et al. (2011) Predictors of radiographic knee osteoarthritis after anterior cruciate ligament reconstruction. Am J Sports Med 39: 2595–2603.
32. Asano H, Muneta T, Ikeda H, Yagishita K, Kurihara Y, et al. (2004) Arthroscopic evaluation of the articular cartilage after anterior cruciate ligament reconstruction: a short-term prospective study of 105 patients. Arthroscopy 20: 474–481.
33. Denhardt DT, Noda M (1998) Osteopontin expression and function: role in bone remodeling. J Cell Biochem Suppl 30–31: 92–102.
34. Xu G, Sun W, He D, Wang L, Zheng W, et al. (2005) Overexpression of osteopontin in rheumatoid synovial mononuclear cells is associated with joint inflammation, not with genetic polymorphism. J Rheumatol 32: 410–416.
35. Courtney P, Doherty M (2009) Joint aspiration and injection and synovial fluid analysis. Best Pract Res Clin Rheumatol 23: 161–192.
36. Mori N, Majima T, Iwasaki N, Kon S, Miyakawa K, et al. (2007) The role of osteopontin in tendon tissue remodeling after denervation-induced mechanical stress deprivation. Matrix Biol 26: 42–53.
37. Toma CD, Ashkar S, Gray ML, Schaffer JL, Gerstenfeld LC (1997) Signal transduction of mechanical stimuli is dependent on microfilament integrity: identification of osteopontin as a mechanically induced gene in osteoblasts. J Bone Miner Res 12: 1626–1636.
38. Dunn WR, Spindler KP, Amendola A, Andrish JT, Kaeding CC, et al. (2010) Which preoperative factors, including bone bruise, are associated with knee pain/symptoms at index anterior cruciate ligament reconstruction (ACLR)? A Multicenter Orthopaedic Outcomes Network (MOON) ACLR Cohort Study. Am J Sports Med 38: 1778–1787.

9

The Treatment Effect of Porous Titanium Alloy Rod on the Early Stage Talar Osteonecrosis of Sheep

Xiao-Kang Li[1]◉, Chao-Fan Yuan[1]◉, Jun-Lin Wang[2]◉, Yong-Quan Zhang[1], Zhi-Yong Zhang[3,4]*, Zheng Guo[1]*

1 Department of Orthopaedics, Xijing Hospital, Fourth Military Medical University, Xi'an, China, **2** School of Stomatology, Fourth Military Medical University, Xi'an, China, **3** Department of Plastic and Reconstructive Surgery, Shanghai 9th People's Hospital, Shanghai Key Laboratory of Tissue Engineering, School of Medicine, Shanghai Jiao Tong University, Shanghai, China, **4** National Tissue Engineering Center of China, Shanghai, China

Abstract

Osteonecrosis of the talus (ONT) may severely affect the function of the ankle joint. Most orthopedists believe that ONT should be treated at an early stage, but a concise and effective surgical treatment is lacking. In this study, porous titanium alloy rods were prepared and implanted into the tali of sheep with early-stage ONT (IM group). The curative effect of the rods was compared to treatment by core decompression (DC group). No significant differences in bone reconstruction were observed between the two groups at 1 month after intervention. After 3 months, the macroscopic view of gross specimens of the IM group showed ordinary contours, but the specimens of the DC group showed obvious partial bone defects and cartilage degeneration. Quantitative analysis of the reconstructed trabeculae by micro-CT and histological study suggested that the curative effect of the IM group was superior to that of the DC group at 3 months after intervention. These favorable short-term results of the implantation of porous titanium alloy rods into the tali of sheep with early-stage ONT may provide insight into an innovative surgical treatment for ONT.

Editor: Paul Eckhard Witten, Ghent University, Belgium

Funding: This work was supported by the National Natural Science Foundation of China (No: 81171773) to Guo Zheng and Xijing Zhutui Project (SJZT10Z09) and National Natural Science Foundation of China (81101353) to Zhang Zhi-Yong. The funders had no role in study design, data collection, decision to publish, or preparation of the manuscript.

Competing Interests: The authors have declared that no competing interests exist.

* E-mail: guozheng@fmmu.edu.cn (ZG); mr.zhiyong@gmail.com (Z-YZ)

◉ These authors contributed equally to this work.

Introduction

Osteonecrosis of the talus (ONT) may be caused by trauma, usage of prednisone, cytostatica treatment or some systematic immune diseases and so on [1–5]. Blockage or disturbance of the blood circulation is thought to be the direct cause of ONT. As a major load-bearing region, the talus provides mechanical support for the whole body weight of a human in the orthostatic state. The development of ONT may substantially alter the structural integrity of the talus and dramatically increase the intraosseous pressure of the talus, which may further disturb blood circulation through the talus [1]. Under the synergetic effects of the increase in intraosseous pressure and decrease in blood supply, without proper therapeutic intervention ONT may rapidly become aggravated and lead to eventual failure of the ankle joint.

Several therapeutic interventions are currently available for the treatment of ONT, including biophosphonate treatments, core decompression, vasotransplantation, and the transposition of vascularized bone flap. Biophosphonate could be used to treat the osteonecrosis, because of their capacity to inhabit the bone resorption. Core decompression and vasotransplantation are traditional approaches to the treatment of early-stage ONT that may help to reduce the intraosseous pressure and improve the blood circulation. However, they do not provide additional mechanical support, which would further reduce the intraosseous talar pressure [3–7]. These approaches also require long-term immobilization of the ankle joint during treatment, which could lead to osteoporosis due to a lack of mechanical stimulation [8]. Therefore, these approaches are associated with very limited success in clinical practice. The transposition of vascularized bone flap aims to treat ONT by reconstructing the bone tissue and providing vascularization. However, this method is associated with an uncertain long-term therapeutic outcome due to the poor survival rate of the implanted bone flap and a lack of sufficient mechanical support [9–11].

To address the decreased mechanical support of the inherent bone tissue associated with osteonecrosis, metal implants have been proposed as a treatment approach, especially for femoral head osteonecrosis [12–16]. Metal implants such as the porous tantalum rod (Trabeculaer Metal, Zimmer, USA) may provide additional mechanical support in the load-bearing region, which may help to maintain the structural integrity of the bone tissue, reduce the intraosseous pressure by creating the implantation canal, and improve blood perfusion for bone regeneration [12–13]. Tantalum rod implantation has been shown to achieve an 80% satisfactory clinical outcome for femoral head osteonecrosis treatment, especially in the early stage, with appropriate mechanical strength and little impingement of the stress shield [12–14]. Furthermore, metal rods can be implanted in a minimally invasive manner, thereby reducing damage to the surrounding tissues, and

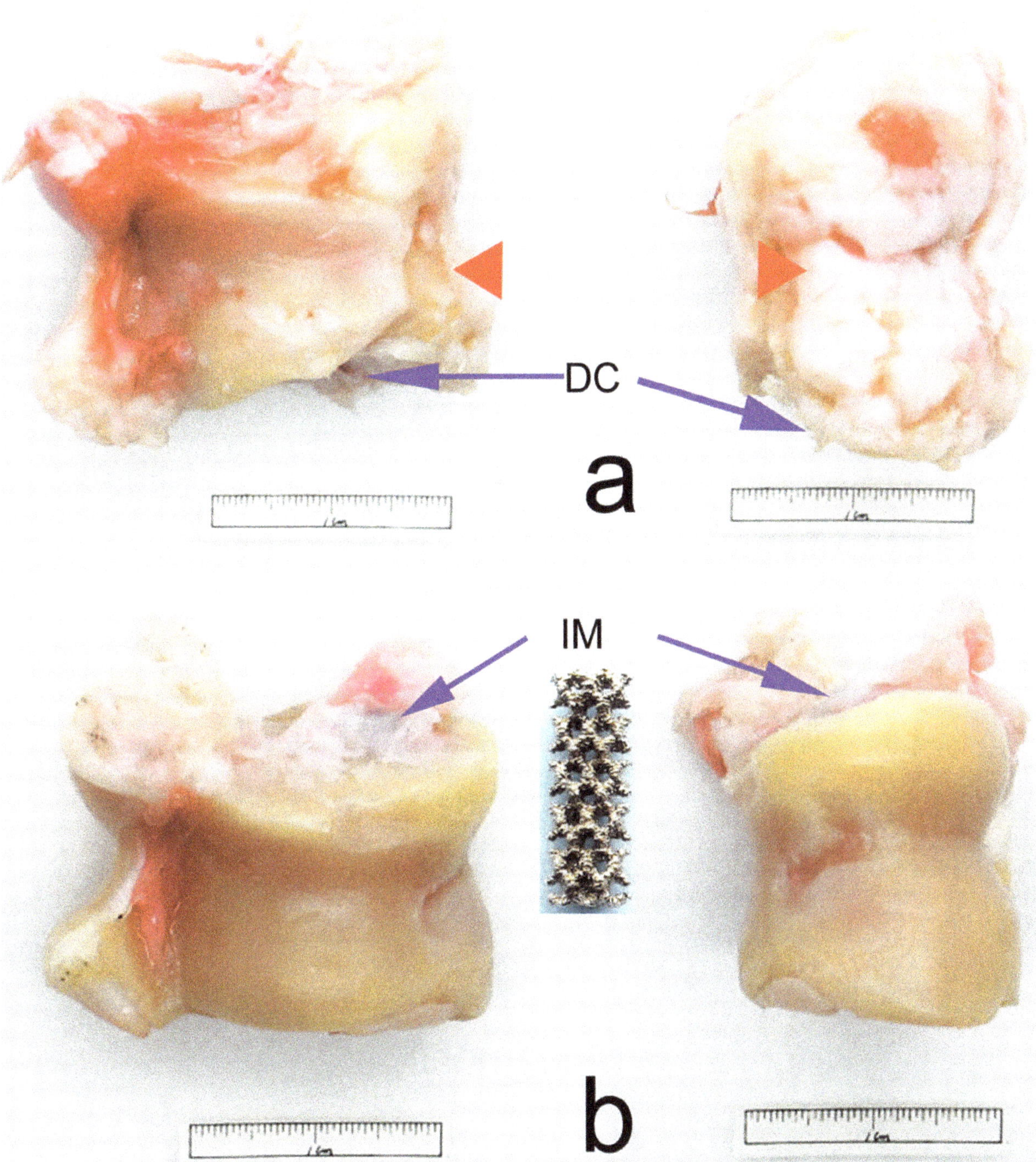

Figure 1. Sample of a porous titanium alloy rod and gross specimens at 3 months after treatment. Blue arrowheads indicate treatment sites.

favoring the rapid regeneration of bone tissue in the later stage [13].

However, the use of metal implants has been limited to femoral head osteonecrosis treatment. To the best of our knowledge, there are no preclinical animal or clinical investigations of their potential use in treating ONT. Therefore, we hypothesized that the implantation of porous metal rods could be an effective surgical intervention for the treatment of ONT by providing sufficient mechanical support to reduce the intraosseous pressure and restore the blood supply, and by acting as a scaffold matrix to promote new bone regeneration. Recently, we have successfully established a preclinical sheep model of ONT with clinical relevance, which provides a good animal model for this hypothesis testing. By using the method of intraosseous injection of pure ethanol in the median talar head, we developed the animal model of ONT with clear sign of stage II osteonecrosis 4 weeks

Table 1. Characteristics of the porous titanium alloy.

Sample mass, m (g)	Sample dimensions, (mm^3)	Density, ρ (g/cm^3)	Relative density, $(\rho/\rho_s)^a$	Porosity (%)	Compressive strength, σ (MPa)
0.45	φ4×12	1.33	0.3	70	36.36

postoperatively, which is considered to be a proper time for surgical intervention [17]. Hence, in the present study, based on the development of this preclinical ONT animal model, we aim to investigate the efficacy of a porous titanium alloy rod, fabricated by the electron beam melting (EBM) technique, for ONT treatment.

Materials and Methods

Animals

All animal experiments were performed according to protocols approved by the Institutional Animal Care Committee of Fourth Military Medical University. Twelve adult female Small Tail Han Sheep (median age: 25 months, range: 20–31 months; median weight: 42.5 kg, range: 35–57 kg) were used in the study. The sheep were housed at the Department of Orthopedics of Xijing Hospital Animal Resources Center in two approved shacks with an average acreage of 18 m^2. All sheep were maintained under routine husbandry.

Fabrication of porous titanium rods using the EBM technique

Porous titanium rods were fabricated by three major procedures. First, the three-dimensional (3-D) rod structure was designed by computer-aided design (CAD). Data were saved in standard template library format and inputted into the EBM S12 system (Acram AB, Sweden). Second, titanium alloy powder (Ti_6Al_4V) was melted layer by layer in the Acram EBM S12 system and the rod structure was remolded according to the CAD model. Third, the residual powder was removed and the products were prepared.

To prepare the products, the titanium alloy powder was made into porous cylinders of 4 mm in diameter and 12 mm in length (IM, Figure 1). The porosity of the cylinders was 70% and the pore size was about 1 mm. The rods had an average compressive strength of 36.36 MPa, which is much higher than that of spongeous bone (Table 1). Based on these data, the elastic modulus of the porous rod as a unit was about 2.2 GPa, according to a previous study [18].

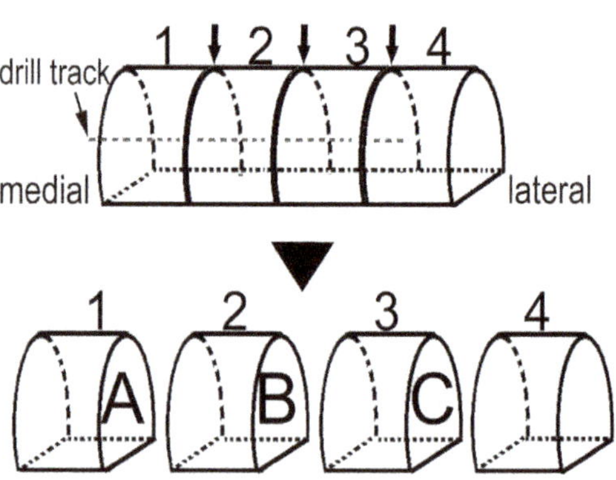

Figure 3. Section design for histology. Sections A, B, and C were prepared for staining.

Experimental design

After the sheep were weighed, they were randomly and evenly divided into two groups. To induce ONT, each talus was administered an intraosseous injection of pure ethanol (Figure 2). At 1 month after ONT induction, the early stage of ONT was confirmed by radiographic and computed tomography (CT) examinations. Porous titanium alloy rods were implanted (group IM), and core decompression surgery was performed (group DC) on the necrotic tali. At 1 month after this intervention, ONT was

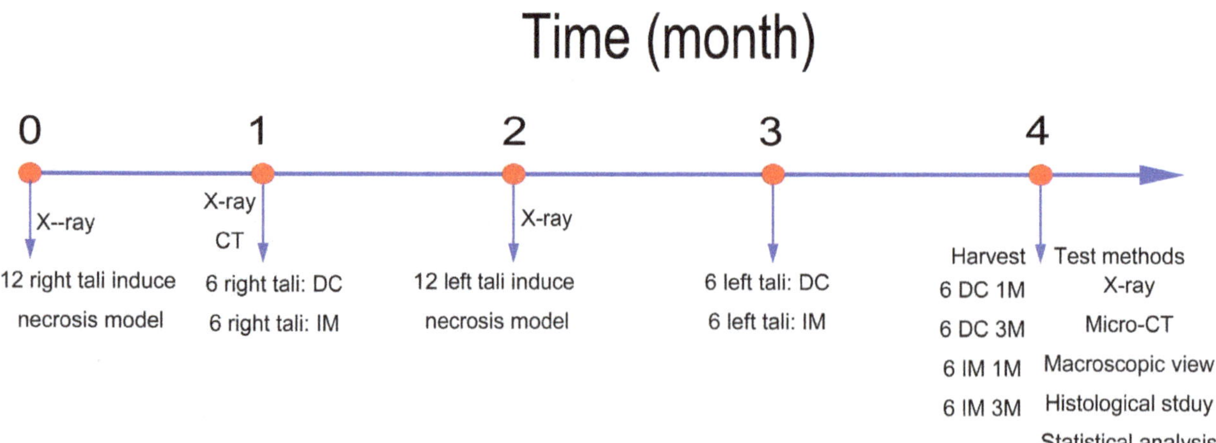

Figure 2. Schematic illustration of experimental design.

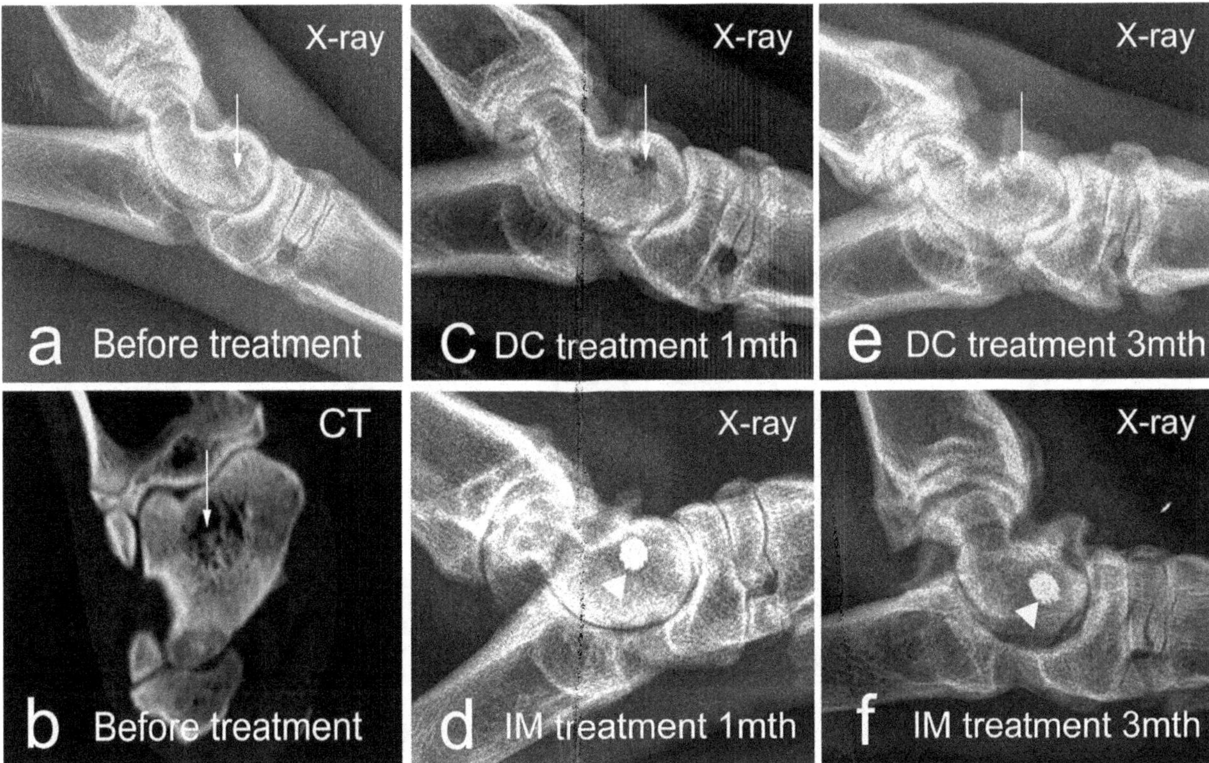

Figure 4. Histological examination of the DC and IM groups. The sections showed that the trabecular reconstruction was remarkable mainly in the IM group at 3 months after treatment, and the combination of the trabeculae and titanium alloy was very tight (Van Gieson stain, original magnification: left ×16; right ×100).

induced in the contralateral tali of the sheep by the same method; rods were implanted, and core decompression was executed on these tali at 1 month after ONT induction. Therefore, six samples with different time points of each kind of treatment were harvested after 4 months.

The testing methods included macroscopic, radiographic, micro-CT, CT, and histological examinations. X-ray photographs were taken at 1 month after inducing the necrotic model, and at 1 and 3 months after the therapeutic treatments. One living sheep was randomly chosen for CT analysis at 1 month after ONT induction for the examination of talus necrosis. Micro-CT (threshold: 500–1400 HU) was performed to observe the 3-D structure inside the bone, with four random samples being taken at 1 and 3 months after intervention. The region of interest (ROI) was chosen as a cylinder (φ4.3×5 mm^3) in the center of the core decompression drill track, which was considered to be the area with the most obvious bone necrosis.

Surgical procedures

All surgical procedures were performed under sterile conditions and followed our previous experiences [17]. The sheep were fasted for 24 hours before the surgery, placed under general anesthesia, and fixed on an operating table in a lateral position. After the skin was shaved and disinfected with iodine solution, a straight incision of about 4 cm was made at the medial ankle. The fascia was separated, and the joint capsule was cut open until the center of the talar head was exposed. A hole (1.2 mm in diameter, 15 mm in depth) was drilled at the center of the medial talar head. Three milliliters of pure ethanol (Fuyu Corporation, Tianjin, China) were instilled into the talar head through the hole at a flow rate of 0.8 mL/min. To prevent liquid reflux, the hole was blocked with bone wax immediately after injection. The wound was then washed and closed in layers.

One month later, therapeutic treatments were performed on the tali in the early stage of necrosis. Under general anesthesia, the center of the medial talar head was exposed as described above, and a hole of approximately 4 mm in diameter and 13 mm in depth was drilled. For the DC group, the debris of the necrotic bone tissue was mostly removed. For the IM group, porous titanium alloy rods were implanted into the hole after removal of the necrotic bone tissue.

Histological examinations

The talar heads of all samples were cut off and fixed in 10% formalin for 2 weeks. Four specimens of each group at each time point were randomly chosen and scanned by micro-CT. All of the specimens were dehydrated for about 20 days and then embedded with synthetic resin. The individual specimens were evenly divided into four parts crossing the drill track, such that three different sections could be observed by histology (Figure 3). The sections (labeled A, B, and C) were cut to 150 μm thick and, after careful sanding, were stained with Van Gieson.

To evaluate and compare the extent of bone reconstruction, a new histological appraisal system was developed. A round ROI that just covered the hole of core decompression was made in the pictures of the tissue slices with a minimum magnification (black circle, magnification: ×16, Figure 4). The average percentage of the trabeculae in this area was calculated.

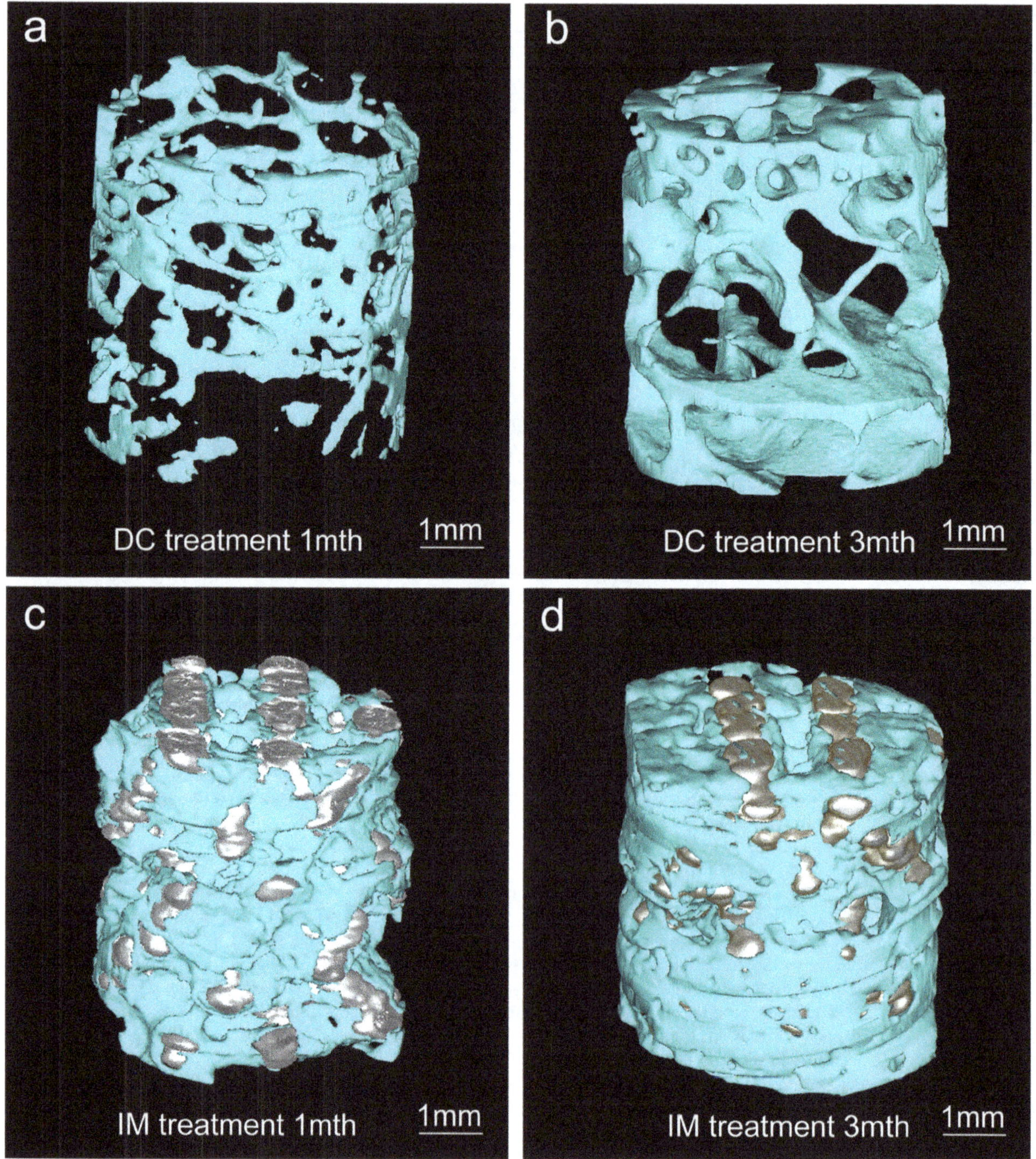

Figure 5. Lateral radiographic images of the ankle at different times. White arrowheads indicate osteolytic changes inside the talus, and white triangles indicate titanium rods.

Statistical analysis

Statistical analyses of samples at different time points (% of reconstructed trabeculae in the ROI) were performed by analysis of variance (ANOVA) with multiple comparisons. The SPSS 16.0 (International Business Machines Corporation, Armonk, New York, USA) program was used for all statistical analyses. Differences were considered significant at a value of $P<0.05$.

Results

The sheep showed good physical conditions after surgery, with complete wound healing by 1 week later, without any complications of infection or pathological bone fracture. The sheep implanted with titanium alloy rods (IM group) regained the normal walking condition, except for a slight degree of lameness in the operated leg in the first 2 weeks post-operatively. The sheep treated by core decompression (DC group) went lame, showing an unwillingness to load the operated leg throughout the whole study.

Table 2. Quantitative analysis of the parameters for reconstructed trabeculae, as calculated by micro-CT.

Time/Treatment	Trabeculae percentage	Trabeculae thickness (mm)	Trabeculae spacing (mm)
Month 1 DC	5%	0.08	1.59
Month 1 IM	20%	0.07	0.26
Month 3 DC	25%	0.18	0.52
Month 3 IM	37%	0.11	0.18

Macroscopic examination

At 1 month after the interventions (i.e., implantation of the titanium alloy rods and core decompression), the tali showed a normal appearance in all gross specimens. At 3 months after core decompression, tali in the DC group showed defects of about 5 mm×6 mm on the cartilage, and the stress-concentrated area of the talar heads had widely degenerated to an enlarged area (red triangle, Figure 1a). However, the tali of the IM group still maintained intact contours (Figure 1b).

X-ray and CT examination

At 1 month after the primary surgery to induce osteonecrosis, X-ray imaging showed an uneven radiographic density of the spongy bone tissue around the drill track, with the lowest density at the center of the talar head (white arrow head, Figure 5a). This finding was further confirmed by CT examination, which showed a necrotic core with a lower density (white arrow head, Figure 5b).

At 1 month after core decompression, the X-ray image of the DC group displayed an empty cavity (white arrow head, Figure 5c). At 3 months after intervention, this region was filled but possessed a lower X-ray density compared to the surrounding tissues (white arrow head, Figure 5e). By contrast, the IM group at 1 and 3 months post-intervention showed homogenous X-ray density of the surrounding bone tissue around the titanium alloy rod (white triangle, Figure 5d and f).

Micro-CT, which was used to discover the visual and 3-D structures of the reconstructed trabeculae, revealed that the quantity and quality of reconstructed trabeculae in the IM group were better than those of the DC group (Figure 6). These findings were further confirmed by a quantitative analysis of the quantity and scale of the reconstructed trabeculae, through the trabeculae percentage and the trabeculae thickness and spacing, respectively (Table 2).

Histological analysis

In the DC group, at 1 month after decompression treatment, the necrotic cavity was obvious, with little bone regeneration and moderate fibrous tissue infiltration (Figure 4a). At 3 months after treatment, the overall structure of the bone trabeculae inside the talus was loose and irregular, and was accompanied by more fibrous tissue (Figure 4b).

By contrast, the implantation of the titanium alloy rod (IM group) allowed much better bone regeneration. At 1 month post-treatment, we observed some fibrous tissue infiltration into the cavity area and a loose trabecular structure around the implanted titanium alloy rod. Nevertheless, bone tissue ingrowth was observed at the edge of the porous titanium alloy rod (blue triangle, Figure 4c), achieving tight integration of the titanium strut with the bone tissue. At 3 months after treatment, porous titanium alloy rod implantation led to robust bone regeneration in the cavity region, with copious bone tissue infiltration within the porous titanium alloy rod (blue triangle, Figure 4d) and the formation of a compact trabeculae structure of bone tissue surrounding the titanium implant. Almost no fibrous tissue was found inside the porous material.

Quantitative analysis

Using the new histological appraisal system and statistical approach, we determined the percentages of reconstructed trabeculae in the ROIs of the two groups (Table 3). In terms of bone tissue regeneration, there was no difference between the DC and IM groups at 1 month post-treatment ($P>0.05$). At 3 months post-treatment, the IM group showed 1.7 times better bone regeneration than the DC group ($P<0.05$).

Discussion

The clinicopathological symptoms of early-stage ONT include a continuous dull pain in the ankle region. The diagnosis may be further validated by magnetic resonance imaging. Late-stage ONT may lead to subchondral collapse of the talus, accompanied by pain and severe dysfunction of the ankle joint [19]. Therapeutic interventions at the early stage of ONT are recommended to prevent subchondral talar collapse, which otherwise may be treated by arthrodesis [2,3,20]. As an early therapeutic intervention strategy, biophosphonates treatment could be utilized, however, its efficacy may be controversial. For instance, Jureus et al. have reported an effectiveness ratio of 57% for the knee osteonecrosis treatment [21], while other studies showed that bisphosphonates treatments may further exacerbate the osteonecrosis through the potential side effect of anti-angiogenic [22].

Alternatively, surgical treatment could be utilized as well.

During the surgical treatment for osteonecrosis, the provision of additional mechanical support to prevent subchondral collapse is highly beneficial [23]. Moreover, Floerkemeier et al. recently suggested that bone reconstruction was possible if the subchondral collapse of the osteonecrotic femoral head had ceased at an early stage [15]. On the basis of these previous findings, we investigated the use of porous titanium alloy rods to treat ONT in a preclinical sheep model. We demonstrated that the porous titanium alloy rods not only provided strong mechanical support for the talus tissue but also worked as a scaffold matrix to promote bone regeneration in the necrotic region.

Several animal models have been established for the study of femoral head osteonecrosis. Methods to induce osteonecrosis include intraosseous injection of pure ethanol or cortical hormone, as well as intraosseous destructive treatment by microwave heating or using a cryogenic reagent (e.g., liquid nitrogen) [24–28]. Nevertheless, to date, no animal model for ONT has been developed before our research research work, which established a clinically relevant animal model to simulate ONT in humans [17]. Sheep were selected because of their similarity to humans in terms of anatomical structure and mechanical loading [29].

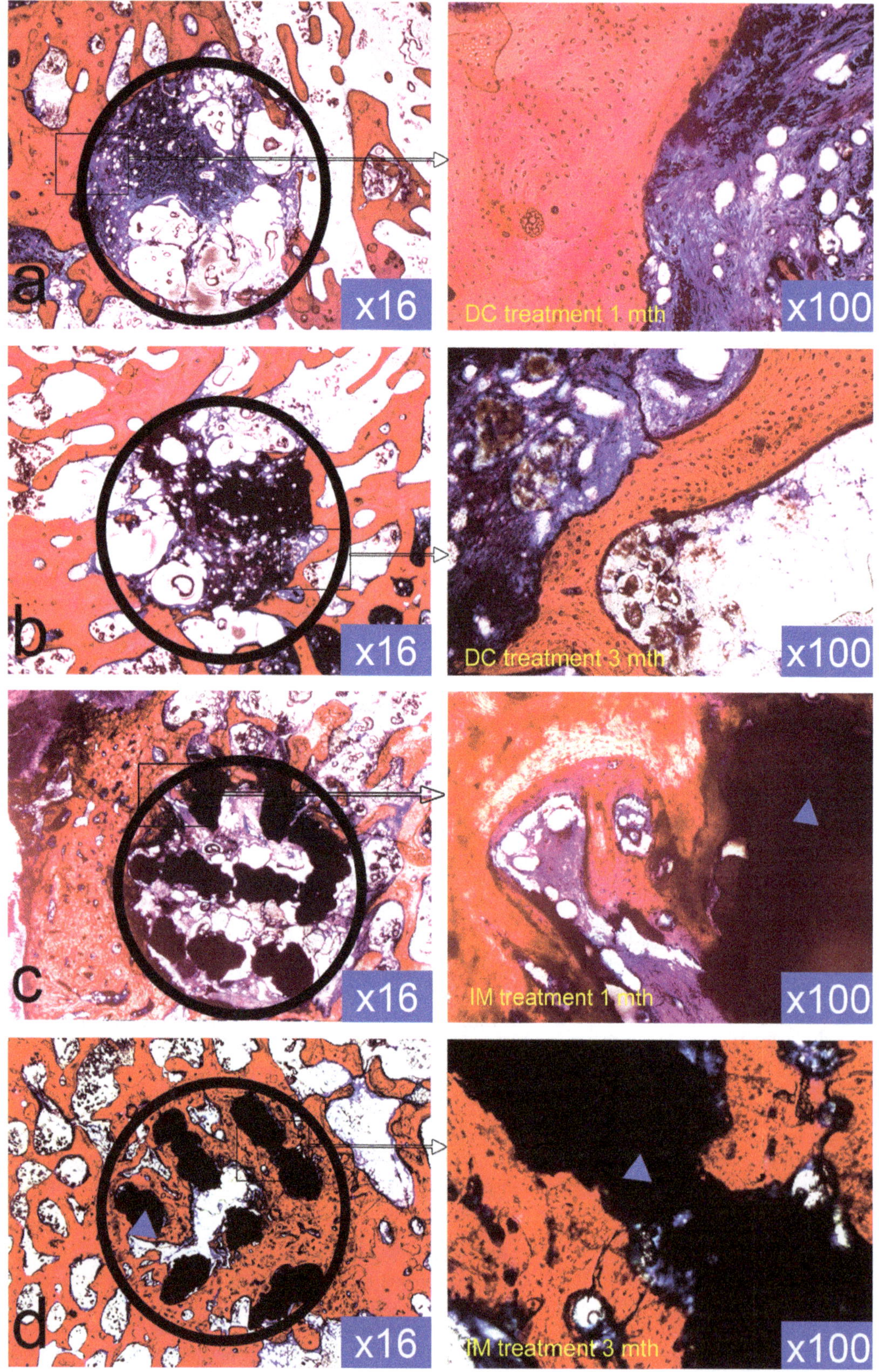

Figure 6. The 3-D reconstruction of talar specimens performed by micro-CT. Quantitative study showed that the trabecular reconstruction of the IM group was prior to that of the DC group at each time point.

Table 3. Percentages of reconstructed trabeculae in the ROIs of the two groups by histological study ($n=6$, x ± s).

Time	DC group	IM group	P
Month 1	0.058±0.015	0.078±0.020	0.482
Month 3	0.250±0.062	0.427±0.070	0.000

The ONT model established in our resent study imitated the pathological characteristics of human ONT in the following two aspects. First, the necrosis originated from the spongy bone area inside the talus and then gradually progressed to the region of cortical bone and cartilage. Second, the pathological progress of the induced ONT was necrobiotic, with obvious osteolytic appearance under radiographic examination at one month after induction [17]. This slower progression of necrosis is closer to the human ONT situation, compared to the rapid osteonecrosis induced by liquid nitrogen or microwave heating [25,28]. Finally, this model preserved the necessary conditions for the subsequent surgical treatment because it did not completely destroy the talar blood circulation.

Using this preclinical ONT model, our study demonstrated that the implantation of a porous titanium alloy rod (IM group) achieved a better therapeutic outcome than the traditional core decompression treatment (DC group), especially in terms of bone tissue regeneration and reconstruction. The trabeculae of bone tissue at the necrotic region was much better restored in the IM group, with larger volume and a thicker and more interconnected structure, as evidenced by micro-CT and histological studies (Tables 2 and 3). By contrast, the trabecular structure in the DC group exhibited many ruptures and irregularities, indicating inferior bone reconstruction. However, the specimen of micro-CT was random chose and the artifact of the metal might influence the result, so we thought the histological data would be more credible. Despite of these positive findings in the current research work, a longer period of study with 6–12 months follow-up investigation may provide a better understanding of the long-term efficacy of this therapeutic strategy.

There are several possible explanations for the observed beneficial therapeutic effects of porous titanium alloy rod implantation. The porous titanium alloy rod provides sufficiently firm mechanical support for the surrounding bone tissue after implantation, which is able to maintain the integrity of the trabecular structure and reduce direct loading on the necrotic bone tissue, favoring bone tissue regeneration [30]. Due to the high elastic modulus of the Ti_6Al_4V material, the titanium alloy rod was fabricated in a porous structure with a porosity of 70%. As a result, the stress shield effect of the titanium alloy rod was greatly depressed [17]. The elastic moduli of the porous titanium alloy rod and trabecular bone were similar, which may enable long-term stability between these structures [31] and ensure the long-term therapeutic utility of this approach.

Moreover, titanium alloy is well known for its long-term in vivo biocompatibility [32]. The implanted porous titanium alloy rod may work as a scaffold matrix, thereby providing the framework with struts for osteogenic cell adhesion, proliferation, and extracellular matrix deposition, and promoting better and faster ingrowth of bone tissue in the necrotic region than the simple core decompression treatment in the DC group. This explanation was evidenced by the histological study, which showed the initial integration of bone tissue with the titanium alloy strut at 1 month, and the rapid infiltration of bone tissue at 3 months post-transplantation (Fig. 4).

In this study, EBM technology was used to fabricate the titanium implant with a precisely controlled porous structure for ONT treatment. EBM technology is widely used in the manufacturing of metal materials with intricate inner or surface structures, and could be used to produce any needed implant to replace a bone defect in orthopedics. As a rapid prototyping technique, EBM technology has many advantages compared to traditional sintering and laser beam fusion techniques, including: (1) its ability to prepare complex and irregular components; (2) its excellent repeatability, due to the use of a computer-controlled process; (3) its ability to manufacture products directly using raw material powder, which could be a high-strength and high-melting metal such as titanium alloy; and (4) its reduced consumption of time and energy [17,33–36]. Therefore, it is both feasible and convenient to produce titanium alloy implants by EBM technology.

Conclusion

The porous titanium alloy rods fabricated by EBM technology possess good characteristics in terms of mechanical properties and biocompatibility, and they show obvious advantages when used to treat early-stage ONT. Although the long-term therapeutic effects need to be tested further, the curative effects of the porous titanium alloy rods appear to arise from their role as a firm scaffold, and their provision of decompression.

Acknowledgments

The authors acknowledge the technical help of Mr. Rong Lv at the Orthopedic Research Laboratory of Xijing Hospital.

Author Contributions

Conceived and designed the experiments: XKL CFY JLW ZG. Performed the experiments: XKL CFY JLW YQZ ZYZ. Analyzed the data: XKL CFY JLW ZG. Contributed reagents/materials/analysis tools: XKL CFY JLW YQZ ZG. Wrote the paper: XKL CFY JLW ZYZ ZG.

References

1. Saini A, Saifuddin A (2004) MRI of osteonecrosis. Clinical Radiology 59:1079–1093.
2. Assouline-Dayan Y, Chang C, Greenspan A, Shoenfeld Y, Gershwin ME (2002) Pathogenesis and natural history of osteonecrosis. Semin Arthritis Rheum 32: 94–124.
3. Delanois RE, Mont MA, Yoon TR, Mizell M, Hungerford DS (1998) Atraumatic osteonecrosis of the talus. J Bone Joint Surg Am 80:529–536.
4. Mont MA, Schon LC, Hungerford MW, Hungerford DS (1996) Avascular necrosis of the talus treated by core decompression. J Bone Joint Surg Br 78: 827–830.
5. Guest M, Binfield PM, O'Doherty D (1999) Core decompression of steroid induced avascular necrosis of the talus. The Foot 9: 44–46.
6. Grice J, Cannon L (2011) Percutaneous core decompression: A successful method of treatment of Stage I avascular necrosis of the talus. Foot Ankle Surg 17: 317–318.
7. Marulanda GA, McGrath MS, Ulrich SD, Seyler TM, Delanois RE, et al. (2010) Percutaneous drilling for the treatment of atraumatic osteonecrosis of the ankle. J Foot Ankle Surg 49: 20–24.
8. Norimatsu H, Mori S, Kawanishi J, Kaji Y, Li J (1997) Immobilization as the pathogenesis of osteoporosis: experimental and clinical studies. Osteoporos Int 7 Suppl 3: S57–62.
9. Rieger UM, Haug M, Schwarzl F, Kalbermatten DF, Hintermann B, et al. (2009) Free microvascular iliac crest flap for extensive talar necrosis–case report with a 16-year long-term follow up. Microsurgery 29: 667–671.

10. Yu XG, Zhao DW, Sun Q, Wang TN, Yu HB, et al. (2010) Treatment of non-traumatic avascular talar necrosis by transposition of vascularized cuneiform bone flap plus iliac cancellous bone grafting. Zhonghua Yi Xue Za Zhi 90: 1035–1038.
11. Hasegawa Y, Iwata H, Torii S, Iwase T, Kawamoto K, et al. (1997) Vascularized pedicle bone-grafting for nontraumatic avascular necrosis of the femoral head: A 5- to 11-year follow-up. Arch Orthop Trauma Surg 116: 251–258.
12. Shuler MS, Rooks MD, Roberson JR (2007) Porous tantalum implant in early osteonecrosis of the hip: preliminary report on operative, survival, and outcomes results. J Arthroplasty 22: 26–31.
13. Nadeau M, Séguin C, Theodoropoulos JS (2007) Short term clinical outcome of a porous tantalum implant for the treatment of advanced osteonecrosis of the femoral head. Mcgill J Med 10: 4–10.
14. Veillette CJ, Mehdian H, Schemitsch EH, McKee MD (2006) Survivorship analysis and radiographic outcome following tantalum rod insertion for osteonecrosis of the femoral head. J Bone Joint Surg Am 88 Suppl 3: 48–55.
15. Floerkemeier T, Thorey F, Daentzer D, Lerch M, Klaqes P, et al. (2011) Clinical and radiological outcome of the treatment of osteonecrosis of the femoral head using the osteonecrosis intervention implant. Int Orthop 35: 489–495.
16. Tanzer M, Bobyn JD, Krygier JJ, Karabasz D (2008) Histopathologic retrieval analysis of clinically failed porous tantalum osteonecrosis implants. J Bone Joint Surg Am 90: 1282–1289.
17. Yuan CF, Wang JL, Li XK, Zhang YQ, Zhang ZY, et al. (2012) Development of a Clinically Relevant Animal Model for The Talar Osteonecrosis in Sheep. Int J Med Sci 9: 816–824.
18. Parthasarathy J, Starly B, Raman S, Christensen A (2010) Mechanical evaluation of porous titanium (Ti6Al4V) structures with electron beam melting (EBM). J Mech Behav Biomed Mater 3: 249–259.
19. Pearce DH, Mongiardi CN, Fornasier VL, Daniels TR (2005) Avascular necrosis of the talus: a pictorial essay. Radiographics 25: 399–410.
20. Kitaoka HB and Patzer GL (1998) Arthrodesis for the treatment of arthrosis of the ankle and osteonecrosis of the talus. J Bone Joint Surg Am 80: 370–379.
21. Jureus J, Lindstrand A, Geijer M, Roberts D, Tägil M. (2012) Treatment of spontaneous osteonecrosis of the knee (SPONK) by a bisphosphonate. Acta Orthop 83: 511–514.
22. Petcu EB, Ivanovski S, Wright RG, Slevin M, Miroiu RI, et al. (2012) Bisphosphonate-related osteonecrosis of jaw (BRONJ): an anti-angiogenic side-effect? Diagn Pathol 7: 78.
23. Kim SY, Kim YG, Kim PT, Ihn JC, Cho BC, et al. (2012) Vascularized compared with nonvascularized fibular grafts for large osteonecrotic lesions of the femoral head. J Bone Joint Surg Am 87: 2012–2018.
24. Zhang P, Liang Y, Kim H, Yokota H (2010) Evaluation of a pig femoral head osteonecrosis model. J Orthop Surg Res 5: 15–21.
25. Li YL, Han R, Geng CK, Wang Y, Wei L (2009) A new osteonecrosis animal model of the femoral head induced by microwave heating and repaired with tissue engineered bone. Int Orthop 33: 573–580.
26. Manggold J, Sergi C, Becker K, Lukoschek M, Simank HG (2002) A new animal model of femoral head necrosis induced by intraosseous injection of ethanol. Lab Anim 36: 173–180.
27. Bekler H, Uygur AM, Gökçe A, Beyzadeoğlu T (2007) The effect of steroid use on the pathogenesis of avascular necrosis of the femoral head: an animal model. Acta Orthop Traumatol Turc 41: 58–63.
28. Vélez R, Soldado F, Hernández A, Barber I, Aguirre M (2011) A new preclinical femoral head osteonecrosis model in sheep. Arch Orthop Trauma Surg 131: 5–9.
29. Wan L, de Asla RJ, Rubash HE, Li G (2006) Determination of in-vivo articular cartilage contact areas of human talocrural joint under weightbearing conditions. Osteoarthritis Cartilage 14: 1294–1301.
30. Bertollo N, Da Assuncao R, Hancock NJ, Lau A, Walsh WR (2012) Influence of Electron Beam Melting Manufactured Implants on Ingrowth and Shear Strength in an Ovine Model. J Arthroplasty [Epub ahead of print]
31. Palmquist A, Snis A, Emanuelsson L, Browne M, Thomsen P (2011) Long-term biocompatibility and osseointegration of electron beam melted, free-form-fabricated solid and porous titanium alloy: Experimental studies in sheep. J Biomater Appl [Epub ahead of print]
32. Rack HJ and Qazi JI (2006) Titanium alloys for biomedical applications. Materials Science and Engineering: C 26: 1269–1277.
33. Bagaria V, Deshpande S, Rasalkar DD, Kuthe A, Paunipagar BK (2011) Use of rapid prototyping and three-dimensional reconstruction modeling in the management of complex fractures. Eur J Radiol 80: 814–820.
34. Comesaña R, Lusquiños F, Del Val J, López-Álvarez M, Quintero F, et al. (2011) Three-dimensional bioactive glass implants fabricated by rapid prototyping based on CO(2) laser cladding. Acta Biomater 7: 3476–3487.
35. Murr LE, Amato KN, Li SJ, Tian YX, Cheng XY, et al. (2011) Microstructure and mechanical properties of open-cellular biomaterials prototypes for total knee replacement implants fabricated by electron beam melting. J Mech Behav Biomed Mater 4: 1396–1411.
36. Heinl P, Müller L, Körner C, Singer RF, Müller FA (2008) Cellular Ti-6Al-4V structures with interconnected macro porosity for bone implants fabricated by selective electron beam melting. Acta Biomater 4: 1536–1544.

10

Coating with a Modular Bone Morphogenetic Peptide Promotes Healing of a Bone-Implant Gap in an Ovine Model

Yan Lu[1,4]*, Jae Sung Lee[2], Brett Nemke[1], Ben K. Graf[4], Kevin Royalty[2], Richard Illgen III[4], Ray Vanderby Jr.[2], Mark D. Markel[1,4], William L. Murphy[2,3,4]*

1 Comparative Orthopaedic Research Laboratory, School of Veterinary Medicine, University of Wisconsin-Madison, Madison, Wisconson, United States of America, **2** Departments of Biomedical Engineering, University of Wisconsin, Madison, Wisconson, United States of America, **3** Pharmacology, University of Wisconsin, Madison, Wisconson, United States of America, **4** Orthopedics and Rehabilitation, University of Wisconsin, Madison, Wisconson, United States of America

Abstract

Despite the potential for growth factor delivery strategies to promote orthopedic implant healing, there is a need for growth factor delivery methods that are controllable and amenable to clinical translation. We have developed a modular bone growth factor, herein termed "modular bone morphogenetic peptide (mBMP)", which was designed to efficiently bind to the surface of orthopedic implants and also stimulate new bone formation. The purpose of this study was to coat a hydroxyapatite-titanium implant with mBMP and evaluate bone healing across a bone-implant gap in the sheep femoral condyle. The mBMP molecules efficiently bound to a hydroxyapatite-titanium implant and 64% of the initially bound mBMP molecules were released in a sustained manner over 28 days. The results demonstrated that the mBMP-coated implant group had significantly more mineralized bone filling in the implant-bone gap than the control group in C-arm computed tomography (DynaCT) scanning (25% more), histological (35% more) and microradiographic images (50% more). Push-out stiffness of the mBMP group was nearly 40% greater than that of control group whereas peak force did not show a significant difference. The results of this study demonstrated that mBMP coated on a hydroxyapatite-titanium implant stimulates new bone formation and may be useful to improve implant fixation in total joint arthroplasty applications.

Editor: Kent Leach, University of California Davis, United States of America

Funding: This study was funded by the Wallace H. Coulter Foundation and by the Wisconsin Alumni Research Foundation: "A Translational Research Partnership Grant from the Wallace H. Coulter Foundation" and "A Technology Accelerator Grant from the Wisconsin Alumni Research Foundation". There is no grant number from either. Smith & Nephew, Inc., provided implants for this study. The funders had no role in study design, data collection and analysis, decision to publish, or preparation of the manuscript.

Competing Interests: Smith&Nephew, Inc., provided titanium implants for this study. There are no further patents, products in development or marketed products to declare.

* E-mail: luy@svm.vetmed.wisc.edu (YL); wlmurphy@wisc.edu (WLM)

Introduction

Total joint replacement surgeries have been performed popularly because these surgeries can successfully relieve pain and improve functional outcomes. However, the failure rate of revision joint replacements is also dramatically higher than primary replacements due primarily to a challenging environment for new bone formation [1]. Therefore, there is a need to develop novel biomaterials to increase replacement success rate and reduce revision rate, and to promote successful bone healing after revision surgery. Besides improving surgery techniques [2], the key factor for successfully improving implant-bone healing in joint replacement is the ability to encourage new bone formation at the implant-native bone interface [3]. Therefore, several groups have begun to explore the use of pro-osteogenic growth factors to induce new bone formation on implant surfaces. For example, Sachse et al recently reported that the recombinant protein bone morphogenetic protein-2 (BMP-2) may foster bone healing on a titanium surface in a sheep model [4]. Further, Lamberg et al stated that transforming growth factor-β1 (TGF-β1) and insulin-like growth factor-1 (IGF-1) enhanced the mechanical fixation and osseointegration of titanium implants in cancellous bone in a dog model [5].

Collectively, previous studies demonstrate the potential for growth factor delivery strategies to promote orthopedic implant healing. However, translation of growth factor delivery to clinical applications is plagued by significant challenges [6]. First, growth factor delivery strategies typically do not use carriers with optimal physical properties. The common strategy instead involves designing a growth factor "carrier", then combining it with a standard orthopedic device with appropriate physical properties. Notable examples include recombinant protein-loaded collagen carriers combined with titanium cages [7,8] or other metallic hardware [9]. Innovative biomaterials for controlled growth factor release [10], ranging from polymer scaffolds to injectable micro- and nano-particles, also typically require combination with a structural device. In addition, existing growth factor carriers contain supraphysiologic doses delivered over relatively short timescales, which has recently led to well-documented side effects including edema [11,12], heterotopic bone formation [13], retrograde ejaculation [14], and potentially increased cancer risk [15].

Bone morphogenetic proteins (BMPs) are the key cytokines in bone formation and repair. A possible strategy to utilize BMPs' activity in clinical applications is to enhance the activity of autologous BMPs. BMP-2 incorporated into biomimetic calcium phosphate coatings has been demonstrated to be capable of inducing bone formation at an ectopic site and sustaining osteogenic activity for a considerable period of time [16,17].

We hypothesized that a modular bone morphogenetic peptide (mBMP) could be used to "dip-coat" the surface of an orthopedic implant, which in turn would be capable of promoting implant-native bone healing. Specifically, we synthesized a peptide with two functional units: i) an osteocalcin-inspired hydroxyapatite (HAP)-binding sequence; and ii) a peptide sequence previously shown to mimic some of the pro-osteogenic properties of the protein BMP-2 [18,19]. We then would perform experiments to determine whether this peptide could "dip-coat" the surface of an orthopedic implant and, in turn, promote bone healing across a well-defined bone gap in a sheep model. The bone-implant gap in the current study was designed into the implant to more effectively mimic the challenging environment that is typically present during revision joint arthroplasty. We hypothesized that an HAP-titanium implant dip-coated with mBMP inserted in cancellous bone would result in improved mechanical implant fixation and induce more bone ingrowth across the defined gap zone.

Materials and Methods

HAP-titanium Implants

Custom implants (diameter: 8 mm, HAP coated length: 14 mm. Smith and Nephew Corp. Andover, MA) were "porous coated", meaning that they incorporate a porous titanium surface that is plasma spray bound with hydroxyapatite. In addition, the implants were designed to include a 1 mm gap all around the perimeter of the cylindrical implants, so that there was a well-defined gap between the native bone and the implant surface (Fig. 1).

Peptide Binding and Release from HAP-titanium Implant

Modular bone morphogenetic peptide (Amino acid sequence of mBMP; KIPKASSVPTELSAISTLYLAAAAγEPRRγEVAγEL) was synthesized using standard Fmoc solid phase peptide synthesis, as reported previously [20,21]. Carboxyfluorescein (Molecular Probes Inc., Eugene, OR) was used to label mBMP to monitor its release from the implants into simulated body fluid (SBF; 136.8 mM NaCl, 3 mM KCl, 0.5 mM Na_2SO_4, 1.5 mM $MgCl_2$, 4.2 mM $NaHCO_3$, 2.5 mM $CaCl_2$, 1.0 mM K_2HPO_4, 50 mM Tris base). First, fluorescently labeled mBMP was bound on implants by incubating each implant in peptide solution (4 mL, 1.9 mM) for 4 hours at 37°C. The mBMP-bound implant was then incubated in 3 mL of SBF solution at 37°C in a static condition to examine the release behavior of peptide. At each time point (day 1, 2, 3, 6, 9, 13, 18, 22 and 28), the fluorescence intensity of release medium was measured and the release medium was replaced with a fresh one. After 4-week release, the mBMP remaining on implant was retrieved by incubating in 0.5 N hydrochloric acid solution overnight. The amount of mBMP was quantified using microBCA (Thermo Fisher Scientific Inc., Rockford, IL) after neutralizing with sodium hydroxide solution, and the amount of initial binding was calculated by adding to that of released peptide.

mBMP Coating of Implants for in vivo Studies

Each experimental HAP-titanium implant was incubated in 4 mL of mBMP solution (1.9 mM) 4 hours at 37°C. The mBMP solution was sterilized by passage through sterile 0.22 μm filters. All incubation procedures were performed in aseptic conditions.

In vivo Experimental Design

Twelve mature female sheep, ranging in age from 3.5 to 5 years and weighing between 70 to 110 kg (82.4±5.6 kg: mean±SD) were utilized in the study. All experimental protocols were approved by the Institutional Animal Use and Care Committee of University of Wisconsin-Madison.

In each of the 12 sheep, one of the stifles was randomized (block design) to receive an mBMP-coated HAP-titanium implant and the other (contralateral) received an un-treated implant (n = 12/ treatment). The sheep were euthanized at 4 weeks after surgery. 8 sheep (16 stifles, 8/group) were subjected to C-arm computed tomography (DynaCT) and biomechanical testing, 4 sheep (8 stifles, 4/group) were used for histologic analysis.

Surgical Procedure

Surgery was carried out under general anesthesia with isoflurane and oxygen inhalation via endotracheal intubation. Procaine Penicillin G (5 mls) was administered via muscle pre-operatively and an additional dose (5 mls) post-operatively. An 8 cm medial incision was made along the anterior edge of medial collateral ligament in one randomly selected stifle. The medial portion of medial condyle was exposed. An 8 mm diameter hole (14 mm deep) was drilled from the medial surface of the condyle near to collateral ligament origin by an 8 mm cannulated drill bit 5 mm proximal to the joint line taking care to avoid the joint. An mBMP-coated HAP-titanium implant was inserted in the hole (Fig. 1). Then the surrounding soft tissue was sutured and the implant was covered. In the contralateral stifle, the identical procedure of exposure was performed with the un-treated implant in the medial condyle. The incision was lavaged by sterile saline. The deep fascia, subcutaneous tissue and skin incision were closed as routine.

After 4 weeks, all sheep were euthanized for biomechanical, DynaCT and histological analyses.

Dyna CT Scan

At the same day of sacrifice, the medial femoral condyles were cut into uniform bone blocks ($3.0\times3.0\times2.0$ cm^3) and imaged using a Siemens Artis Zeego (Siemens Healthcare, Erlangen, Germany) C-arm computed tomography (DynaCT), which has a wide angle cone-beam x-ray tube and 40 cm × 30 cm flat-panel detector integrated with a robotic C-arm gantry. The acquisition parameters for DynaCT were as follows: 86 kV tube voltage, automatic tube current ranging from 70 to 125 mA, a 20 s rotation time (total of 496 projections over 200 degree sweep angle). The projection images were acquired in a 2 × 2 binning mode, providing a 154 μm detector element resolution. Acquired images were then transferred to a dedicated post-processing workstation (*syngo* X-Workplace, Siemens Healthcare, Erlangen, Germany) where a volume data set was reconstructed to a 512×512 matrix and 306–328 slices with an isotropic voxel size of 140 μm using a sharp bone kernel for visualization of the bony structure.

The Dyna CT image of each specimen was analyzed with Image J software (National Institutes of Health, Bethesda, MA). The area of bone ingrowth in the gap between the implant and hosting bone was calculated and compared between mBMP-coated and control groups.

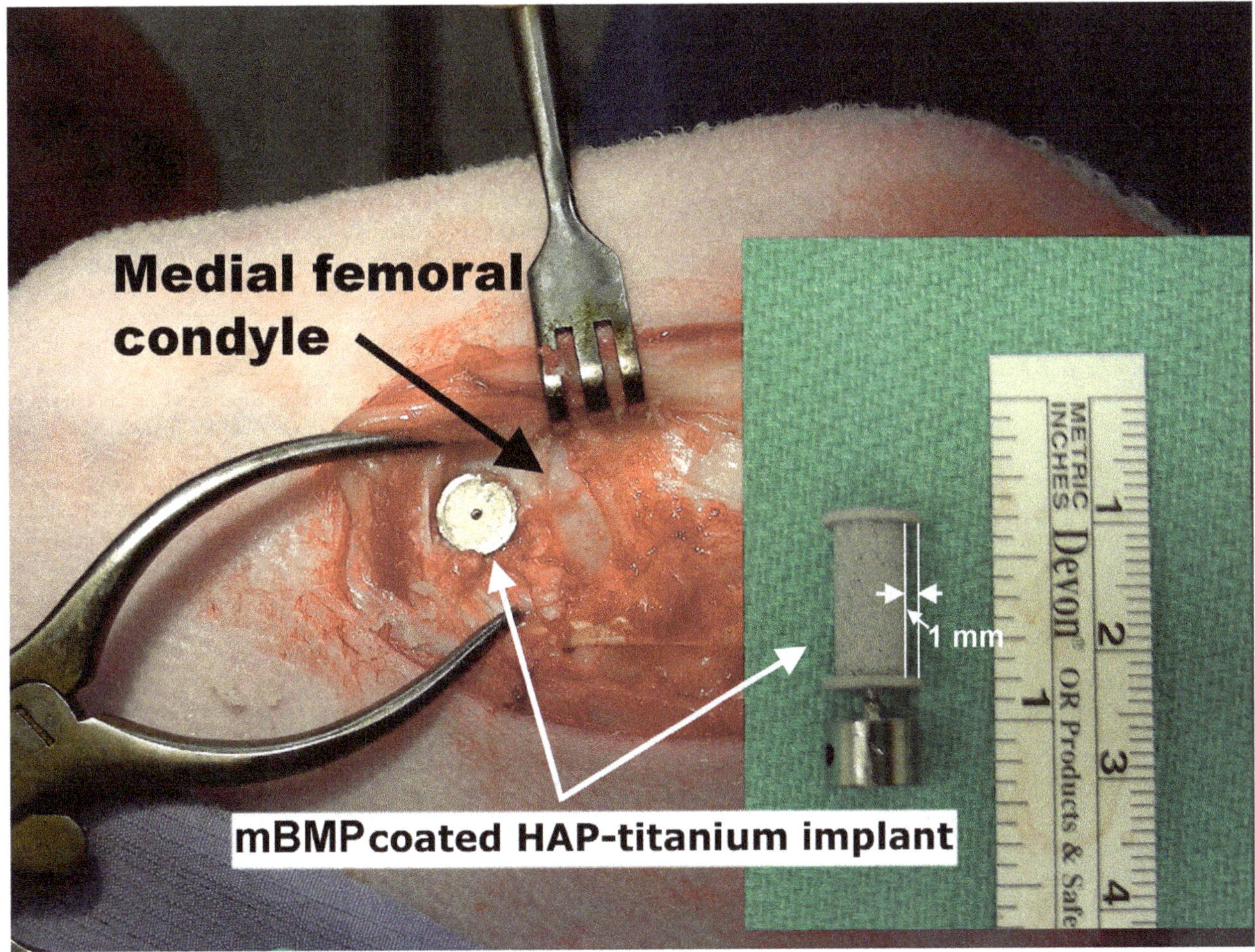

Figure 1. Image of mBMP coated HAP-titanium implant and surgical implantation in sheep medial femoral condyle.

Biomechanical Testing

After DynaCT scan, the femoral condylar bone blocks were used for push out mechanical testing. The specimen was placed in a MTS 858 BIONIX Test System (MTS Systems Corp., Eden Prairie, MN) with a 1500 lb load cell. The titanium implant in the specimen was precisely aligned with a pushing shaft. A linear extensometer was attached to measure the displacement of the implant. The displacement rate was 5.0 mm/min as previously described [22]. A 50 N preload was applied. Peak force at failure (N) and stiffness (N/mm) were measured and recorded. Peak force was determined from the load-displacement curve. Stiffness was calculated by measuring the slope from the linear portion of the curve.

Histological Analysis

The remaining 8 condyles in 4 sheep were used for histological analysis. The specimens were fixed in neutral buffered 10% formalin for 1 week. The medial condyle was sectioned sagitally into 3 equal sections crossing the implant axis. The undecalcified specimens were embedded in polymethylmethacrylate (PMMA), sectioned (100 μm) and stained with Goldner's Trichrome for the evaluation of implant to bone healing. The sections from each specimen were examined by three senior researchers blinded to group assignments. Fine detail contact microradiography (Hewlett-Packard Faxitron, McMinnville, OR. USA) combined with vacuum technique was also performed on 3 sections of each specimen as previously described. [23] The 3 sections were defined as "outer" (near to cortex), "middle", and "inner" (farther to cortex). Bone density in the implant-bone gap region of each 3 section levels and total bone density of 3 sections [(sum of bone-occupied area of "inner", "middle" and "outer" groups)/(sum of area of interest of "inner", "middle" and "outer" groups)*100] were quantified using Image J software for both histological and microradiographical images.

Statistical Analysis

The Shapiro-Wilk Test was first used to determine the normal distribution (Gaussian distribution) of histological, microradiographic, DynaCT and mechanical testing data sets. If the data sets were normally distributed, the Student's Paired t-test was used for statistical analysis for histology, microradiography, DynaCT and mechanical testing data between the two treatment groups. If the data sets were detected to be not normally distributed, the Mann-whitney U test was used to compare these differences. Differences were considered to be significant at a probability level of 95% ($p<0.05$). All statistical analyses were performed with a commercially available software program (SAS Version 8e, SAS Institute Inc., Cary, NC).

Results

In Vitro

The amount of mBMP initially bound to a HAP-titanium implant was 414.4±22.8 µg. The release profile of mBMP in SBF showed large initial release 51.1±2.9% of initially bound mBMP during first two days (Fig. 2A). Afterwards, the mBMP was released in a nearly linear fashion for 4 weeks with total release of 263.1±20.7 µg (63.4±1.8% of initially bound mBMP). As evidenced in Figure 2B, a significant amount of mBMP molecules still resides on HAP-implant surface after 28-day release.

In Vivo

No postoperative complications were seen and all sheep were fully weight-bearing at the same day after surgery. No signs of infection were observed at the time of euthanasia.

CT Results

DynaCT analysis demonstrated that the mBMP-treated group (4.7±2.0 mm^2) had a significantly higher density of mineralized bone tissue filling the 1 millimeter bone-implant gap than the control group (3.7±2.0 mm^2) ($p<0.05$) (Fig. 3).

Histological Results

Microradiographical data analyses showed the mBMP-coated HAP-titanium implants had significantly greater area of higher bone density in the bone-implant gaps compared to the controls ($p<0.05$) (Fig. 4). This increased bone formation was observed throughout the bone-implant interface - at outer, middle, and inner section levels. Microradiographical images also demonstrated that the control group had significantly less new bone formation in the bone-implant gap than the mBMP-coated implant group (Fig. 5 A and B). Histological analysis further demonstrated significantly greater new bone formation in the bone-implant gap in the mBMP-coated implant conditions (Fig. 5 C and D). Specifically, calculation of new bone formation in Goldner's trichrome stained images demonstrated a significant increase in new bone formation in the middle section and in the inner/middle/outer section levels combined for mBMP coated implants when compared to controls ($p<0.05$) (Fig. 6).

Mechanical Testing Results

The results of mechanical push-out testing demonstrated that the stiffness of the mBMP-treated group (2157±651.9 N/mm) was significantly greater than that of control group (1545±480.5 N/mm) ($p<0.05$), whereas there was no significant difference in peak force between the mBMP-treated group (1022±371.4 N) and the control group (682.2±269.3 N) groups ($p>0.05$).

Discussion

The mBMP peptides were efficiently bound to a HAP-titanium implant and released over 28 days in simulated body fluid. *In vivo* results of this study demonstrated that mBMP-coated HAP-titanium implant increased implant fixation and stimulated bone formation in the gap between implant and surrounding host cancellous bone after 4 weeks post-surgery compared to the control.

mBMP release kinetics showed a substantial initial release of over 50% during the initial 2 days, followed by minimal release kinetics over more than 28 days. These distinct regimes of mBMP release can be attributed to an initial release of poorly bound peptide due to surface saturation, followed by slower release of mBMP that was strongly bound to the hydroxyapatite surface. In particular, the solution concentration used for mBMP binding here (1.9 mM) was much higher than the concentration previously shown to saturate binding to a hydroxyapatite surface [20,24], which likely explains the rapid initial release kinetics. The minimal mBMP release after the first two days is indicative of the high mBMP-implant binding affinity, as demonstrated previously [20]. The observation that nearly 40% of the initially bound mBMP remained on the implant surface after 4 week incubation is potentially interesting in the context of contemporary growth factor delivery strategies. Rapid and poorly-localized bone growth factor delivery can lead to significant clinical side effects, as demonstrated by recent clinical analyses of BMP-2-releasing implants [13,14,25]. Although further studies will be needed to demonstrate control over mBMP dosage on the implant surface, our previous studies have demonstrated that mBMP dosage can be controlled by simply varying the mBMP concentration in solution during implant dip-coating [20,21,24].

Sheep were selected for this study because they provide similar bone density and weight to humans, and they have been widely used for evaluation implant-bone healing in previous studies [4,26–29]. The sheep femoral condyle was particularly used as a model in this study because it is rich in high quality cancellous bone with ample blood supply, which is suitable for an evaluation of early implant bone healing [22]. In addition, it is also

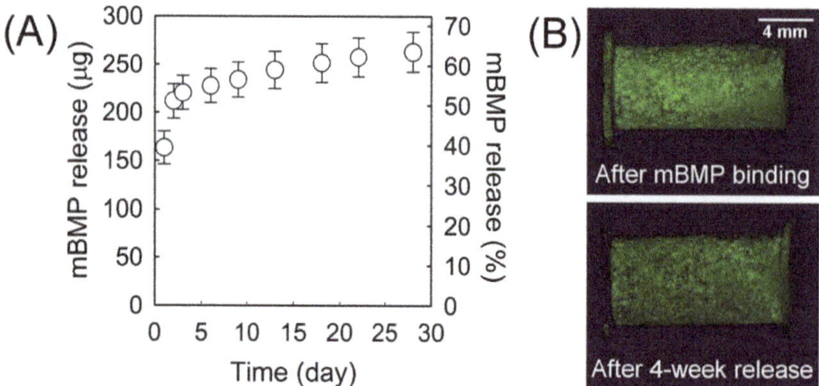

Figure 2. Images of release profile of mBMP in vitro. (A) Cumulative release of mBMP from HAP-titanium implant in SBF is over 60% at 4 weeks. (B) Fluorescent images of an implant after incorporation with fluorescently labeled mBMP (top) and after 4-week incubation in simulated body fluid (SBF) (bottom).

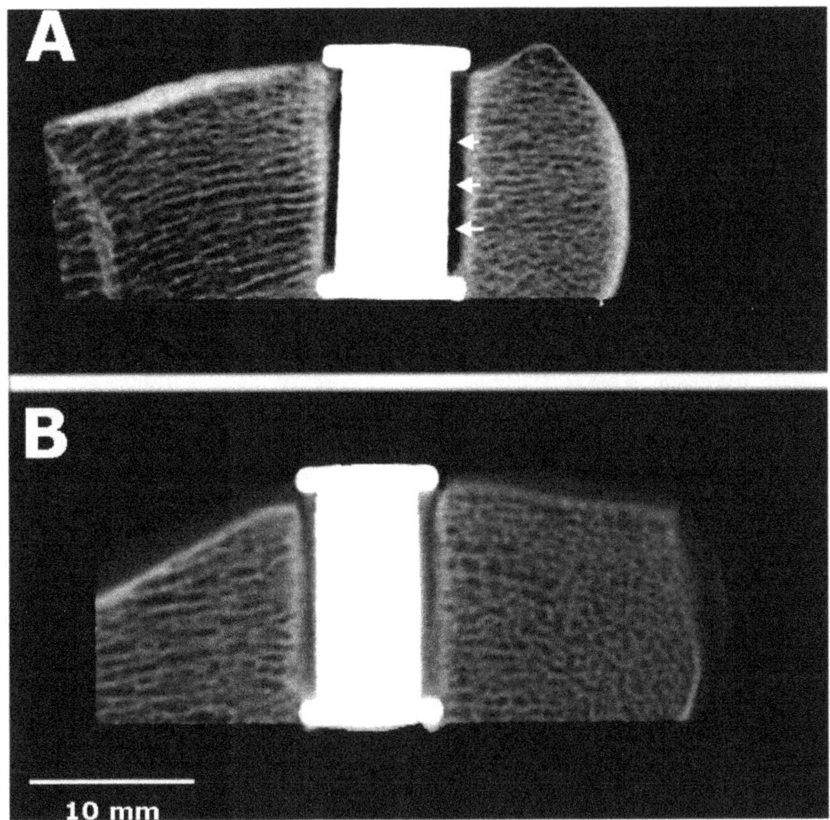

Figure 3. Images of Dyna CT results between control and mBMP coated implants. A: Control, DynaCT demonstrating that gap between the implant and host bone was still visible (white arrows). B: The gap between mBMP coated HAP-implant and host bone was filled with high density mineralized tissue.

representative of the bony fixation regions, such as proximal femoral prostheses in humans. The gap size (1.0 mm) selected for this study was defined as critical size under non-loading condition based on a previous study [22]. The sacrifice time at 4 weeks post-surgery was selected for monitoring early stage of bone ingrowth in the gap between the titanium implant and host bone. Several previous studies have used the same time point to evaluate bone ingrowth in bone-implant gaps in animal models [22,30,31].

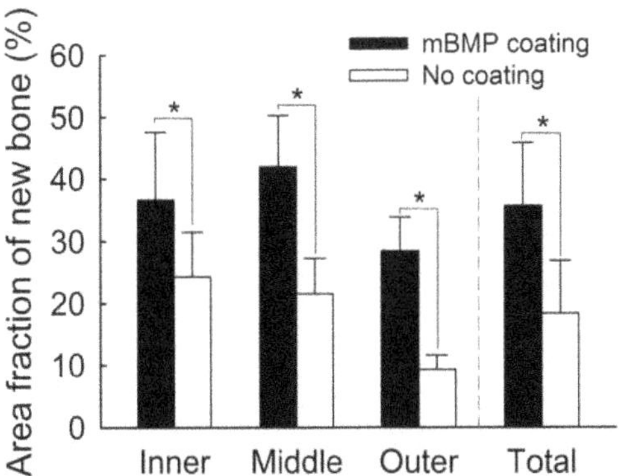

Figure 4. Microradiographic calculation of new bone formation in the gap demonstrating mBMP group had significantly more new bone ingrowth than non-mBMP group at 3 levels of the implant and in total amount. "*" means significant difference between treatments ($p<0.05$).

DynaCT, histological and microradiographical results of this study demonstrated that significantly higher density tissue and new bone formation was present in the gap between mBMP-coated HAP-titanium implant and condylar bone compared to control. An interesting observation here was that endochondral ossification with the formation of cartilaginous tissues was not observed at 4 weeks post-surgery. Instead, it appeared that direct ossification of mesenchymal tissue as intramembraneous ossification was taking place, as reported in a previous study [4].

New bone formation in the gap between the implant and native host bone can also increase rigidity and fixation of an implant, which has been validated in the current study. The push-out stiffness of mBMP coated HAP-titanium implant group was significantly greater than that of control although the peak force did not reveal a statistically significant difference. Few studies to date have performed mechanical push-out testing on HAP-titanium implants treated with biologic molecules. Elmengaard et al evaluated the effects of an Arg-Gly-Asp (RGD) peptide coating on tissue integration and titanium implant fixation across a bone-implant gap in dogs [22]. At 4 weeks post-surgery, it was reported that RGD-coated implants had significantly greater push-out stiffness compared to controls, whereas the peak strength was not significant different [22]. Sachse et al performed a study to evaluate HAP-titanium implants in sheep and reported that implants treated with BMP-2 displayed 50% higher pull-out force than controls at 20 weeks post-surgery [4]. Relative to these

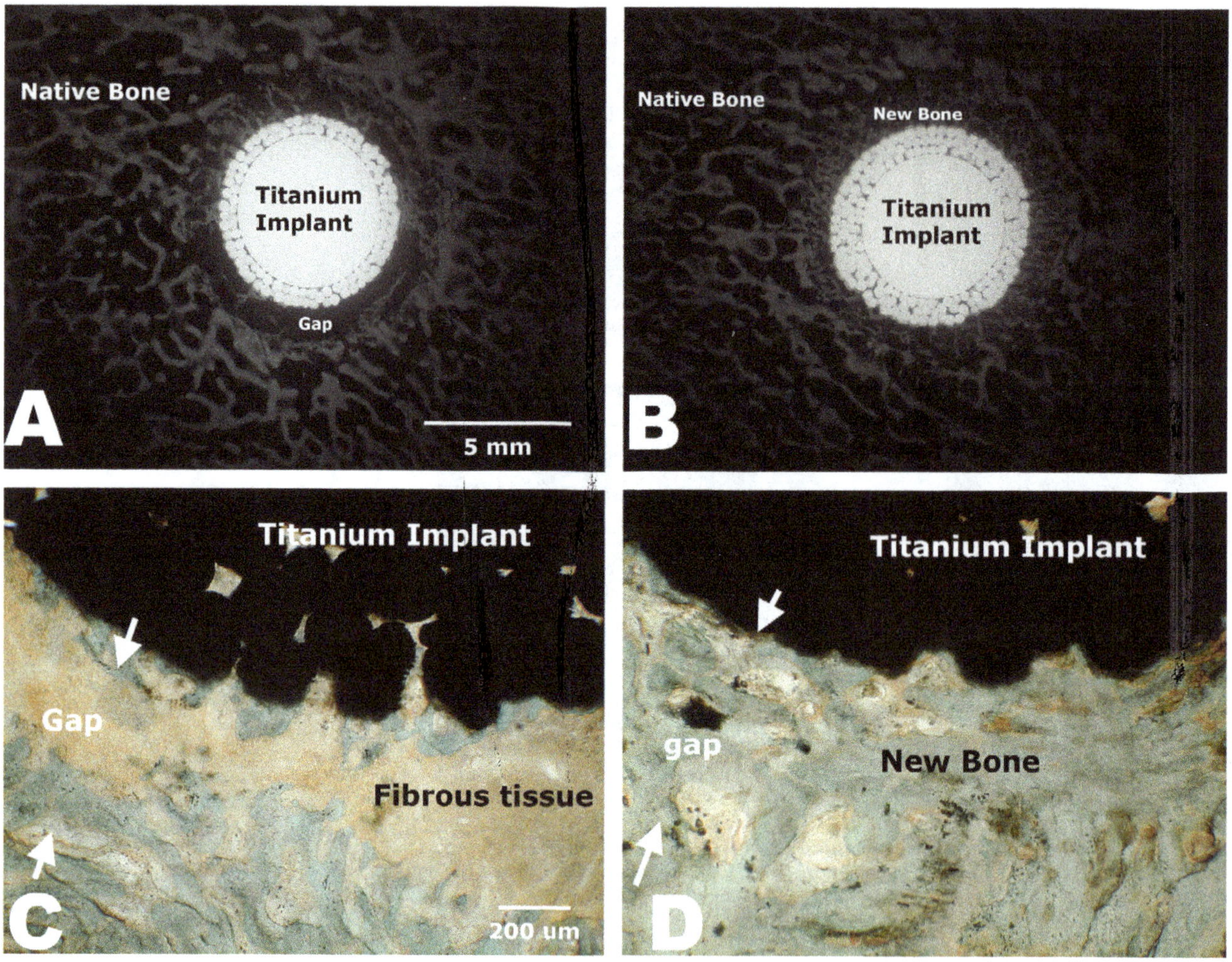

Figure 5. High detailed radiograph (A, B) and histologic section (C, D) of non-mBMP coated HAP-implants (A, C) and mBMP-coated implants (B, D). In C and D, areas between white arrows highlighted original 1-mm gap between the implant and host bone.

previous studies, the current study indicates that the modular peptide mBMP may also be useful in total joint arthoplasty, and other orthopedic implant applications. In addition, the ability of mBMP to bind with high efficiency to hydroxyapatite-containing implants may be particularly advantageous, as our previous studies have shown that efficient binding results in controllable dosages and localized release [20,21,24,32]. In addition, we have recently shown that mBMP can be modified to control the release rate from hydroxyapatite substrates [20,21,32]. Finally, recent studies indicate that the approach described here can be applied to other biologically active molecules, such as vascular endothelial growth factor (VEGF) [33]. Collectively, these studies suggest that the current approach may be useful in a range of orthopedic implant applications.

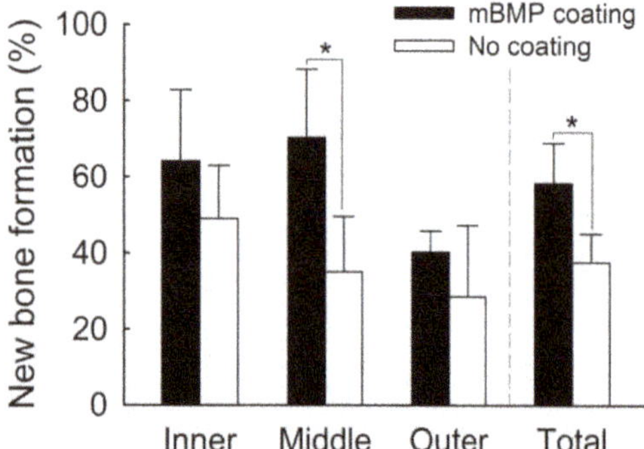

Figure 6. Histologic calculation of new bone formation in the implant-bone gap on the Goldner's trichrome staining slides demonstrated that middle section and total 3 sections of mBMP coated implant had significantly more new bone formation compared to control. "*" means significant difference between treatments ($p<0.05$).

It is noteworthy that specific aspects of this study were designed for relevance to potential clinical applications of these biomaterials. First, the bone-implant gap size of implant selected for this study (1 mm) was a critical size, which may be larger than the gap in actual human clinical applications, but may represent a challenging scenario for bone-implant healing in revision joint arthroplasty. Second, the four week evaluation time is a relatively early time point to characterize new bone formation, and may provide particular insights into the degree of accelerated bone formation. A later time point could provide insight into the ability of mBMP to promote stable long-term implant fixation, but would not indicate an ability to promote the rapid fixation that is needed. The purpose of this study was to characterize a challenging bone-implant gap and an early time point, to more directly represent the challenging environment present during revision arthroplasty, and the need to accelerate fixation and avoid development of fibrous tissue that can lead to pain and implant instability.

Conclusions

The mBMP peptides were efficiently bound to a HAP-titanium implant and released over 28 days in a sustained manner *in vitro. In vivo* results demonstrated that mBMP-coated HAP-titanium implants increased implant fixation and stimulated bone formation in a well-defined, critical gap between the implant and surrounding host cancellous bone after 4 weeks post-surgery compared to untreated HAP-titanium implants. This technique may be beneficial for human clinical applications, such as mBMP-coating on the stem of prosthesis, to enhance new bone formation at early stages.

Acknowledgments

The authors thank Vicki Kalscheur and Kari A. Pulfer for their technical support and Smith&Nephew Corp. for its providing HAP-titanium implants.

Author Contributions

Conceived and designed the experiments: YL JSL BKG RI RV MDM WLM. Performed the experiments: YL JSL BN. Analyzed the data: YL JSL KR RV MDM WLM. Contributed reagents/materials/analysis tools: JSL KR MDM WLM. Wrote the paper: YL. Proofread the manuscript: MDM, WLM.

References

1. Bozic KJ, Kurtz SM, Lau E, Ong K, Chiu V et al. (2010) The epidemiology of revision total knee arthroplasty in the United States. Clin Orthop Relat Res 468: 45–51.
2. Elmengaard B, Bechtold JE, Chen X, Soballe K (2009) Fixation of hydroxyapatite-coated revision implants is improved by the surgical technique of cracking the sclerotic bone rim. J Orthop Res 27: 996–1001.
3. Daugaard H, Elmengaard B, Bechtold JE, Soballe K (2008) Bone growth enhancement in vivo on press-fit titanium alloy implants with acid etched microtexture. J Biomed Mater Res A 87: 434–440.
4. Sachse A, Wagner A, Keller M, Wagner O, Wetzel WD et al. (2005) Osteointegration of hydroxyapatite-titanium implants coated with nonglycosylated recombinant human bone morphogenetic protein-2 (BMP-2) in aged sheep. Bone 37: 699–710.
5. Lamberg A, Schmidmaier G, Soballe K, Elmengaard B (2006) Locally delivered TGF-beta1 and IGF-1 enhance the fixation of titanium implants: a study in dogs. Acta Orthop 77: 799–805.
6. Hollister SJ, Murphy WL (2011) Scaffold translation: barriers between concept and clinic. Tissue Eng Part B Rev 17: 459–474.
7. Peng S, Zhou G, Luk KD, Cheung KM, Li Z et al. (2009) Strontium promotes osteogenic differentiation of mesenchymal stem cells through the Ras/MAPK signaling pathway. Cell Physiol Biochem 23: 165–174.
8. Boden SD, Zdeblick TA, Sandhu HS, Heim SE (2000) The use of rhBMP-2 in interbody fusion cages. Definitive evidence of osteoinduction in humans: a preliminary report. Spine (Phila Pa 1976) 25: 376–381.
9. Kanayama M, Hashimoto T, Shigenobu K, Yamane S, Bauer TW et al. (2006) A prospective randomized study of posterolateral lumbar fusion using osteogenic protein-1 (OP-1) versus local autograft with ceramic bone substitute: emphasis of surgical exploration and histologic assessment. Spine (Phila Pa 1976) 31: 1067–1074.
10. Govender S, Csimma C, Genant HK, Valentin-Opran A, Amit Y et al. (2002) Recombinant human bone morphogenetic protein-2 for treatment of open tibial fractures: a prospective, controlled, randomized study of four hundred and fifty patients. J Bone Joint Surg Am 84: 2123–2134.
11. Cahill KS, Chi JH, Day A, Claus EB (2009) Prevalence, complications, and hospital charges associated with use of bone-morphogenetic proteins in spinal fusion procedures. JAMA 302: 58–66.
12. Shields LB, Raque GH, Glassman SD, Campbell M, Vitaz T et al. (2006) Adverse effects associated with high-dose recombinant human bone morphogenetic protein-2 use in anterior cervical spine fusion. Spine (Phila Pa 1976) 31: 542–547.
13. Wong DA, Kumar A, Jatana S, Ghiselli G, Wong K (2008) Neurologic impairment from ectopic bone in the lumbar canal: a potential complication of off-label PLIF/TLIF use of bone morphogenetic protein-2 (BMP-2). Spine J 8: 1011–1018.
14. Carragee EJ, Mitsunaga KA, Hurwitz EL, Scuderi GJ (2011) Retrograde ejaculation after anterior lumbar interbody fusion using rhBMP-2: a cohort controlled study. Spine J 11: 511–516.
15. Carragee EJ, Hurwitz EL, Weiner BK (2011) A critical review of recombinant human bone morphogenetic protein-2 trials in spinal surgery: emerging safety concerns and lessons learned. Spine J 11: 471–491.
16. Liu Y, de Groot K, Hunziker EB (2005) BMP-2 liberated from biomimetic implant coatings induces and sustains direct ossification in an ectopic rat model. Bone 36: 745–757.
17. Liu Y, Enggist L, Kuffer AF, Buser D, Hunziker EB (2007) The influence of BMP-2 and its mode of delivery on the osteoconductivity of implant surfaces during the early phase of osseointegration. Biomaterials 28: 2677–2686.
18. Saito A, Suzuki Y, Ogata S, Ohtsuki C, Tanihara M (2003) Activation of osteo-progenitor cells by a novel synthetic peptide derived from the bone morphogenetic protein-2 knuckle epitope. Biochim Biophys Acta 1651: 60–67.
19. Saito A, Suzuki Y, Kitamura M, Ogata S, Yoshihara Y et al. (2006) Repair of 20-mm long rabbit radial bone defects using BMP-derived peptide combined with an alpha-tricalcium phosphate scaffold. J Biomed Mater Res A 77: 700–706.
20. Lee JS, Lee JS, Wagoner-Johnson A, Murphy WL (2009) Modular peptide growth factors for substrate-mediated stem cell differentiation. Angew Chem Int Ed Engl 48: 6266–6269.
21. Lee JS, Lee JS, Murphy WL (2010) Modular peptides promote human mesenchymal stem cell differentiation on biomaterial surfaces. Acta Biomater 6: 21–28.
22. Elmengaard B, Bechtold JE, Soballe K (2005) In vivo effects of RGD-coated titanium implants inserted in two bone-gap models. J Biomed Mater Res A 75: 249–255.
23. Faria ML, Lu Y, Heaney K, Uthamanthil RK, Muir P et al. (2007) Recombinant human bone morphogenetic protein-2 in absorbable collagen sponge enhances bone healing of tibial osteotomies in dogs. Vet Surg 36: 122–131.
24. Lu Y, Markel MD, Nemke B, Lee JS, Graf BK et al. (2009) Influence of hydroxyapatite-coated and growth factor-releasing interference screws on tendon-bone healing in an ovine model. Arthroscopy 25: 1427–1434.
25. Shields LB, Raque GH, Glassman SD, Campbell M, Vitaz T et al. (2006) Adverse effects associated with high-dose recombinant human bone morphogenetic protein-2 use in anterior cervical spine fusion. Spine 31: 542–547.
26. Campbell AW, Bain WE, McRae AF, Broad TE, Johnstone PD et al. (2003) Bone density in sheep: genetic variation and quantitative trait loci localisation. Bone 33: 540–548.
27. Fini M, Giavaresi G, Greggi T, Martini L, Aldini NN et al. (2003) Biological assessment of the bone-screw interface after insertion of uncoated and hydroxyapatite-coated pedicular screws in the osteopenic sheep. J Biomed Mater Res A 66: 176–183.
28. Lu Y, Nemke B, Lorang DM, Trip R, Kobayashi H et al. (2009) Comparison of a new braid fixation system to an interlocking intramedullary nail for tibial osteotomy repair in an ovine model. Vet Surg 38: 467–476.
29. Rammelt S, Heck C, Bernhardt R, Bierbaum S, Scharnweber D et al. (2007) In vivo effects of coating loaded and unloaded Ti implants with collagen, chondroitin sulfate, and hydroxyapatite in the sheep tibia. J Orthop Res 25: 1052–1061.
30. Elmengaard B, Bechtold JE, Soballe K (2005) In vivo study of the effect of RGD treatment on bone ongrowth on press-fit titanium alloy implants. Biomaterials 26: 3521–3526.
31. Kessler S, Mayr-Wohlfart U, Ignatius A, Puhl W, Claes L et al. (2003) [The impact of bone morphogenetic protein-2 (BMP-2), vascular endothelial growth factor (VEGF) and basic fibroblast growth factor (b-FGF) on osseointegration, degradation and biomechanical properties of a synthetic bone substitute]. Z Orthop Ihre Grenzgeb 141: 472–480.
32. Suarez-Gonzalez D, Barnhart K, Migneco F, Flanagan C, Hollister SJ et al. (2012) Controllable mineral coatings on PCL scaffolds as carriers for growth factor release. Biomaterials 33: 713–721.
33. Lee JS, Wagoner Johnson AJ, Murphy WL (2010) A modular, hydroxyapatite-binding version of vascular endothelial growth factor. Adv Mater 22: 5494–5498.

11

Enhanced Periosteal and Endocortical Responses to Axial Tibial Compression Loading in Conditional Connexin43 Deficient Mice

Susan K. Grimston[1,3]*, Marcus P. Watkins[1,3], Michael D. Brodt[2,3], Matthew J. Silva[2,3], Roberto Civitelli[1,3]

1 Division of Bone and Mineral Diseases, Department of Internal Medicine, Washington University in St. Louis, St. Louis, Missouri, United States of America, **2** Department of Orthopedic Surgery, Washington University in St. Louis, St. Louis, Missouri, United States of America, **3** Musculoskeletal Research Center, Washington University in St. Louis, St. Louis, Missouri, United States of America

Abstract

The gap junction protein, connexin43 (Cx43) is involved in mechanotransduction in bone. Recent studies using in vivo models of conditional Cx43 gene (*Gja1*) deletion in the osteogenic linage have generated inconsistent results, with *Gja1* ablation resulting in either attenuated or enhanced response to mechanical load, depending upon the skeletal site examined or the type of load applied. To gain further insights on Cx43 and mechanotransduction, we examined bone formation response at both endocortical and periosteal surfaces in 2-month-old mice with conditional *Gja1* ablation driven by the *Dermo1* promoter (cKO). Relative to wild type (WT) littermates, it requires a larger amount of compressive force to generate the same periosteal strain in cKO mice. Importantly, cKO mice activate periosteal bone formation at a lower strain level than do WT mice, suggesting an increased sensitivity to mechanical load in Cx43 deficiency. Consistently, trabecular bone mass also increases in mutant mice upon load, while it decreases in WT. On the other hand, bone formation actually decreases on the endocortical surface in WT mice upon application of axial mechanical load, and this response is also accentuated in cKO mice. These changes are associated with increase of *Cox-2* in both genotypes and further decrease of *Sost* mRNA in cKO relative to WT bones. Thus, the response of bone forming cells to mechanical load differs between trabecular and cortical components, and remarkably between endocortical and periosteal envelopes. Cx43 deficiency enhances both the periosteal and endocortical response to mechanical load applied as axial compression in growing mice.

Editor: Ryan K. Roeder, University of Notre Dame, United States of America

Funding: This work was supported by National Institutes of Health/National Institute of Arthritis and Musculoskeletal Skin Diseases grants AR041255 (RC), AR047867 (MJS), P30AR057235 (Washington University Core Center for Musculoskeletal Biology and Medicine) and funds from the Barnes Jewish Hospital Foundation. The funders had no role in the study design, data collection and analysis, decision to publish, or preparation of the manuscript.

Competing Interests: Roberto Civitelli has a material transfer agreement with Zealand Pharma (Glostrup, Denmark) for the use of gap junction-modifying peptides but receives no honoraria or research funds from Zealand. He receives consultant fees from Novartis and Amgen, grant support from Eli-Lilly and Pfizer, and owns stock of Eli-Lilly, Merck, and Amgen. All other authors state they have no conflict of interest.

* E-mail: Sgrimsto@dom.wustl.edu

Introduction

Connexin43 (Cx43) is the predominant gap junction protein present in bone cells, particularly in cells of the osteoblast lineage [1–3]. The importance of Cx43 for bone homeostasis is demonstrated by the skeletal abnormalities present in mice with ablation of the Cx43 gene (*Gja1*) [4], and further underscored by the skeletal malformations described in patients with the autosomal dominant disorder oculodentodigital dysplasia, a disease linked to *Gja1* mutations [5–7].

We have previously reported that mice with conditional deletion of *Gja1* in cells of the osteogenic lineage have enlarged marrow cavities, thin cortices and hypomineralized long bones [8–11]. We also find that activation of endocortical bone formation by application of mechanical load in vivo by a 3-point bending regimen is attenuated in Cx43 deficient mice driven by a 2.3 kb fragment of the *Col1a1* promoter [9]. In that study, periosteal response to the mechanical load was not quantifiable because of exuberant production of woven bone on the periosteal surface of both Cx43 deficient and wild type mice, likely representing a reaction to compressive pressure generated by the device used to produce the load [9]. More recently, others have used cantilever bending to apply load in vivo, and found actually enhanced periosteal bone formation response in *Gja1* deleted mice driven by the *Bglap* promoter [12]. Endocortical response was not reported in that study. While the different methods used to apply skeletal load, the different anatomical locations studied, and perhaps even the slightly different genetic models of *Gja1* ablation may contribute to explain the apparently discrepant result, it is also quite conceivable that endocortical and periosteal bone cells respond differently to mechanical load, a discrepancy that may be affected or even enhanced by Cx43 deficiency.

In this study, we addressed this issue by applying a more physiologic loading regime, axial tibial compression, and evaluated the bone formation response at both periosteal and endocortical surfaces. We also tested whether the altered response of Cx43 deficient bones is related to abnormal sensitivity to load, and examined the gene expression profile in bones before and after loading to garner some insights on the potential mechanisms of

Cx43 modulation of mechanical skeletal responses. For these studies, we used mice in which the *Dermo1* promoter drives *Gja1* deletion in the chondro-osteogenic lineage, and whose phenotype of larger but thinner cortical bone is accentuated relative to other genetic models of more restricted *Gja1* deletion. We reasoned that any roles that Cx43 may have in mediating the osteo-anabolic response to mechanical load should be more evident in these mice with a broader *Gja1* ablation.

Our results indicate that Cx43 deficiency alters the endocortical and periosteal responses to mechanical load, resulting in enhanced activation of periosteal bone formation and further decrease in endocortical bone formation induced by axial tibial compression. We also find Cx43-dependent altered expression of selected genes involved in mechanotransduction in bone.

Methods

Ethics Statement

This study was carried out in strict accordance with the recommendations in the Guide for the Care and Use of Laboratory Animals of the National Institutes of Health. All procedures were approved by the Animal Studies Committee of Washington University in St. Louis (protocol number 20090128).

Transgenic Mice

Mice were generated as described previously [10]. Briefly, mice harboring a mutant "floxed" *Gja1* allele were mated to mice expressing *Cre* under the control of the *Dermo1/Twist2* promoter resulting in *Cre*-mediated gene replacement of the entire *Gja1* reading frame with the *LacZ* reporter cassette. One Gja1 null allele was also introduced to generate *DM1-Cre;Gja1*$^{flox/-}$ conditional knockout (cKO) mice. *Gja1*$^{flox/+}$ were used as wild type equivalent (WT) mice. The *DM1-Cre* transgene effectively deletes *Gja1* in osteoblasts on the endocortical surface, osteocytes [10], as well as periosteal cells (Figure S1). Genotyping was performed by PCR on genomic DNA extracted from mouse tails using the HotSHOT method [13]. Primers and conditions have been described previously [10]. All mouse lines were developed in a mixed C57BL/6-C129/J background and cKO and WT littermates were used. Mice were fed regular chow and water ad libitum and housed communally in a room maintained at a constant temperature (25°C) on a 12 hour light/dark schedule. Mice were weighed daily during the loading phase of the study as an index of overall body health.

Strain Gauge Analysis

Strain-force relationship studies were performed on 2-month-old male cKO (n = 8) and WT (n = 6) mice using tibial compression loading as described previously [14]. Briefly, after euthanasia 1 mm strain gauges (Tokyo Sokki Kenkyujo Co., Japan) were placed along the longitudinal axis of the antero-medial surface of the right tibia, at a point 5 mm proximal to the distal tibiofibular junction (TFJ). Previous analysis indicated that the site of peak axial tensile strain is at this location [15]. Because of the curvature of the tibia axial compression generates combined compression-bending at the aforementioned point. Mice were positioned in a servohydraulic materials testing machine (Instron; Dynamite) such that the loading piston applied a compressive load through contacts at the knee and ankle (foot up, knee down) [14]. After application of a 0.5 N compressive pre-load, a trapezoidal waveform was applied to generate peak forces of 4 N up to a maximum of 14 N, at 2 N intervals. A 10 sec rest interval was allowed between each of 8 loading cycles for each force tested. Strains were recorded through a signal conditioning amplifier system (SCX1-1001; National Instruments), with 160 secs recovery interval between each set of eight cycles. Peak strains were determined for cycles 4–8, and the average computed. The region of the bone at the gauge site, with the strain gauge attached was scanned using µCT (µCT- 40; Scanco, Basserdorf, Switzerland) to assess the location of the strain gauge and the accuracy of its placement relative to the TFJ. From cross sectional images, the bone centroid, area, and moment of inertia about the neutral axis were determined as well as the distance from the centroid to the gauge location (y_{gauge}) and the predicted site of peak periosteal strain (y). Based on beam theory [16], we then extrapolated the strain-gauge data to estimate strain values at the site of maximal tensile periosteal strain (ε) using the relation $\varepsilon = \varepsilon_{gauge}(y/y_{gauge})$.

In Vivo Axial Compression Loading

Mice (2 month old) were loaded in axial tibial compression using the Instron Dynamite, 5 consecutive days, 60 cycles per day, with a 10 sec rest interval inserted between each loading cycle, as described previously [14]. After a 0.5 N pre-load was applied, a trapezoidal waveform was applied at 40 N/sec. Peak forces were chosen based on the strain analysis (see Results). The controlateral tibia was used as an internal, non-loaded control in all cases. Mice were loaded under isofluorane and were kept in isolation until full recovery from anesthesia. Mice were given a subcutaneous injection of Buprenex (0.1 ml/25 mg) following each loading session; they were allowed normal ambulatory cage activity between loading sessions and from the end of the loading period until sacrifice. Mice were injected with calcein on day 4 (4 µl/g body weight) and with Alizarin Red (6 µl/g body weight) on day 9, and were sacrificed on day 11. For gene expression analysis, 2-month-old WT and cKO mice were all loaded at a force of 7 N, using 120 cycles with a 10 second rest interval between cycles. Mice were sacrificed 2 hours after the loading session for RNA extraction (see below).

In Vivo µCT

In vivo µCT scans were performed as described previously [11,14], using a VivaCT 40 scanner (Scanco Medical). Briefly, mice were anesthetized with isoflurane and positioned in a specifically designed fixture providing for reliable placement of the leg. Scan settings were 70 KVp, 109 µA and 21.5 µm voxel resolution. Cortical bone parameters were assessed at a point 5 mm proximal to the TFJ (25 slices); trabecular bone was analyzed as the area immediately distal to the growth plate (100 slices) in the metaphysis. Contours were drawn manually of the area encompassing the trabecular bone and excluding the cortical shell.

Histomorphometry

Bone formation indices were assessed using standard histomorphometric techniques [17]. Tibiae were fixed in 10% buffered formalin for up to 24 hours, dehydrated and embedded in methyl methacrylate as described previously [9]. Triplicate 100 µm thick transverse sections were cut (Leica 1600SP, Wetzlar, Germany) from each tibia 5 mm proximal to the TFJ. Sections were mounted on glass and polished to a thickness of approximately 30 µm. Two color fluorescent images were taken (calcein – green, and alizarin – red) using a confocal microscope (LSM 510, Axiovert 200 M, Plan-Neofluar Carl Zeiss, Jena, Germany). Dynamic histomorphometry analysis was performed using commercially available software (OSTEO II, Bioquant, Nashville, TN, USA). Single and double labeling surface (sLS/BS, dLS/BS), mineral apposition rate (MAR) and bone formation rate (BFR/BS) were determined as defined previously [9,17]. Endocortical and periosteal surfaces were analyzed separately. Single labeled surface was defined as any surface with green, red, or yellow (no separation between green and red). Double labeled surface was any surface with green and red separated by a measureable distance. MS/BS was calculated as 0.5× sLS/BS + dLS/BS for all samples. Based on a previously published recommendation [18] samples with no dLS/BS were coded as "no data" for MAR and BFR/BS. Some sections were decalcified and processed for β-galactosidase staining as detailed [8], with the addition of 100 mM galactose to the staining solution to quench non-specific staining.

Gene Expression Analyses

Tibiae were cleaned of all connective tissue and after dissection of the distal epiphysis, the bone marrow was removed by centrifugation (10,000 rpm for 15 sec). Tibiae were then flash frozen in liquid nitrogen for storage at −80°C. The bones were pulverized using a Braun Mikrodismembranator (Sartorius BBI Systems Inc., Bethlehem, PA) and total RNA was extracted using Trizol reagent (Invitrogen, Carlsbad, CA) and purified using Phase-Lock gel tubes (5 Prime, Hamburg, Germany) and the RNeasy Mini Kit (Qiagen) according to the manufacturer's directions. DNA was removed using the RNase-free DNase set (Qiagen, Valencia, CA). Messenger RNA was measured and 1 µg total RNA was reverse transcribed using a superscript VILO cDNA synthesis kit (Invitrogen, Carlsbad, CA). The SYBR green (Applied Biosystems, Foster City, CA) realtime PCR method was used in an Applied Biosystem 7500 Fast detector system, as described previously [19,20]. PCR products were normalized to cyclophilin (*Ppib*). Primer sets are detailed in Table S1.

Statistical Analysis

Differences between groups were assessed by paired t-tests (two-tailed). Effects of load and genotype were assessed using two-way ANOVA, with post-hoc comparisons using the Bonferroni multiple t-test (SigmaPlot Version 11.0; Systat Software GmbH, Germany). Where the data indicated, one-way ANOVA was applied to test for differences among groups. Significant differences between slopes of Force-Strain regression lines were determined using the Test for Parallelism. Differences were defined as statistically significant at $p<0.05$. Values are expressed as the mean ± standard error of the mean unless otherwise specified.

Results

Since cKO mice have abnormal cortical structure and biomechanical properties, we first experimentally determined the relationships between applied force and strain generated at the bone surface by axial loading for WT and cKO mice. To this end, the force applied was plotted against the strain detected by strain gauges placed on the surface of the tibia. A regression line was calculated by fitting all experimental data points obtained for each animal in each genotype group. The slope of this regression line was significantly lower for cKO than for WT mice ($t=4.328$; $p<0.01$), implying that cKO bones require greater force to generate the same peak tensile periosteal strain relative to WT mice (Figure 1A, B).

Based on the force-strain plots we used a periosteal strain of 1200 µε for the following studies. This level of strain represents a good compromise between the need of generating an anabolic stimulus and delivering submaximal force. To achieve a periosteal strain of 1200 µε required an axial load of 8 N in the WT (WT-1200 µε) and 12 N in the cKO (cKO-1200 µε). As additional control, a second group of WT mice was loaded at the same force as the cKO, i.e. 12 N, resulting in a periosteal strain magnitude of approximately 1900 µε (WT-1900 µε). Unilateral tibial loading was applied daily (60 cycles for 5 days). Perhaps because of reduced bone strength in cKO mice application of 12 N force in axial compression resulted in tibial fractures in 7 out of 15 cKO mice. Notably, this occurred in mice weighing less than 15 g and these mice were excluded from the analyses. Indeed, *Gja1* cKO mice weighed significantly less than WT mice (16.69±2.77 g vs. 24.54±2.30 g, respectively; $p<0.001$). The WT-1900 µε mice lost body weight over the 5 day period (−4.53±1.89%; $p=0.047$), while the weight loss in the cKO-1200 µε group barely missed the significance level (−7.19±2.55%; $p=0.054$). Such degree of weight loss is consistent with a previous study using the same loading regime [14]. There was no significant weight change in the group of WT mice loaded at 1200 µε (0.14±0.81%; $p>0.05$).

Assessment of trabecular parameters at baseline by in vivo µCT revealed no significant differences between right and left tibiae within each genotype, or between genotypes (not shown). On the other hand, analysis of cortical bone at baseline confirmed the larger marrow (Ma.Ar) and total tissue (Tt.Ar) areas, and decreased cortical bone volume (Ct.BV) and cortical tissue area fraction (Ct.Ar/Tt.Ar) in cKO relative to WT littermates, while there were no differences between controlateral tibiae in each genotype group (Figure S2). Also as previously noted [10], the calculated area moment of inertia was significantly greater in the cKO compared to WT mice (0.106±0.004 mm^4 vs. 0.069±0.006 mm^4, respectively; $p<0.001$).

Application of axial loads that produced either 1200 or 1900 µε strain in WT mice had no stimulatory effect on trabecular bone volume; indeed, we detected a paradoxical decrease in BV/TV at the higher strain. By contrast, 1200 µε was sufficient to generate a significant increase in BV/TV in cKO mice (Figure 2A). No effects of axial load on trabecular number was recorded at 1200 µε in either WT or cKO mice, but there was a decrease at 1900 µε (Figure 2B) consistent with the decrease in BV/TV. In contrast we observed an increase in trabecular thickness in WT mice at 1200 µε, but no effects at the higher strain. Since the latter is the only significant difference in the WT-1200 group, it most likely represents a random finding rather than an effect of load. On the other hand, trabecular thickness increased significantly in the cKO group (Figure 2C).

There was a significant stimulatory effect of loading on cortical bone volume in the WT-1900 and cKO-1200 groups, but not in the WT-1200 group, relative to their respective non-loaded control limbs (Figure 3A). Changes in marrow area and total tissue area after loading followed a similar pattern, with significant increases only in the WT-1900 and cKO-1200 groups and not in the WT-1200 group (Figure 3B, C). These relative changes indicated accrual of periosteal bone with resorption of endocortical bone in the WT-1900 and cKO-1200 groups.

Consistent with increased cortical bone volume and cortical total bone area, we detected significant effects of load on periosteal mineralizing surfaces and bone formation rate in the WT-1900 and cKO-1200 groups, but not in the WT-1200 group (Figure 4A–C). On the other hand, at the endocortical surface both indices of bone formation paradoxically decreased after load in both WT groups and such decrease was of significantly larger magnitude in cKO relative to the WT-1200 group (Figures 4D–E and S3). We observed only upward trends in periosteal mineral apposition rate in WT-1900 and cKO-1200, but the differences with control tibiae failed to reach significance; and endocortical mineral apposition rate decreased only in cKO- 1200 but not in WT mice (Figure S4A, B). There were no significant differences in bone formation

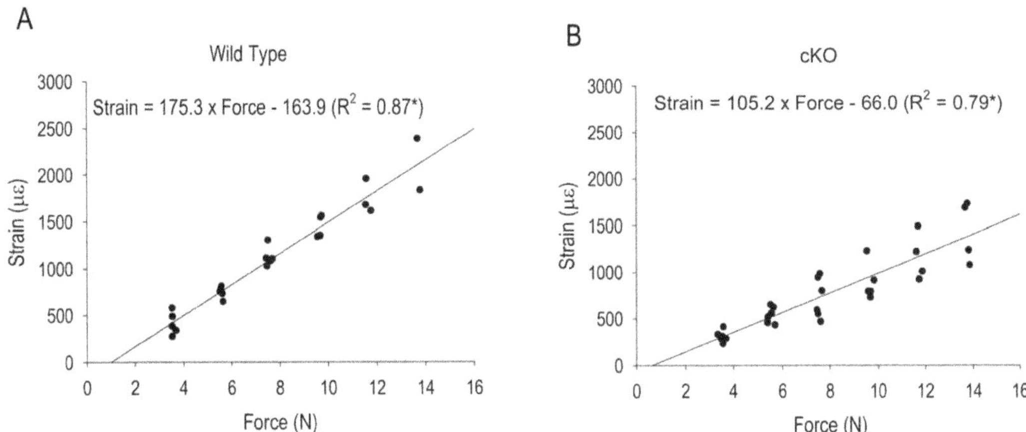

Figure 1. Relationship between applied force and strain measured at the bone surface in (A) wild type and (B) *Gja1* conditional knockout (cKO) mice. Regression equations are given for each genotype, and the slopes of the Regression lines were compared using the test for Parallelism; $p<0.05$.

indices at either periosteal or endocortical surfaces in control tibiae among all groups (Figures 4B–D, and S4).

We next explored expression of genes that had been previously shown to be altered by mechanical load in vitro or in vivo [21–23]. Considering the high frequency of fractures in the cKO at 12 N of axial load, we chose to use a lower force, on the assumption that changes in gene expression would be easier to detect at lower loads than changes in osteoblast activity. Thus, we applied a force of 7 N, which generated an estimated periosteal strain of 1063 με in WT and 670 με in the cKO. As shown in Fig. 5, we verified that *Gja1* mRNA was barely detectable in the cKO bones using qPCR in marrow-free whole bone extracts. In WT mice the abundance of *Cox-2* mRNA increased 3-fold compared to a doubling in cKO mice, whereas *β-catenin* and *Nfat-C1* mRNA were only marginally increased after mechanical stimulation in both genotypes (Figure 5). Importantly, *Sost* mRNA abundance was dramatically down-regulated by mechanical loading in the WT mice. In cKO mice, *Sost* mRNA was already 50% lower relative to WT at baseline and it was further down-regulated by mechanical load. *Bmp4* mRNA was also significantly down-regulated by mechanical loading in both genotypes, while only negative, non-significant trends were observed for *Bmp2* and *Smad2* mRNA.

Discussion

This study demonstrates that mice with *Gja1* ablation in the osteogenic lineage activate periosteal bone formation at a lower level of strain than do WT mice, suggesting an increased sensitivity to mechanical load in Cx43 deficiency. Consistently, trabecular bone mass also increases in mutant mice upon load, while it decreases in WT. On the other hand, bone formation actually decreases on the endocortical surface in WT mice upon application of axial mechanical load, and this response is also accentuated in cKO mice. Thus, the response of bone forming cells to mechanical load differs between trabecular and cortical components, and remarkably between endocortical and periosteal envelopes. Cx43 deficiency enhances both the periosteal and endocortical response to mechanical load applied as axial compression in growing mice.

The greater load required in conditional Cx43 deficient mice to generate a specific strain relative to WT mice is consistent with a previous finding using a 3-point bending method to apply load [9]; a finding later confirmed by other groups using different promoters to delete *Gja1* [12,24]. The abnormal force-strain relationship is most likely related to both the different geometry and altered bone matrix and mineralization of Cx43 deficient bones. The typical phenotype of expanded marrow cavity and periosteal perimeter, particularly evident in the cKO model used in this study, result in a greater area moment of inertia [9,11], hence a greater resistance to bending in the anterior/posterior direction and lower values of strain for a given compressive load. Strain values upon loading also depend on the bone modulus, which is a function of both the mineral and collagen phases of bone, and both mineral content and collagen fiber organization are abnormal in cKO compared to WT mice [10]. Finally, cKO bones are slightly shorter than WT bones [10], and this could affect response to load. Nonetheless, because we physically measured strains using strain gauges, both geometric and material property differences should be accounted for.

Our data demonstrate that different responses to mechanical loading occur on the periosteal and endocortical bone surfaces. In particular, we find that Cx43 deficiency enhances the periosteal bone formation response to loading (for equivalent strains) and further decreases bone formation on the endocortical response relative to WT bones in growing mice. This differential response explains the apparently discordant results obtained by independent studies that have examined the different cortical envelopes [9,12]. The characteristics of the loading regime may result in different strain stimuli at different sites and thus in different outcomes. Axial tibial compression loading produces both a compressive and bending load on the tibia due to the curvature of the bone. Although a bit surprising, a negative effect of axial mechanical load on trabecular bone of WT mice is consistent with previous studies from our group in aged mice, showing that trabecular bone volume actually decreases in young adult (7 months) mice upon axial compression using the waveform used here [14]. This is in contrast to findings from other groups who have used tibial compression under different loading regimes [25–27]. Preliminary results from our laboratory suggest this discrepancy may depend on the waveform and cycle number. On the other hand, BV/TV significantly increased in cKO mice with 1200 με load, further suggesting that Cx43 is involved in response to load, though the trabecular compartment in the cKO may

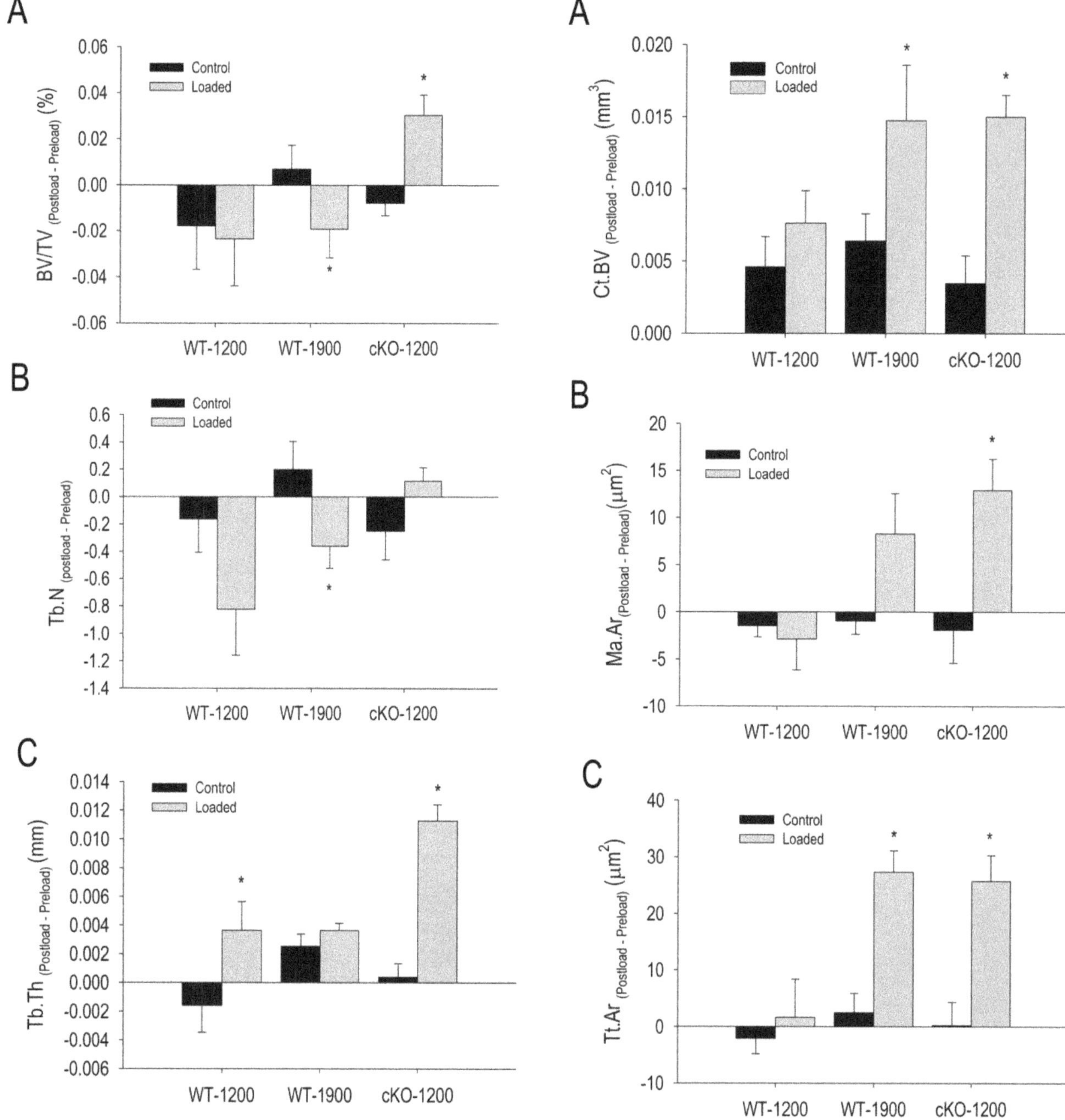

Figure 2. Effect of axial tibial loading on trabecular bone parameters in wild type (WT) and *Gja1* conditional knockout (cKO) mice. The right tibia was subjected to forces generating 1200 με or 1900 με in WT, or 1200 με in cKO, as noted, while the left was used as non-loaded control. (A) Trabecular bone volume (BV/TV); (B) Trabecular Number (Tb.N); (C) Trabecular thickness (Tb.Th). Data are expressed as absolute difference between post- and pre-load for each parameter. *$p<0.05$ vs. respective non-loaded control; two-tailed t-test.

Figure 3. Effect of axial tibial loading on cortical parameters in wild type (WT) and *Gja1* conditional knockout (cKO) mice. The right tibia was subjected to forces generating 1200 με or 1900 με in WT, or 1200 με in cKO, as noted, while the left was used as non-loaded control. (A) Cortical bone volume (Ct.BV). (B) Marrow area (Ma.Ar). (C) Total tissue area (Tt.Ar). Data are expressed as absolute difference between post- and pre-load for each parameter. *$p<0.05$ vs. respective control; two-tailed t-test.

experience greater compressive strains than WT due to the altered architecture.

Interestingly, axial load increased periosteal formation rate in cKO loaded at 1200 με as well as in WT loaded at 1900 με; however, periosteal mineral apposition rate did not significantly change in either group. Such a discrepancy implies a higher number of osteoblasts depositing new bone, rather than increased activity of existing osteoblasts. Thus, these results are consistent with the notion that axial compression loading promotes osteoblast recruitment and differentiation on the periosteal surface, an effect enhanced by Cx43 deficiency. It is possible that signaling from osteocytes to the periosteal surface is enhanced in the cKO. However, since periosteal cells in cKO mice are exposed to a lower degree of strain for a given force (based on our force-strain

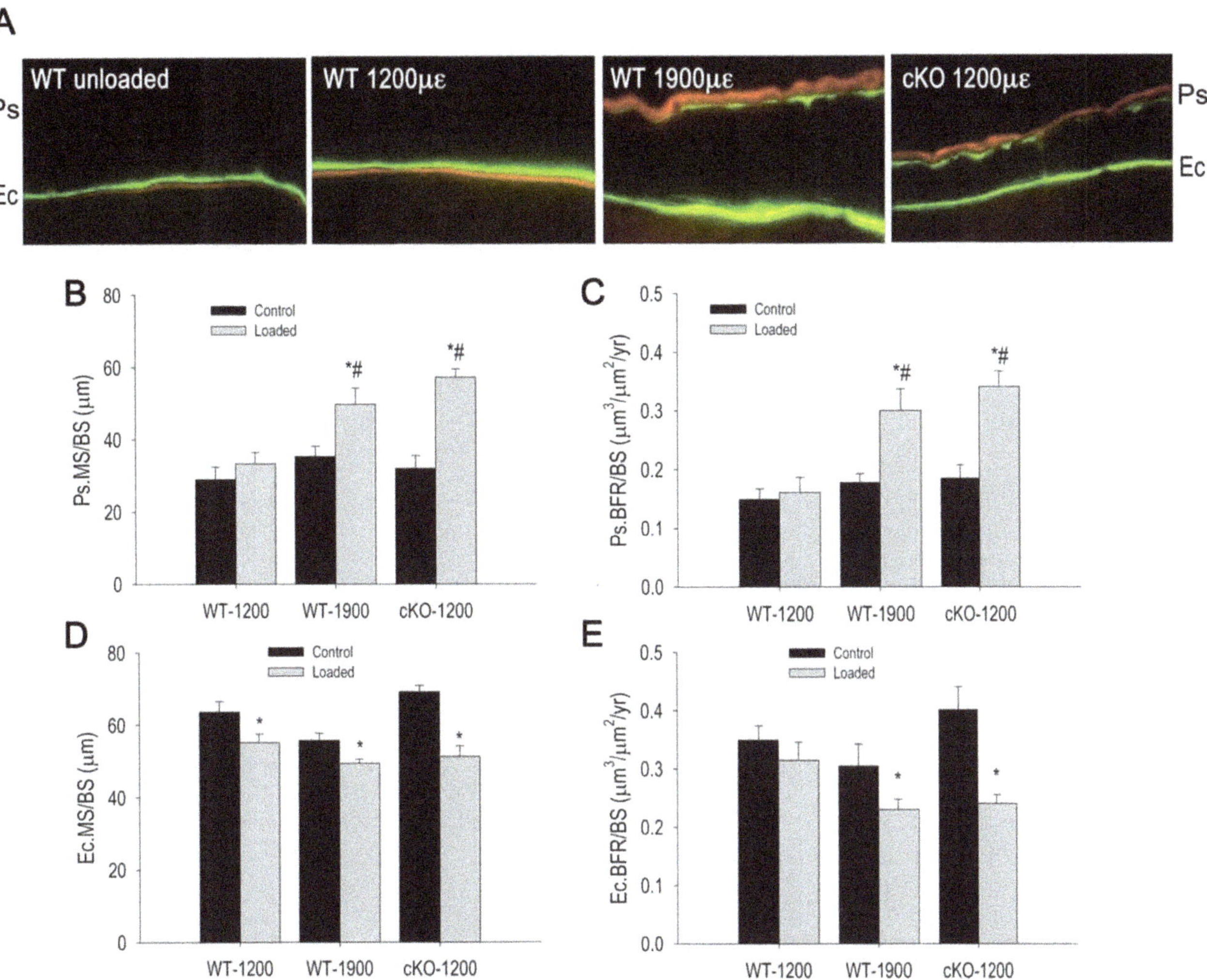

Figure 4. Effect of axial tibial loading on periosteal and endocortical bone formation in wild type (WT) and *Gja1* conditional knockout (cKO) mice. The right tibia was subjected to forces generating 1200 με or 1900 με in WT, or 1200 με in cKO, as noted, while the left was used as non-loaded control. (A) Double calcein/alizarin red labels on cortical sections of tibiae from the different groups, showing both periosteal (Ps) and endocortical (Ec) surfaces. (B) Periosteal mineralizing surfaces per bone surface (Ps.MS/BS) and (C) periosteal bone formation rate per bone surface (Ps.BFR/BS). (D) Endocortical MS/BS (Ec.MS/BS), and (E) endocortical BFR/BS (Ec.BFR/BS). * $p<0.05$ vs respective Control; # $p<0.05$ vs WT-1200 Loaded; ANOVA.

analysis), the fact that periosteal bone formation is increased in Cx43 deficient bones relative to WT bone even in animals living under normal loading conditions [24] strongly suggests that periosteal cells from cKO are more sensitive to mechanical strain than are periosteal WT cells. This conclusion is fully consistent with one of the main findings of this study demonstrating that 1200 με was sufficient in cKO to elicit the same bone formation response as did 1900 με in WT animals. Notably, a periosteal increase in bone diameter contributes more to load bearing strength than do increases in cortical thickness associated with endocortical apposition [28]. Thus, the increased periosteal bone formation observed in the cKO may be related to the need for generating bone at the diaphysis to withstand loads that are sensed as abnormally higher than they actually are.

Increased periosteal bone apposition but decreased endosteal formation after mechanical loading had been previously reported in 9 week old C3H/HeJ mice [29]. Such a paradoxical effect on the endocortical surface may reflect the young age of the mice used in these studies, and the decrease in bone formation rate may represent a slowing of the rapid bone formation rate occurring in growing mice. Since such an effect is more pronounced in mice with an osteoblast/osteocyte specific deletion of *Gja1*, it can be concluded that Cx43 deficiency also increases (in this case in a negative direction) the sensitivity of the endocortical cells to mechanical loading.

Decreased endocortical bone formation by axial load is in apparent contrast with our previous study showing increased endosteal bone formation after application of a 3-point bending load [9]. Aside the different loading approaches, other differences in the experimental settings may contribute to the discrepancy, including a substantially larger strain (1600 με at the anterior-lateral endocortical surface, corresponding to 3774 με at the periosteal surface) and older mice (4-month-old) used in the 3-point bending experiment relative to the present study, as well as different promoters used to drive *Gja1* ablation. In both cases, however, Cx43 deficiency reduces bone formation at the endocortex upon mechanical loading. Lack of differences in periosteal bone formation between WT and cKO at baseline is

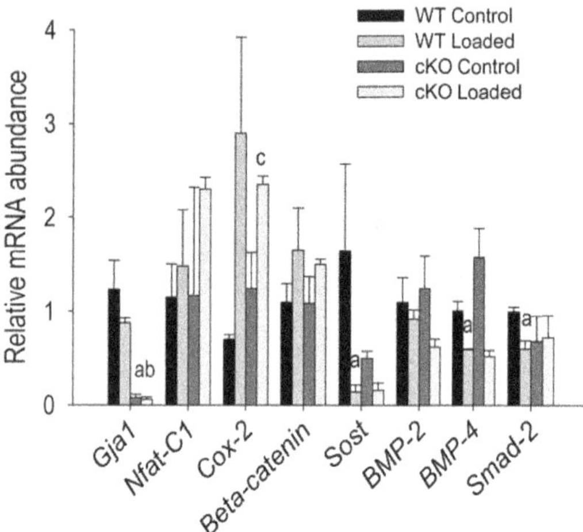

Figure 5. Effect of axial tibial loading on gene expression in vivo. Mice were sacrificed 2 hours after load (120 cycles, 10 sec interval between cycles), and mRNA extracted from whole bone extracts before qPCR analyses for the genes of interest. a: $p<0.05$ vs WT control; b: $p<0.05$ vs WT Loaded and c: $p<0.05$ vs cKO Control; one-way ANOVA.

also in apparent contrast with our previous report [10]. However in that study surface labeling was assessed from the proximal to distal ends of the tibia, whereas in the present experiments cross sections were cut close to the mid-diaphysis – the location at which there is least bone formation activity, and thus genotype differences may be minimized. Consistent with a previous study from our groups using the same loading regime [14], there was a modest weight loss at the end of the study, but this was only significant in one group, WT-1900, which also lost cancellous bone mass. However, cortical bone mass and bone formation rates increased in these mice, and trabecular bone volume increased in the cKO-1200 group, which experienced an even higher weight loss. Therefore it is unlikely that weight loss may have substantially affected changes in bone mass.

While the mechanisms underlying the enhanced periosteal sensitivity require more in-depth investigation, our gene expression studies point to a potentially significant role of sclerostin, the product of *Sost*, a paracrine inhibitor of Wnt signaling. The robust down-regulation of *Sost* expression, among all the genes we investigated, in both WT and cKO implies activation of Wnt signaling by mechanical load. Indeed, the anabolic response to mechanical load is dependent on an intact Lrp5/β-catenin signaling system [21,30], and β-catenin abundance or activity is affected by mechanical stimulation [31,32]. Furthermore, *Sost* is up-regulated by skeletal unloading [33]. Hence, *Sost* down-regulation in Cx43 deficient animals, a finding we had already reported [10], and recently confirmed by others [24], perfectly fits with the model of increased sensitivity of Cx43 deficient bones to mechanical load. On the other hand, this model does not explain the decreased endocortical bone formation upon loading and the further decrease in cKO mice. A very recent study proposes that sclerostin production is altered by Cx43 deficiency specifically in osteocytes in close proximity to the periosteal surface [24]. However, unless one postulates a selective flow of sclerostin from matrix embedded osteocytes to the periosteal surface, an autonomous defect in mechanosensing by periosteal and endocortical cells remains a viable hypothesis.

We also observed the expected increase in *Cox2* expression after axial tibial compression, and this effect was attenuated in Cx43 cKO mice. Although this might reflect a low degree of strain applied to the cKO bones, it is very likely that the cycloxygenase pathway is integrated in the mechanotransduction mechanism modulated by Cx43 [34]. Recent work from our group suggests that the Wnt and BMP signaling systems reciprocally control cell proliferation in bone [35]; thus, the decrease of *Bmp4*, and to a lesser extent *Bmp2*, together with *Sost* down-regulation we observed in this study might be seen as part of a general response to mechanical loading, resulting in expansion of bone forming cells and increased periosteal bone formation.

In summary, we show that Cx43 deficiency in bone cells alters the relationship between mechanical force applied as axial compression and strain produced on the bone surface, so that a higher force is required to generate the same amount of strain compared to WT bones. Importantly, we demonstrate that a lower degree of strain is required to stimulate periosteal bone formation in Cx43 deficient mice, and that this is associated with profound down-regulation of *Sost* and increased *Cox2* mRNA expression. Furthermore, we find that contrary to the stimulatory effect on the periosteal surface, axial tibial mechanical load does not activate endocortical bone formation, and it actually decreases it in conditions of Cx43 deficiency. Thus, Cx43 regulates cortical bone remodeling in part by modulating bone cell sensitivity to mechanical load.

Supporting Information

Figure S1 X-gal stained, paraffin-embedded section of the diaphysis of *Gja1* conditional knockout mouse, counterstained with H&E. Strong β-galactosidase activity is evident in periosteal cells and, to a lesser degree, in osteocytes.

Figure S2 Baseline cortical bone morphology of wild type (WT) and *Gja1* conditional knockout mice (cKO). The right tibia was subjected to forces generating 1200 με or 1900 με in WT, or 1200 με in cKO, as noted, while the left was used as non-loaded control. (A) Marrow area (Ma.Ar). (B) Total tissue area (Tt.Ar). (C) Cortical bone volume (Ct.BV). (D) Cortical area/total tissue area (Ct.Ar/Tt.Ar). * $p<0.05$ vs WT-1200 and WT-1900 (one-way ANOVA).

Figure S3 Percent changes in endocortical bone formation rate per bone surface (Ec.BFR/BS) in loaded relative to control bones after application of axial load. The decrease in Ec.BFR/BS was significantly larger in the *Gja1* conditional knockout (cKO) than in the WT-1200 group ($p<0.05$; two-tailed t-test); whereas the difference between WT-1900 and cKO-1200 was not statistically significant.

Figure S4 Effect of axial tibial loading on periosteal (A) and endocortical (B) mineral apposition rate (MAR) in wild type (WT) and *Gja1* conditional knockout (cKO) mice. The right tibia was subjected to forces generating 1200 με or 1900 με in WT, or 1200 με in cKO, as noted, while the left was used as a non-loaded control. *$p<0.05$ vs. respective control; two-tailed t-test.

Table S1 Forward and reverse primers used for real time PCR in the gene expression analyses for wild type (WT) and *Gja1* conditional knockout (cKO) mice loaded at 7 N in axial tibial compression loading.

Acknowledgments

Part of this work was presented at the 33rd Annual Meeting of the American Society for Bone and Mineral Research, San Diego, California, 2011.

Author Contributions

Conceived and designed the experiments: SKG MJS RC. Performed the experiments: SKG MDB MPW. Analyzed the data: SKG RC MJS. Wrote the paper: SKG MPW MDB MJS RC.

References

1. Civitelli R, Beyer EC, Warlow PM, Robertson AJ, Geist ST, et al. (1993) Connexin43 mediates direct intercellular communication in human osteoblastic cell networks. J Clin Invest 91: 1888–1896.
2. Van der Molen MA, Rubin CT, McLeod KJ, McCauley LK, Donahue HJ (1996) Gap junctional intercellular communication contributes to hormonal responsiveness in osteoblastic networks. J Biol Chem 271: 12165–12171.
3. Civitelli R (2008) Cell-cell communication in the osteoblast/osteocyte lineage. Arch Biochem Biophys 473: 188–192.
4. Lecanda F, Warlow PM, Sheikh S, Furlan F, Steinberg TH, et al. (2000) Connexin43 deficiency causes delayed ossification, craniofacial abnormalities, and osteoblast dysfunction. J Cell Biol 151: 931–944.
5. Paznekas WA, Boyadjiev SA, Shapiro RE, Daniels O, Wollnik B, et al. (2003) Connexin 43 (GJA1) mutations cause the pleiotropic phenotype of oculodentodigital dysplasia. AmJHumGenet 72: 408–418.
6. Kjaer KW, Hansen L, Eiberg H, Leicht P, Opitz JM, et al. (2004) Novel Connexin 43 (GJA1) mutation causes oculo-dento-digital dysplasia with curly hair. AmJMedGenet 127A: 152–157.
7. Malone AM, Anderson CT, Tummala P, Kwon RY, Johnston TR, et al. (2007) Primary cilia mediate mechanosensing in bone cells by a calcium-independent mechanism. Proc Natl Acad Sci U S A 104: 13325–13330.
8. Chung DJ, Castro CH, Watkins M, Stains JP, Chung MY, et al. (2006) Low peak bone mass and attenuated anabolic response to parathyroid hormone in mice with an osteoblast-specific deletion of connexin43. J Cell Sci 119: 4187–4198.
9. Grimston SK, Brodt MD, Silva MJ, Civitelli R (2008) Attenuated response to in vivo mechanical loading in mice with conditional osteoblast ablation of the connexin43 gene (Gja1). J Bone Miner Res 23: 879–886.
10. Mahajan G, Kotru M, Batra M, Gupta A, Sharma S (2011) Usefulness of histopathological examination in uterine prolapse specimens. The Australian & New Zealand journal of obstetrics & gynaecology 51: 403–405.
11. Grimston SK, Goldberg DB, Watkins M, Brodt MD, Silva MJ, et al. (2011) Connexin43 deficiency reduces the sensitivity of cortical bone to the effects of muscle paralysis. J Bone Miner Res.
12. Zhang Y, Paul EM, Sathyendra V, Davison A, Sharkey N, et al. (2011) Enhanced osteoclastic resorption and responsiveness to mechanical load in gap junction deficient bone. PLoS One 6: e23516.
13. Truett GE, Heeger P, Mynatt RL, Truett AA, Walker JA, et al. (2000) Preparation of PCR-quality mouse genomic DNA with hot sodium hydroxide and tris (HotSHOT). Biotechniques 29: 52, 54.
14. Brodt MD, Silva MJ (2010) Aged mice have enhanced endocortical response and normal periosteal response compared with young-adult mice following 1 week of axial tibial compression. J Bone Miner Res 25: 2006–2015.
15. Christiansen BA, Bayly PV, Silva MJ (2008) Constrained tibial vibration in mice: a method for studying the effects of vibrational loading of bone. J Biomech Eng 130: 044502.
16. Silva MJ, Brodt MD, Hucker WJ (2005) Finite element analysis of the mouse tibia: estimating endocortical strain during three-point bending in SAMP6 osteoporotic mice. AnatRecA DiscovMolCell EvolBiol 283: 380–390.
17. Parfitt AM, Drezner MK, Glorieux FH, Kanis JA, Malluche H, et al. (1987) Bone histomorphometry: standardization of nomenclature, symbols, and units. Report of the ASBMR Histomorphometry Nomenclature Committee. J Bone Miner Res 2: 595–610.
18. Foldes J, Shih MS, Parfitt AM (1990) Frequency distributions of tetracycline-based measurements: implications for the interpretation of bone formation indices in the absence of double-labeled surfaces. J Bone Miner Res 5: 1063–1067.
19. Stains JP, Civitelli R (2003) Genomic approaches to identifying transcriptional regulators of osteoblast differentiation. Genome Biol 4: 222.
20. Mbalaviele G, Sheikh S, Stains JP, Salazar VS, Cheng SL, et al. (2005) β-catenin and BMP-2 synergize to promote osteoblast differentiation and new bone formation. J Cell Biochem 94: 403–418.
21. Robinson JA, Chatterjee-Kishore M, Yaworsky PJ, Cullen DM, Zhao W, et al. (2006) Wnt/beta-catenin signaling is a normal physiological response to mechanical loading in bone. J Biol Chem 281: 31720–31728.
22. Forwood MR (1996) Inducible cyclo-oxygenase (COX-2) mediates the induction of bone formation by mechanical loading in vivo. J Bone Miner Res 11: 1688–1693.
23. Gluhak-Heinrich J, Gu S, Pavlin D, Jiang JX (2006) Mechanical loading stimulates expression of connexin 43 in alveolar bone cells in the tooth movement model. Cell CommunAdhes 13: 115–125.
24. Bivi N, Condon KW, Allen MR, Farlow N, Passeri G, et al. (2011) Cell autonomous requirement of connexin 43 for osteocyte survival: consequences for endocortical resorption and periosteal bone formation. J Bone Miner Res 27: 374–389.
25. Fritton JC, Myers ER, Wright TM, van der Meulen MC (2005) Loading induces site-specific increases in mineral content assessed by microcomputed tomography of the mouse tibia. Bone 36: 1030–1038.
26. Fritton JC, Myers ER, Wright TM, van der Meulen MC (2008) Bone mass is preserved and cancellous architecture altered due to cyclic loading of the mouse tibia after orchidectomy. J Bone Miner Res 23: 663–671.
27. Sugiyama T, Saxon LK, Zaman G, Moustafa A, Sunters A, et al. (2008) Mechanical loading enhances the anabolic effects of intermittent parathyroid hormone (1–34) on trabecular and cortical bone in mice. Bone 43: 238–248.
28. De Souza RL, Matsuura M, Eckstein F, Rawlinson SC, Lanyon LE, et al. (2005) Non-invasive axial loading of mouse tibiae increases cortical bone formation and modifies trabecular organization: a new model to study cortical and cancellous compartments in a single loaded element. Bone 37: 810–818.
29. Wyatt SS, Price RA, Holthouse D, Elsaleh H (2001) Choroid plexus carcinoma in an adult. Australasian radiology 45: 369–371.
30. Sawakami K, Robling AG, Ai M, Pitner ND, Liu D, et al. (2006) The Wnt co-receptor LRP5 is essential for skeletal mechanotransduction but not for the anabolic bone response to parathyroid hormone treatment. J Biol Chem 281: 23698–23711.
31. Norvell SM, Alvarez M, Bidwell JP, Pavalko FM (2004) Fluid shear stress induces beta-catenin signaling in osteoblasts. Calcif Tissue Int 75: 396–404.
32. Hens JR, Wilson KM, Dann P, Chen X, Horowitz MC, et al. (2005) TOPGAL mice show that the canonical Wnt signaling pathway is active during bone development and growth and is activated by mechanical loading in vitro. J Bone Miner Res 20: 1103–1113.
33. Lin C, Jiang X, Dai Z, Guo X, Weng T, et al. (2009) Sclerostin mediates bone response to mechanical unloading through antagonizing Wnt/beta-catenin signaling. J Bone Miner Res 24: 1651–1661.
34. Bonewald LF, Johnson ML (2008) Osteocytes, mechanosensing and Wnt signaling. Bone 42: 606–615.
35. Salazar V, Zarkadis N, Huang L, Mbalaviele G, Civitelli R (2011) Smad4 Antagonizes Osteoblast Proliferation via Competitive Recruitment of beta-catenin. 33rd Annual Meeting of the American Society for Bone and Mineral Research, San Diego, California, USA.

12

Role of Tachykinin 1 and 4 Gene-Derived Neuropeptides and the Neurokinin 1 Receptor in Adjuvant-Induced Chronic Arthritis of the Mouse

Éva Borbély[1,2], Zsófia Hajna[1,2], Katalin Sándor[1], László Kereskai[3], István Tóth[1], Erika Pintér[1,2], Péter Nagy[1,2], János Szolcsányi[1], John Quinn[4], Andreas Zimmer[5], James Stewart[6], Christopher Paige[7,8], Alexandra Berger[7,8], Zsuzsanna Helyes[1,2]*

1 Department of Pharmacology and Pharmacotherapy, Faculty of Medicine, University of Pécs, Pécs, Hungary, **2** János Szentágothai Research Center, University of Pécs, Pécs, Hungary, **3** Department of Pathology, Faculty of Medicine, University of Pécs, Pécs, Hungary, **4** Department of Molecular and Clinical Pharmacology, Institute of Translational Medicine Liverpool University, Liverpool, United Kingdom, **5** Laboratory of Molecular Neurobiology, Department of Psychiatry, University of Bonn, Bonn, Germany, **6** School of Infection and Host Defense, University of Liverpool, Liverpool, United Kingdom, **7** Ontario Cancer Institute, University Health Network, Toronto, Canada, **8** Department of Immunology, University of Toronto, Toronto, Canada

Abstract

Objective: Substance P, encoded by the Tac1 gene, is involved in neurogenic inflammation and hyperalgesia via neurokinin 1 (NK1) receptor activation. Its non-neuronal counterpart, hemokinin-1, which is derived from the Tac4 gene, is also a potent NK1 agonist. Although hemokinin-1 has been described as a tachykinin of distinct origin and function compared to SP, its role in inflammatory and pain processes has not yet been elucidated in such detail. In this study, we analysed the involvement of tachykinins derived from the Tac1 and Tac4 genes, as well as the NK1 receptor in chronic arthritis of the mouse.

Methods: Complete Freund's Adjuvant was injected intraplantarly and into the tail of Tac1$^{-/-}$, Tac4$^{-/-}$, Tacr1$^{-/-}$ (NK1 receptor deficient) and Tac1$^{-/-}$/Tac4$^{-/-}$ mice. Paw volume was measured by plethysmometry and mechanosensitivity using dynamic plantar aesthesiometry over a time period of 21 days. Semiquantitative histopathological scoring and ELISA measurement of IL-1β concentrations of the tibiotarsal joints were performed.

Results: Mechanical hyperalgesia was significantly reduced from day 11 in Tac4$^{-/-}$ and Tacr1$^{-/-}$ animals, while paw swelling was not altered in any strain. Inflammatory histopathological alterations (synovial swelling, leukocyte infiltration, cartilage destruction, bone damage) and IL-1β concentration in the joint homogenates were significantly smaller in Tac4$^{-/-}$ and Tac1$^{-/-}$/Tac4$^{-/-}$ mice.

Conclusions: Hemokinin-1, but not substance P increases inflammation and hyperalgesia in the late phase of adjuvant-induced arthritis. While NK1 receptors mediate its antihyperalgesic actions, the involvement of another receptor in histopathological changes and IL-1β production is suggested.

Editor: Oliver Frey, University Hospital Jena, Germany

Funding: Funding provided by Developing Competitiveness of Universities in the South Transdanubian Region (SROP-4.2.2.A-11/1/KONV-2012-0024, SROP-4.2.1.B-10/2/KONV-2010-0002, SROP-4.2.2.B-10/1/2010-0029), OTKA-NK78059, OTKA-K81984, Terry Fox Program Project Grant (National Cancer Institute of Canada #015005), and the Canadian Institute of Health Research (#9862). The funders had no role in study design, data collection and analysis, decision to publish, or preparation of the manuscript.

Competing Interests: The authors have declared that no competing interests exist.

* E-mail: zsuzsanna.helyes@aok.pte.hu

Introduction

Rheumatoid arthritis (RA) is a progressive, systemic auto-immune disease. Among adult Western white populations its prevalence is approximately 1% [1]. Pain and inflammation are the initial symptoms, followed by various degrees of joint destruction. In RA, pain is generally perceived to arise directly from inflammatory processes, as well as from the activation of central and peripheral neuronal mechanisms [2,3]. The peripheral sensory nervous system with special emphasis on the capsaicin-sensitive peptidergic terminals densely innervating the joints, participates in inflammatory and pain processes. Proinflammatory sensory neuropeptides, such as tachykinins and calcitonin-gene related peptide (CGRP) in the target organs induce vasodilatation and recruitment of inflammatory cells to sites of inflammation [4,5]. Increased sensory neuropeptide levels have been demonstrated in the serum and synovial fluid taken from RA patients [6,7] and arthritic animals [8]. More recently Tac1 has been demonstrated to be transiently expressed in non- neuronal cells in response to challenge including chondrocytes and epithelical cells. In several models such expression is implicated in the initiation and progression of the inflammatory process [9,10,11].

Mammalian tachykinins are 10–12 amino acid peptides sharing the hydrophobic C-terminal region FXGLM-NH_2. Substance P (SP) and neurokinin A (NKA), encoded by the preprotachykinin A (Tac1) gene, are expressed predominantly in capsaicin-sensitive primary sensory neurones of the dorsal root ganglia, although transient expression in response to challenge is seen in a variety of non-neuronal cells. Neurokinin B (NKB), derived from the preprotachykinin B (Tac3) gene, is found predominantly in the central nervous system. The newest member of the tachykinin gene family is the preprotachykinin C (Tac4) gene discovered in 2000 [12]. Tac4 encodes hemokinin-1 (HK-1) in mice and its equivalent peptides, endokinins, in human predominantly in immune cells, but also in various brain regions [13].

Three G-protein-coupled mammalian receptors have been identified, to which tachykinins have different affinities [4]. SP binds predominantly to the NK1 tachykinin receptor localized mainly on neuronal, endothelial and immune cells. NKA shows the greatest affinity to NK2 receptors, while NKB to NK3 receptors in the brain. HK-1 is very similar to SP regarding its structure and pharmacology, it has similar receptor binding and preference for NK1 [13,14,15,16,17]. However, some data on the basis of different actions compared to SP, strongly suggest that there might be a specific HK-1 receptor [18].

Tachykinins are conserved in mammalian species, and they are involved in several biological actions, such as smooth muscle contraction, vasodilation, pain transmission, inflammation, haematopoiesis, activation of the immune and endocrine system, and emotional behaviour [19,20,21]. In contrast to other tachykinins, HK-1 is mainly expressed in non-neuronal tissues. Tac4 expression levels are significantly lower in most neuronal, but higher in peripheral tissues compared to Tac1 [13]. Since Tac4 mRNA expression has been detected in a variety of immune cells, such as T and B lymphocytes, macrophages and dendritic cells, [12,22,23] HK-1 may have an important role in immune regulation.

Tachykinin research was florishing 15–20 years ago, and NK1 receptor antagonists were suggested as potential anti-inflammatory and analgesic agents according to their efficacy in animal experiments. However, most clinical trials did not reflect that promise [24,25]. This might have been due to species differences in biology or pharmacodynamics of specific antagonists, but also to the fact that these agents were designed to block SP binding. The recent discovery of Tac4-derived tachykinins and evidence on the transient expression of Tac1 in non-neuronal cells revived the

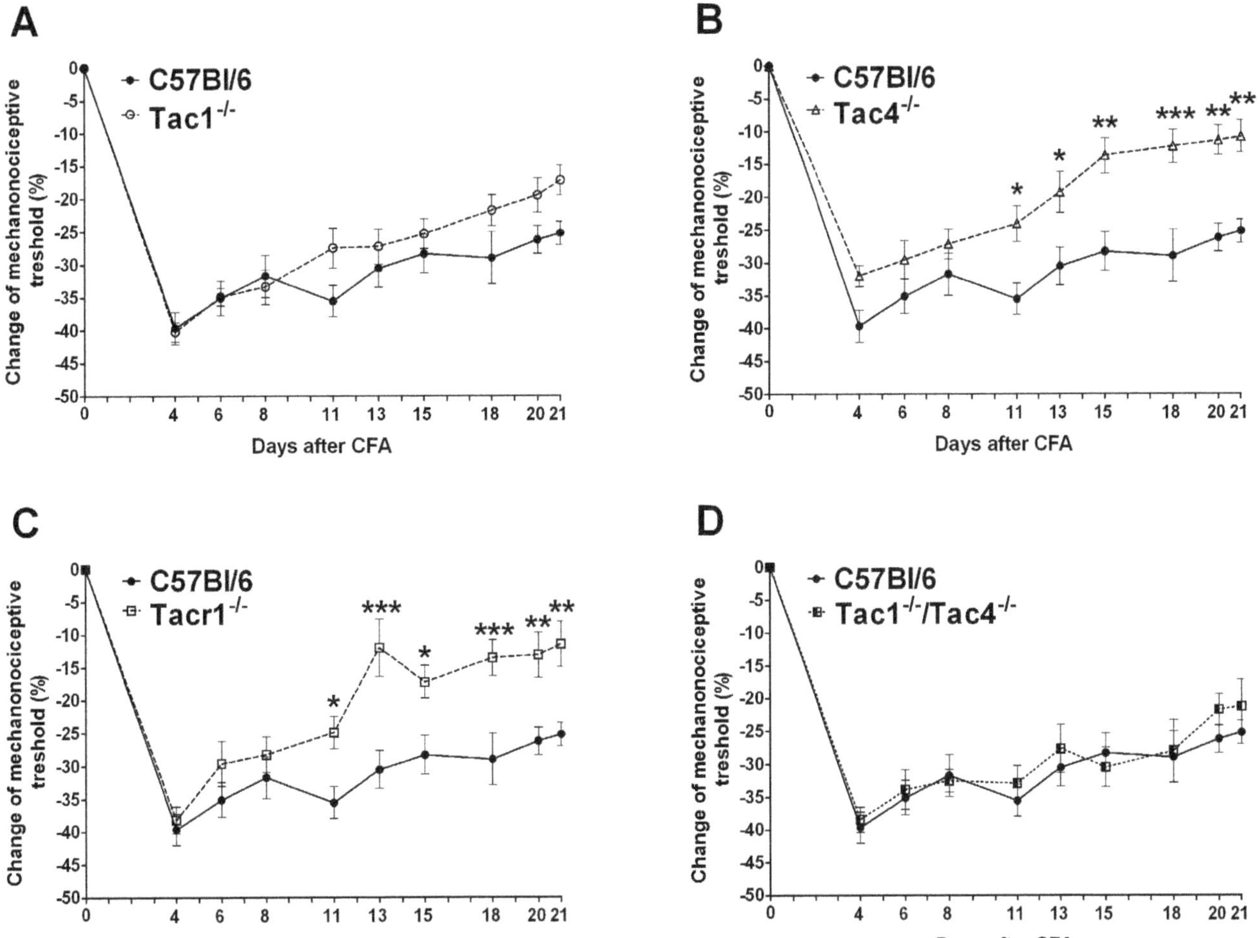

Figure 1. Adjuvant-induced mechanical hyperalgesia throughout the 21-day experimental period. Each data point represents the mean ± SEM of the percentage decrease of the mechanonociceptive threshold of (**A**) Tac1$^{-/-}$, (**B**) Tac4$^{-/-}$, (**C**) Tacr1$^{-/-}$, (**D**) Tac1$^{-/-}$/Tac4$^{-/-}$ mice compared to the initial control values (n = 9–24 mice per group; *p<0.05, **p<0.01, ***p<0.001 vs. C57Bl/6; two-way ANOVA followed by Bonferroni's modified t-test).

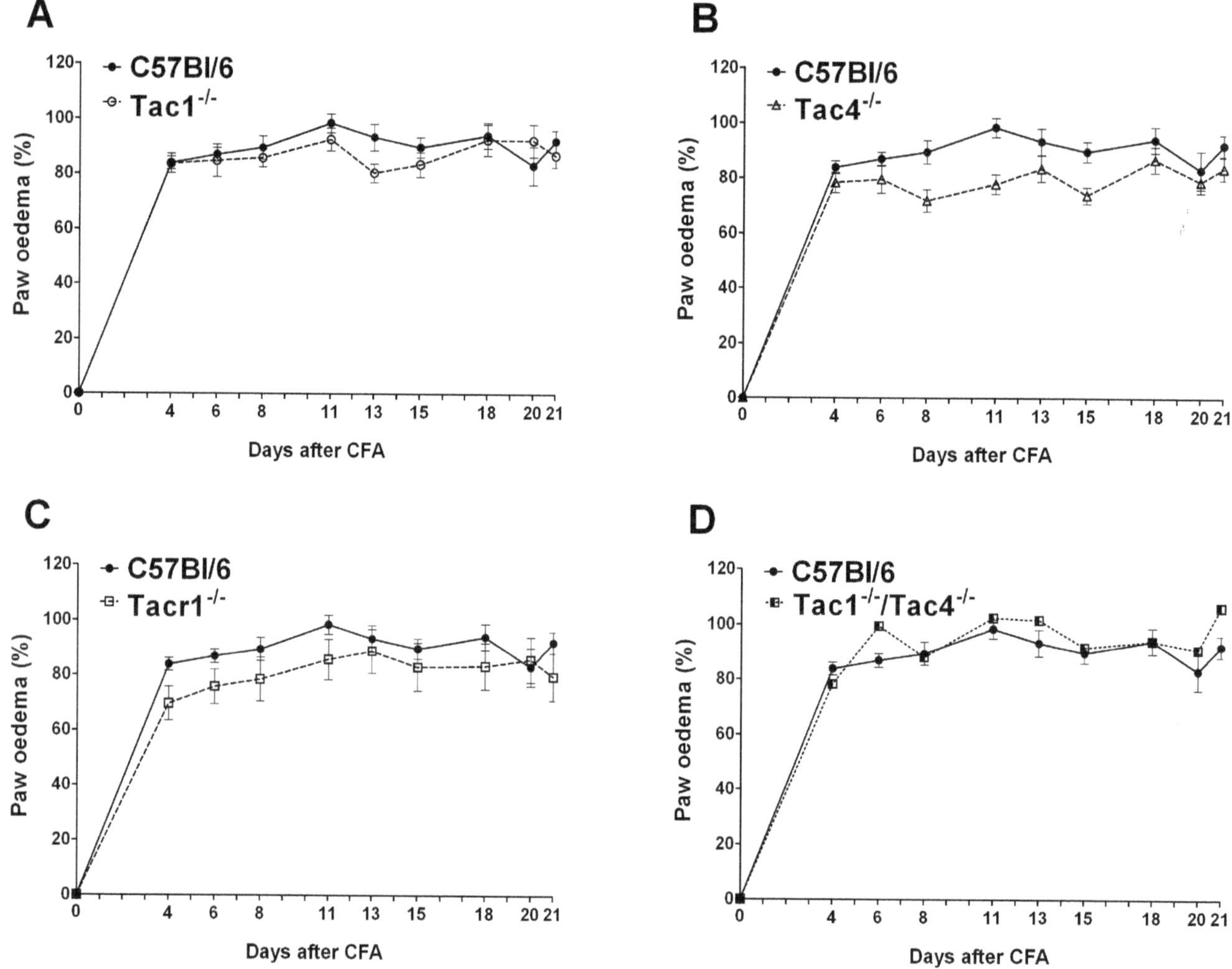

Figure 2. Adjuvant-induced oedema throughout the 21-day experimental period. Each data point represents the mean ± SEM of the percentage increase of the paw volume of (**A**) Tac1$^{-/-}$, (**B**) Tac4$^{-/-}$, (**C**) Tacr1$^{-/-}$, (**D**) Tac1$^{-/-}$/Tac4$^{-/-}$ mice compared to the initial control values (n = 9–24 mice per group, two-way ANOVA followed by Bonferroni's modified t-test).

tachykinin research field [10]. Our present study represents an integrative analysis of the role and complexity of the tachykinin system in a murine model of chronic arthritis evoked by the administration of complete Freund's adjuvant using genetically manipulated tachykinin and receptor knockout mouse strains.

Methods

Ethics Statement

All experimental procedures were carried out according to the 1998/XXVIII Act of the Hungarian Parliament on Animal Protection and Consideration Decree of Scientific Procedures of Animal Experiments (243/1988) and complied with the recommendations of the International Association for the Study of Pain and the Helsinki Declaration. The studies were approved by the Ethics Committee on Animal Research of University of Pécs according to the Ethical Codex of Animal Experiments and licence was given (licence No.: BA 02/2000–2/2012).

Experimental Animals

Experiments were performed on male NK1 receptor (Tacr1$^{-/-}$), Tac1$^{-/-}$, Tac4$^{-/-}$ and Tac1$^{-/-}$/Tac4$^{-/-}$ gene-deficient mice backcrossed for 8–10 generations to C57Bl/6 mice. C57Bl/6 mice were used as wildtype (WT) controls and the original breeding pairs were purchased from Charles-River Ltd. (Hungary). Tac1$^{-/-}$ and Tacr1$^{-/-}$ mice were generated at the University of Liverpool as previously described [26,27,28,29]. Tac4$^{-/-}$ and Tac1$^{-/-}$/Tac4$^{-/-}$ mice were obtained from Berger et al. [30,31]. The animals were bred and kept in the Laboratory Animal House of the Department of Pharmacology and Pharmacotherapy of the University of Pécs at 24–25°C, provided with standard mouse chow and water ad libitum and maintained under a 12-h light-dark cycle.

Induction of Arthritis

We have previously adapted the adjuvant-induced arthritis originally developed in Lewis rats [29] to mice to create a suitable experimental model for the examination of long-term joint inflammation in genetically manipulated animals [32]. Chronic arthritis of mice weighing 20–22 g (C57Bl/6 n = 24, Tac1$^{-/-}$ n = 22, Tac4$^{-/-}$ n = 18, Tacr1$^{-/-}$ n = 19, Tac1$^{-/-}$/Tac4$^{-/-}$ n = 9; since there were 4 different gene-deleted strains and the study was performed in 5 experimental series in order to be able to precisely carry out all measurements, wildtypes were investigated

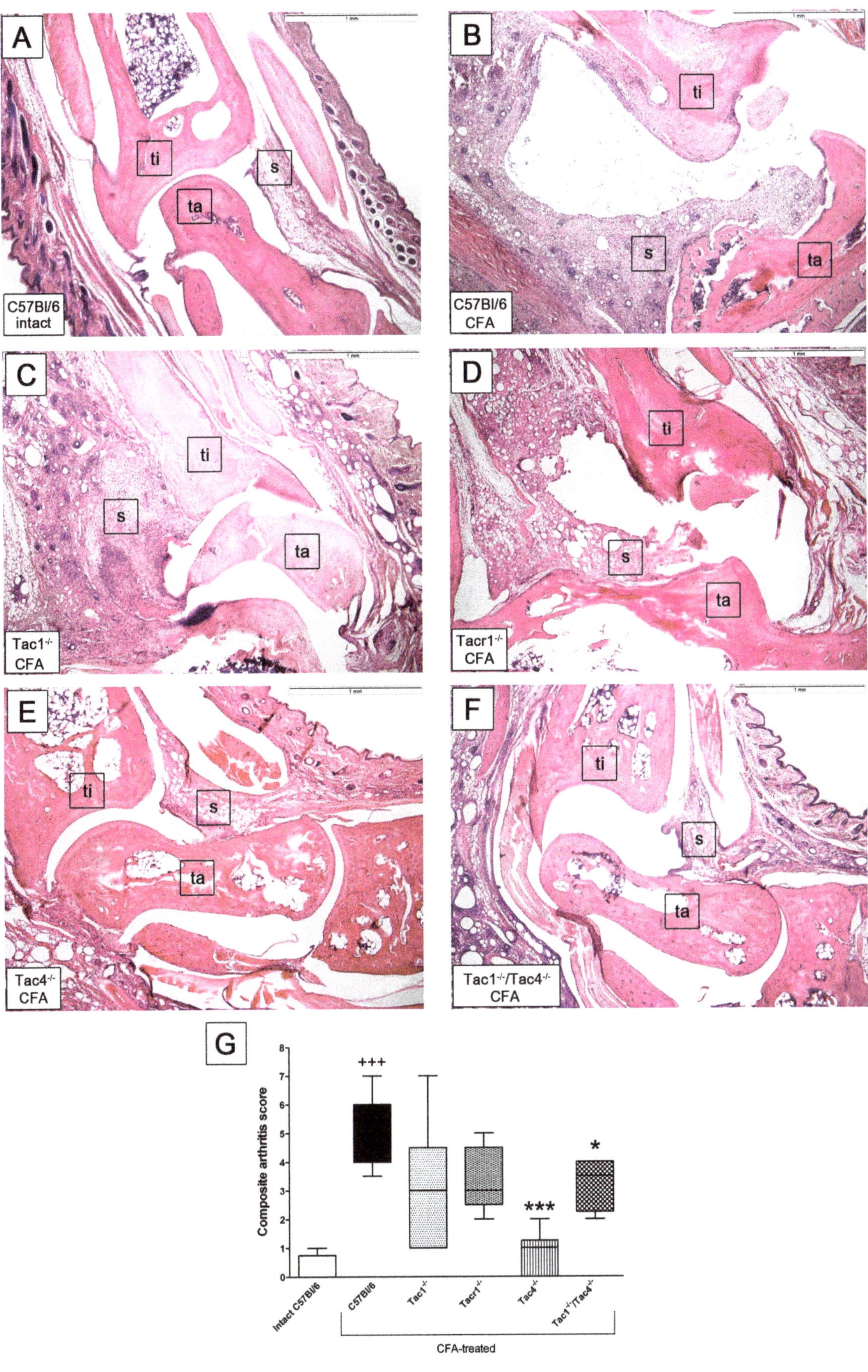
A
ti
s
ta
C57Bl/6
intact
B
ti
s
ta
C57Bl/6
CFA
C
ti
s
ta
Tac1-/-
CFA
D
ti
s
ta
Tacr1-/-
CFA
E
ti
s
ta
Tac4-/-
CFA
F
ti
s
ta
Tac1-/-/Tac4-/-
CFA
G
Composite arthritis score
+++
*
***
Intact C57Bl/6
C57Bl/6
Tac1-/-
Tacr1-/-
Tac4-/-
Tac1-/-/Tac4-/-
CFA-treated

Figure 3. Histopathological changes of the paws on day 21. Panel **A** shows a representative histopathological picture of an intact tibiotarsal joint and panel **B** demonstrates the joint structure of an adjuvant-treated C57Bl/6 wildtype mouse with remarkable synovial swelling, leukocyte infiltration, cartilage damage, and bone destruction. The lower panes demonstrate the joint structures of adjuvant-treated (**C**) Tac1$^{-/-}$, (**D**) Tacr1$^{-/-}$, (**E**) Tac4$^{-/-}$, and (**F**) Tac1$^{-/-}$/Tac4$^{-/-}$ mice, decreased inflammatory parameters can be observed in the latter two groups. Hematoxylin-eosin staining, 40x magnification (ti: tibia, ta: tarsus, s: synovium). (**G**) Semiquantitative histopathological scoring on the basis of inflammatory cell accumulation, synovial enlargement, cartilage destruction and bone erosion. Box plots represent the composite scores (n=4–12 mice per group,$^{+++}$p<0.001 vs. intact C57Bl/6, *p<0.05, ***p<0.001 vs. C57Bl/6 CFA-treated, Kruskal-Wallis followed by Dunn's post test).

in each series to minimize potential bias and differences induced by environmental changes.) was induced by intraplantar injection of 50 µl of Complete Freund's Adjuvant (CFA, killed Mycobacteria suspended in paraffin oil, 1 mg/ml; Sigma, St. Louis, MO) into the right hind paw and s.c. into the root of the tail. An additional s.c. injection was given on the following day into the tail in order to potentiate the systemic effects and to make our model more similar to the human disease, as described in our earlier studies [32,34].

Measurement of Touch Sensitivity of the Paw

Touch sensitivity of the plantar surface of the paw was determined by dynamic plantar aesthesiometry (Ugo Basile 37400, Comerio, Italy) before and 4, 6, 8, 11, 13, 15, 18, 20 and 21 days after CFA administration. This device is a modified, electronic von Frey technique, which is used to assess mechanonociception. Mechanical hyperalgesia was expressed as % of control mechanonociceptive threshold compared to the initial values [29,32,33].

Measurement of the Paw Volume

Paw volume was measured by plethysmometry (Ugo Basile Plethysmometer 7140, Comerio, Italy) [29,32]. Volumes were measured prior to CFA-injection, and 4, 6, 8, 11, 13, 15, 18, 20 and 21 days after CFA administration. Oedema was expressed in percentage compared to the initial values [34].

Histological Processing and Assessment of Joint Inflammation

Mice were anaesthetized with ketamine (100 mg/kg, i.p., Richter Gedeon Plc., Hungary) and xylazine (10 mg/kg, i.m., Lavet Ltd., Hungary), then sacrificed by cervical dislocation on day 21 after CFA administration and the paws were excised. After formaldehyde fixation, decalcification and dehydration the samples were embedded in paraffin, sectioned (5 µm) and stained with hematoxylin and eosin [29,32].

Arthritic changes were scored by an observer blinded from the treatment the animals received using a grading scale of 0 to 3 according to the 1) proportion of the areolar tissue, infiltration by mononuclear cells, synovial lining cell hyperplasia, 2) the number of leukocytes observed in the synovial tissue, 3) cartilage destruction and 4) bone erosion. The score values given for these four different histopathological features were added to generate a composite arthritis score ranging between 0 and 12 [29,32].

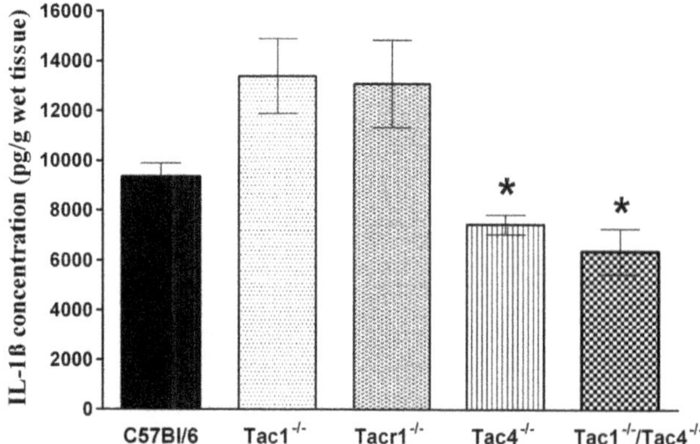

Figure 4. Concentrations of the inflammatory cytokine interleukin-1β (IL-1β) in the joint homogenates on day 21. Each bar represents the mean ± SEM of each group (n=5–12 mice per group, *p<0.05 vs. C57Bl/6; Kruskal-Wallis followed by Dunn's post test).

Determination of IL-1β Concentrations in Tissue Homogenates

Excised paws were frozen in liquid nitrogen and kept at −80°C until further processing. Samples were homogenized in 1 ml buffer containing 990 µl RPMI 1640 medium and 10 µl PMSF (phenyl-methyl-sulphonyl-fluoride) protease inhibitor for 2 min at 21,000 rpm with Miccra D-9 Digitronic device (Art-moderne Laborteknik, Germany), centrifuged for 10 min at 5°C at 12,500 rpm, and the supernatants were stored at −20°C. The concentrations of the inflammatory cytokine IL-1β were measured by ELISA using IL-1β OptEIA set (BD Biosciences, USA).

Statistical Analysis

All data were carefully tested for normal distribution (GraphPad Prism). Since hyperalgesia and oedema values followed normal distribution, they were evaluated by repeated measures two-way analysis of variance (ANOVA) followed by Bonferroni's modified t-test in order to be able to compare the results at distinct timepoints. Since cytokine concentrations and semiquantitative composite arthritis scores were not normally distributed, they were analysed by the non-parametric Kruskal-Wallis test followed by Dunn's post test to evaluate the differences between gene-deleted and WT mice. In all cases P<0.05 was considered to be significant, which are indicated in the graphs, where applicable.

Results

Role of Tachykinins in Adjuvant-induced Inflammatory Mechanical Hyperalgesia

In WT mice an approximately 40% decrease of the mechanonociceptive threshold developed 4 days after adjuvant injection, which gradually decreased to 20% by the end of the study (Figure 1). Significantly reduced mechanical hyperalgesia was observed in the Tac4 and Tacr1 gene-deleted groups starting on day 11 of the experiment (Figures 1B, C). In contrast, no significant difference in pain thresholds was detected in either Tac1$^{-/-}$ or Tac1$^{-/-}$/Tac4$^{-/-}$ mice (Figures 1A, D).

Tachykinins are not Involved in Adjuvant-induced Oedema

In control animals, the volume of the CFA-injected paws increased to about 90% within 4 days post adjuvant injection, reaching a maximal swelling of approximately 98% 11 days after

Table 1. Summary of functional, morphological and immunological alterations in gene-deleted mouse strains compared to the C57Bl/6 WT group.

Mouse strain	Hyperalgesia	Oedema formation	Histopathological alterations	IL-1β
Tac1$^{-/-}$	–	–	–	–
Tacr1$^{-/-}$	↓	–	–	–
Tac4$^{-/-}$	↓	–	↓	↓
Tac1$^{-/-}$/Tac4$^{-/-}$	–	–	↓	↓

Mechanical hyperalgesia was significantly attenuated in Tac4$^{-/-}$ and Tacr1$^{-/-}$ animals, while oedema formation did not differ in any strain. Inflammatory reactions characterised by the histological alterations and changes of cytokine levels were significantly reduced in Tac4$^{-/-}$ and Tac1$^{-/-}$/Tac4$^{-/-}$ groups.

the induction of inflammation. No significant differences were observed in any knockout strains compared to controls (Figure 2).

Role of Tachykinins in Adjuvant-induced Arthritic Histopathological Alterations

There was no difference between the intact joint structures of C57Bl/6 WT (Figure 3A) and any gene-deleted mice (data not shown). Meanwhile, the right tibiotarsal joints of adjuvant-injected WT mice were damaged by expanding synovial pannus. Widening of the synovial cavity, synovial hyperplasia and its infiltration with inflammatory cells, as well as cartilage destruction and minimal bone erosion were apparent (Figure 3B). There were only mild inflammatory changes, such as synovial swelling and inflammatory cell influx on the contralateral side showing systemic manifestations of the disease (picture not shown). Histopathological alterations typically seen in arthritic joints of the WT mice were not altered in Tac1$^{-/-}$ and Tacr1$^{-/-}$ mice (Figures 3C, D), while they were reduced in the Tac4$^{-/-}$ and Tac1$^{-/-}$/Tac4$^{-/-}$ groups: synovial swelling, lymphocyte accumulation and cartilage erosion were diminished and signs of bone destruction were not detectable (Figures 3E, F). The semiquantitative scoring obtained from measuring the characteristic inflammatory parameters demonstrates the significantly decreased severity of arthritis in Tac4$^{-/-}$ and Tac1$^{-/-}$/Tac4$^{-/-}$ mice (Figure 3G).

Role of Tachykinins in Adjuvant-induced IL-1β Production in the Joints

The IL-1β concentration in the intact tibiotarsal joint homogenates of all mouse groups was below the detection limit of the ELISA technique. Adjuvant administration induced an approximately 9000 pg/g production of this inflammatory cytokine in WT control mice. In accordance with the histopathological scoring, IL-1β production was significantly lower in the joints of Tac4$^{-/-}$ and Tac1$^{-/-}$/Tac4$^{-/-}$ double knockout mice compared to WT controls (Figure 4).

Discussion

The present study provides the first evidence that HK-1 increases inflammatory pain in the chronic phase of CFA-induced arthritis. Although it does not perfectly mimic all pathophysiological processes of rheumatoid arthritis, but is a widely used, well-defined and internationally accepted model with several similarities in the mechanisms (T cell dominant immune response with increase of TNFα, IL-1β, IFNγ, IL-6, IL-17 levels) and symptoms (synovial hyperplasia, inflammatory cell accumulation, cartilage destruction and bone erosion) of the human disease. In addition in several cases results of this model were reliable indicators of efficacy and toxicity of new therapeutics [35,36,37]. HK-1 also plays a predominant role in the development of inflammatory morphological alterations and inflammatory cytokine production in the joint. Interestingly, our data reveals for the first time that HK-1 exerts different effects through different mechanisms. While the development of mechanical hyperalgesia involves NK1 receptors, the development of arthritic histopathological changes are not NK1 receptor mediated (Table 1).

Joints are innervated by capsaicin-sensitive afferents that are not only responsible for nociception and pain sensation, but also exert local and systemic effector functions through the released sensory neuropeptides [4,5]. Neurogenic inflammatory component defined as vasodilatation, plasma protein extravasation and inflammatory cell recruitment in response to the activation of sensory fibres plays a significant role in rheumatoid arthritis [38]. Transection of sensory nerves reduces hyperalgesia, swelling and joint destruction in artritis models [2]. Our previous results with Transient Receptor Potential Vanilloid 1 (TRPV1) capsaicin receptor deficient mice revealed that the activation of this ion channel by bradykinin, lipoxygenase products and prostanoids enhances the adjuvant-induced oedema, mechanical hyperalgesia and inflammatory reaction in this murine model of arthritis [32]. The release of pro-inflammatory neuropeptides, such as tachykinins (e.g. SP, NKA and NKB), as well as CGRP from these fibers results in neurogenic inflammation around the site of activation. CGRP induces local vasodilatation and SP evokes plasma protein extravasation through NK1 receptor activation on vascular endothelial cells, modulate inflammatory and immune cell functions [4,5], as well as its central release in the spinal dorsal horn activates the pain pathway [27,39]. Furthermore, there is a significant number of SP-positive sensory fibres in the synovial tissue. In a healthy joint both the cell lining layer and some nerves branching towards the synovial space are SP-containing [27,40]. The density of SP-positive sensory fibres is increased in the synovium of RA patients, but decreased in osteoarthritis [41].

Although the patterns and levels of expression of Tac1- and Tac4-derived peptides at early time points prior to the immune response initiation is not known, the present results outline the complexity of the tachykinin system in different mechanisms in arthritis and arthritis-related pain [10,11]. For decades, SP was the only tachykinin known to be detected by anti-SP antibodies, and a positive readout in a SP radioimmunassay was interpreted as SP immunoreactivity. However the discovery of Tac4 gene-derived peptides changed the interpretation of this paradigm. Since hemokinins and endokinins exhibit structural homology, this consequently results in immunological crossreactivity with anti-SP antibodies. Thus, to date SP and HK-1 cannot be differentiated by radioimmunoassay [16]. It has therefore been suggested, that in several experimental layouts the measured SP-like immunoreactivity reflects both SP and HK-1 contents. Hemokinins were first classified as tachykinins derived from hematopoietic cells [12], but recently they have been shown in immune cells e.g. T and B lymphocytes, macrophages and dendritic cells in the periphery, mediating a broad range of hematopoietic and inflammatory actions [12,22,23,42]. A recent paper has reported that SP and HK-1 are similarly involved in the differentiation of memory CD4+ T cells into Th17 cells via NK1 receptor activation and production of certain cytokines, indicating that SP and HK-1 may act locally on memory T cells to amplify inflammatory responses and could be critical targets in several inflammatory disorders. The other members of the tachykinin family, neurokinins A and B, have no effect on the differentiation of naive and memory T cells [43]. However, HK-1 is also expressed in the sensory nervous system and has a remarkable selectivity and potency for the NK1 receptors [13]. These characteristics allow HK-1 to participate in pain mediation. Nevertheless, HK-1 might have different binding sites on the NK1 receptors, distinct receptor activation mechanisms and signal transduction pathways compared to SP [44]. Furthermore, Endo and colleagues have raised the possibility of a presently unidentified proper receptor related to HK-1 on the basis of several actions of hemokinins different from that of SP [18].

Besides, similarly to SP, HK-1 was also found to enhance the induction of scratching behavior by resiniferatoxin, a TRPV1 agonist, indicating that both HK-1 and SP modulate the response to TRPV1 receptor activation [45].

Concerning chronic autoimmune/inflammatory diseases in human, a recent publication has suggested that HK-1 may be involved in the pathophysiology of inflammatory bowel diseases, such as ulcerative colitis [46], but no data are available on its role in arthritic diseases. However, promising approaches highlight the importance of B cell targeting in arthritis therapy [47]. Since B cells are an important source of HK-1, decreased HK-1 production and release might be an explanation for the efficacy of rituximab, the anti-CD20 monoclonal anibody inducing B cell depletion in rheumatoid arthritis patients [48].

In contrast, the role of NK1 receptors in inflammatory joint diseases has been investigated for decades and a lot of information is available for various disease models and clinical trials. NK1 receptor mRNA is highly expressed in the synovia of RA patients, which is downregulated by tumor necrosis factor alpha [49]. Intraarticular pretreatment with of the NK1 receptor antagonist L-703,606, reduces carrageenan-evoked inflammatory pain, but not oedema in the rat knee [50]. Intaarticular injection of another NK1 receptor antagonist (RP67580) improved the efficacy of dexamethasone to attenuate knee oedema and arthritic allodynia during the experimental period of 7 days of CFA-induced arthritis [51]. Both intraarticular and intraplantar injection of NK1 receptor antagonists 2 days after arthritis induction, reduced pain, oedema and progressive joint destruction in the rat [52].

Adjuvant-induced inflammatory mechanical hyperalgesia, was significantly and similarly reduced from the 11th day of the experiment in $Tac4^{-/-}$ and $Tacr1^{-/-}$ animals, but not in the other knockouts compared to wildtypes suggesting that HK-1 induces hyperalgesia through NK1 receptor activation on sensory neurons. Besides peripheral mechanisms at the nerve terminals, central sensitization in the spinal cord also plays a predominant role in this process.

Although we do not have a precise explanation for why the hyperalgesic action of HK-1 presumably at the NK1 receptors is not observed when SP and NKA are also missing from the system, some hypothesis can be made: a) HK-1 exerts its hyperalgesic effect in the nociceptive pathway through the NK1 tachykinin receptor, but it is counteracted by NKA acting at NK2 receptors in the central nervous system [53], b) HK-1 and SP act at the same receptors (NK1), but they might have different binding sites, affinities and intinsinc efficacies, as well as distinct activation mechanisms and signalling pathways. When both are removed from the system, the inhibition observed in case of the HK-1 absence, might be counteracted via intracellular molecular mechanisms.

There are contradictory data on the role of the tachykinin system in joint swelling. Only some, but not all NK1 receptor antagonists attenuate oedema [50,51]. Our data also suggest that tachykinins and NK1 receptors are not involved in aduvant-induced swelling.

The inflammatory changes in the joint were also significantly decreased in Tac4 gene-deleted mice, but in contrast to hyperalgesia there were no changes in Tacr1 knockouts. Therefore, a different mechanism seems to mediate the inflammatory functions of HK-1, and a role for a putative HK receptor can be proposed. There are data showing interactions between the tachykinin system and cytokines in rheumatoid arthritis. Monocytes of RA patients secrete greater amounts of TNFα after SP-treatment, compared to monocytes of healthy controls [54]. Reduced substance P release and disease severity were observed after the TNFα inhibitor etanercept treatment in RA patients [55]. Although RA is known as a TNFα dominant disease, other interleukines are also involved in chronic joint destruction. IL-1β plays a role in the immune response modulation and osteoclast activation [56]. In agreement with the histopathological findings, IL-1β decrease in joint homogenates of Tac4 and double gene-deleted mice also suggest that HK-1 acts at another receptor, not the NK1.

In summary, we provided the first evidence for inflammatory and nociceptive roles of HK-1 in a mouse model of chronic arthritis. However, the mechanisms of these actions are different: the peripheral inflammatory effects are not NK1 receptor-mediated, but mechanical hyperalgesia involving central sensitization is dependent on NK1 activation. Based on the present results, identification of the target and the precise signalling pathways, then antagonizing the actions of HK-1 might be a new perspective for the treatment of arthritis.

Acknowledgments

The authors are grateful to Anikó Perkecz for her expert help in histological processing and for Dr. Ágnes Kemény for editing Fig. 3.

Author Contributions

Conceived and designed the experiments: Z. Helyes EP J. Szolcsányi. Performed the experiments: ÉB KS LK IT PN. Analyzed the data: ÉB KS. Contributed reagents/materials/analysis tools: AB JQ AZ J. Stewart CP. Wrote the paper: ÉB Z. Hajna AB Z. Helyes.

References

1. Abdel-Nasser AM, Rasker JJ, Valkenburg HA (1997) Epidemiological and clinical aspects relating to the variability of rheumatoid arthritis. Seminars in Arthritis & Rheumatism 27: 123–140.
2. Levine JD, Collier DH, Basbaum AI, Moskowitz MA, Helms CA (1986) Hypothesis: the nervous system may contribute to the pathophysiology of rheumatoid arthritis. J Rheumatol 12: 406–11.

3. Schaible HG, von Banchet GS, Boettger MK, Bräuer R, Gajda M, et al. (2010) The role of proinflammatory cytokines in the generation and maintenance of joint pain. Ann N Y Acad Sci. 1193: 60–9.
4. Maggi CA (1995) Tachykinins and calcitonin gene-related peptide (CGRP) as cotransmitters released from peripheral endings of sensory nerves. Prog Neurobiol. 45: 1–98.
5. Szolcsanyi J (1996) Capsaicin-sensitive sensory nerve terminals with local and systemic efferent functions: facts and scopes of an unorthodox neuroregulatory mechanism. Prog Brain Res. 113: 343–59.
6. Anichini M, Cesaretti S, Lepori M, Maddali Bongi S, Maresca M, et al. (1997) Substance P in the serum of patients with rheumatoid arthritis. Rev Rhum Engl Ed. 64: 18–21.
7. Larsson J, Ekblom A, Henriksson K, Lundeberg T, Theodorsson E (1991) Concentration of substance P, neurokinin A, calcitonin generelated peptide, neuropeptide Y and vasoactive intestinal polypeptide in synovial fluid from knee joints in patients suffering from rheumatoid arthritis. Scand J Rheumatol 20: 326–35.
8. Bileviciute I, Lundeberg T, Ekblom A, Theodorsson E (1993) Bilateral changes of substance P-, neurokinin A-, calcitonin gene-related peptide- and neuropeptide Y-like immunoreactivity in rat knee joint synovial fluid during acute monoarthritis. Neurosci Lett 153: 37–40.
9. Stewart JP, Kipar A, Cox H, Payne C, Vasiliou S, et al. (2008) Induction of tachykinin production in airway epithelia in response to viral infection. PLoS ONE 3: e1673.
10. Millward-Sadler SJ, Mackenzie A, Wright MO, Lee HS, Elliot K, et al. (2003) Tachykinin expression in cartilage and function in human articular chondrocyte mechanotransduction. Arthritis Rheum 48: 146–156.
11. Howard MR, Millward-Sadler SJ, Vasilliou AS, Salter DM, Quinn JP (2008) Mechanical stimulation induces preprotachykinin gene expression in osteoarthritic chondrocytes which is correlated with modulation of the transcription factor neuron restrictive silence factor. Neuropeptides 42: 681–686.
12. Zhang Y, Lu L, Furlonger C, Wu GE, Paige CJ (2000) Hemokinin is a hematopoietic-specific tachykinin that regulates B lymphopoiesis. Nat Immunol 1: 392–397.
13. Duffy RA, Hedrick JA, Randolph G, Morgan CA, Cohen-Williams ME, et al. (2003) Centrally administered Hemokinin-1 (HK-1), a neurokinin NK1 receptor agonist, produces substance P-like behavioral effects in mice and gerbils. Neuropharmacology 45: 242–250.
14. Berger A, Paige CJ (2005) Hemokinin-1 has substance P-like function in U-251 MG astrocytoma cells: a pharmacological and functional study. J. Neuroimmunol 164: 48–56.
15. Kurtz MM, Wang R, Clements MK, Cascieri MA, Austin CP, et al. (2002) Identification, localization and receptor characterization of novel mammalian substance P-like peptides. Gene 296: 205–212.
16. Page NM (2004) Hemokinins and endokinins. Cell Mol Life Sci. 61: 1652–63.
17. Page NM (2006) Characterization of the gene structures, precursor processing and pharmacology of the endokinin peptides. Vascul Pharmacol 45: 200–208.
18. Endo D, Ikeda T, Ishida Y, Yoshioka D, Nishimori T (2006) Effect of intrathecal administration of hemokinin-1 on the withdrawal response to noxious thermal stimulation of the rat hind paw. Neurosci Lett 392: 114–117.
19. Graham GJ, Stevens JM, Page NM, Grant AD, Brain SD, et al. (2004) Tachykinins regulate the function of platelets. Blood 104: 1058–1065.
20. Longmore J, Hill RG, Hargreaves RJ (1997) Neurokinin-receptor antagonists: pharmacological tools and therapeutic drugs. Can J Physiol Pharmacol 75: 612–621.
21. Pernow B. (1983) Substance P – a putative mediator of antidromic vasodilation. Gen Pharmacol 14: 13–16.
22. Metwali A, Blum AM, Elliott DE., Setiawan T, Weinstock JV (2004) Cutting edge: Hemokinin has substance P-like function and expression in inflammation. J Immunol 172: 6528–6532.
23. Nelson DA, Bost KL (2004) Non-neuronal mammalian tachykinin expression. Front Biosci 9: 2166–2176.
24. Hill R (2000) NK1 (substance P) receptor antagonists–why are they not analgesic in humans? Trends Pharmacol Sci. 7: 244–6.
25. Urban LA, Fox AJ (2000) NK1 receptor antagonists–are they really without effect in the pain clinic? Trends Pharmacol Sci. 12: 462–4.
26. Zimmer A, Zimmer AM, Baffi J, Usdin T, Reynolds K, et al. (1998) Hypoalgesia in mice with a targeted deletion of the tachykinin 1 gene. Proc Natl Acad Sci U S A. 3: 2630–5.
27. De Felipe C, Herrero JF, O'Brien JA, Palmer JA, Doyle CA, et al. (1998) Altered nociception, analgesia and aggression in mice lacking the receptor for substance P. Nature. 26: 394–7.
28. Laird JM, Olivar T, Roza C, De Felipe C, Hunt SP, et al. (2000) Deficits in visceral pain and hyperalgesia of mice with a disruption of the tachykinin NK1 receptor gene. Neuroscience. 98: 345–52.
29. Helyes Zs, Szabó Á, Németh J, Jakab B, Pintér E, et al. (2004) Anti-inflammatory and analgesic effect of somatostatin released from capsaicin-sensitive sensory nerve terminals in Freund's adjuvant-induced chronic arthritis model of the rat. Arthritis Rheum 50: 1677–85.
30. Berger A, Benveniste P, Corfe SA, Tran AH, Barbara M, et al. (2010) Targeted deletion of the tachykinin 4 gene (TAC4−/−) influences the early stages of B lymphocyte development. Blood 116: 3792–801.
31. Berger A, Tran AH, Dida J, Minkin S, Gerard NP, et al. (2012) Diminished pheromone-induced sexual behavior in neurokinin-1 receptor deficient (TACR1(−/−)) mice. Genes Brain Behav. 11: 568–76.
32. Szabó Á, Helyes Zs, Sándor K, Bite A, Pintér E, et al. (2005) Role of TRPV1 receptors in adjuvant-induced chronic arthritis: in vivo study using gene-deficient mice. J Pharmacol Exp Ther 314: 111–9.
33. Bölcskei K, Helyes Zs, Szabó Á, Sándor K, Pethő G, et al. (2005) Investigation of the role of TRPV1 receptors in acute and chronic nociceptive processes using genedeficient mice. Pain 117: 368–76.
34. Helyes Zs, Pintér E, Németh J, Sándor K, Elekes K, et al. (2006) Effects of the somatostatin receptor subtype 4 selective agonist J-2156 on sensory neuropeptide release and inflammatory reactions in rodents. Br J Pharmacol 149: 405–15.
35. Bevaart L, Vervoordeldonk MJ, Tak PP (2010) Evaluation of therapeutic targets in animal models of arthritis: how does it relate to rheumatoid arthritis? Arthritis Rheum. 62: 2192–205.
36. Billiau A, Matthys P (2001) Modes of action of Freund's adjuvants in experimental models of autoimmune diseases. J Leukoc Biol. 70: 849–60.
37. Hegen M, Keith JC, Collins M, Nickerson-Nutter CL (2008) Utility of animal models for identification of potential therapeutics for rheumatoid arthritis. Ann Rheum Dis. 67: 1505–15.
38. Jorgensen C, Sany J (1994) Modulation of the immune response by the neuroendocrine axis in rheumatoid arthritis. Clin Exp Rheumatol. 12: 435–41.
39. Ribeiro-da-Silva A, Hökfelt T (2000) Neuroanatomical localisation of Substance P in the CNS and sensory neurons. Neuropeptides 34: 256–271.
40. Keeble JE, Brain SD (2004) A role for substance P in arthritis? Neurosci Lett. 6: 176–9.
41. Weidler C, Holzer C, Harbuz M, Hofbauer R, Angele P, et al. (2005) Low density of sympathetic nerve fibres and increased density of brain derived neurotrophic factor positive cells in RA synovium. Ann Rheum Dis. 64: 13–20.
42. Tran AH, Berger A, Wu GE, Paige CJ (2009) Regulatory mechanisms in the differential expression of Hemokinin-1. Neuropeptides. 43: 1–12.
43. Cunin P, Caillon A, Corvaisier M, Garo E, Scotet M, et al. (2011) The tachykinins substance P and hemokinin-1 favor the generation of human memory Th17 cells by inducing IL-1β, IL-23, and TNF-like 1A expression by monocytes. J Immunol. 186: 4175–82.
44. Kurtz MM, Wang R, Clements MK, Cascieri MA, Austin CP, et al. (2002) Identification, localization and receptor characterization of novel mammalian substance P-like peptides. Gene. 296: 205–12.
45. Naono-Nakayama R, Sunakawa N, Ikeda T, Nishimori T (2010) Differential effects of substance P or hemokinin-1 on transient receptor potential channels, TRPV1, TRPA1 and TRPM8, in the rat. Subcutaneous injection of endokinin C/D attenuates carrageenan-induced inflammation. Neuropeptides. 44: 57–61.
46. Liu L, Markus I, Saghire HE, Perera DS, King DW, et al. (2011) Distinct differences in tachykinin gene expression in ulcerative colitis, Crohn's disease and diverticular disease: a role for hemokinin-1? Neurogastroenterol Motil. 23: 475–83.
47. Chen DR, Cohen PL (2012) Living life without B cells: is repeated B-cell depletion a safe and effective long-term treatment plan for rheumatoid arthritis? Int J Clin Rheumtol. 2: 159–166.
48. Popa C, Leandro MJ, Cambridge G, Edwards JC (2007) Repeated B lymphocyte depletion with rituximab in rheumatoid arthritis over 7 yrs. Rheumatology (Oxford). 4: 626–30.
49. Krause JE, DiMaggio DA, McCarson KE (1995) Alterations in neurokinin 1 receptor gene expression in models of pain and inflammation. Can J Physiol Pharmacol. 73: 854–9.
50. Hong SK, Han JS, Min SS, Hwang JM, Kim YI, et al. (2002) Local neurokinin-1 receptor in the knee joint contributes to the induction, but not maintenance, of arthritic pain in the rat. Neurosci Lett. 322: 21–4.
51. Lam FF, Ng ES (2010) Substance P and glutamate receptor antagonists improve the anti-arthritic actions of dexamethasone in rats. Br J Pharmacol. 159: 958–69.
52. Uematsu T, Sakai A, Ito H, Suzuki H (2011) Intra-articular administration of tachykinin NK_1 receptor antagonists reduces hyperalgesia and cartilage destruction in the inflammatory joint in rats with adjuvant-induced arthritis. Eur J Pharmacol. 668: 163–8.
53. Tauer U, Zhao Y, Hunt SP, Culman J (2012) Are biological actions of neurokinin A in the adult brain mediated by a cross-talk between the NK1 and NK2 receptors? Neuropharmacology. 63: 958–65.
54. Lavagno L, Bordin G, Colangelo D, Viano I, Brunelleschi S (2001) Tachykinin activation of human monocytes from patients with rheumatoid arthritis: in vitro and ex-vivo effects of cyclosporin A. Neuropeptides. 35: 92–9.
55. Origuchi T, Iwamoto N, Kawashiri SY, Fujikawa K, Aramaki T, et al. (2011) Reduction in serum levels of substance P in patients with rheumatoid arthritis by etanercept, a tumor necrosis factor inhibitor. Mod Rheumatol. 21: 244–50.
56. Gonzalez-Rey E, Chorny A, Delgado M (2007) Regulation of immune tolerance by anti-inflammatory neuropeptides. Nat Rev Immunol. 7: 52–63.

13

Three Groups in the 28 Joints for Rheumatoid Arthritis Synovitis – Analysis Using More than 17,000 Assessments in the KURAMA Database

Chikashi Terao[1,2]*, Motomu Hashimoto[2,3], Keiichi Yamamoto[4], Kosaku Murakami[2], Koichiro Ohmura[2], Ran Nakashima[2], Noriyuki Yamakawa[2], Hajime Yoshifuji[2], Naoichiro Yukawa[2], Daisuke Kawabata[2], Takashi Usui[2], Hiroyuki Yoshitomi[5], Moritoshi Furu[3,5], Ryo Yamada[1,6], Fumihiko Matsuda[1,7,8], Hiromu Ito[3,5], Takao Fujii[2,3], Tsuneyo Mimori[2,3]

1 Center for Genomic Medicine, Kyoto University Graduate School of Medicine, Kyoto, Japan, **2** Department of Rheumatology and Clinical Immunology, Kyoto University Graduate School of Medicine, Kyoto, Japan, **3** Department of the Control for Rheumatic Diseases, Kyoto University Graduate School of Medicine, Kyoto, Japan, **4** Department of Clinical Trial Design and Management, Translational Research Center, Kyoto University Hospital, Kyoto, Japan, **5** Department of Orthopaedic Surgery, Kyoto University Graduate School of Medicine, Kyoto, Japan, **6** Unit of Statistical Genetics Center for Genomic Medicine, Kyoto University Graduate School of Medicine, Kyoto, Japan, **7** Institut National de la Sante et de la Recherche Medicale (INSERM) Unite U852, Kyoto University Graduate School of Medicine, Kyoto, Japan, **8** CREST Program, Japan Science and Technology Agency, Kawaguchi, Saitama, Japan

Abstract

Rheumatoid arthritis (RA) is a joint-destructive autoimmune disease. Three composite indices evaluating the same 28 joints are commonly used for the evaluation of RA activity. However, the relationship between, and the frequency of, the joint involvements are still not fully understood. Here, we obtained and analyzed 17,311 assessments for 28 joints in 1,314 patients with RA from 2005 to 2011 from electronic clinical chart templates stored in the KURAMA (Kyoto University Rheumatoid Arthritis Management Alliance) database. Affected rates for swelling and tenderness were assessed for each of the 28 joints and compared between two different sets of RA patients. Correlations of joint symptoms were analyzed for swellings and tenderness using kappa coefficient and eigen vectors by principal component analysis. As a result, we found that joint affected rates greatly varied from joint to joint both for tenderness and swelling for the two sets. Right wrist joint is the most affected joint of the 28 joints. Tenderness and swellings are well correlated in the same joints except for the shoulder joints. Patients with RA tended to demonstrate right-dominant joint involvement and joint destruction. We also found that RA synovitis could be classified into three categories of joints in the correlation analyses: large joints with wrist joints, PIP joints, and MCP joints. Clustering analysis based on distribution of synovitis revealed that patients with RA could be classified into six subgroups. We confirmed the symmetric joint involvement in RA. Our results suggested that RA synovitis can be classified into subgroups and that several different mechanisms may underlie the pathophysiology in RA synovitis.

Editor: Bernhard Kaltenboeck, Auburn University, United States of America

Funding: This study was supported by research grants from Mitsubishi Tanabe Pharma Corporation (http://www.mt-pharma.co.jp/e/), Eisai Co., Ltd. (http://www.eisai.co.jp/index.html), Abbott Japan Co., Ltd. (http://www.abbott.co.jp/), Chugai Pharmaceutical Co., Ltd. (http://www.chugai-pharm.co.jp/hc/ss/english/index.html), Pfizer Japan Inc. (http://www.pfizer.co.jp/pfizer/english/company/), and Bristol-Myyers K.K. (http://www.bms.co.jp/). The funders had no role in study design, data collection and analysis, decision to publish, or preparation of the manuscript. No additional external funding was received for this study.

Competing Interests: The KURAMA database was supported by funding from Mitsubishi Tanabe Pharma Corporation, Eisai Co., Ltd., Abbott Japan Co., Ltd., Chugai Pharmaceutical Co., Ltd., Pfizer Japan Inc. and Bristol-Myyers.

* E-mail: a0001101@kuhp.kyoto-u.ac.jp

Introduction

Rheumatoid arthritis (RA) is the most frequent inflammatory arthritis worldwide affecting 0.5 to 1% of the population [1]. As RA is a bone-destructive disease and functional impairment caused by joint damage is well correlated with swelling and tenderness of joints [2–3], the evaluation of joints in patients with RA is very important to assess disease activity and predict the risk of future joint deformity. ACR core set [4] and DAS (disease activity score) [5–6] were developed for evaluation of disease activity in RA. Recently, the three composite indices, namely, DAS28 [5], simplified disease activity index (SDAI) [7] and clinical disease activity index (CDAI) [8] are frequently used for disease activity evaluation among rheumatologists. All of the three indices are shown to be well correlated with future joint destruction [7,9]. These three methods include the same 28 joints for evaluation of disease activity, namely, bilateral wrist, 1st to 5th metacarpal (MCP) joints and proximal interphalangeal (PIP) joints, elbow, shoulder, and knee joints. Though RA is known to show symmetric joint symptoms [10], the frequency of bilateral joint symptoms and the correlations between each joint symptom are not fully analyzed by using large numbers of joint assessments. There are several reports of successful prediction of joint damage using a reduced number of joints for evaluation by ultrasonography [11–12]. These reports raise the possibility that some of the 28 joints are less frequently involved, and are less informative for disease activity. Analyses for characterization of joint symptoms would uncover correlations of unexpected joint symptoms and distribution of synovitis in RA.

Here, we analyzed the distribution of affected joints in the 28 joints in patients with RA using more than 17,000 joint assessments from 1,314 patients with RA and showed that synovitis in RA patients can be classified into three groups. We also showed that affected rates of the 28 joints greatly vary in RA patients, and that RA patients could be classified into subgroups based on the distribution of joint synovitis.

Table 1. Summary of the KURAMA database.

	The KURAMA database
RA patients	1314
Age (mean±SD)	60.2±15.1
female ratio	81.70%
disease duration (years)	12.2±9.8
Stage*	2.75±1.17
Class*	1.87±0.69

*Stage and Class represent Steinbrocker's stage and class, respectively.
SD: standard deviation.

Results

Frequency order of joints involvement

We recruited 17,311 assessments for the 28 joints in 1,314 patients with RA from 2005 to 2011. A summary of the registered patients is listed in Table 1. The distribution of the number of patients with RA in each year and the number of joint assessments for each patient are shown in Figure S1. We analyzed how often each of the 28 joints was tender or swollen in patients with RA in 2011. From the analysis of 735 patients, we found that the frequency of joint swelling and tenderness in the 28 joints is widely different from joint to joint (Figure 1 and Table S1). The wrist joints were the most frequently affected joints for swelling and tenderness. The frequency of the right wrist joint being affected was more than four times as high as the least frequently affected joint. Many of the joints showed right-dominant tenderness (eleven of fourteen joints, $p = 0.057$, binomial test), indicating mostly right-handedness. We found strong correlations for the affected rates of each joint between swellings and tenderness except for shoulder joints (Spearman's rank-sum coefficient, $rho = 0.70$ and $p = 3.8\times10^{-5}$, Figure 1, Table S1). Shoulder joints showed much higher frequencies of tenderness than those of swellings.

Next, we tried to replicate the order of affected frequencies of the 28 joints and the correlation between tenderness and swellings in different RA patients. We obtained 579 patients whose joints data were not available for 2011, indicating we analyzed independent RA patients. We found that the order of the affected joint frequencies were well correlated for both swelling and tenderness among different sets of RA patients (Spearman's rank-sum coefficient, rho:0.815 and 0.904, $p = 1.3\times10^{-7}$ and $p = 4.6\times10^{-11}$ for swelling and tenderness, respectively, Figure S2). We also confirmed that rates of tenderness were well correlated with those of swellings in the 28 joints in the 579 patients (rho:0.604). These results indicate that some of the 28 joints are more likely to develop arthritis than the others in RA patients. The swelling and tenderness correlate with each other except for shoulder joints.

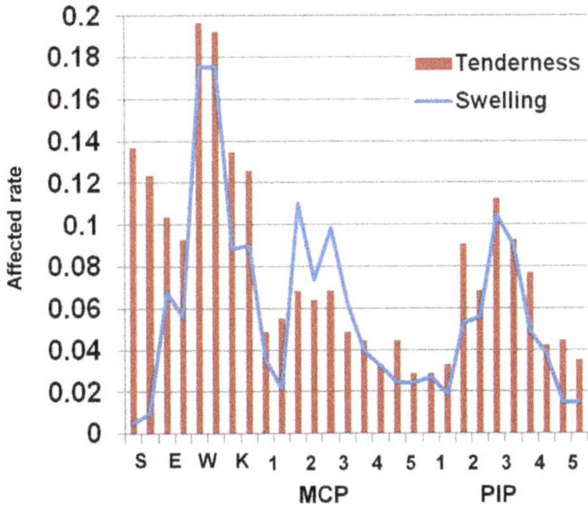

Figure 1. Affected rate of joint symptoms. Affected rate of joint symptoms. Each joint is arranged in the order of right and left. S:shoulder, E:elbow, W:wrist, K:knee.

Whether the right-dominant involvement of joints in patients with RA is associated with joint destruction was analyzed. Joint destruction in the hand was evaluated for 246 patients with RA by modified Sharp score [13]. The six elements of the scores were separately analyzed, namely erosion of PIP, MCP, and wrist joints (we defined as joints other than MCP and PIP in hand) and narrowing of PIP, MCP, and wrist joints. We found that five out of six elements showed right-dominant destruction. In particular, narrowing and erosion of MCP joints showed a statistically significant right-dominance in binomial test ($p <= 0.0050$, Table S2).

Three groups of 28 joints in RA synovitis

Next we analyzed correlations of joint symptoms between the 28 joints. We randomly picked up one assessment from each of the 1,314 patients to maximize the power. When the correlation of tenderness of the 28 joints was analyzed with kappa coefficient, we confirmed that each joint showed a symmetric involvement (Figure 2A). The results also showed that the tenderness of large joints and wrist joints are not correlated with the tenderness of PIP and MCP joints. We found that the tenderness of MCP joints was especially well correlated with each other and that PIP joints tenderness was well correlated with each other. The correlation of swelling in the 28 joints showed the same tendency as that of tenderness, namely, symmetric joint involvement, correlations between large joints and wrist joints, and no strong correlations between wrist joints and other small joints (Figure 2B).

Next we used eigen vectors of principal component analysis to assess the correlations of the 28 joints involvement. When we analyzed correlations of tenderness, eigen vectors revealed that PIP and MCP joints can be clearly distinguished from large joints and wrist joints (Figure 3A). PIP joints and MCP joints turned out to make independent groups after excluding large joints and wrist joints (Figure 3B). These three groups of affected joints were found both for tenderness and swelling (Figure 3C and 3D). We confirmed these three correlation groups in four independent resampling analyses by randomly picking up one assessment from each of the 1,314 patients four times (data not shown). The three groups were observed in the two independent sets of RA patients which were used in the analysis of joints involvement frequency

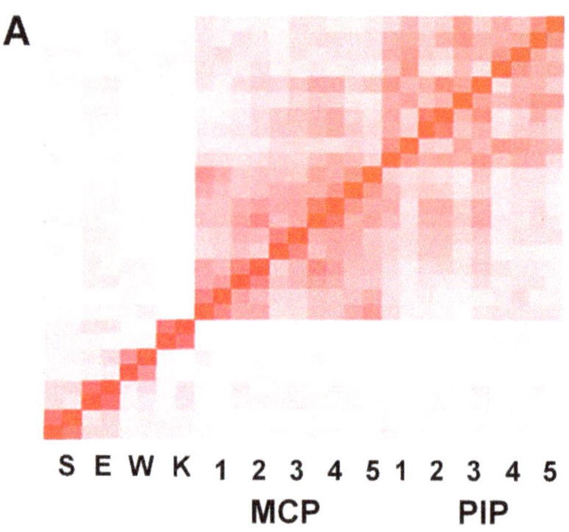

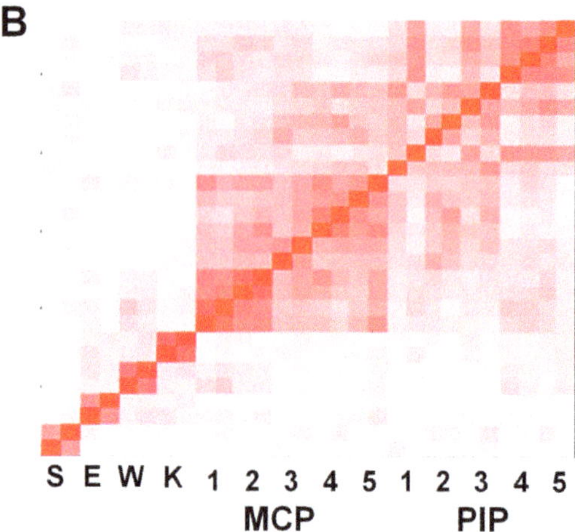

Figure 2. Correlations between the 28 joint symptoms. Brightness of the red color corresponds to the strength of correlations between joint tenderness (A) or swellings (B), using the Kappa coefficient. Each joint is arranged in the order of right and left. The joint order in the y axis is the same as the x axis. The result is a representative of five analyses based on resampled assessments. S:shoulder, E:elbow, W:wrist, K:knee.

(Figure S3). In addition, no significant difference was observed in the relationship of the three groups of joint involvement when we divided the 1,314 patients into two groups according to the patients' caring physicians (Figure S4). We confirmed the three groups by resampling four times for each analysis (data not shown). These results indicate that these three groups were not due to specific patients, examiners, or time of evaluation.

Taken together, the correlation analyses using kappa coefficient and eigen vectors in principal component analysis indicated that there are three correlated groups of joints in RA synovitis, namely, large joints with wrist joints (which we express as "large and wrist joints"), PIP joints, and MCP joints.

Subgroups of patients with RA

We performed a clustering analysis of 5,383 evaluations of 28 joints from 1,314 patients with RA. Six subgroups of evaluations of 28 joints were observed (Figure 4). Each of the subgroups was characterized by 1) no synovitis (34.6%), 2) mild activity with dominant involvement of large and wrist joints (17.4%), 3) dominant involvement of MCP joints (18.3%), 4) dominant involvement of PIP joints (9.3%), 5) active synovitis (4.1%), and 6) moderate activity with dominant involvement of large and wrist joints (16.4%) (Table S3). Whether patients with RA are classified into the same subgroups was analyzed. There were 998 patients with four or five evaluations, and of these, 734 were categorized into the regular groups across different evaluations, indicating that the patterns of synovitis in the same patients were stable. Analysis of joint destruction in each subgroup revealed that the sixth subgroup demonstrated dominant destruction of large and wrist joints compared with MCP and PIP joints ($p<=2.8\times10^{-5}$, Figure S5 and Figure S6).

Discussion

Since RA is a joint destructive autoimmune arthritis and joint damage occurs rapidly in the early stages of the disease course [14], the development of a quantitative scale which assesses disease activity and predicts joint damage is very important. After DAS and ACR core sets were introduced, DAS28, SDAI, and CDAI were developed to evaluate disease activity and easily calculate the disease activity score in patients with RA. All three indices were shown to be well correlated with future joint destruction and they share the same 28 joints for evaluation. Joint symptoms especially joint swelling is known to correlate with future joint damage [3]. While these indices were developed for use in clinical trials such as responsiveness to treatment, they are used by rheumatologists in daily clinical practice and they are reported to coincide very well among different examiners [9]. Characterizing the relative affected frequency of each joint and analysis of correlation between joint symptoms are important to analyze the basic mechanisms of synovitis and to efficiently select the joints to predict future joint destruction. However, there is no detailed analysis to address the correlations between the 28-joint symptoms.

In the current study, we characterized the 28-joint symptoms using large numbers of joint assessments. While we reported the affected rates of each joint in the 28 joints for tenderness and swelling of RA patients registered in the KURAMA database in 2011 as a representative (Table S1), these rates should not be generalized considering large effects of treatment especially biologics agents on joint symptoms. Thus, we focused on relative frequencies of joint involvement for the 28 joints. The affected frequency pattern was compared between the two sets of RA patients, and there were no apparent differences between the two sets for both tenderness and swelling. We also showed that joint symptoms in RA could be classified into three groups both for tenderness and swelling. Our analysis also demonstrated that patients with RA can be regularly classified into six subgroups based on patterns of joint symptoms. These results suggest that regular RA joint involvement pattern, including relative frequency and groups of joints, is largely maintained in RA patients. In addition, we confirmed that these patterns of joint involvement were not attributed to evaluators and fractions of RA patients.

It is interesting that the affected frequencies greatly varied from joint to joint, and the rate of the most highly affected joint was more than four times as high as the least-affected joint. The affected frequencies indicated that wrist joints were the most frequently affected. It should be noted that surface area may have influenced the sensitivity of detecting synovitis in physical exams when different joints were compared. The relatively high frequency of tenderness and swelling in large and wrist joints compared with MCP and PIP joints can be explained by this difference in surface area. However, surface area cannot fully explain the highest frequency of wrist involvement and different frequencies within the MCP or PIP joints. A dominant involve-

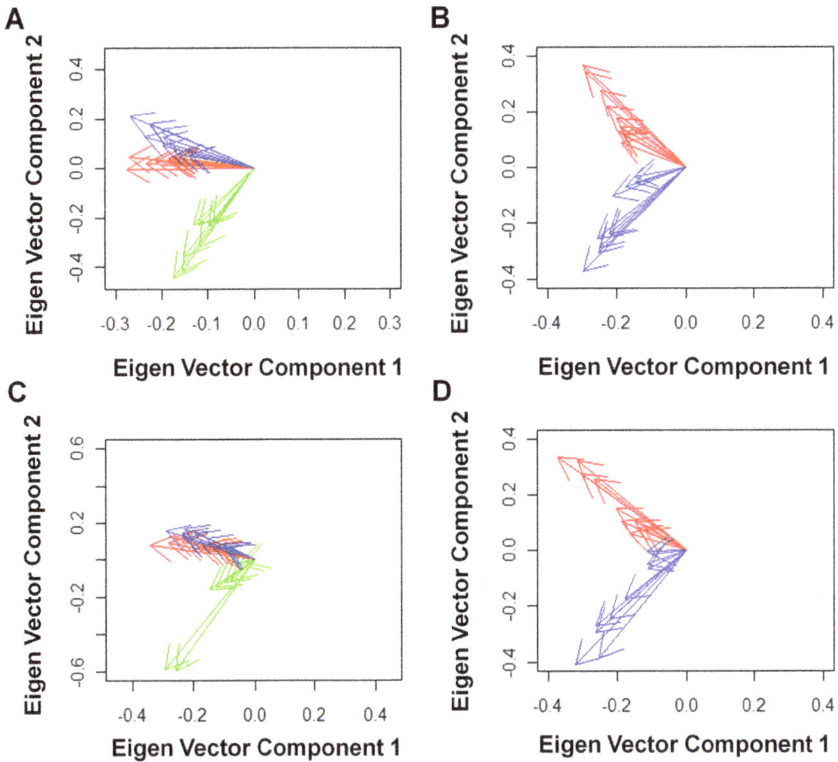

Figure 3. Relationship of the 28-joint involvement. The 1st and 2nd components of eigen vectors of the joint symptoms are plotted, using principal component analysis of the 28 joint involvement for tenderness (A) and swelling (C) or using that of the 20 joint involvement other than large and wrist joints for tenderness (B) and swelling (D). The results are representatives of five analyses based on resampled assessments. Green: large and wrist joints. Red: MCP joints. Blue: PIP joints.

ment of right joints seemed to indicate a majority of the study population being right-handed in spite of the small difference of affected rates between bilateral joints. We also demonstrated that the right dominant involvement was also true for joint destruction. We could not compare the joint involvement and joint destruction between right-handed patients and left-handed patients due to a lack of information regarding handedness of patients.

Correlation analysis confirmed the well-known symmetric joint involvement in patients with RA. Strong correlations of tenderness and swelling in the same joints except for shoulder joints may indicate low sensitivity of shoulder swelling in the physical exams and common mechanisms of swelling and tenderness. It is striking that joint symptoms can be classified into three groups based on correlation analysis and principal component analysis. The

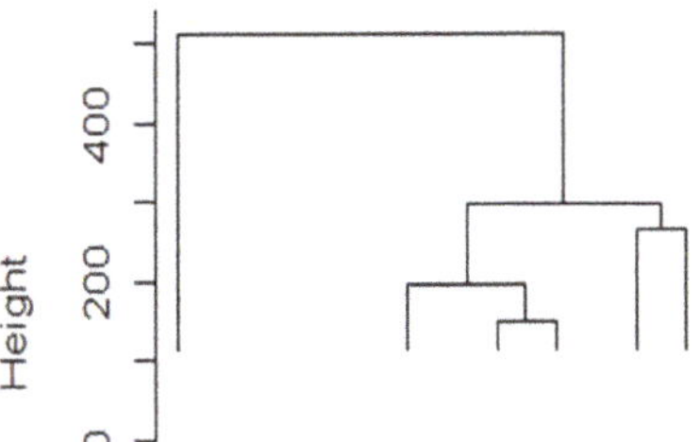

Figure 4. Six subgroups of evaluations of the 28 joints in RA. Results of clustering analysis with Ward method using randomly obtained 5,383 evaluations of the 28 joints in 1,314 patients were plotted.

association observed between the symptoms in the wrist joints and the large joints is worth noting, since wrist joints are regarded as small joints according to ACR/EULAR criteria set in 2010. As wrist joints are much closer to other small joints than large joints, the relationship between wrist joints and large joints cannot be explained by the distance of joints. The distance of joints cannot explain the two different groups of MCP and PIP joints either. While symptoms of large and wrist joints are not related with those of MCP and PIP joints, they were not very strongly correlated with each other, compared with correlations among PIP joints or MCP joints. This may indicate that there are no common strong factors which predispose large and wrist joints to swelling and tenderness in patients with RA.

We also showed that patients with RA can be divided into six subgroups based on these three groups of joint involvement. More than 70% of patients are classified into regular subgroups, indicating that the pattern of synovitis in a patient with RA is stable. When patients who were regularly classified into the first subgroup of patients characterized by no synovitis were removed, more than 60% of patients were still classified into regular subgroups (data not shown), indicating that the stable patterns were observed regardless of activity of RA. As joint destruction was influenced by disease duration, disease activity, and treatment, we analyzed the relative distribution of joint destruction between the three joint groups in a patient with RA. We found that the sixth subgroup of patients, characterized by moderate activity with dominant involvement of large and wrist joints, demonstrated dominant destruction of wrist joints. This suggests that classifying patients with RA into appropriate subgroups would lead to prediction of patterns of joint destruction.

There are reports that evaluating fraction of joints by ultrasonography is a good way to predict future joint damage [11–12]. One study reported that 5 of the 28 joints with MTP2 and MTP5 joints, namely, wrist, MCP2, MCP3, PIP2, and PIP3 joints, are enough for ultrasonography evaluation [12]. Their data seems to be consistent with our results as they selected at least two joints from three different groups into which the 28-joint symptoms were classified. As ultrasonography usually surpasses physical examination in terms of the sensitivity to detect synovitis, it is interesting to analyze whether the assessments of synovitis using ultrasonography show the same pattern of synovitis over the 28 joints in RA.

Our results indicate that RA does not develop synovitis in the 28 joints with the same frequency and that the affected rate of each joint greatly varies from joint to joint. These different distributions of joint synovitis would lead to different distribution of joint destruction. Based on our results, the 28 joints can be categorized into three groups, and it is possible that some fractions of the 28 joints are less informative to assess disease activity than others. It would be interesting to develop a novel simplified joint core set, and analyze the correlation between joint damage and activity score based on this. It would be also interesting to characterize each of RA subsets in more detail.

Materials and Methods

Ethics Statement

Written informed consent to enroll in the database described below was obtained from most of the patients, but for some patients the information regarding the construction of this database was disclosed instead of obtaining written informed consent. Participants who were informed regarding the construction of the database (instead of obtaining written informed consent) were allowed to withdraw from the study if desired.

All data were de-identified and analyzed anonymously. This study was designed in accordance with the Helsinki Declaration. This study including the consent procedure was approved by the ethics committee of Kyoto University Graduate School and Faculty of Medicine.

The KURAMA database

The KURAMA (Kyoto University Rheumatoid Arthritis Management Alliance) database was established in 2011 at Kyoto University to store detailed clinical information and specimens from patients with arthritis and arthropathy. The alliance is composed of rheumatic disease-associated departments in Kyoto University Hospital as well as its allied, integrating previous database and specimen collections in each department and allied. A template for electronic clinical charts developed at Kyoto University Hospital in 2004 to evaluate joint involvements in RA patients was used to obtain joint assessments. Rheumatologists evaluated swelling and tenderness of the 28 joints in patients with RA on each visit and filled in the template. The synovitis information of the 28 joints and data for C-reactive protein and erythrocyte sedimentation rate were extracted from electronic clinical charts [15] and stored in the KURAMA database.

Patients and data of joint assessment

A total of 17,311 joint assessments from 1,314 patients with RA from 2005 to 2011 were obtained in a retrospective manner from the KURAMA database. All of the patients fulfilled ACR revised criteria for RA in 1987 [10] or ACR and EULAR classification criteria for RA in 2010 [16–17].

Analysis of affected frequencies in the 28 joints

RA patients were subdivided depending on whether their data were available in 2011 or not, and the affected frequency in each of the 28 joints was calculated. We compared the order of the affected frequency in the 28 joints between the two patient sets with Spearman's rank-sum coefficient. We separately analyzed the affected rates of joints for swelling and tenderness. When multiple joint assessments in different visits were available in the same patient with RA, we randomly selected one of the assessments as representative in the patient. We compared frequencies between tenderness and swellings for the 28 joints with Spearman's rank-sum coefficient.

Clustering of patients with RA

Clustering analyses were performed by Ward method, using randomly-selected 5,383 evaluations of the 28 joints from 1,314 patients with RA. These evaluations did not contain more than six assessments from each patient to avoid excess influence of particular patients. Affected rates were calculated for the three groups of joints (namely PIP joints, MCP joints and large and wrist joints) in this clustering analysis. For example, when a patient showed tenderness and swelling for all PIP joints, the affected rate of PIP joints in the patient is 2. When a patient showed tenderness for four MCP joints, the affected rate of MCP joints is 0.4.

RA patients were regarded as belonging to a particular group when more than 60% of evaluations belonging to the same patients with four or five evaluations were classified into the same group.

Analysis between RA subgroups and joint destruction

Joint destruction of hand joints in 246 patients with RA was evaluated by modified Sharp score by a trained rheumatologist who was not informed of the patients' characteristics (KM). Joint destruction rates were defined for the three groups of joints as a sum of scores divided by the full score in the joints group. For example, when a patient shows 50 as a sum of scores in the large and wrist group, the patient's joint destruction rate for the group is 0.463 (50/108).

Correlation of the 28 joints and statistical analysis

Correlations of joint symptoms among the 28 joints were estimated separately for tenderness and swelling. We randomly obtained one assessment of the 28 joints in each patient as a representative of the patient's joint assessments for maximization of the power. Kappa coefficient was used to analyze coincidence of joint symptoms in each pair of the 28 joints. Eigen vectors obtained in principal component analysis were used to analyze the deviation of joint symptoms. We resampled joint assessments for each patient and created four other sets of joint assessments. The same correlation analyses were performed using the four resampled assessments to confirm the correlation shown in the first assessment set. Right dominance of the synovitis and joint destruction was analyzed by binomial test. Dominant destruction of joints was evaluated by paired-t test. Statistical analysis was performed by R software or SPSS (ver18).

Supporting Information

Figure S1 Distribution of joint evaluation counts and patients across different years. A) Distribution of number of RA patients according to numbers of 28-joint assessments. B) Distribution of number of patients with RA whose joint assessment data were available from 2005 to 2011 in the KURAMA database.

Figure S2 Good correlations between joint involvement rates in different sets of RA patients. Rates of joint involvement for A) swelling and B) tenderness were compared between the two different sets of RA patients. X and Y axes represent rates in the first set of RA patients in 2011 and those in the second set in 2005 to 2010, respectively.

Figure S3 Three groups of joints regardless of different sets of RA patients. Analysis using one of four resampled assessments in one of the two sets of RA patients is shown as a representative. The 1st and 2nd components of eigen vectors of the joint symptoms are plotted, using principal component analysis of the 28 joint involvement for tenderness (A) and swelling (C) or using that of the 20 joint involvement other than large and wrist joints for tenderness (B) and swelling (D). Green: large and wrist joints. Red: MCP joints. Blue: PIP joints.

Figure S4 Three groups of joints regardless of different evaluators. Analysis using one of five resampled assessments by one of the two groups of medical doctors is shown as a representative. The 1st and 2nd components of eigen vectors of the joint symptoms are plotted, using principal component analysis of the 28 joint involvement for tenderness (A) and swelling (C) or using that of the 20 joint involvement other than large and wrist joints for tenderness (B) and swelling (D). Green: large and wrist joints. Red: MCP joints. Blue: PIP joints.

Figure S5 Dominant destruction of large and wrist joints in the sixth subgroup of patients with RA. Box plots indicating the joint destruction rates in the three joint groups in subjects belonging to the sixth subgroup.

Figure S6 Destruction of large and wrist joints among the six subgroups of RA. Differences in destruction rates were plotted for each subject in the six subgroups. The difference was defined as: A) destruction rate of group of large and wrist joints – destruction rate of MCP joints and B) destruction rate of group of large and wrist joints – destruction rate of PIP joints.

Table S1 Rate of joint involvement for 28 joints in RA.

Table S2 Right-dominant joint destruction in RA. Patients who showed unilateral higher or lower scores in each element were analyzed.

Table S3 Mean affected rates of the three joint groups in the six subgroups of patients with RA.

Acknowledgments

We would like to thank to Mr. Wataru Yamamoto at Kurashiki Kosai Hospital for his excellent support to establish and maintain the KURAMA database. We also thank Drs Hisashi Yamanaka, Katsunori Ikari, and Ayako Nakajima at Institute of Rheumatology, Tokyo Women's Medical University for their kind instruction and advice for management of rheumatic diseases database.

Author Contributions

Evaluation of joint X-rays: KM. Conceived and designed the experiments: CT MH KO RY FM HI TF TM. Analyzed the data: CT. Contributed reagents/materials/analysis tools: CT MH KO RN KM N. Yamakawa H. Yoshifuji N. Yukawa DK TU H. Yoshitomi MF HI TF TM KY. Wrote the paper: CT.

References

1. Firestein GS (2003) Evolving concepts of rheumatoid arthritis. Nature 423: 356–361.
2. Drossaers-Bakker KW, de Buck M, van Zeben D, Zwinderman AH, Breedveld FC, et al. (1999) Long-term course and outcome of functional capacity in rheumatoid arthritis: the effect of disease activity and radiologic damage over time. Arthritis and Rheumatism 42: 1854–1860.
3. Smolen JS, Van Der Heijde DM, St Clair EW, Emery P, Bathon JM, et al. (2006) Predictors of joint damage in patients with early rheumatoid arthritis treated with high-dose methotrexate with or without concomitant infliximab: results from the ASPIRE trial. Arthritis and Rheumatism 54: 702–710.
4. Felson DT, Anderson JJ, Boers M, Bombardier C, Chernoff M, et al. (1993) The American College of Rheumatology preliminary core set of disease activity measures for rheumatoid arthritis clinical trials. The Committee on Outcome Measures in Rheumatoid Arthritis Clinical Trials. Arthritis and Rheumatism 36: 729–740.
5. van der Heijde DM, van 't Hof MA, van Riel PL, Theunisse LA, Lubberts EW, et al. (1990) Judging disease activity in clinical practice in rheumatoid arthritis: first step in the development of a disease activity score. Annals of the Rheumatic Diseases 49: 916–920.
6. van der Heijde DM, van't Hof MA, van Riel PL, van Leeuwen MA, van Rijswijk MH, et al. (1992) Validity of single variables and composite indices for measuring disease activity in rheumatoid arthritis. Annals of the Rheumatic Diseases 51: 177–181.
7. Smolen JS, Breedveld FC, Schiff MH, Kalden JR, Emery P, et al. (2003) A simplified disease activity index for rheumatoid arthritis for use in clinical practice. Rheumatology 42: 244–257.
8. Aletaha D, Smolen JS (2007) The Simplified Disease Activity Index (SDAI) and Clinical Disease Activity Index (CDAI) to monitor patients in standard clinical care. Best Pract Res Clin Rheumatol 21: 663–675.
9. Salaffi F, Cimmino MA, Leardini G, Gasparini S, Grassi W (2009) Disease activity assessment of rheumatoid arthritis in daily practice: validity, internal consistency, reliability and congruency of the Disease Activity Score including 28 joints (DAS28) compared with the Clinical Disease Activity Index (CDAI). Clinical and Experimental Rheumatology 27: 552–559.
10. Arnett FC, Edworthy SM, Bloch DA, McShane DJ, Fries JF, et al. (1988) The American Rheumatism Association 1987 revised criteria for the classification of rheumatoid arthritis. Arthritis Rheum 31: 315–324.
11. Scheel AK, Hermann KG, Kahler E, Pasewaldt D, Fritz J, et al. (2005) A novel ultrasonographic synovitis scoring system suitable for analyzing finger joint inflammation in rheumatoid arthritis. Arthritis and Rheumatism 52: 733–743.
12. Backhaus M, Ohrndorf S, Kellner H, Strunk J, Backhaus TM, et al. (2009) Evaluation of a novel 7-joint ultrasound score in daily rheumatologic practice: a pilot project. Arthritis and Rheumatism 61: 1194–1201.
13. van der Heijde D (2000) How to read radiographs according to the Sharp/van der Heijde method. Journal of Rheumatology 27: 261–263.
14. Machold KP, Stamm TA, Eberl GJ, Nell VK, Dunky A, et al. (2002) Very recent onset arthritis – clinical, laboratory, and radiological findings during the first year of disease. Journal of Rheumatology 29: 2278–2287.
15. Yamamoto K, Yamanaka K, Hatano E, Sumi E, Ishii T, et al. (2012) An eClinical trial system for cancer that integrates with clinical pathways and electronic medical records. Clin Trials 9: 408–417.
16. Aletaha D, Neogi T, Silman AJ, Funovits J, Felson DT, et al. (2010) 2010 Rheumatoid arthritis classification criteria: an American College of Rheumatology/European League Against Rheumatism collaborative initiative. Arthritis and Rheumatism 62: 2569–2581.
17. Aletaha D, Neogi T, Silman AJ, Funovits J, Felson DT, et al. (2010) 2010 rheumatoid arthritis classification criteria: an American College of Rheumatology/European League Against Rheumatism collaborative initiative. Annals of the Rheumatic Diseases 69: 1580–1588.

14

Joint Loads in Marsupial Ankles Reflect Habitual Bipedalism versus Quadrupedalism

Kristian J. Carlson[1,2]*, Tea Jashashvili[1,3], Kimberley Houghton[1], Michael C. Westaway[4], Biren A. Patel[5]

1 Institute for Human Evolution, University of the Witwatersrand, Johannesburg, South Africa, **2** Department of Anthropology, Indiana University, Bloomington, Indiana, United States of America, **3** Department of Geology and Paleontology, Georgian National Museum, Tbilisi, Georgia, **4** Cultures and Histories Program, Queensland Museum, Brisbane, Australia, **5** Department of Cell and Neurobiology, Keck School of Medicine, University of Southern California, Los Angeles, California, United States of America

Abstract

Joint surfaces of limb bones are loaded in compression by reaction forces generated from body weight and musculotendon complexes bridging them. In general, joints of eutherian mammals have regions of high radiodensity subchondral bone that are better at resisting compressive forces than low radiodensity subchondral bone. Identifying similar form-function relationships between subchondral radiodensity distribution and joint load distribution within the marsupial postcranium, in addition to providing a richer understanding of marsupial functional morphology, can serve as a phylogenetic control in evaluating analogous relationships within eutherian mammals. Where commonalities are established across phylogenetic borders, unifying principles in mammalian physiology, morphology, and behavior can be identified. Here, we assess subchondral radiodensity patterns in distal tibiae of several marsupial taxa characterized by different habitual activities (e.g., locomotion). Computed tomography scanning, maximum intensity projection maps, and pixel counting were used to quantify radiodensity in 41 distal tibiae of bipedal (5 species), arboreal quadrupedal (4 species), and terrestrial quadrupedal (5 species) marsupials. Bipeds (*Macropus* and *Wallabia*) exhibit more expansive areas of high radiodensity in the distal tibia than arboreal (*Dendrolagus*, *Phascolarctos*, and *Trichosurus*) or terrestrial quadrupeds (*Sarcophilus*, *Thylacinus*, *Lasiorhinus*, and *Vombatus*), which may reflect the former carrying body weight only through the hind limbs. Arboreal quadrupeds exhibit smallest areas of high radiodensity, though they differ non-significantly from terrestrial quadrupeds. This could indicate slightly more compliant gaits by arboreal quadrupeds compared to terrestrial quadrupeds. The observed radiodensity patterns in marsupial tibiae, though their statistical differences disappear when controlling for phylogeny, corroborate previously documented patterns in primates and xenarthrans, potentially reflecting inferred limb use during habitual activities such as locomotion. Despite the complex nature of factors contributing to joint loads, broad observance of these patterns across joints and across a variety of taxa suggests that subchondral radiodensity can be used as a unifying form-function principle within *Mammalia*.

Editor: Andrew A. Farke, Raymond M. Alf Museum of Paleontology, United States of America

Funding: Funding for the project was provided by the African Origins Platform of the Department of Science and Technology (South Africa), the National Research Foundation of South Africa, and the University of the Witwatersrand. The funders had no role in the study design, data collection and analysis, decision to publish, or preparation of the manuscript.

Competing Interests: The authors have declared that no competing interests exist.

* E-mail: kristian.carlson@wits.ac.za

Introduction

Eutherian and metatherian (marsupials) lineages diverged approximately 160 million years ago [1]. The latter often serve as phylogenetic controls for understanding morphology-behavior relationships in the former [2–5]. Where consistent form-function relationships appear in both groups, unifying principles in mammalian physiology, morphology and behavior can be established [6]. For example, arboreal quadrupedal marsupials, such as opossums [4,7] and the tree kangaroo (*Dendrolagus*; [8]) converge on aspects of gait (e.g., compliancy) that are exhibited by arboreal quadrupedal eutherian mammals, such as primates [9–10]. Inconsistencies, however, are to be found as well. Some bipedal macropods (e.g., a few kangaroos and wallabies) are uniquely specialized compared to quadrupedal mammals, including the only living arboreal macropod (*Dendrolagus*), in that the former are able to decouple speed and cost of transport [11–12]. Moreover, the hind limbs of bipedal macropods appear to experience peak vertical components of the substrate reaction force (SRF) that are twice those experienced by hind limbs of quadrupeds trotting at physiologically equivalent speeds [13].

Eutherian mammals and marsupials [14–17] have postcranial morphologies that reflect how they use their skeletons during habitual activities such as locomotion. Direct quantification of loads imposed on articular surfaces during locomotion, however, is problematic because the requisite experimental procedures (e.g., load cells, strain gages) necessitate disruption of joint integrity, which in turn causes abnormal movement. Internal characteristics of the bone that occurs in joints, such as radiodensity of subchondral bone lining some articular surfaces, offer a non-invasive alternative for estimating joint loads [18–23], providing otherwise unobtainable information on the form-function relationships expressed in the skeleton of free-ranging mammals. Marsupial joint loads in comparison to those of eutherian mammals are poorly documented, despite the mechanics of some marsupial gaits, particularly hopping, being well-studied [2,5–8,11,24–29]. Data on marsupial joint loads would provide crucial insight into their intertwined morphology and behavior (e.g., locomotion). Here, we test whether radiodensity patterns in the subchondral bone of marsupial distal tibiae differ in a predictable fashion by evaluating a number of marsupial species characterized by different habitual behavioral activities.

Compressive strength of subchondral bone is determined by mineral content and porosity [30], which can be cumulatively quantified as radiodensity using radiographic-based techniques, such as computed tomography (CT). Higher radiodensity indicates higher apparent density, whether it is through lower porosity, higher mineral content, or a combination of both. When a joint is congruent its articular surfaces are subjected to trivial bending loads; though joint surfaces may experience shear forces, subchondral radiodensity is a reasonable estimator of compressive loads in habitual joint loading regimes in such cases [31–32]. Joint congruency is relative and can be dynamic over a range of motion (e.g., close-packed versus not close-packed), with examples such as the humeroulnar joint considered relatively incongruent [32] compared to other joints (e.g., wrist, ankle, and knee joints). Subchondral bone in relatively congruent diarthrodial joints experiences compression from joint reaction forces during behaviors in which the limbs are used, most often during locomotor activities [33]. When limbs are weight-bearing and positioned beneath the body, these joints experience reaction forces that are largely axially-directed and proportional to body weight. Vertical shifts in the center of mass result in accelerations or decelerations of body weight; are partly a function of limb kinematics, substrate use, and speed [34]; and can influence joint loads. Musculotendon complexes bridging a joint also contribute to compressive loads experienced in subchondral bone whenever muscles contract. Studies of cat or rabbit [35] and human knees [36] demonstrate that muscle contractile forces contribute more to overall knee joint loads than body weight. Interestingly, studies of subchondral radiodensity in the distal radius of suspensory and quadrupedal primates and xenarthrans [18–20] suggest that muscle contractile forces may contribute less to overall wrist joint loads than body weight [18–20]. To date, these relationships providing information about bone functional adaptations are unassessed in the ankle joint. Adding data from the ankle to the burgeoning literature on joint loading, therefore, could help to understand these differences.

Primates and xenarthrans exhibit subchondral radiodensity patterns that corroborate theoretical expectations of limb loading according to their habitual activity patterns (e.g., distributions in forelimbs and hind limbs distinguish bipeds, suspensory, and arboreal or terrestrial quadrupeds). Human distal radii exhibit lower weight-bearing (compressive) loads compared to suspensory and quadrupedal primates, as would be expected since human forelimbs no longer have an active weight-bearing role in locomotion [18]. Suspensory primates, such as orangutans, load their distal radii during locomotion, but since pronograde quadrupedalism comprises such a small percentage of total locomotor repertoires of orangutans compared to percentage of below-branch activity (e.g., suspension) in which the center of mass is below the handhold [37], compressive forces through the orangutan forelimb likely reflect predominantly muscle contractile forces maintaining joint integrity. A similar trend has been documented in xenarthran distal radii when comparing suspensory sloths and quadrupedal anteaters [20]. Quadrupedal primates exhibit the most extensive distribution of high radiodensity in their distal radii, even differing in predictable ways according to hand postures habitually adopted during quadrupedalism [19]. Similarly, the distribution of high radiodensity areas in the primate foot (e.g., calcaneocuboid joint) corroborates theoretical differences in loading arising from overall foot mobility and habitual foot postures adopted during quadrupedalism [22].

The goals of this study are two-fold. First, we aim to document whether a form-function relationship exists in radiodensity patterns in subchondral bone of marsupial distal tibiae. Second, we evaluate whether radiodensity patterns of subchondral bone exhibit a unifying form-function principle within *Mammalia.* In order to achieve these aims, we test two predictions. First, bipedal marsupials should exhibit significantly more expansive high radiodensity area in the distal tibia compared to quadrupedal marsupials because of the unique mechanics of their hopping gait, and because they carry body weight only through the hind limbs rather than all four limbs (i.e., we hypothesize compressive loads in ankles should be proportionately higher in the former group). Second, high radiodensity area in distal tibiae of terrestrial quadrupedal marsupials should exceed high radiodensity area in distal tibiae of arboreal quadrupedal marsupials because the latter may systematically adopt a more compliant gait, and/or systematically use more compliant arboreal substrates (i.e., we hypothesize compressive loads in ankles should be proportionately higher in the former group). If observed relationships between high radiodensity patterns and limb use in marsupials are consistent with previously documented relationships in eutherian mammals (e.g., primates and xenarthrans), it would be reasonable to elevate these relationships to unifying form-function principles throughout *Mammalia.*

Materials and Methods

The study sample consists of data derived from 41 marsupial tibiae housed in collections curated at the: Australian Museum (AM), Australian National Wildlife Collection (ANWC), Queensland Museum (QM), and Tasmanian Museum (TM) (see Table S1 for specimen information). Either a left or a right tibia was used without preference, often the choice being dictated by availability. We excluded tibiae that originated from known captive individuals in order to avoid sampling idiosyncratic locomotor activities or possibly implicating the use of artificial substrates (e.g., floors of captive enclosures). Data were acquired from specimens only when they lacked obvious visible evidence of trauma or pathology on limb bones, since this could signal potentially altered gait patterns or bone density (e.g., degenerative joint disease), respectively. Institutions allowed short-term loans (e.g., a few hours) for the purposes of transporting specimens to and from scanning facilities, in some cases with a museum representative assisting with the scanning.

We acquired image data from distal tibiae using CT osteoabsorptiometry (Table 1). The data acquisition protocol and rationale have been published elsewhere [18–19]. Briefly, tibiae were aligned with their longitudinal axis perpendicular to the scan plane, usually with the anterior surface facing upwards and the tibial plafond positioned in the coronal plane. In some cases, it was necessary to place a tibia with a different surface facing upwards in order to achieve a stable resting position on the CT scanner bed. Such alignment changes have trivial affects since specimens can be repositioned in a virtual 3D environment [18–19], but were necessary to avoid movement artifacts that can result from poor stability during CT scanning. To the extent permitted by CT manufacturer and model differences, we attempted to use similar scan parameters in each facility: tube voltage = 120 kV; tube current = 200–300 mA; slice thickness = 0.5–0.625 mm; field

Table 1. Sample (n = 41).

Genus	Species	Common name	Tibiae	Source[1]	Gait category
Macropus	*giganteus*	Eastern Grey Kangaroo	5	AM, ANWC, QM, TM	Bipedal
Macropus	*fuliginosus*	Western Grey Kangaroo	2	ANWC	Bipedal
Macropus	*eugenii*	Tammar Wallaby	4	AM, ANWC	Bipedal
Macropus	*parma*	Parma Wallaby	1	AM	Bipedal
Wallabia	*bicolor*	Swamp Wallaby	2	AM	Bipedal
Dendrolagus	*dorianus*	Doria's Tree-kangaroo	1	ANWC	Arboreal quadrupedal
Dendrolagus	*lumholtzi*	Lumholtz's Tree kangaroo	1	QM	Arboreal quadrupedal
Phascolarctos	*cinereus*	Koala	9	AM, ANWC, QM	Arboreal quadrupedal
Trichosurus	*vulpecula*	Common Brushtail Possum	6	AM, ANWC, QM	Arboreal quadrupedal
Lasiorhinus	*krefftii*	Northern Hairy-nosed Wombat	2	QM	Terrestrial quadrupedal
Lasiorhinus	*latifrons*	Southern Hairy-nosed Wombat	1	QM	Terrestrial quadrupedal
Sarcophilus	*harrisii*	Tasmanian Devil	1	AM	Terrestrial quadrupedal
Thylacinus	*cynocephalus*	Tasmanian Wolf	3	TM	Terrestrial quadrupedal
Vombatus	*ursinus*	Common Wombat	3	ANWC, QM, TM	Terrestrial quadrupedal

[1]AM: Australian Museum (Sydney); ANWC: Australian National Wildlife Collection (Canberra); QM: Queensland Museum (Brisbane); TM: Tasmanian Museum (Hobart). See Table S1 for specimen numbers.

of view (FOV) = 180–285; reconstruction increment = 0.4 mm; 512×512 voxel matrix. Image data were reconstructed from raw CT data using standard and bone (e.g., edge-enhanced) filters to produce two sets of DICOM files for each specimen. Image data can be obtained by contacting the corresponding author.

We generated maximum intensity projection (MIPs) maps from the standard reconstructions and fitted them to 3D renderings of distal tibiae generated from the bone reconstructions [18–19]. During fitting procedures, we excluded regions of the distal articular surface that descended inferiorly onto the medial malleolus because theoretically this region should not experience substantial axial compressive loading during body weight support by the hind limb (Figure 1). In some cases when this surface is more obliquely oriented rather than vertically oriented, it is reasonable to assume that this surface may experience a relatively small component of axial compressive loading accompanying shear loading. An element of compressive loading also may be experienced by this part of the articular surface due to non-trivial mediolaterally-directed forces during locomotion [38], for example, those possibly arising during movement across uneven terrain. In order to simplify our model of the distal tibia, we focus on the horizontally-positioned portion of the tibiotalar joint, specifically the tibial plafond, and assume that axial loading of the distal tibial articular surface is the primary contributing factor to its compressive loading. Fitting MIPs to 3D renderings was performed in Adobe Photoshop (5.0; Adobe Systems Incorporated). Fitted MIPs represent a 3D voxel matrix that is condensed into a 2D pixel matrix (an 8-bit image) containing the highest radiodensity value extracted from a column of voxels following a line of sight through the depth of the subchondral bone. Pixels in fitted MIPs were binned into eight groups according to gray values, from which false color maps were generated to visualize radiodensity patterns (Figure 1).

Following field observations and locomotor descriptions [39], taxa were parsed into one of three habitual gait categories: bipedal, arboreal quadrupedal (AQ), and terrestrial quadrupedal (TQ). In order to control for potential body size-related differences in pixel counts (i.e., larger specimens potentially have more pixels per bin overall than smaller specimens), we created ratios between the number of pixels in each bin and the total number of pixels in the fitted MIP (i.e., the entire articular surface). Only ratios from the maximum and second highest bins were reported (Table 2), since other bins are less informative to compressive loading patterns [18].

Ratio distributions for gait groups did not differ significantly from normal distributions according to a series of Kolmogorov-Smirnov Tests ($p > 0.05$). Thus, we applied a series of one-way ANOVAs in order to statistically evaluate observed differences between gait group means (Table 2). Gait group variances did not differ significantly according to Levene tests for homogeneity of variances ($p > 0.05$). Thus, in order to evaluate the statistical significance of pairwise comparisons, we applied a series of Tukey Honestly Significant Difference post-hoc tests. We used SPSS (v. 16.0.1) for these statistical analyses.

In our sample, some marsupial taxa representing gait groups are also closely related (e.g., bipeds are all macropods). In order to tease apart the extent to which observed gait group differences may have reflected phylogeny and function, we performed a second set of ANOVAs in which we accounted for phylogenetic effects (pANOVAs). We constructed a phylogenetic tree with known divergence dates (Figure 2) for taxa in the sample based on recent molecular studies of marsupials [40–41]. The tree file was created with Mesquite software (Table S2). For pANOVAs and post-hoc analyses, we used R software and the *phytools* package [42]. In all statistical testing, significance was established at $p < 0.05$.

Results

Prediction 1: Bipedal Marsupials>Quadrupedal Marsupials

Ratios of maximum radiodensity area to total articular surface area differ between groups. As predicted, bipeds exhibit the largest ratios (Figure 3, Tables 2 and 3), regardless of whether they are small-bodied (wallaby mean = 0.184, n = 7: Tables 1 and 3) or large-bodied (kangaroo mean = 0.243, n = 7: Tables 1 and 3).

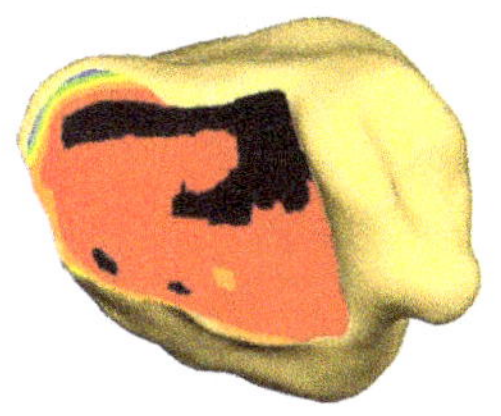

Macropus eugenii (**Bipedal**)

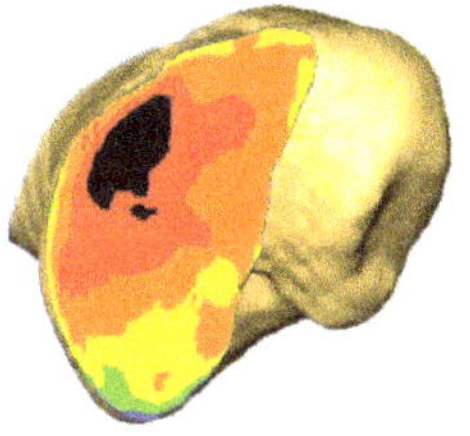

Phascolarctos cinereus (**AQ**)

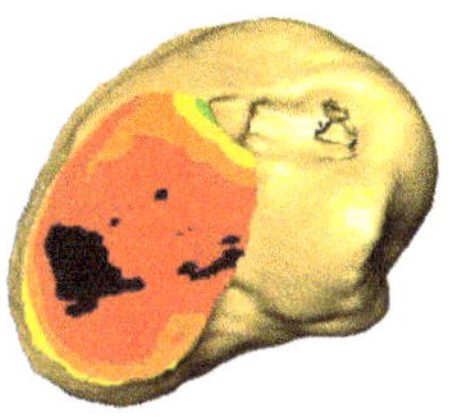

Lasiorhinus krefftii (**TQ**)

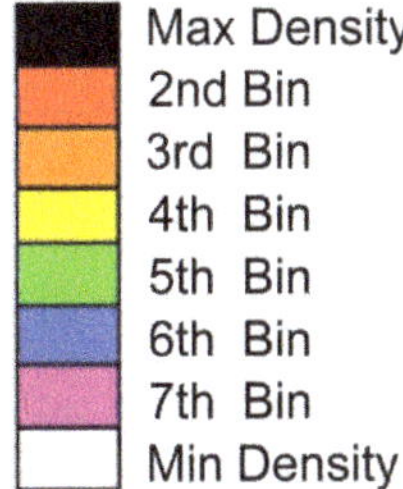

Figure 1. Maximum intensity projection (MIP) maps of marsupials representing gait categories. For each of the distal tibiae, its anterior surface faces upwards and its medial surface faces to the right. AQ = Arboreal quadrupedal, TQ = Terrestrial quadrupedal.

Biped ratios are significantly higher than ratios of quadrupeds, whether they are arboreal or terrestrial (Table 4). Interestingly, the only arboreal macropod (*Dendrolagus*) has a comparatively low mean ratio of 0.017 (n = 2). When accounting for phylogeny, the comparison of species means eliminates statistical significance (Table 4).

Ratios of the second highest radiodensity area to total articular surface area differ between groups in a way that is consistent with differences in maximum-to-total ratios. Bipeds again exhibit the largest ratios (Figure 3, Tables 2 and 3), regardless of whether they are small-bodied (wallaby mean = 0.558, n = 7: Tables 1 and 3) or large-bodied (kangaroo mean = 0.488, n = 7: Tables 1 and 3). The biped ratio is significantly higher than the quadruped ratio, but only the difference between bipeds and arboreal quadrupeds is significant while the difference between bipeds and terrestrial quadrupeds is borderline non-significant (Table 4). The only arboreal macropod (*Dendrolagus*) again has a comparatively low mean ratio of 0.300 (n = 2) compared to other macropods. When accounting for phylogeny, the comparison of species means eliminates statistical significance (Table 4).

Prediction 2: Terrestrial Quadrupedal Marsupials>Arboreal Quadrupedal Marsupials

As predicted, arboreal quadrupeds exhibit the smallest maximum radiodensity area relative to total articular surface area of any group (Figure 3, Tables 2 and 3). However, differences between terrestrial quadruped and arboreal quadruped ratios are small and non-significant (Table 4). When accounting for phylogeny, the comparison of species means remains non-significant (Table 4).

Arboreal quadrupeds also exhibit the smallest ratios of second highest radiodensity area to total articular surface area of any group in a way that is consistent with maximum-to-total ratios (Figure 3, Tables 2 and 3). As was observed in comparisons of maximum radiodensity area ratios, however, differences between terrestrial quadruped and arboreal quadruped ratios are small and non-significant (Table 4). When accounting for phylogeny, the comparison of species means remains non-significant (Table 4).

Discussion

As predicted, bipedal marsupials such as kangaroos and wallabies exhibit distal tibiae with more expansive maximum radiodensity areas than the distal tibiae of quadrupedal marsupials investigated in this study. It appears that compressive loads borne through hind limbs are more substantial in bipeds than quadrupeds, possibly due to more body weight support per hind limb generating higher vertical components of SRFs experienced in the former [13]. While we did not exhaustively sample bipedal and quadrupedal marsupials, the extent of the observed differences in representative taxa (Tables 1 and 3) strongly suggests that this may be a common trend amongst marsupials. The statistical significance of this trend disappears when accounting for

Table 2. Descriptive statistics for ANOVA.

		Max/total pixels	Max/total pixels	Second/total pixels	Second/total pixels
Gait category[1]	**n**	**Mean (1 SD)**	**Range**	**Mean (1 SD)**	**Range**
Bipedal	14	0.214 (0.151)	0.045–0.567	0.523 (0.156)	0.253–0.799
AQ	17	0.080 (0.103)	0.000–0.352	0.289 (0.158)	0.013–0.580
TQ	10	0.083 (0.077)	0.000–0.174	0.364 (0.203)	0.094–0.667

[1]AQ = Arboreal quadrupedal; TQ = Terrestrial quadrupedal. SD = standard deviation.

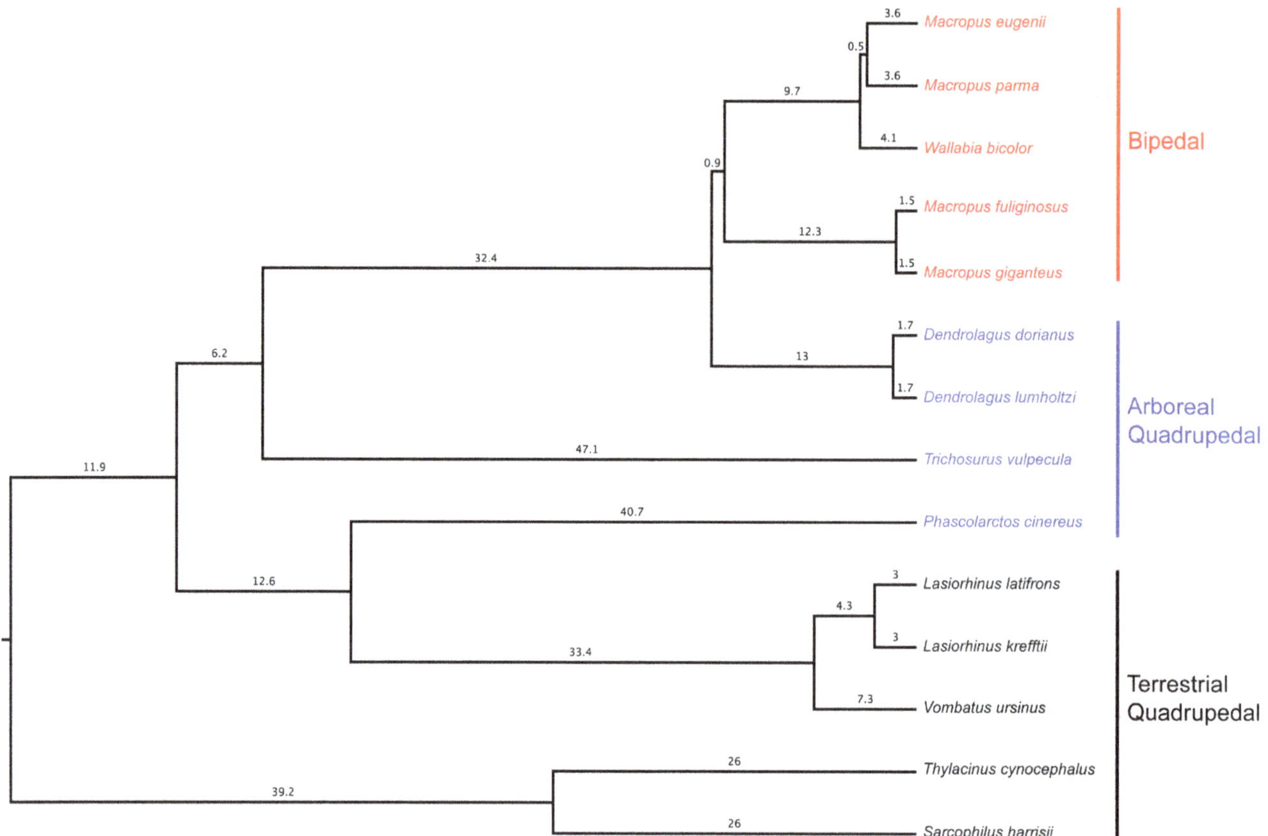

Figure 2. Phylogenetic tree and divergence times of marsupial species included in the study. Branch lengths indicate millions of years based on molecular analyses [40–41]. Colors distinguish between groups characterized by different habitual locomotor activities (red: bipedal; blue: arboreal quadruped; black: terrestrial quadruped).

phylogeny (Table 4). However, it is noteworthy in support of a functional basis to the observed trend that two species of *Dendrolagus*, the tree kangaroo, and the only living arboreal macropod, exhibit substantially lower mean ratios compared to mean ratios of closely related bipedal macropods (Figure 2 and Table 3). This suggests a functional signal in macropod distal tibiae is not completely obscured by phylogeny. Moreover, the phylogenetically-controlled ANOVAs, which utilize species means and thus do not account for intraspecific biological variation, are hampered by small sample sizes in several cases. In our study, *Macropus parma*, *Sarcophilus harrisii*, and *Lasiorhinus latifrons*, each represented by only one individual per species, have notably low values compared to related taxa that are represented by multiple individuals (Table 4). Investigation of radiodensity patterns within primate distal tibiae would be a worthwhile investigation as an independent test of the bipedal versus quadrupedal signal that is observed in the present study. While there are clear differences between the mechanics of macropod and human bipedalism, based on the present results we would predict that patterns in primate distal tibiae should mirror those in marsupials, specifically, that bipedal humans should be unique (and more expansive) in relative maximum radiodensity area compared to quadrupedal primates.

The distinctiveness of distal tibiae of bipedal marsupials corroborates findings of others who have noted distinctiveness of the calcaneus of bipedal marsupials [43]. Functional anatomy of the marsupial calcaneus, including its dimensions, would seem strongly integrated with functional anatomy of the ankle joint. Serving as the insertion point for the Achilles tendon, and thus operating as the moment arm for ankle plantar flexors such as the triceps surae, the calcaneus plays a key role in foot function. Among several hind limb joints of tammar wallabies (*Macropus eugenii*), the ankle was observed to be the greatest contributor to whole limb work and power over a range of accelerations and decelerations [44]. The present study provides supporting evidence for the ankle joint playing a central role in the distinctiveness of macropod hopping gaits versus gaits of other marsupials. In addition to the distal tibia, it would be worthwhile to assess the articulating component of the ankle joint (i.e., the talar trochlea) for concordant or discrepant trends, as has been done in some primates [23].

It was unexpected that mean radiodensity ratios of arboreal and terrestrial quadruped marsupials did not differ significantly. Arboreal quadrupedal primates exhibit gait compliancy compared to terrestrial quadrupedal primates, and thus limbs of the former experience lower peak vertical components of SRFs [9–10,45]. A convergent pattern in aspects of gait compliancy has been demonstrated in at least one arboreal quadrupedal marsupial [4]. Arboreal substrates usually are more compliant and more susceptible to movement (i.e., instability) compared to terrestrial substrates, which could favor reduced peak compressive loading experienced through limb joints because of higher duty factors when moving on branches [46]. One possible explanation for this unexpected result amongst marsupials could be that gait compliancy is more effective at reducing compressive loads in forelimb joints rather than hind limb joints, as appears to be the case in

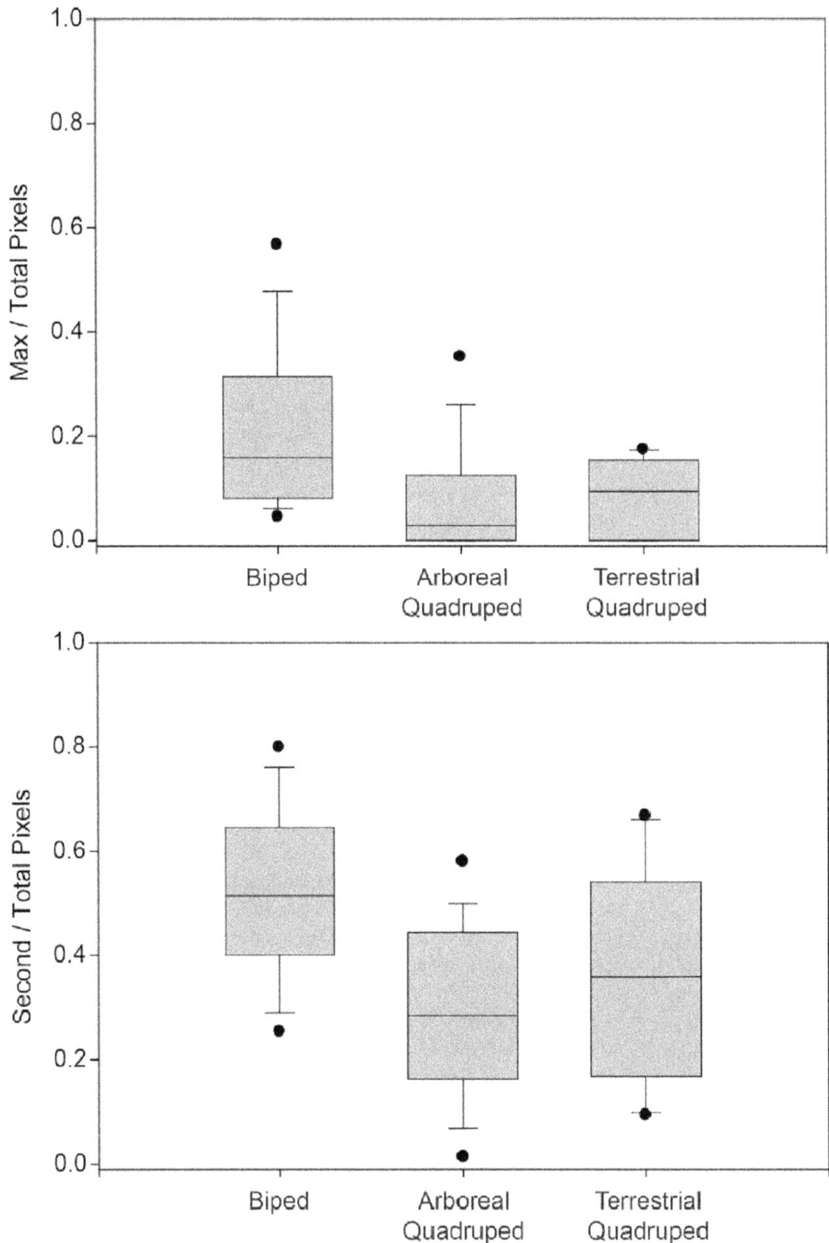

Figure 3. Box plots of pixel ratios in articular surfaces. Top row indicates ratios of pixels in the maximum bin to total pixels, while the bottom row indicates ratios of pixels in the second highest bin to total pixels. These values are derived from distal tibiae, excluding the region of the articular surface that descends onto the lateral aspect of the medial malleolus. Horizontal lines within each box indicate medians, while the entire box envelops the interquartile range of the distribution (i.e., 50% of values), and whiskers encompass the remaining range, excluding outliers. Filled circles beyond whiskers indicate outliers.

some primates. In capuchin monkeys, for example, peak vertical components of SRFs experienced by their forelimbs during walks, runs, and gallops were significantly lower on simulated arboreal supports than on a wooden runway, while hind limb peak vertical forces did not differ significantly between substrates during as many of these gaits [47]. It would be worthwhile, in this regard, to compare marsupial distal radii from the same locomotor groups and document whether bipeds exhibit the smallest areas of maximum radiodensity and terrestrial quadrupeds the largest.

A second potential explanation for the unexpected non-significant difference between arboreal and terrestrial marsupial quadrupeds could be related to the application of such rigid gait and substrate use categories in the first place. There are a wealth of primate observational data on locomotor activities and substrate use [48]. Similar data from free-ranging marsupials are not as widely documented. For example, some primates traditionally recognized as quadrupeds also have been observed habitually using suspensory behaviors [49]. Primates typically categorized as digitigrade or palmigrade have been shown to dynamically switch between both hand postures, depending on speed, gait, and substrate used during quadrupedal gaits [50–54]. Because of the relative paucity of quantitative observational data on marsupial

Table 3. Descriptive statistics for pANOVA.

			Max/total pixels	Second/total pixels
Genus[1]	**Species**	**n**	**Mean (1 SD)**	**Mean (1 SD)**
Macropus	*giganteus*	5	0.298 (0.203)	0.470 (0.104)
Macropus	*fuliginosus*	2	0.107 (0.043)	0.532 (0.271)
Macropus	*eugenii*	4	0.149 (0.077)	0.562 (0.229)
Macropus	*parma*	1	0.076 (−)	0.668 (−)
Wallabia	*bicolor*	2	0.307 (0.003)	0.495 (0.018)
Bipedal species		**5**	**0.187 (0.108)**	**0.545 (0.077)**
Dendrolagus	*dorianus*	1	0.029 (−)	0.144 (−)
Dendrolagus	*lumholtzi*	1	0.005 (−)	0.457 (−)
Phascolarctos	*cinereus*	9	0.110 (0.127)	0.272 (0.145)
Trichosurus	*vulpecula*	6	0.058 (0.065)	0.309 (0.188)
AQ species		**4**	**0.051 (0.045)**	**0.296 (0.129)**
Lasiorhinus	*krefftii*	2	0.138 (0.019)	0.635 (0.046)
Lasiorhinus	*latifrons*	1	0.000 (−)	0.094 (−)
Sarcophilus	*harrisii*	1	0.000 (−)	0.153 (−)
Thylacinus	*cynocephalus*	3	0.133 (0.060)	0.355 (0.155)
Vombatus	*ursinus*	3	0.051 (0.086)	0.353 (0.167)
TQ species		**5**	**0.064 (0.068)**	**0.318 (0.212)**

[1]AQ = Arboreal quadrupedal; TQ = Terrestrial quadrupedal. SD = standard deviation. See Table 1 for common names.

locomotor behavior and substrate use, the possibility exists that there could be an underappreciated amount of crossover in gait and substrate use amongst the marsupial quadrupeds included in this study. If arboreal and terrestrial quadrupedal marsupials differ less in substrate preference than presently assumed, it could explain the greater than expected similarity exhibited in their relative maximum radiodensity areas. It is worth noting that compliant gait has been proposed as a solution for additional challenges besides those arising during arboreal locomotion [55]. With additional data on substrate use, reassessing quadrupedal marsupials (or primates) according to terrain unevenness and compliant gait, irrespective of whether they are presently characterized as arboreal or terrestrial, could provide interesting insights for the observed variation in subchondral radiodensity areas and estimated compressive loads of marsupial (or primate) distal tibiae.

Expanding samples of fossorial (i.e., *Vombatus* and *Lasiorhinus*) and non-fossorial terrestrial quadrupeds (i.e., *Sarcophilus* and *Thylacinus*) would facilitate another potentially interesting comparison within marsupials. Wombats are described as emphasizing forelimbs during digging, while their hind limbs are primarily relegated to clearing accumulated sediment [43]. Thus, wombat hind limbs may be less functionally specialized away from the limbs of other terrestrial quadrupeds compared to wombat forelimbs. External calcaneal morphology of fossorial and non-fossorial quadrupeds supports this possibility since their calcanei could not be differentiated in a morphometric analysis of calcaneal shape and dimension [43]. As noted previously, investigating the distal radius of bipedal and different forms of quadrupedal marsupials could prove especially illuminating. We would predict that fossorial taxa may show evidence of elevated compressive loading of the wrist compared to all other marsupial taxa, if digging indeed fosters more morphological specialization in the forelimb than the hind limb.

We are aware of only one published study that has focused on quantifying similar radiodensity patterns in joints of the foot. Nowak et al. [22] observed the predicted correspondence between presumed joint loading patterns and locations of maximum radiodensity areas in primates that experience a "mid-tarsal break" versus humans that typically do not, but that may in small frequencies [56]. Observation of the predicted distinctiveness of bipedal marsupials in the extent of maximum radiodensity area in their distal tibiae also accords well with predicted patterns of radiodensity distribution observed in the forelimb joints of primates and xenarthrans. Quadrupedal primates exhibit more expansive areas of high radiodensity in their distal radius compared to the distal radii of bipedal and suspensory primates [18], while quadrupedal xenarthrans exhibit more expansive areas of high radiodensity in their distal radius compared to the distal radii of suspensory sloths [20]. In each case, it is reasonable to conclude that the quadrupedal group experiences compressive loading during forelimb use resulting from the *additive* effects of body weight support and musculotendon contractile forces from complexes that bridge joints, while the other groups may experience the former contributing factor to a lesser degree. Teasing apart the relative contribution of the two factors is complex, however, as demonstrated by a recent study of joint forces in the human knee showing that a muscle can contribute to

Table 4. ANOVA and pANOVA results.

		ANOVA				pANOVA			
Ratio	**Comparison[1]**	**df**	**F**	**p**	**Post hoc analyses**	**df**	**F**	**p**	**Post hoc analyses**
Max bin/total	B v. AQ v. TQ	2, 38	5.920	0.006**	B v. AQ: p = 0.008**	2, 11	4.152	0.045*	B v. AQ = 0.342
					B v. TQ: p = 0.027*			0.422[2]	B v. TQ: p = 0.698
					AQ v. TQ: p = 0.998				AQ v. TQ: p = 0.903
Second bin/total	B v. AQ v. TQ	2, 38	7.492	0.002**	B v. AQ: p = 0.001**	2, 11	3.948	0.051	B v. AQ = 0.441
					B v. TQ: p = 0.072			0.410[2]	B v. TQ: p = 0.760
					AQ v. TQ: p = 0.511				AQ v. TQ: p = 0.907

[1]B = Bipedal; AQ = Arboreal quadrupedal; TQ = Terrestrial quadrupedal.
[2]Phylogenetic p-value. df = Degrees of Freedom;
*denotes statistical significance at 0.05 level;
**denotes statistical significance at 0.01 level.

overall joint force via its contribution to the substrate reaction force even when the muscle does not cross the joint in question [57].

Despite the limitations of this study (e.g., small samples of some species, relative lack of quantitative data on marsupial behavior and substrate use, and the complexity of musculotendon loading of joints), the observed trend exhibited by bipedal and quadrupedal marsupials adds to the accumulating evidence suggesting that the relationship between relative area of maximum radiodensity and joint compressive loads in limbs may be a unifying form-function principle amongst eutherian and metatherian mammals. By demonstrating how behavior influences morphology in a variety of mammals, these unifying principles support the existence of form-function signals in skeletal tissues that often elude comparative functional anatomists.

Supporting Information

Table S1 Specimen information and raw data used in analyses.

Table S2 Nexus tree file used in the pANOVA. The phylogenetic tree with known divergence dates for taxa in the sample is based on recent molecular studies of marsupials [40–41]. The tree file was created with Mesquite software.

Acknowledgments

We thank several museums and their respective curators and staff for assistance: Dr. Sandy Ingleby and Dr. Anja Divljan (Australian Museum, Sydney); Dr. Leo Joseph and Robert Palmer (Australian National Wildlife Collection, Canberra); Heather Janetzki and Nicholas Hadnutt (Queensland Museum, Brisbane); and Kathryn Medlock, Nikki Kingsmith, and Nicole Zehntner (Tasmanian Museum, Hobart). We thank Claire Da Deppo, Dr. Ross O'Neil, Stephen Hamilton, Bede Yates, Josh Crockett, and Anita Lee for assistance with CT scanning specimens in the various collections. We thank Matt Borths and Dr. Steve Van Dyck for their assistance in formulating and constructing the phylogenetic tree used in this study.

Author Contributions

Conceived and designed the experiments: KJC BAP. Performed the experiments: KJC. Analyzed the data: KJC TJ. Contributed reagents/materials/analysis tools: KJC TJ KH MCW BAP. Wrote the paper: KJC BAP.

References

1. Luo Z, Yuan C, Meng Q, Ji Q (2011) A Jurassic eutherian mammal and divergence of marsupials and placentals. Nature 476: 442–445.
2. Garland T Jr, Geiser F, Baudinette RV (1988) Comparative locomotor performance of marsupial and placental mammals. J Zool Lond 215: 505–522.
3. Pridmore PA (1992) Trunk movements during locomotion in the marsupial *Monodelphis domestica (Didelphidae)*. J Morphol 211: 137–146.
4. Schmitt D, Lemelin P (2002) Origins of primate locomotion: gait mechanics of the woolly opossum. Am J Phys Anthropol 118: 231–238.
5. Shapiro LJ, Young JW (2012) Kinematics of quadrupedal locomotion in sugar gliders (*Petaurus breviceps*): effects of age and substrate size. J Exp Biol 215: 480–496.
6. Bennett MB (2000) Unifying principles in terrestrial locomotion: do hopping Australian marsupials fit in? Physiol Biochem Zool 73: 726–735.
7. Lammers AR, Biknevicius AR (2004) The biodynamics of arboreal locomotion: the effects of substrate diameter on locomotor kinetics in the gray short-tailed opossum (*Monodelphis domestica*). J Exp Biol 207: 4325–4336.
8. Windsor DE, Dagg AI (1971) The gaits of the *Macropodinae* (*Marsupialia*). J Zool Lond 163: 165–175.5.
9. Schmitt D (1999) Compliant walking in primates. J Zool Lond 248: 149–160.
10. Larney E, Larson SG (2004) Compliant walking in primates: elbow and knee yield in primates compared to other mammals. Am J Phys Anthropol 125: 42–50.
11. Dawson TJ, Taylor CR (1973) Energetic cost of locomotion in Kangaroos. Nature 246: 313–314.
12. Baudinette RV, Snyder GK, Frappell PB (1992) Energetic cost of locomotion in the Tammar wallaby. Am J Physiol 262: R771–778.
13. Farley CT, Glasheen J, McMahon TA (1993) Running springs: speed and animal size. J Exp Biol 185: 71–86.
14. Szalay FS (2006) Evolutionary history of the marsupials and an analysis of osteological characters. Cambridge: Cambridge University Press. 496 p.
15. Szalay FS, Sargis EJ (2001) Model-based analysis of postcranial osteology of marsupials from the Palaeocene of Itaborai (Brazil) and the phylogenetics and biogeography of *Metatheria*. Geodiversitas 23: 139–302.
16. Argot C (2001) Functional-adaptive anatomy of the forelimb in the *Didelphidae*, and the paleobiology of the Paleocene marsupials *Mayulestes ferox* and *Pucadelphys andinus*. J Morphol 247: 51–79.
17. Argot C (2002) Functional-adaptive analysis of the hindlimb anatomy of extant marsupials and the paleobiology of the Paleocene marsupials *Mayulestes ferox* and *Pucadelphys andinus*. J Morphol 253: 76–108.
18. Carlson KJ, Patel BA (2006) Habitual use of the primate forelimb is reflected in the material properties of subchondral bone in the distal radius. J Anat 208: 659–670.
19. Patel BA, Carlson KJ (2007) Material properties of the distal radius reflect habitual hand postures adopted by quadrupedal primates. J Hum Evol 52: 130–141.
20. Patel BA, Carlson KJ (2008) Apparent density patterns in subchondral bone of the sloth and anteater forelimb. Biol Lett 4: 486–489.
21. Polk JD, Blumefeld J, Ahluwalia K (2008) Knee posture predicted from subchondral apparent density in the distal femur: an experimental validation. Anat Rec 291: 293–302.
22. Nowak MG, Carlson KJ, Patel BA (2010) Apparent density of the primate calcaneo-cuboid joint and its association with locomotor mode, foot posture, and the "midtarsal break." Am J Phys Anthropol 142: 180–193.
23. Su A (2011) The functional morphology of subchondral and trabecular bone in the hominoid tibiotalar joint. PhD Dissertation. Stony Brook University.
24. Alexander RM, Vernon A (1975) The mechanics of hopping by kangaroos (*Macropodidae*). J Zool Lond 177: 265–303.
25. Cavagna GA, Heglund NC, Taylor CR (1977) Mechanical work in terrestrial locomotion: two basic mechanisms for minimizing energy expenditure. Am J Physiol 233: R243–R261.
26. Baudinette RV (1994) Locomotion in macropodoid marsupials: gaits, energetic, and heat balance. Aust J Zool 42: 103–23.
27. Biewener AA, Baudinette RV (1995) *In vivo* muscle force and elastic energy storage during steady-speed hopping of Tammar wallabies (*Macropus eugenii*). J Exp Biol 198: 1829–1841.
28. Kram R, Dawson TJ (1998) Energetics and biomechanics of locomotion by red kangaroos (*Macropus rufus*). Comp Biochem Physiol, Part B 120: 41–49.
29. McGowan CP, Baudinette RV, Biewener AA (2008) Differential design for hopping in two species of wallabies. Comp Biochem Physiol, Part A 150: 151–158.
30. Currey JD (1984) Comparative mechanical properties of histology of bone. Am Zool 24: 5–12.
31. Müller-Gerbl M, Putz R, Kenn R (1992) Demonstration of subchondral bone density patterns by three-dimensional CT osteoaborptiometry as a non-invasive method for *in vivo* assessment of individual long-term stresses in joints. J Bone Miner Res 7: S411–S418.
32. Eckstein F, Merz B, Schön M, Jacobs CR, Putz R (1999) Tension and bending, but not compression alone determine the functional adaptation of subchondral bone in incongruous joints. Anat Embryol 199: 85–97.
33. Radin EL, Paul IL, Lowy M (1970) A comparison of the dynamic force transmitting properties of subchondral bone and articular cartilage. J Bone Joint Surg 52A: 444–456.
34. Biewener AA (2003) Animal locomotion. Oxford: Oxford University Press. 296 p.
35. Herzog W, Longino D, Clark A (2003) The role of muscles in joint adaptation and degeneration. Langenbecks Arch Surg 288: 305–315.
36. Winby CR, Lloyd DG, Besier TF, Kirk TB (2009) Muscle and external load contribution to knee joint contact loads during normal gait. J Biomech 42: 2294–2300.
37. Thorpe SKS, Crompton RH (2006) Orangutan positional behavior and the nature of arboreal locomotion in Hominoidea. Am J Phys Anthropol 131: 384–401.
38. Carlson KJ, Demes B, Franz TM (2005) Mediolateral forces associated with quadrupedal gaits of lemurids. J Zool Lond 266: 261–273.
39. Jones C, Parish S (2010) Field guide to Australian mammals. Archerfield, Queensland: Steve Parish Publishing Pty Ltd. 216 p.
40. Beck MD (2008) A dated phylogeny of marsupials using a molecular supermatrix and multiple fossil constraints. J Mamm 89: 175–189.
41. Meredith RW, Westerman M, Springer MS (2009) The phylogeny of Diprotodontia (*Marsupialia*) based on sequences for five nuclear genes. Mol Phylogenet Evol 51: 554–571.

42. Revell LJ (2012) Phytools: an R package for phylogenetic comparative biology (and other things). Meth Ecol Evol 3: 217–223.
43. Bassarova M, Janis CM, Archer M (2009) The calcaneum – on the heels of marsupial locomotion. J Mammal Evol 16: 1–23.
44. McGowan CP, Baudinette RV, Biewener AA (2005) Joint work and power associated with acceleration and deceleration in tammar wallabies (*Macropus eugenii*). J Exp Biol 208: 41–53.
45. Schmitt D, Hanna JB (2004) Substrate alters forelimb to hindlimb peak force ratios in primates. J Hum Evol 46: 239–254.
46. Stevens NJ (2006) Stability, limb coordination and substrate type: the ecorelevance of gait sequence pattern in Primates. J Exp Zool 305A: 953–963.
47. Carlson KJ, Demes B (2010) Gait dynamics of *Cebus apella* during quadrupedalism on different substrates. Am J Phys Anthropol 142: 273–286.
48. Hunt KD, Cant JGH, Gebo DL, Rose MD, Walker S (1996) Standardized descriptions of primate locomotor and postural modes. Primates 37: 363–387.
49. Byron C, Covert HH (2004) Unexpected locomotor behaviour: brachiation by an Old World monkey from Vietnam. J Zool Lond 263: 101–106.
50. Patel BA (2009) Not so fast: speed effects on forelimb kinematics in cercopithecine monkeys and implications for digitigrades postures in primates. Am J Phys Anthropol 140: 92–112.
51. Patel BA (2010) The interplay between speed, kinetics, and hand postures during primate terrestrial locomotion. Am J Phys Anthropol 141: 222–234.
52. Patel BA, Polk JD (2010) Distal forelimb kinematics in *Erythrocebus patas* and *Papio anubis* during walking and galloping. Int J Primatol 31: 191–207.
53. Patel BA, Wunderlich R (2010) Dynamic pressure patterns in the hands of olive baboons (*Papio anubis*) during terrestrial locomotion: implications for cercopithecoid primate hand morphology. Anat Rec 293: 710–718.
54. Patel BA, Larson SG, Stern JT Jr (2012) Electromyography of wrist and finger flexor muscles in olive baboons (*Papio anubis*). J Exp Biol 215: 115–123.
55. Daley MA, Usherwood JR (2010) Two explanations for the compliant running paradox: reduced work of bouncing viscera and increased stability in uneven terrain. Biol Lett 6: 418–421.
56. Crompton RH, Pataky TC, Savage R, D'Août K, Bennett MR, et al. (2011) Human-like external function of the foot, and fully upright gait, confirmed in the 3.66 million year old Laetoli hominin footprints by topographic statistics, experimental footprint-formation and computer simulation. J R Soc Interface 9: 707–719.
57. Sasaki K, Neptune RR (2010) Individual muscle contributions to the axial knee joint contact force during normal walking. J Biomech 43: 2780–2784.

15

Trabecular Bone Adaptation to Low-Magnitude High-Frequency Loading in Microgravity

Antonia Torcasio[1], Katharina Jähn[2], Maarten Van Guyse[1], Pieter Spaepen[1], Andrea E. Tami[2], Jos Vander Sloten[1], Martin J. Stoddart[2], G. Harry van Lenthe[1,3*]

1 Biomechanics Section, KU Leuven, Leuven, Belgium, **2** AO Research Institute, Davos, Switzerland, **3** Institute for Biomechanics, ETH Zurich, Zurich, Switzerland

Abstract

Exposure to microgravity causes loss of lower body bone mass in some astronauts. Low-magnitude high-frequency loading can stimulate bone formation on earth. Here we hypothesized that low-magnitude high-frequency loading will also stimulate bone formation under microgravity conditions. Two groups of six bovine cancellous bone explants were cultured at microgravity on a Russian Foton-M3 spacecraft and were either loaded dynamically using a sinusoidal curve or experienced only a static load. Comparable reference groups were investigated at normal gravity. Bone structure was assessed by histology, and mechanical competence was quantified using μCT and FE modelling; bone remodelling was assessed by fluorescent labelling and secreted bone turnover markers. Statistical analyses on morphometric parameters and apparent stiffness did not reveal significant differences between the treatment groups. The release of bone formation marker from the groups cultured at normal gravity increased significantly from the first to the second week of the experiment by 90.4% and 82.5% in response to static and dynamic loading, respectively. Bone resorption markers decreased significantly for the groups cultured at microgravity by 7.5% and 8.0% in response to static and dynamic loading, respectively. We found low strain magnitudes to drive bone turnover when applied at high frequency, and this to be valid at normal as well as at microgravity. In conclusion, we found the effect of mechanical loading on trabecular bone to be regulated mainly by an increase of bone formation at normal gravity and by a decrease in bone resorption at microgravity. Additional studies with extended experimental time and increased samples number appear necessary for a further understanding of the anabolic potential of dynamic loading on bone quality and mechanical competence.

Editor: Ali Al-Ahmad, University Hospital of the Albert-Ludwigs-University Freiburg, Germany

Funding: This study was financially supported by grant C90346 (Belgium PRODEX-9 project) and the ESA MAP grant #AO99-122. The funders had no role in study design, data collection and analysis, decision to publish, or preparation of the manuscript.

Competing Interests: The authors have declared that no competing interests exist.

* E-mail: harry.vanlenthe@mech.kuleuven.be

Introduction

One of the effects resulting from the exposure to microgravity is the loss of bone mass in the lower limbs and spine in some astronauts [1,2]. Data from spaceflights on the Russian space station Mir and the International Space Station ISS have demonstrated the impact of weightlessness on bone volume. During a space mission at the Mir, areal bone mineral density (aBMD) of some astronauts was reduced by a monthly rate of 0.3% from the total skeleton, with 97% of that loss occurring in the pelvis and legs [3]. These measurements varied largely between astronauts; some individuals incurred losses equivalent to one-half the bone mineral they would lose in a lifetime of normal aging, while others experienced only a small BMD reduction.

In the spine and hip, relevant areas of frequently seen osteoporotic bone fractures in the elderly, a decrease in aBMD of 0.9% and 1.5% per month respectively was found in ISS crew members [4]. Computed Tomography (CT) measurements in combination with DXA (dual energy X-ray absorptiometry) revealed that bone is lost in cancellous as well as in cortical bone volumes. These effects on bones might not have immediate implications for the astronauts, but could lead to increased fracture risk because of an associated loss in bone strength as well as to an early onset of age-related osteoporosis in the more advanced age.

As a potential countermeasure to prevent bone loss, mechanical stimulation has attracted much attention in recent years. It is well known that bone is capable of adapting its mass and structure in response to mechanical loading. The nature of the mechanical stimulus for bone adaptation has been debated for over 100 years [5]. Researchers initially showed that the adaptive response of bone to loading is influenced by the mechanical strain magnitude and demonstrated that bone formation is initiated when a certain strain threshold is surpassed. An important contribution was made in 1971 by Hert and co-workers when they showed that dynamic, but not static, strains increased bone formation in rabbits [6]. Dynamic strains thus appeared to be the primary stimulus of bone adaptation. O'Connor et al [7] emphasized the influence of the rate of strain, more specifically that high frequency components of the loading cycle were important for maximal bone response. With incremental increases in strain, bone responds with further increases in formation activity [8]. By decomposing the mechanical stimulus into constituent components, researchers have subsequently identified several mechanical parameters that influence the anabolic response to loading. Among these are strain rate, strain distribution, local strain gradients [9], number of cycles [10], and resting periods [11,12]. Strain rate can be further decomposed into strain magnitude and loading frequency. Low-amplitude high-frequency loading in bone has been shown to occur more often in normal daily activities in vivo [13] and has been investigated as a loading regime to promote adaptive bone formation. Specifically, it has been demonstrated that low-amplitude high-frequency stimuli (500 microstrains at 30 Hz) were sufficient to stimulate new bone formation in experimental animals, whereas high-amplitude low-frequency (3000 microstrains at 1 Hz) was insufficient [14]. The tissue's sensitivity to low-amplitude high-frequency loading suggests an interesting potential pathway for therapeutic intervention, as the adaptive capacity of bone in response to such loading could be considered as a potential countermeasure to prevent bone loss under weightlessness conditions.

For the present study we hypothesized that low-amplitude (apparent strain <500 microstrains) high-frequency (30 Hz) mechanical loading would influence the bone remodelling processes in microgravity conditions also. In addition, we addressed the question whether the amount of bone adaptation is related to strain magnitude. In order to test these hypotheses, an explant culture system that provides mechanical loading, in addition to managing nutrition and waste products [15,16] was used for the first time in space.

Materials and Methods

Fully automated microgravity experiments were conducted on board of the unmanned Russian Foton-M3 spacecraft, launched from Kazakhstan on September 14, 2007. When Foton-M3 was in orbit, a reference experiment at 1 g was conducted on ground. The mission duration was 12 days. After the experiments, the bone samples and perfusion media were collected. First, bone turnover markers (C-terminal propeptide of type I collagen and N-terminal telopeptide of type I collagen) were quantified to analyse whether trabecular bone adapts to dynamic loading at normal and microgravity. Second, histological evaluation of the bone was performed to investigate the morphology of the bone tissue and determine the presence of osteoblasts and osteoclasts. Third, we evaluated bone quality, in terms of its micro-architecture and mechanical stiffness, in response to mechanical loading at normal and microgravity. Finally, we investigated whether the bone adaptation processes may be linked to strain levels within the trabeculae.

The FreqBone experiment

Four different groups each containing six bovine cancellous bone explants were taken from the sternum of a 1-year old cow. Given the restrictions related to performing an experiment in space, only a limited number of specimens per group was investigated. All samples were obtained from one animal in order to avoid any inter-individual variations. The sternum was ordered from a local butcher (Van den Berg, Voorhout, the Netherlands). Animal euthanasia was performed in order to guarantee the quality of the tissue. Procedures were checked in person by a veterinary of the Netherlands Food and Consumer Product Safety Authority. The sternum was considered a normal product of slaughter; hence, no ethics approval was required. Two groups were cultured at microgravity and were either loaded dynamically using a sinusoid curve (30 N peak to peak amplitude and 30 Hz frequency), or experienced only a static load of 30 N. Two reference groups were cultured at normal gravity and experienced either static or dynamic load identical to the groups at microgravity.

The preparation of the cylindrical bone explants (diameter = 10 mm, height = 5 mm), as well as the culture medium (Dulbecco's Modified Eagle Medium DMEM +10% Fetal Calf Serum FCS) was performed at the European Space Agency (ESA) Research and Technology Centre in Noordwijk (Netherlands).

The bovine sternum was cleaned of remaining soft tissues. With the use of an 'Exakt 300' band saw (Exakt Apparatebau GmbH & Co. KG) the bone was cut into 7 mm-thick sections. Cancellous bone cores were drilled out from these sections using an EcoMac 212 bench drill containing a Synthes drill bit (Ref: 387.661, Synthes, Bettlach, Switzerland), resulting in 10 mm diameter cancellous bone cores. Cores were then grounded parallel to 5 mm height. During all cutting and drilling procedures, the bone explants were irrigated with sterile pre-cooled (4°C) saline (0.9% sodium chloride solution) to reduce the formation of bone debris and heat-induced cell death. Adherent bone debris was removed by washing each explant three times in 10 ml HBSS (Hank's Buffered Salt Solution) for 30 min each at 4°C. Each cancellous bone explant was then inserted inside a culture chamber (Mathys, CH) under sterile conditions. The FreqBone culture and bioreactor system containing the bone samples was brought to Baikonur (Kazakhstan). The normal gravity experiment with the reference samples was performed in Leuven (Belgium). All bone explants and culture media were kept at 10°C for 4.5 days prior to the start of the experiment. The experiment was started on board of the spacecraft immediately after launch by raising the temperature of the explants from 10°C to 37°C; the temperature of the explants was maintained at 37°C for the duration of the flight. The explants were subjected to mechanical loading for 12 days continuously. The FreqBone bioreactor and culture system had been developed on the basis of the technology previously used in the 'Zetos' system [17]. Extensive cell viability investigations on the Zetos system have been reported [17,18]. In short, the culture chambers containing the bone explants were perfused with a pump system connected to the culture medium reservoirs. For mechanical stimulation, the chambers were in circular arrangement with a circulating loading stack in the centre [19] (Figure 1).

At two different time points of the FreqBone experiment, bone explants were perfused with fluorescent labels in order to detect small changes in bone formation. Specifically, calcein green was applied prior to launch and alizarin complexon was given after the mission. The labelling was performed at 10°C to avoid high metabolic activity of the explants and, therefore, uptake of the dye at active surfaces [20]. Each label was applied for 24 h.

The culture medium was exchanged once after 6 days, hence, two medium samples per explant (day 6 and day 12) were used for analyses. Media were kept at 10°C and were heated to 37°C just prior to bone explant contact. Each explant was cultured with 20 ml medium for 6 days prior to exchange. When the 12-day spaceflight was over, bone explants were stored for 2 days at 10°C prior to fixation in 70% ethanol. Culture media collected at day 6 and day 12 were frozen and stored for further analysis. All reference specimens were treated the same as experimental group specimens with the exception that the reference specimens were not flown to Kazakhstan.

Culture medium analyses

The soluble products in the culture medium that arise from matrix breakdown and formation were quantified. All medium investigations were performed on one day to avoid repeated freezing and thawing of the samples and to keep analyses consistency. Analyses of the medium samples involved the detection of the C-terminal propeptide of type I collagen (ProCI)

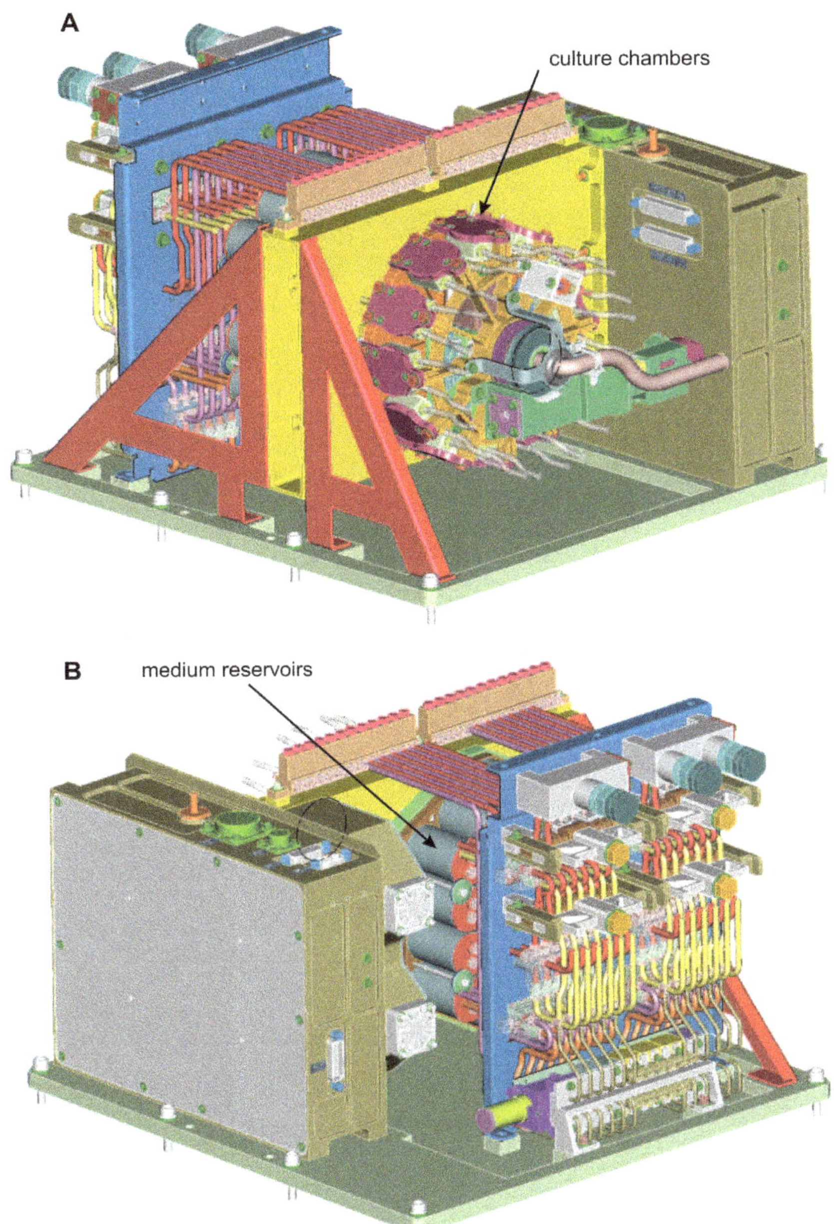

Figure 1. Schematic illustration of the FreqBone bioreactor and culture system. A) The front side shows the culture chambers that are arranged in a circle with a rotating loading stack in the centre; B) The medium reservoirs and the pump system are visible on the back side.

as a bone formation marker, and of N-terminal telopeptide of type I collagen (NTx) as indicator of bone resorption.

The release of ProCI was quantified using the "Procollagen Type I C-Peptide Enzyme Immunoassay Kit" (Takara Bio Inc., Shiga, Japan) according to manufacturer's instructions. Briefly, 20 µl sample or standard (with a range from 0–640 ng ProCI/ml were used in this assay per 96-well. The absorbance of the final product was measured at 450 nm using a "HTS 7000 Bio Assay Reader" (Perkin Elmer Perkin-Elmer, Shelton, CT).

The osteoclast-dependent release of NTx was quantified using the "OSTERMARK® NTx-Serum" (Ostex International Inc., Seattle, WA) according to manufacturer's instructions. The culture medium samples were diluted 1:1 in "specimen diluent". Samples, "assay calibrators", and reference samples were used at 100 µl per well in 96-well plates. The optical density of the colour reaction was determined at 450 nm using a "HTS 7000 Bio Assay Reader" (Perkin Elmer Perkin-Elmer, Shelton, CT).

Histological Analyses

Bone explants were dehydrated in a gradient of ethanol and embedded in Technovit ('Technovit 9100 New' kit, Kulzer GmbH) according to manufacturer instructions. Thick sections were prepared from embedded tissue blocks using a Leitz 1600 saw microtome. Grinding and polishing of the sections was performed until a final section thickness of 100 µm was reached. Visualisation of calcein and alizarin fluorescent labelling was performed using an 'Axioplan 2' microscope (Zeiss). The analysis of bone formation rate was not possible, due to a lack of a distinct

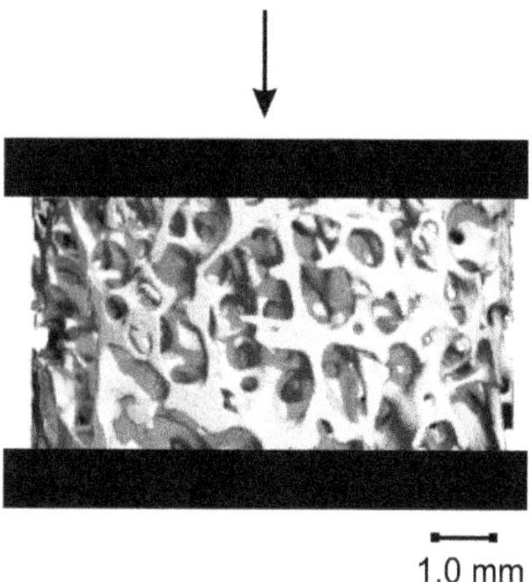

Figure 2. μCT-based model. μCT-based model (diam. = 8 mm, height = 4 mm) of bovine trabecular bone to which 1% deformation in compression is applied.

double label. Only single bands of either fluorochrome or a yellow band created by the overlapping of both fluorochrome bands could be detected. Nevertheless, labelling fluorescence indicated the presence of free calcium binding sites either created by osteoblasts or osteoclasts activity. To evaluate cell activity of cells inside the bone explants label penetration into the bone explants was measured. Therefore, fluorescent micrographs from the whole area of the centre section from each explant were stitched together to represent this section of each explant. The maximal label penetration was measured both from the upper and lower surfaces, as well as from the circumference edge. To investigate the morphological state of the cultured bone explants, the same sections used for the visualisation of the fluorescent double labelling were stained with Giemsa and eosin.

Micro-computed tomography (μCT)

The ethanol-fixed bone explants were imaged using a μCT-40 apparatus (Scanco Medical, Brüttisellen, Switzerland) with a nominal resolution of 10 μm. The X-ray tube was operated at 70 kV and 114 μA. Three-fold oversampling was used with an integration time of 300 ms.

The μCT data of each sample were filtered using a constrained three-dimensional Gaussian filter ($\sigma = 1.2$, support = 2), to partially suppress the noise in the volumes. Bone tissue was separated from marrow using a global threshold (22.4% of maximal gray value). The edge regions containing bone debris derived from sample preparation were excluded from the

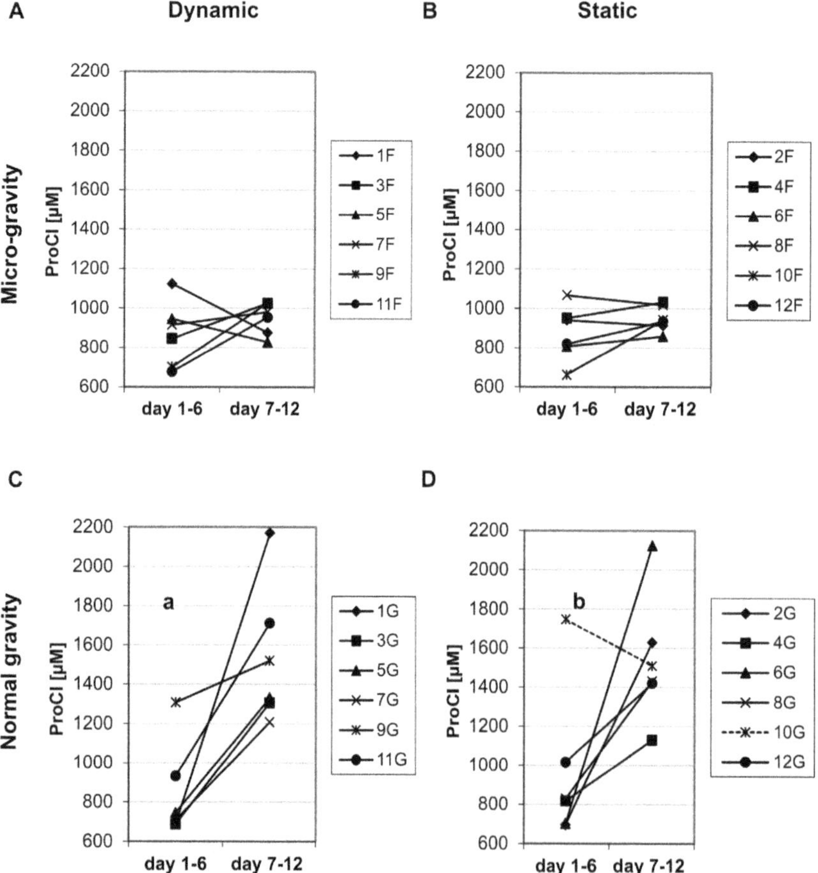

Figure 3. ProCl (μM) released by each bone sample. ProCl (μM) released by each sample in the culture medium during the first week (medium analyzed at the 6th day) and the second week (medium analyzed at the 12th day) of the experiment for the four groups of samples. A) Data relative to the samples dynamically loaded at micrograviy; B) Data relative to the samples statically loaded at microgravity; C) Data relative to the samples dynamically loaded at normal gravity; D) Data relative to the samples statically loaded at normal gravity. $^{a}p<0.05$, n = 6. $^{b}p<0.05$, n = 5 (sample '10G' is an outlier and was excluded for statistical analyses).

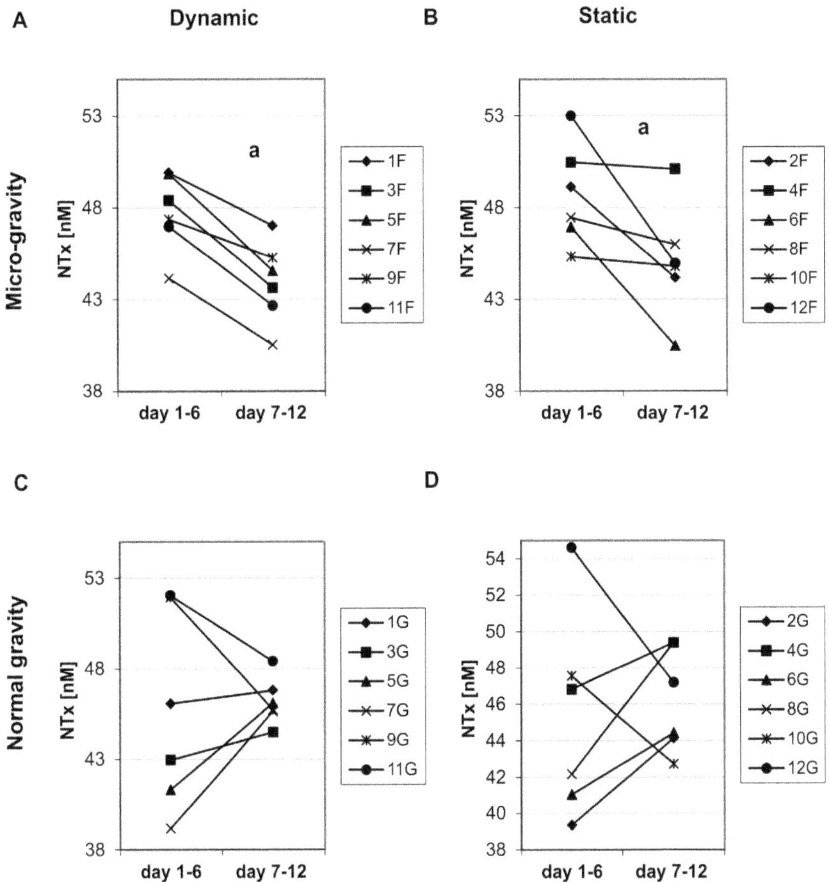

Figure 4. NTx (nM BCE) released by each bone sample. NTx (nM BCE) released by each sample in the culture medium during the first week (medium analyzed at the 6th day) and the second week (medium analyzed at the 12th day) of the experiment for the four groups of samples. A) Data relative to the samples dynamically loaded at microgravity; B) Data relative to the samples statically loaded at microgravity; C) Data relative to the samples dynamically loaded at normal gravity; D) Data relative to the samples statically loaded at normal gravity. [a]$p<0.05$, n = 6.

segmented data resulting in a cylindrical volume of interest with 8 mm diameter and 4 mm height. Image processing was performed using IPL (Scanco Medical, Brüttisellen, Switzerland).

3D morphometry

For each model, standard morphometric indices were assessed ([21]). Bone surface area (BS), bone volume (BV) and total volume (TV) were calculated using the software program IPL (Scanco, Brüttisellen, Switzerland). From these, bone volume fraction (BV/TV) and bone surface density (BS/TV) were derived. Further morphometry parameters included trabecular thickness (Tb.Th.), trabecular separation (Tb. Sp.), trabecular number (Tb. N.), connectivity density (Conn. D.) and Structure Model Index (SMI), an estimation of the plate-rod characteristic of the structure.

μCT based finite element models (μFE)

Detailed microstructural finite element (μFE) models (element size of 10 μm) were created by a direct conversion of bone voxels to linear hexahedral elements. The number of degrees of freedom in the models ranged from 32 to 60 million.

Linear and isotropic material behaviour was assumed for bone tissue in accordance to previous studies aimed at determining the apparent Young's modulus in trabecular bone by using micro-FE analyses [22]. As the analyses were linear-elastic and we were interested in assessing differences between groups rather than absolute values of apparent elastic modulus, all elements in the μFE models were given an arbitrary tissue modulus of 15 GPa and a Poisson ratio of 0.3.

Boundary conditions that simulated the real loading situation were defined. An arbitrary displacement of 1% strain was applied to the top surface of the models without constraining the displacement in the other two directions. Only the vertical displacement of the bottom surface was constrained to simulate a friction-less contact between the specimen and the plate (Figure 2). The models were solved using ParFE, a dedicated large-scale finite element solver using 1024 cores on a Cray XT5 system [23].

The apparent elastic modulus E of each model was calculated as:

$$E = \frac{FL}{\Delta u \times A} \tag{1}$$

where F is the calculated reaction force at the top surface while the applied displacement on the top surface (Δu), the length (L) and cross-sectional area of the sample (A), were equal to 0.04 mm, 4 mm and 50.2 mm^2 respectively for all the models.

Effective strains corresponding to an applied load of 30 N were calculated in all elements of each sample. Effective strain, also known as "equivalent strain", is a scalar value which summarizes

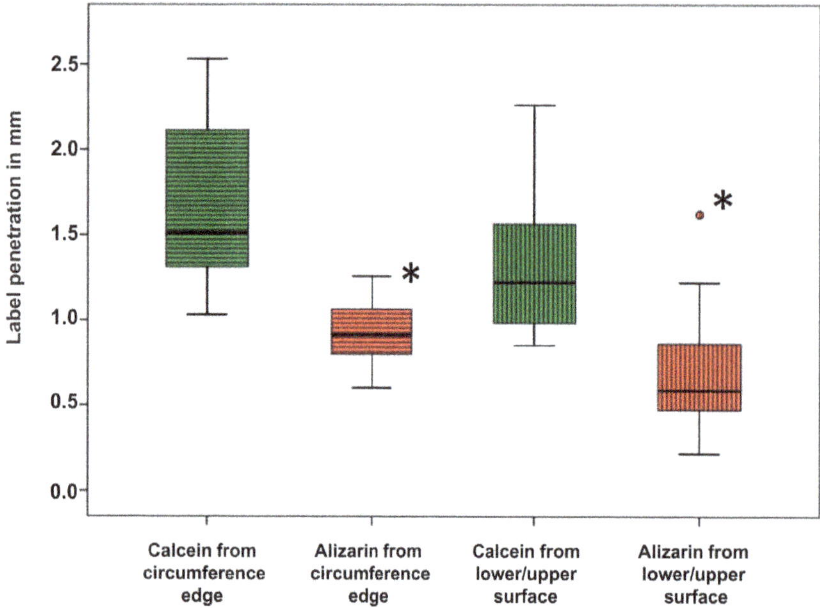

Figure 5. Label penetration depth at two penetration sites (from lower and upper surfaces, and from circumference edge). Calcein green penetration, which can be defined as time point zero, was significantly increased (*$p<0.01$) compared to the alizarin complexon penetration (end time point). Box plots show the median line, the 25% and the 75% quartiles which define the box, the 1.5x interquartile-range whiskers, as well as outliers (○).

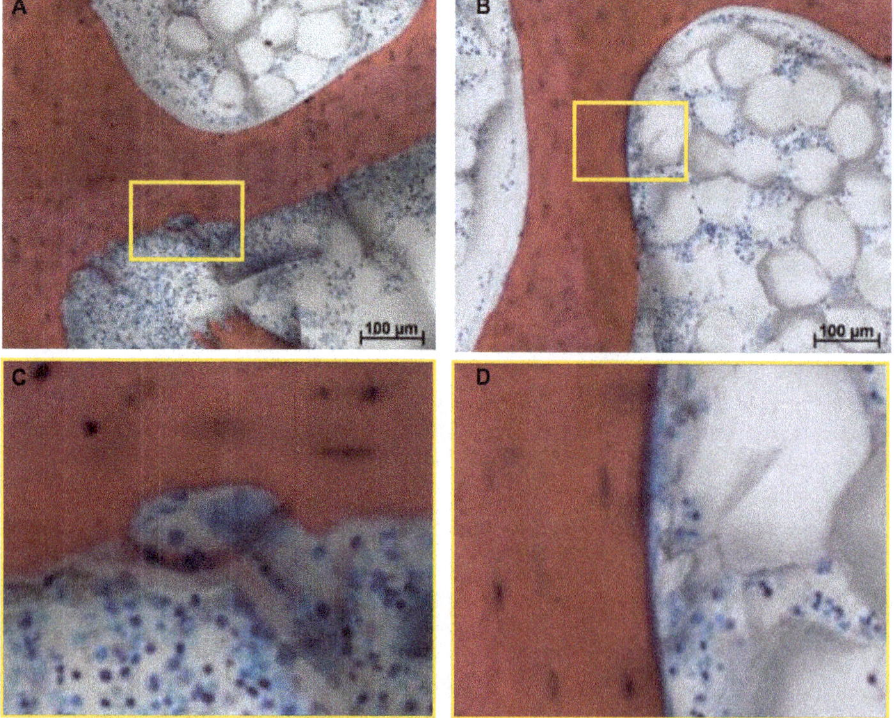

Figure 6. Light microscopic micrographs of Giemsa and eosin stained sections of the bone explants. A) Micrograph shows bone matrix labelled (red), haematopoietic bone marrow (blue), and the presence of a multinucleated osteoclast (blue) lying in its resorption lacunae; B) Micrograph shows bone matrix (red), haematopoietic bone marrow (blue), and the presence of an osteoid seam (blue); C) Close-up of osteoclast; D) Close-up of osteoid. Close-up scale bar represents 25 µm.

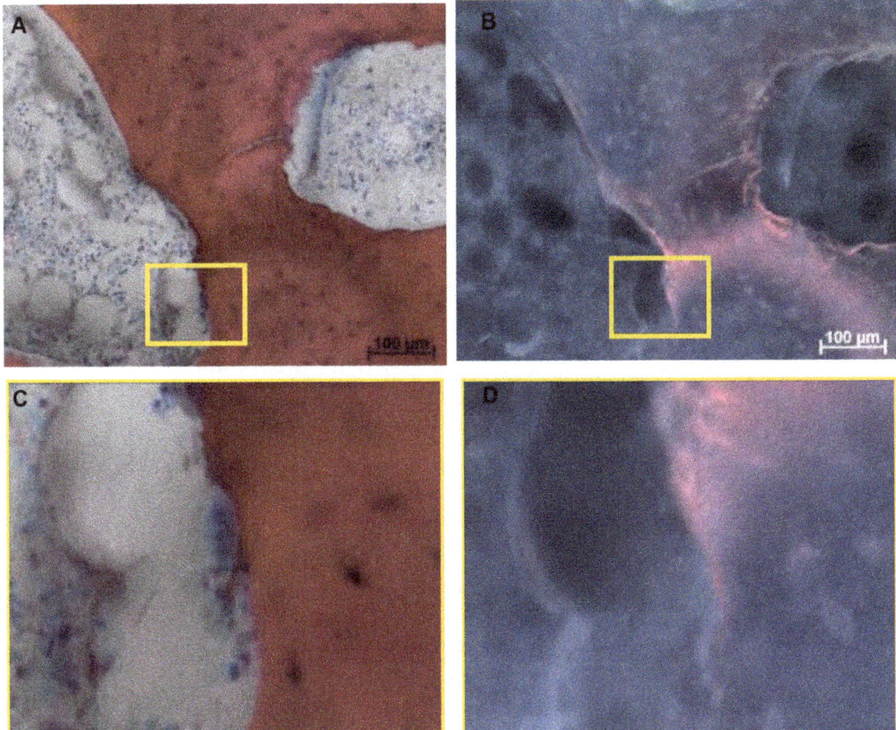

Figure 7. Light microscopy and fluorescence micrographs of sections of a bone explant dynamically loaded at micro-gravity. A) Light microscopic image showing an osteoclast within its resorption lacunae; B) Fluorescence micrograph showing the same area of cell activity with the corresponding alizarin bone surface labelling. C) Close-up of osteoclast as visualized by light microscopy; D) Close-up of the same area of cell activity as visualized by fluorescence labelling. Close-up scale bar represents 25 µm.

the strain tensor and it has been shown to be one of the most relevant measures for predicting the bone remodeling process [24,25]. Strain histograms (percentage of bone volume versus effective strain) for all the samples were computed.

Statistics

A single factor analysis of variance (ANOVA) followed by a post-hoc Tukey test was performed to examine differences in label penetration, as well as morphometric and mechanical parameters between groups. Data are presented as mean $\pm$ SD and $p<0.05$ was accepted as significant.

The change in bone turnover release between the first and the second week of the experiment was analysed by means of paired t-tests ($p<0.05$ accepted as significant).

Nonparametric analyses using Spearman's rank correlation coefficient were performed to correlate the percentage of total volume experiencing high strains to the release of bone formation and resorption markers within each group of samples. For each test, a significance level of $p<0.05$ was applied. Spearman's rank correlation coefficient r_s were calculated to reflect the trends in the relationships. All statistical analyses of the data were performed using the statistical software package SPSS (SPSS Inc., Chicago, IL, USA).

Results

Bone turnover biomarkers

Both the ProCI and NTx intra-assay variation between two repeated measurements on the same sample was lower than 5%. The inter-assay variation between two measurements performed on the same sample by two different kits was lower than 8%.

The biomarker data of the statically loaded group at normal gravity showed the presence of one potential outlier relative to the release of bone formation marker in the first week (Figure 3 D). The specific value was 115% higher than the average of the remaining values. The interquartile range rule confirmed this to be an outlier; hence, this value ("10G") was removed from all further analyses in this study.

The bone formation marker ProCI showed an increased release from the first to the second week of the experiment in response to static and dynamic loading at normal gravity (by 90.4% and 82.5% in average, respectively) (Figure 3). The change in ProCI release at microgravity was not significant (Figure 3). The bone resorption data (Figure 4) indicated a decrease in NTx release in the second week from the explants cultured at microgravity in response to static and dynamic loading; on average, the decrease was 7.5% and 8.0% for the static and dynamic loading group, respectively; the change in NTx release from explants cultured at normal gravity was not significant.

Bone histology

The comparison of label penetration of the single labels (calcein green or alizarin complexon) at either penetration site (upper and lower surface, or circumference edge) showed no significant differences between the experimental groups. However, the overall calcein penetration depth at either penetration site was significantly greater than alizarin penetration (p = 0.001) (Figure 5). Specifically, the penetration for calcein and alizarin from the circumference edge was 1.65 mm (+/−0.45 mm) and 0.93 mm

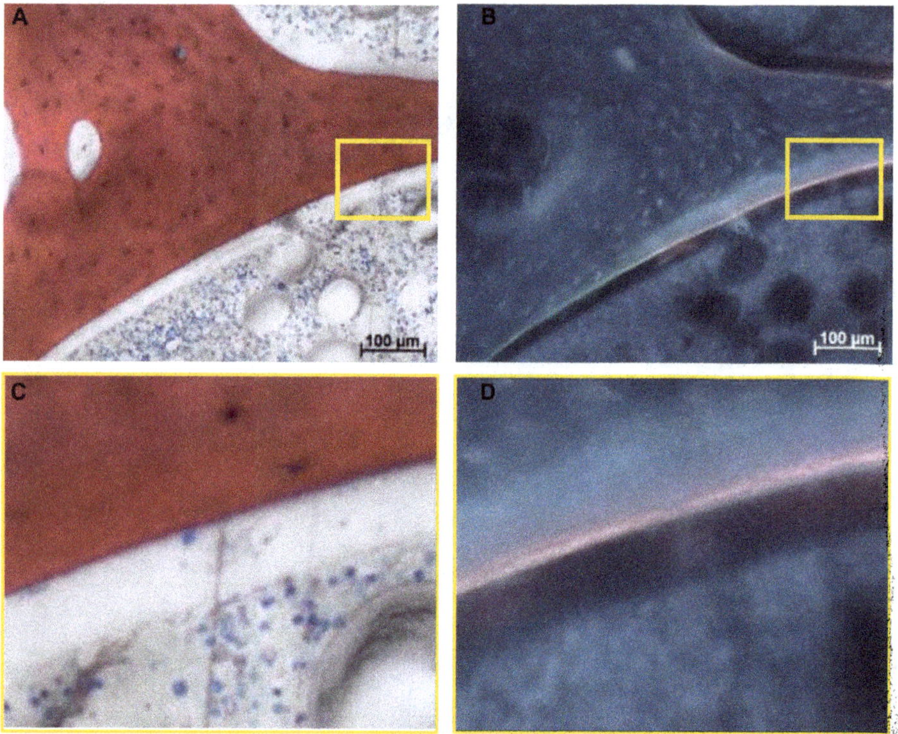

Figure 8. Light microscopic and fluorescence micrographs of sections of a bone explant dynamically loaded at micro-gravity. A) Light microscopic image showing an osteoid seam; B) Fluorescence micrograph showing the same area of cell activity with the corresponding alizarin bone surface labelling. C) Close-up of osteoclast as visualized by light microscopy; D) Close-up of the same area of cell activity as visualized by fluorescence labelling. Close-up scale bar represents 25 µm.

(+/−0.18 mm), respectively; penetration of the labels from the upper and lower surfaces was lower with 1.33 mm (+/−0.39 mm) on average for calcein green and 0.69 mm (+/−0.33 mm) for alizarin complexon ($p<0.0001$).

To investigate the morphological state of the cultured bone explants, Giemsa and eosin staining was performed. The presence of mainly red bone marrow was detected in the samples (Figure 6 A). Furthermore, several intact osteoclasts were detected after 20 days experimental culture time (Figure 6 A, C). Osteoclasts as multinucleated mature bone-resorbing cells have a life span of only 12.5 days *in vivo* [26]. The presence of osteoid seams - newly deposited, non-mineralised matrix – could also be visualised (Figure 6 B, D).

It was possible, to correlate areas of bone formation and resorption activities seen by the detection of osteoid seams and intact osteoclasts respectively with fluorescent double labelling in order to demonstrate that labelling was specific to the cellular activity during the mission. Both applied labels bind to all 'free calcium binding sites', therefore, labels can bind during bone formation but also during bone resorption processes when free

Table 1. Bone structure and mechanical competence for the 4 groups of samples.

	Microgravity		Normal gravity	
Variable	dynamic	static	dynamic	static
BV/TV (%)	16.50±2.80	14.58±2.48	15.61±2.44	14.83±1.76
BS/TV (1/mm)	3.02±0.31	2.83±0.29	2.92±0.20	2.82±0.33
Tb.Th. (mm)	0.15±0.014	0.14±0.007	0.15±0.01	0.15±0.012
Tb. N. (1/mm)	1.39±0.11	1.34±0.09	1.35±0.09	1.33±0.15
Tb. Sp. (mm)	0.65±0.07	0.68±0.06	0.68±0.057	0.70±0.09
Conn. D. (1/mm3)	6.07±1.31	5.33±0.48	5.59±0.58	5.21±1.06
SMI	0.85±0.25	0.94±0.30	0.85±0.25	0.97±0.20
E app (MPa)	940.60±637.95	560.90±171.50	733.13±195.50	636.27±270.53

Morphometric parameters (BV/TV = bone volume fraction, BS/TV = bone surface density, Tb.Th. = trabecular thickness, Tb.N. = trabecular number, Tb.Sp. = trabecular separation, Conn. D. = connectivity density, SMI = structure model index) and calculated apparent Young's modulus (E app) for the 4 groups of samples are indicated. No statistical differences were found. Values are expressed as mean ± standard deviation (n = 6 samples/group).

Table 2. Outcomes of the correlation analyses between the bone turnover markers (ProCI and NTx) released by the samples with the volume (expressed in percentage) strained above different strain effective levels.

		ProCI *versus* volume percentage strained above threshold			NTx *versus* volume percentage strained above threshold		
		strain threshold (μstrains)	R^2	Direction	strain threshold (μstrains)	R^2	Direction
Microgravity	**dynamic**	-	-	-	373	0.60	↓[a]
Microgravity	**static**	1090	0.80	↑[a]	-	-	-
Normal gravity	**dynamic**	191	0.45	↓[a]	222	0.94	↓[a]
Normal gravity	**static**	-	-	-	-	-	-

Reported are the strain thresholds for which the coefficient of determination R^2 was maximum (only when the *p*-value associated with the Spearman correlation analyses was significant). 'Direction' indicates whether the bone markers were increasing (↑) or decreasing (↓) with increasing the strained bone volume.

[a], $p<0.05$.

calcium binding sites are made available by the activity of osteoclasts. Direct labelling of resorption sites can thus come about because the osteoclasts expose binding sites for the fluorochromes. Labelled resorption lacunae remain visible in the section, but only when the resorption process does not proceed further after application of the fluorochrome [27,28]. The four micrographs in figure 7 show the overlapping osteoclast presence inside its resorption lacuna and alizarin complexon labelling, demonstrating that bone resorption can be correlated with the labelling. The presence of osteoid and overlapping alizarin complexon labelling (Figure 8) highlights the localisation of calcium label to bone forming sites.

Bone quality

No statistically significant differences were found for any of the morphometric and mechanical properties for the four groups of sample (Table 1).

Strain distribution versus bone turnover

Bone turnover in the second week was associated with the volume of highly strained bone (Table 2). In the dynamically loaded groups NTx levels were negatively correlated to the percentages bone strained above 222 ($r_s = -1$) and 373 microstrains ($r_s = -0.812$) at normal and microgravity, respectively. For the statically loaded groups no statistically significant correlations between the volume of loaded bone and NTx were found.

ProCI levels were decreasing with the volume of highly strained bone for the group dynamically loaded at normal gravity; the highest linearity was detected at 191 microstrains ($r_s = -0.829$). In the statically loaded group at microgravity ProCI levels were positively correlated to the percentages bone strained above 1090 microstrains ($r_s = 0.829$). No statistically significant correlations between the volume of highly strained bone and ProCI were found for the statically loaded at normal gravity and the dynamically loaded group at microgravity.

Discussion

In this study we evaluated bone quality of the trabecular bone samples after being cultured in normal and microgravity and being subjected to either a static or a dynamic load. Statistical analyses on morphometric parameters and apparent stiffness did not reveal significant differences between the treatment groups.

Histological analysis demonstrated structural maintenance of the tissue specimens throughout the experimental procedure with the presence of red bone marrow and morphological intact osteoclasts. Fluorescent labelling with calcein green and alizarin complexon showed correlation with osteoclast and osteoblast activity; yet this was found in a few samples only (Fig. 6, 7, and 8). Label penetration analysis showed significant differences. Both labels represent experimental time points, calcein green specifies the time point zero prior to launch, while alizarin complexon specifies the end point of the experiment after explant recovery. Therefore, the decrease in label penetration of alizarin complexon in comparison to calcein green describes a reduction in label penetration over time.

The analysis of the bone turnover markers showed an increase in bone formation marker (ProCI) release from the first to the second week of the experiment at normal gravity; this suggested that both static and dynamic loading stimulated the bone formation processes in the cancellous bone samples. In addition, it appeared that mechanical stimulation was less effective in inducing bone formation at microgravity compared to normal gravity. The changes in bone resorption marker (NTx) release indicated that bone resorption is reduced at microgravity in response to both static and dynamic loading. Overall, the effect of mechanical loading appeared regulated mainly by an increase of bone formation at normal gravity and by a decrease in bone resorption at microgravity.

Previous studies have revealed that bone formation can decrease and bone resorption can increase during space flight [29] and bed rest conditions [30]. The precise bone response cannot be compared directly to our findings, as these studies referred to bone remodeling processes at microgravity *in vivo*, which were quantified by serum or urinary assays, hence, included the influence of the systemic regulations. Moreover, our study concentrated on the comparison of dynamic versus static loading and lacks a true disuse group due to space constraints on the spacecraft. Yet, our study fills a gap in the understanding of the bone adaptive responses to microgravity. Specifically, in addition to the experiments mentioned above, demonstrating decreased bone formation in humans due to microgravity, it has been demonstrated that dissected bones, i.e. without the influence of systemic signals, also experience less osteoblast activity under microgravity [31]. In addition, it has been shown that osteoblast cultures show reduced activity under microgravity with respect to normal gravidty conditions [32,33]. The present study showed microgravity to be inhibitory towards bone cell function too as confirmed by the reduction of osteoblast activity from day 6 to day 12 of the experiment in bones subject to mechanical loading.

The third and final goal of this study was to investigate whether a strain threshold would exist above which bone response was activated. In the group dynamically loaded at normal gravity, strains of similar order of magnitude appeared to regulate bone formation and resorption processes (191 microstrains and 222 microstrains, respectively). The group dynamically loaded at microgravity showed significance for bone resorption only and for a strain threshold of 373 microstrains. These results might confirm bone adaptation to be driven by tissue strain magnitude lower than 500 microstrains applied at 30 Hz [14] and this to be valid both at normal and microgravity.

Also in the group statically loaded at microgravity, we found that a strain threshold existed at which the change in bone formation with the percentage volume was significant; this value was substantially higher (1090 microstrains) compared to the dynamically loaded groups. This implicates that bone responds to static mechanical strain and that higher strain magnitudes will be necessary when the complementary effect of loading frequency is missing. Whether this bone response may lead to a net anabolic or catabolic effect requires additional investigation, e.g. comparisons with data relative to reference (unloaded) bone samples.

Several limitations can be identified for this study. First, we used six samples per group. A proper prospective power analysis was not possible because of the lack of comparable studies. From a post-hoc power analysis of the morphometric data we determined that at least 25 samples per group had been needed in order to detect statistically significant differences with $p<0.05$ at a statistical power of at least 0.81. Due to limitations related to volume as well as weight and power consumption, this amount of samples would have not been realistic to include in the mission [34]. The challenges of performing bioreactor experiments under microgravity are immense as there are severe restrictions on the access to the device and limitations on its size and weight. This reduces the potential sample size to the minimum and eliminates the possibilities for repeats, hence making statistical analysis almost impossible. It also requires careful experimental design to obtain as much data as possible from a limited sample set. Nevertheless, in this study, valuable data was obtained which provides insights into the behavior of cyclically loaded samples cultured under this very challenging environment. Recent developments in *in* vivo micro-CT scanning would allow for pre-flight scanning of the samples. That could reduce the required number of samples, because each sample would act as its own control [35].

Second, we used cancellous bone taken from the bovine sternum based on the finding that sternum cancellous bone explants do respond to dynamic loading [15]. Yet, it is questionable whether this is the bone with the best adaptive response as the negative changes in BMD during weightlessness and microgravity have primarily been detected in weight-bearing bones [36] found in the lower extremities and the pelvis.

Third, although the computational analyses provided information about the local mechanical stimuli (effective strain magnitude) that would occur in the samples at day 12 of the experiment, the release of bone markers that might have been driven by such stimuli remained unknown. In this study we hypothesized that the release of bone turnover markers from day 6 – day 12 would be indicative for the bone turnover at day 12. Unfortunately, no data are available that may support this assumption.

In conclusion, we found mechanical loading to affect trabecular bone remodelling by different mechanisms at normal and microgravity. Additional studies with extended experimental time and increased samples number appear necessary for a further understanding of the anabolic potential of dynamic loading on bone quality and mechanical competence. We found low strain magnitudes to drive bone turnover when applied at high frequency, and found this to be valid at normal as well as at microgravity. Further investigations are indispensable for better understanding the linkage between mechanical stimuli and bone tissue response at normal and microgravity.

Acknowledgments

The flight opportunity was offered by ESA (the European Space Agency). The experimental hardware was developed by Verhaert Space (Kruibeke, Belgium). Computational time was provided by the Swiss National Supercomputing Centre (CSCS). We thank Rene Demets (Estec/ESA) for providing critical input to this paper. The data relative to this study have been published in the PhD theses of A.Torcasio and K. Jähn, and made publicly available.

Author Contributions

Conceived and designed the experiments: AT KJ MVG PS AET JVS MJS GHVL. Performed the experiments: AT KJ MVG PS AET. Analyzed the data: AT KJ. Contributed reagents/materials/analysis tools: AT KJ. Wrote the paper: AT KJ MJS GHVL.

References

1. Vico L, Collet P, Guignandon A, Lafage-Proust MH, Thomas T, et al. (2000) Effects of long-term microgravity exposure on cancellous and cortical weight-bearing bones of cosmonauts. Lancet 355: 1607–1611.
2. LeBlanc A, Lin C, Shackelford L, Sinitsyn V, Evans H, et al. (2000) Muscle volume, MRI relaxation times (T2), and body composition after spaceflight. J Appl Physiol 89: 2158–2164.
3. Lang T, LeBlanc A, Evans H, Lu Y, Genant H, et al. (2004) Cortical and trabecular bone mineral loss from the spine and hip in long-duration spaceflight. Journal of Bone and Mineral Research 19: 1006–1012.
4. Lang T, LeBlanc A, Evans H, Lu Y, Genant H, et al. (2004) Cortical and trabecular bone mineral loss from the spine and hip in long-duration spaceflight. J Bone Miner Res 19: 1006–1012.

5. Roux W (1881) Der Kampf der Theile im Organismus. Ein Beitrag zur vervollständigung der mechanischen Zweckmässigkeitslehre, von Wilhelm Roux. Leipzig: W. Engelmann.
6. Liskova M, Hert J (1971) Reaction of bone to mechanical stimuli. 2. Periosteal and endosteal reaction of tibial diaphysis in rabbit to intermittent loading. Folia Morphol (Praha) 19: 301–317.
7. O' Connor JA, Lanyon LE, Macfie H (1982) The Influence of Strain Rate on Adaptive Bone Remodeling. J Biomech 15: 767–781.
8. Rubin CT, Lanyon LE (1984) Regulation of bone formation by applied dynamic loads. J Bone Joint Surg Am 66: 397–402.
9. Judex S, Boyd S, Qin Y-X, Turner S, Ye K, et al. (2003) Adaptations of Trabecular Bone to Low Magnitude Vibrations Result in More Uniform Stress and Strain Under Load. Annals of Biomedical Engineering 31: 12–20.
10. Kaspar D, Seidl W, Neidlinger-Wilke C, Beck A, Claes L, et al. (2002) Proliferation of human-derived osteoblast-like cells depends on the cycle number and frequency of uniaxial strain. J Biomech 35: 873–880.
11. Srinivasan S, Weimer DA, Agans SC, Bain SD, Gross TS (2002) Low-magnitude mechanical loading becomes osteogenic when rest is inserted between each load cycle. Journal of Bone and Mineral Research 17: 1613–1620.
12. LaMothe JM, Zernicke RF (2004) Rest insertion combined with high-frequency loading enhances osteogenesis. J Appl Physiol 96: 1788–1793.
13. Fritton SP, McLeod KJ, Rubin CT (2000) Quantifying the strain history of bone: spatial uniformity and self-similarity of low-magnitude strains. J Biomech 33: 317–325.
14. Sun YQ, Mcleod KJ, Rubin CT (1995) Mechanically Induced Periosteal Bone-Formation Is Paralleled by the up-Regulation of Collagen Type One Messenger-Rna in Osteocytes as Measured by in-Situ Reverse Transcript Polymerase Chain-Reaction. Calcif Tissue Int 57: 456–462.
15. David V, Guignandon A, Martin A, Malaval L, Lafage-Proust MH, et al. (2008) Ex vivo bone formation in bovine trabecular bone cultured in a dynamic 3D bioreactor is enhanced by compressive mechanical strain. Tissue Engineering Part A 14: 117–126.
16. Richards RG, Simpson AE, Jaehn K, Furlong PI, Stoddart MJ (2007) Establishing a 3D ex vivo culture system for investigations of bone metabolism and biomaterial interactions. ALTEX 24 Spec No: 56–59.
17. Davies CM, Jones DB, Stoddart MJ, Koller K, Smith E, et al. (2006) Mechanically loaded ex vivo bone culture system 'Zetos': Systems and culture preparation. European Cells & Materials 11: 57–75.
18. Simpson AE, Stoddart MJ, Davies CM, Jahn K, Furlong PI, et al. (2009) TGFbeta3 and loading increases osteocyte survival in human cancellous bone cultured ex vivo. Cell Biochem Funct 27: 23–29.
19. Van Guyse M, Spaepen P, Vander Sloten J, Jones D (2006) Freqbone, a perfused and dynamically loaded bioreactor for culture of trabecular bone in microgravity. Proceedings of IEEE/EMBS Benelux Symposium 59.
20. Harris WH, Jackson RH, Jowsey J (1962) The in vivo distribution of tetracyclines in canine bone. J Bone Joint Surg Am 44-A: 1308–1320.
21. Bouxsein ML, Boyd SK, Christiansen BA, Guldberg RE, Jepsen KJ, et al. (2010) Guidelines for Assessment of Bone Microstructure in Rodents Using Micro-Computed Tomography. Journal of Bone and Mineral Research 25: 1468–1486.
22. van Lenthe GH, van den Bergh JP, Hermus AR, Huiskes R (2001) The prospects of estimating trabecular bone tissue properties from the combination of ultrasound, dual-energy X-ray absorptiometry, microcomputed tomography, and microfinite element analysis. J Bone Miner Res 16: 550–555.
23. Arbenz P, van Lenthe GH, Mennel U, Muller R, Sala M (2008) A scalable multi-level preconditioner for matrix-free mu-finite element analysis of human bone structures. International Journal for Numerical Methods in Engineering 73: 927–947.
24. Szwedowski TD, Taylor WR, Heller MO, Perka C, Muller M, et al. (2012) Generic Rules of Mechano-Regulation Combined with Subject Specific Loading Conditions Can Explain Bone Adaptation after THA. Plos One 7.
25. Taylor WR, Warner MD, Clift SE (2003) Finite element prediction of endosteal and periosteal bone remodelling in the turkey ulna: effect of remodelling signal and dead-zone definition. Proceedings of the Institution of Mechanical Engineers Part H-Journal of Engineering in Medicine 217: 349–356.
26. Hill PA (1998) Bone remodelling. Br J Orthod 25: 101–107.
27. Hulth A, Olerud S (1962) Tetracycline labelling of growing bone. Acta Soc Med Ups 67: 219–231.
28. Olerud S, Lorenzi GL (1970) Triple fluorochrome labeling in bone formation and bone resorption. J Bone Joint Surg Am 52: 274–278.
29. Smith SM, Wastney ME, O'Brien KO, Morukov BV, Larina IM, et al. (2005) Bone markers, calcium metabolism, and calcium kinetics during extended-duration space flight on the mir space station. Journal of Bone and Mineral Research 20: 208–218.
30. LeBlanc AD, Spector ER, Evans HJ, Sibonga JD (2007) Skeletal responses to space flight and the bed rest analog: a review. J Musculoskelet Neuronal Interact 7: 33–47.
31. Demets R, Jansen WH, Simeone E (2002) Biological experiments on the Bion-10 satellite. Noordwijk: ESA publ. division.
32. Vico L, Lafage-Proust MH, Alexandre C (1998) Effects of gravitational changes on the bone system in vitro and in vivo. Bone 22: 95s–100s.
33. Genty C, Palle S, Alexandre C (1993) First osteoblast culture in space: cellular response to unloading. J. Bone and Mineral Research. pp. S367.
34. Loomer PM (2001) The Impact of Microgravity on Bone Metabolism in vitro and in vivo. Critical Reviews in Oral Biology & Medicine 12: 252–261.
35. Boyd SK, Davison P, Muller R, Gasser JA (2006) Monitoring individual morphological changes over time in ovariectomized rats by in vivo micro-computed tomography. Bone 39: 854–862.
36. Trappe S, Costill D, Gallagher P, Creer A, Peters JR, et al. (2009) Exercise in space: human skeletal muscle after 6 months aboard the International Space Station. J Appl Physiol 106: 1159–1168.

16

Unique Suites of Trabecular Bone Features Characterize Locomotor Behavior in Human and Non-Human Anthropoid Primates

Timothy M. Ryan[1,2]*, Colin N. Shaw[1,2,3]

1 Department of Anthropology, Pennsylvania State University, University Park, Pennsylvania, United States of America, 2 Center for Quantitative Imaging, EMS Energy Institute, Pennsylvania State University, University Park, Pennsylvania, United States of America, 3 PAVE Research Group and The McDonald Institute for Archaeological Research, Department of Archaeology and Anthropology, University of Cambridge, Cambridge, United Kingdom

Abstract

Understanding the mechanically-mediated response of trabecular bone to locomotion-specific loading patterns would be of great benefit to comparative mammalian evolutionary morphology. Unfortunately, assessments of the correspondence between *individual* trabecular bone features and inferred behavior patterns have failed to reveal a strong locomotion-specific signal. This study assesses the relationship between inferred locomotor activity and a *suite* of trabecular bone structural features that characterize bone architecture. High-resolution computed tomography images were collected from the humeral and femoral heads of 115 individuals from eight anthropoid primate genera (*Alouatta, Homo, Macaca, Pan, Papio, Pongo, Trachypithecus, Symphalangus*). Discriminant function analyses reveal that subarticular trabecular bone in the femoral and humeral heads is significantly different among most locomotor groups. The results indicate that when a suite of femoral head trabecular features is considered, trabecular number and connectivity density, together with fabric anisotropy and the relative proportion of rods and plates, differentiate locomotor groups reasonably well. A similar, yet weaker, relationship is also evident in the trabecular architecture of the humeral head. The application of this multivariate approach to analyses of trabecular bone morphology in recent and fossil primates may enhance our ability to reconstruct locomotor behavior in the fossil record.

Editor: Fred H. Smith, Illinois State University, United States of America

Funding: This project was supported by National Science Foundation grant number BCS-0617097 (to TMR). The funders had no role in study design, data collection and analysis, decision to publish, or preparation of the manuscript.

Competing Interests: The authors have declared that no competing interests exist.

* E-mail: tmr21@psu.edu

Introduction

Trabecular bone plays a significant structural role in the skeletal system [1–10] and has been shown to respond to the loading environment throughout ontogeny [10–13]. Despite its clearly mechanical function, attempts to identify locomotion-specific architectural characteristics in the postcranial trabeculae of primates have produced largely mixed results [11,13–31]. While a few studies have found structural differences apparently related to divergent locomotor loading patterns [17,19,26], others have failed to detect significantly different structural characteristics across groups [16,20,24,32]. Variation in data collection methods, quantification procedures, sample selection, sample size, anatomical location, and volume of interest (VOI) selection may all influence the detection of a 'locomotor signal' in trabecular bone. The fundamental question of whether trabecular bone architecture in complex postcranial joints, such as the proximal femur and humerus, reflects a strong locomotion-specific signal remains unresolved. Demonstration of a strong functional signal within trabecular bone would aid reconstructions of locomotor behaviors in the fossil and archaeological record.

Shaw and Ryan [32] recently compared subarticular humeral and femoral head trabecular bone morphology as well as humeral and femoral mid-diaphysis cortical bone structure among eight anthropoid genera. In contrast to comparisons of inter-limb diaphyseal bone robusticity, which display a strong locomotor signal [33], femoral head trabecular bone was significantly more robust (higher bone volume fraction, lower trabecular spacing) than humeral head trabecular bone in all taxa. Comparisons revealed an osteological 'locomotor signal' indicative of differential use of the forelimb and hind limb in diaphyseal cortical bone geometry, but not in subarticular trabecular bone.

Analyses of interspecific variation using single morphometric variables alone (e.g., bone volume fraction, trabecular number, degree of anisotropy) may be inadequate for identifying morphological patterns that reflect adaptation to habitual locomotor loading. Studies addressing the interrelationships among trabecular bone features have demonstrated a strong correlation between the various morphometric variables and bone volume fraction [2,22,34]. Mittra et al. [2,34], using samples from sheep and humans, found strong relationships between bone volume fraction and trabecular thickness, spacing, number, connectivity, and structure model index, a measure of the relative proportion of plate-like and rod-like trabeculae. Cotter et al. [22] found similar relationships in the vertebral bodies of apes and humans with the notable exceptions of trabecular thickness and degree of anisotropy, neither of which correlated significantly with bone volume fraction in their sample. The results from these studies suggest that as bone volume fraction increases, trabeculae become more numerous, more plate-like, less widely spaced, and more interconnected. The strength of the interrelationships among other structural features varies, but is generally less robust. Trabecular thickness and anisotropy do not correlate strongly with many other variables, aside from bone volume fraction and structure model index, while features such as trabecular number, connectivity, and spacing display strong correlations with each other. Considering these structural relationships, analyses that account for variation within an entire suite of trabecular bone properties (multiple architectural variables) might be more appropriate, and indeed may prove more accurate for identifying locomotor and functional signals.

By partitioning trabecular bone architecture into its component parts and focusing on pairwise comparisons among taxa, previous studies may have inadvertently atomized the complex inter-dependent structure of trabecular bone and consequently precluded identification of a relevant locomotor signal. This approach of examining individual morphological features is appropriate for analyses of cortical bone cross-sectional geometry, for example, because each measureable cortical bone feature (i.e. cortical area, torsional rigidity) has a direct and well-understood biomechanical implication [35–41]. A more accommodating paradigm for analyses of trabecular bone architecture may be to apply the principle of *Holism*, and consider whether 'the whole is greater than the sum of its parts' [42].

The goal of this study is to assess whether variation in features of subarticular trabecular bone morphology, taken as a collective suite, accurately reflects differences in locomotor patterns across anthropoid primate taxa. This question is addressed using eight anthropoid genera that can be coarsely differentiated into separate locomotor categories. The first hypothesis is that groups with more derived locomotor patterns such as bipeds (*Homo*) and brachiators (*Symphalangus*) will express trabecular bone patterns that are significantly different from one another, while groups with more similar locomotor patterns, such as arboreal quadrupeds (*Alouatta*, *Macaca*, *Trachypithecus*) and terrestrial quadrupedal climbers (*Pan*), will express more similar trabecular bone architecture. Secondly, because the primate forelimb is used less extensively for propulsion during locomotion and is often used to perform more diverse manipulative behaviors, it is hypothesized that humeral head trabecular architecture will display less variation among locomotor groups.

Materials and Methods

Sample

The skeletal sample used in the current study consisted of one femur and one humerus from a total of 115 individuals from eight anthropoid genera (Table 1). All non-human specimens were wild-shot adults and exhibited no external signs of pathology or trauma. Age at death was estimated only for *Homo*. Individuals who displayed external signs of osteological senescence (i.e. osteoarthritis, eburnation) were excluded from the study. Bones from both right and left sides were used in the sample, one femur and humerus per specimen, but only elements from the same side were used for a single individual.

Trabecular Bone Structural Analysis

All bones were scanned on the OMNI-X HD-600 High-Resolution X-ray computed tomography (HRCT) scanner (Varian Medical Systems, Lincolnshire, IL) at the Center for Quantitative Imaging (CQI) at The Pennsylvania State University (PSU). Each specimen was mounted in foam and positioned vertically in the scanner to collect transverse slices through the long bones. Serial cross-sectional scans were collected beginning in the shaft and proceeding proximally to cover the entire femoral or humeral head. For the femur, scans were collected beginning at or near the level of the lesser trochanter. In the humerus, scans were collected beginning just below the surgical neck and progressing proximally. All HRCT scans were collected using source energy settings of

Table 1. Attributes of the taxonomic sample used in the current study.

Genus	Species	Museum	Locomotor Category	Demographics	Estimated Body Mass (kg)
Alouatta	*caraya*	AMNH	arboreal quadruped, climber	M: 4, F: 9	5.79 (0.96)[a]
Homo	*sapiens*	PSU	biped	M: 10, F: 10	60.86 (6.41) [b]
Macaca	*fascicularis*	MCZ	arboreal quadruped	I:19	4.07 (0.92) [c]
Pan	*troglodytes, verus, schweinfurthii*	AMNH	terrestrial quadruped, climber	M: 11, F: 4, I: 2	50.13 (10.22) [d]
Papio	*anubis, cynocephalus, hamadryas, ursinus*	AMNH, NMNH	terrestrial quadruped	M: 2, F: 4, I: 5	18.25 (4.72) [c]
Pongo	*pygmaeus, abelii*	NMNH	quadrumanous, climber	M: 5, F: 2	65.70 (21.50) [e]
Trachypithecus	*cristatus*	MCZ	arboreal quadruped	I: 21	5.92 (0.80) [f]
Symphalangus	*syndactylus*	NMNH	brachiator	M: 3, F: 4	10.77 (2.48) [e]

Length and body mass data presented as: mean (standard deviation).
NMNH: National Museum of Natural History (Smithsonian Museum), Washington, USA; American Museum of Natural History, New York, USA; PSU: Norris Farms Collection, Pennsylvania State University, Department of Anthropology, MCZ: Museum of Comparative Zoology, Harvard University.
M: Male, F: Female, I: Indeterminate.
Body Mass Estimation Equations:
[a]Haplorhine: 2.729*LN(FemHeadSI)+1.42) (SEE =0.239) [66].
[b]Female: (2.426*FemHeadAP-35.1)*0.9 (SEE =17.5); Male: (2.741*FemHeadAP-54.9)*0.9 (SEE =13.7) [68].
[c]Cercopithecine: (2.389*LN(FemHeadSI)-4.541))*1.014 (SEE =0.1670) [67].
[d]All hominoids: (3.019*LN(FemHeadSI)-6.668))*1.006 (SEE =0.1137) [67].
[e]Asian ape: (3.024*LN(FemHeadSI)-6.718))*1.008 (SEE =0.1309) [67].
[f]Colobines: (2.424*LN(FemHeadSI)-4.684))*1.01 (SEE =0.1385) [67].

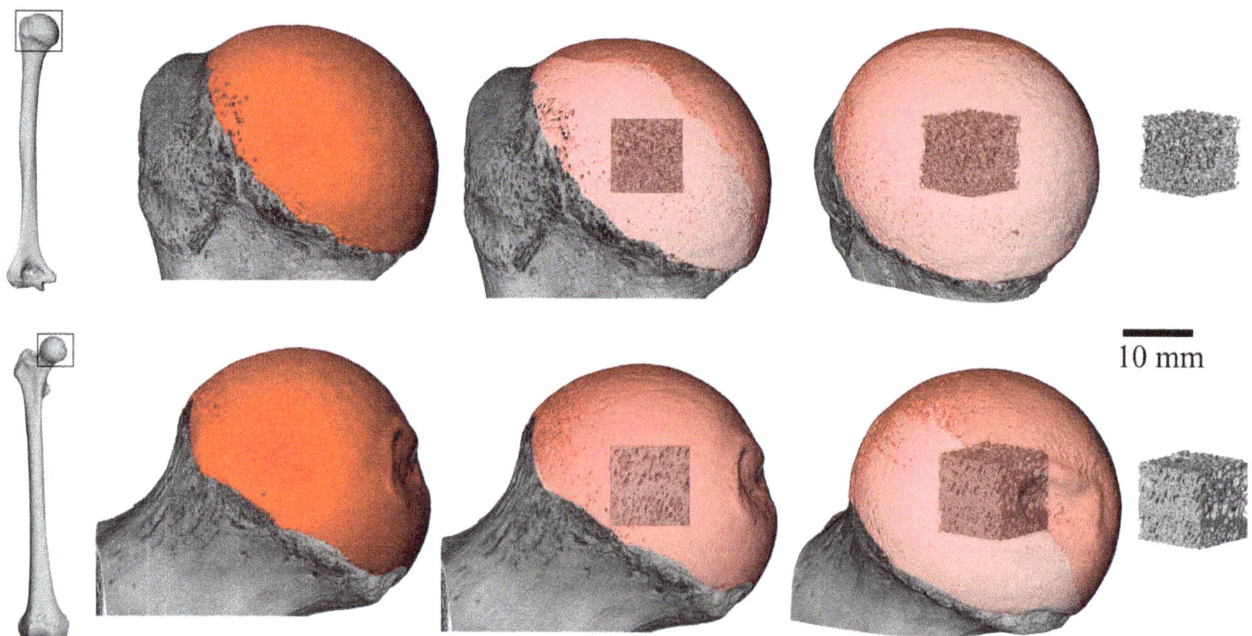

Figure 1. Volume of interest (VOI) selection method. The articular surface of the humeral and femoral heads (shown in red) were extracted from a three-dimensional isosurface reconstruction. The volume of interest was scaled based on the size of a best-fit cube for the articular surface and was positioned in the center of the humeral or femoral head.

either 180 kV/0.11 μA or 150 kV/0.2 μA, between 2800 and 4800 views, and a Feldkamp reconstruction algorithm. The differences in energy settings resulted from a refinement of bone scanning protocols at the PSU CQI over the last 6 years and are unlikely to have an effect on the evaluation of trabecular structure in this study. For each scan, between 41 and 100 slices were collected during each rotation. Voxel sizes ranged between 0.027 and 0.0687 mm depending on the size of the femoral or humeral head. In all cases, the highest-resolution images were obtained given the size of the specimen. The images were reconstructed as 16-bit TIFF grayscale images with a 1024×1024 pixel matrix.

Table 2. K-statistic calculated for select femoral head and humeral head trabecular bone measurements.

Variable	K
Fem Conn.D	0.2614
Fem SMI	0.4219
Fem Tb.N	0.5308
Fem Tb.Th	0.5033
Fem Tb.Sp	0.5234
Fem DA	0.2928
Hum Conn.D	0.4121
Hum SMI	0.2987
Hum Tb.N	0.5551
Hum Tb.Th	0.5933
Hum Tb.Sp	0.5479
Hum DA	0.4416

A single cubic volume of interest (VOI) was extracted from the center of the femoral and humeral heads for each individual (Figure 1). The method for determining the size and position of the

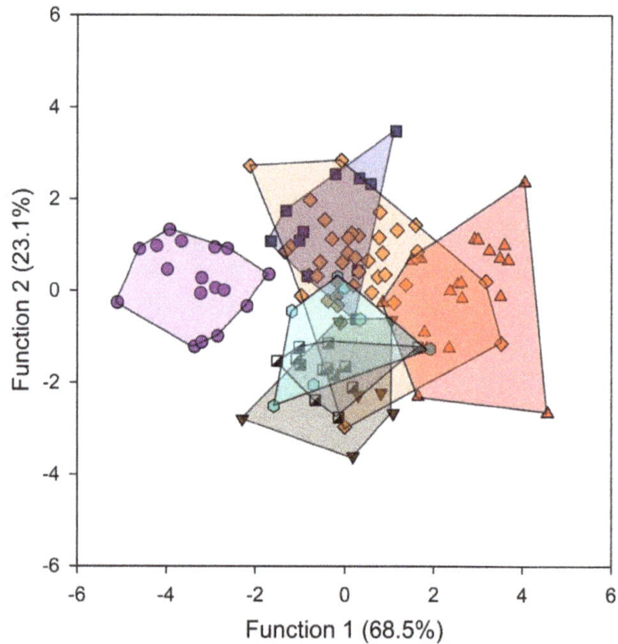

Figure 2. Results of multivariate discriminant function analyses for the femoral head. Symbols: red triangles, bipeds; blue squares, terrestrial quadrupeds; orange diamonds, arboreal quadrupeds; black and white squares, arboreal quadruped-climbers; cyan hexagons, quadrumanous climbers; brown triangles, brachiators; purple circles, terrestrial quadruped-climbers.

Table 3. Stepwise discriminant function analysis for locomotor group using five femoral head trabecular bone variables.

		Predicted group membership							
Locomotor group	**n**	**Biped**	**Terrestrial quad**	**Arboreal quad**	**Arboreal quad-climber**	**Quadrumanous climber**	**Brachiator**	**Terrestrial quad-climber**	**% correct**
Biped	20	17	0	2	1	0	0	0	85.0
Terrestrial quad	11	0	8	1	1	1	0	0	72.7
Arboreal quad	40	4	8	22	1	5	0	0	55
Arboreal quad-climber	13	0	0	0	12	0	1	0	92.3
Quadrumanous, climber	7	1	0	1	1	4	0	0	57.1
Brachiator	7	0	0	1	0	1	5	0	71.4
Terrestrial quad-climber	17	0	0	0	0	0	0	17	100.0

Classification results (total correct = 73.9%).
Biped: *Homo*; Terrestrial quadruped: *Papio*; Arboreal quadruped: *Macaca, Trachypithecus*; Arboreal quadruped-climber: *Alouatta*; Quadrumanous climber: *Pongo*; Brachiator: *Symphalangus*; Terrestrial quadruped-climber: *Pan*.

VOIs using Avizo 6.3 (Visualization Sciences Group, Inc., Burlington MA) is detailed in Ryan and Walker [20] and described briefly here. The articular surface of the femoral or humeral head was defined for each specimen by manually selecting the surface triangles from a three-dimensional isosurface reconstruction. Because a precise division between articular and non-articular regions is not possible to obtain from HRCT data alone (i.e. without other visual and physical clues present on the bones), a conservative approach was taken for all specimens to ensure that non-articular bone was not included in the articular surface selection. The bounding box of the triangulated articular surface shell was defined as the maximum and minimum extents of the articular surface in each of the three orthogonal axes. The center of the bounding box, defined for the purposes of the current analysis as the center of the articular region, was determined by calculating the midpoints of the x, y, and z dimensions of the bounding box.

The center of the VOI was placed at the calculated center of the articular surface bounding box and the edge length of the cube was equal to 1/6 the proximodistal height of the articular surface. This VOI selection protocol ensured that each VOI was positioned homologously (at the center of the joint), and was scaled to the size of the individual joint being analyzed. All measured variables were calculated on a sphere centered within the cubic VOI to avoid corner effects [43]. The VOIs ranged in size from approximately 2.5 to 14 mm in diameter for the humerus, and 2.3 to 15 mm in diameter for the femur. When analyzing trabecular structure in small animals using VOIs scaled by joint size, it is possible that the continuum assumption of Harrigan et al. [44] may not be fully satisfied. Visual inspection of the smallest VOIs used in this study ensured that each one included a minimum of three to five intertrabecular lengths, thereby satisfying this assumption.

Table 4. Pooled within-group correlations (r) between functions and variables.

Variable	Function 1	Function 2
Conn.D	0.024	0.256
SMI	0.329	−0.160
Tb.N	−0.374	0.802
Tb.Th	−0.136	−0.003
DA	0.761	0.569

The trabecular bone morphometric variables quantified included degree of anisotropy (DA), trabecular number (Tb.N), trabecular thickness (Tb.Th), connectivity density (Conn.D), and structure model index (SMI). Due to strong correlations with other variables and thus the potential to erroneously inflate differences among taxa, some important trabecular bone features typically analyzed in interspecific studies, including bone volume fraction and trabecular spacing, were excluded from the current analysis.

All trabecular bone morphometric analyses were performed using the Scanco Image Processing Language (IPL; Scanco Medical AG, Brüttisellen, Switzerland). The HRCT images were segmented using a threshold value calculated from the iterative segmentation algorithm of Ridler and Calvard [45,46], based on the grayscale values of the VOI only. This localized segmentation approach ensured appropriate definition of the trabecular bone in the VOI. Segmented data were inspected to ensure appropriate thresholding, and the same threshold value was used for all subsequent morphometric analyses for each individual VOI. Trabecular thickness and number were calculated using model-independent distance transform methods [47]. The structure model index measures the proportion of rod-like and plate-like trabeculae and was calculated following Hildebrand and Ruegsegger [48]. Connectivity density reflects the number of interconnections among trabeculae per unit volume and was calculated following the topological approach of Odgaard and Gunderson [49]. Degree of anisotropy was calculated using the mean intercept length (MIL) method on the three-dimensional volume [50–52].

Resolution Dependency of Trabecular Bone Variables

The spatial resolution (voxel dimensions) of the HRCT datasets used in the current study differs due to the large variation in body sizes, and therefore humeral and femoral head size, across the taxa in the sample. To ensure that this variation in voxel dimensions did not affect the trabecular bone measurements, the resolution dependency of each trabecular bone variable was determined

Table 5. F-test results between groups (DF = 3, 106) for stepwise discriminant function analyses for locomotor group using five femoral head trabecular bone variables.

	Biped	Terrestrial quad	Arboreal quad	Arboreal quad-climber	Quadrumanous climber	Brachiator	Terrestrial quad-climber
Biped	X	<0.001	<0.001	<0.001	<0.001	<0.001	<0.001
Terrestrial quad	22.73	X	NS	<0.001	<0.001	<0.001	<0.001
Arboreal quad	25.02	2.58	X	<0.001	<0.01	<0.001	<0.001
Arboreal quad-climber	31.16	20.23	19.58	X	NS	<0.01	<0.001
Quadrumanous, climber	14.30	8.33	5.46	2.00	X	NS	<0.001
Brachiator	22.59	18.31	16.66	5.14	2.19	X	<0.001
Terrestrial quad- climber	106.05	24.50	51.32	31.39	20.55	29.54	X

Upper half of plot: p-values, lower half of plot: F-scores.
Stepwise analyses included DA, Tb.N. and ConnD in the final 'best fit' solution (thus excluding SMI and Tb.Th.), the results for which are presented here.

prior to interspecific analysis. The femoral heads of fifteen specimens from five separate species were scanned at an isotropic spatial resolution of 0.014 mm following the same scanning protocols used for the current analysis. The taxa used in this resolution dependency assessment were mostly small-bodied primates due to the need for small limb elements to obtain high resolution. The species included *Galago senegalensis* (n = 5), *Loris tardigradus* (n = 2), *Hapalemur griseus* (n = 1), *Saimiri boliviensis* (n = 2), and *Macaca fascicularis* (n = 5). A cubic VOI was extracted from each specimen following the same VOI sampling procedures used for the current study. Each VOI was then down-sampled to six lower spatial resolutions – isotropic voxel dimensions of 0.02, 0.03, 0.04, 0.05, 0.06, 0.07 mm – using the Resample module in Avizo 6.3 with a Lanczos filter. Trabecular bone structure was quantified at each resolution, for each individual. Least squares linear regression analyses were conducted for each variable to test the relationship with voxel size. The only variable to display a statistically significant relationship ($p<0.001$) was Tb.Th. While re-sampling to lower spatial resolutions may produce different values than actually re-scanning at those same lower resolutions [53], the 'corrected' Tb.Th values obtained in this study are comparable to those found in the literature [11].

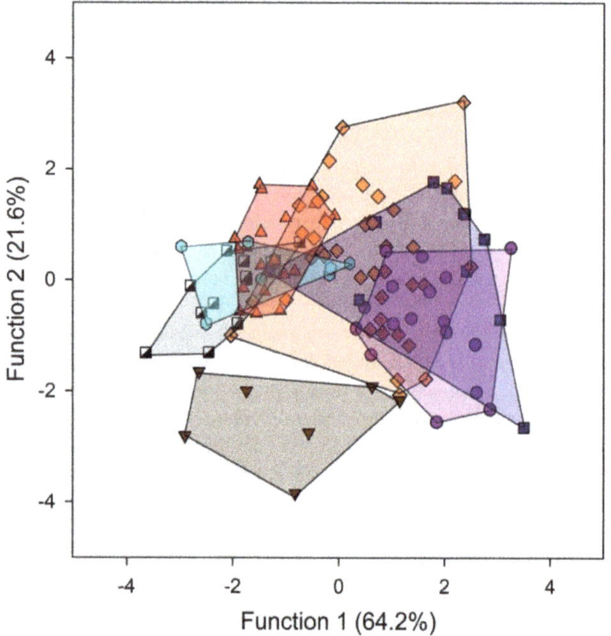

Figure 3. Results of multivariate discriminant function analyses for the humeral head. Symbols as in Figure 2.

A corrected trabecular thickness (Tb.Th.corr) value was calculated to account for the observed voxel size dependency. The Tb.Th calculated from the highest resolution images (voxel size of 0.014 mm) was considered the most accurate value for Tb.Th. For each of the 15 individuals the $Tb.Th_{0.014}$ value was divided by the Tb.Th value calculated at each of the six down-sampled spatial resolutions (i.e., 0.02, 0.03, 0.04, 0.05, 0.06, 0.07 mm). The mean ratio ($Tb.Th_{0.014}/Tb.Th_x$) at each voxel resolution was then calculated using all 15 individuals included in the resolution dependency analysis sample (*Galago senegalensis, Loris tardigradus, Hapalemur griseus, Saimiri boliviensis,* and *Macaca fascicularis*). Values for these ratios ranged from 0.995 (for the 0.02 mm voxel size) to 0.770 (for the 0.07 mm voxel size). A voxel size correction equation was developed by inputting these six values into a least squares linear regression. The resulting regression equation for Tb.Th (correction factor = $-4.4856 * \text{voxel size} + 1.0805$; $R^2 = 0.998$; $p<0.001$) was then applied to the measured Tb.Th values. The resulting Tb.Th.corr values were then used for all subsequent analyses.

Test for Phylogenetic Signal

Previous tests for a phylogenetic signal in primate long bone structure have demonstrated a significant effect on raw data uncorrected for variation in body size [54]. The influence of phylogeny on trabecular bone structure was tested in this study using the K statistic method [55]. This approach uses generalized least squares to characterize phylogenetic signal given relationships among taxa. The K statistic characterizes phylogenetic signal in a comparative dataset as the ratio between the observed level of phylogenetic covariance in tip data and the expected level of covariance under a Brownian motion model of character evolution. As defined by Blomberg et al. [55], a K statistic less than 1 indicates that close relatives resemble each other less than expected. Conversely, a K value greater than 1 indicates that closely related taxa are more similar than expected under Brownian motion. While 8 taxa are adequate for the calculation of K [56], at least 20 taxa are required to calculate the statistical significance of a phylogenetic signal using randomization tests [55]. As a result, statistical differences were not calculated here.

Table 6. Stepwise discriminant function analyses for locomotor group using seven humeral head trabecular bone variables.

		Predicted group membership							
Locomotor group	**n**	**Biped**	**Terrestrial quad**	**Arboreal quad**	**Arboreal quad-climber**	**Quadrumanous climber**	**Brachiator**	**Terrestrial quad-climber**	**% correct**
Biped	20	14	0	1	1	4	0	0	70
Terrestrial quad	11	0	6	2	1	0	0	2	54.5
Arboreal quad	40	4	6	18	2	2	1	7	45
Arboreal quad-climber	13	1	0	0	11	1	0	0	84.6
Quadrumanous, climber	7	1	0	3	1	2	0	0	28.6
Brachiator	7	0	0	0	1	0	1	1	71.4
Terrestrial quad-climber	17	0	3	3	0	0	11	11	64.7

Classification results (total correct = 58.3%).
Biped: *Homo*; Terrestrial quadruped: *Papio*; Arboreal quadruped: *Macaca, Trachypithecus*; Arboreal quadruped-climber: *Alouatta*; Quadrumanous climber: *Pongo*; Brachiator: *Symphalangus*; Terrestrial quadruped-climber: *Pan*.

Phylogenetic signal was calculated for each trabecular bone variable as follows. The $\log_{10}$ transformed values for each trabecular bone variable for each individual were regressed against $\log_{10}$ transformed estimates of body mass for each individual (see below) using ordinary least squares regression. The unstandardized residuals from each of these regression analyses were calculated and represented a body mass-standardized variable. The specialized Matlab code PHYSIG was used to calculate the strength of the phylogenetic signal for the species mean of each body mass-standardized variable [55]. The phylogenetic tree for the 8 taxa (Information S1) used estimated divergence dates as branch lengths and was based on published phylogenetic analyses [57–62]. For each variable, K is much less than 1, indicating less phylogenetic signal than expected under a Brownian motion model of character evolution (Table 2). While these tests do not necessarily indicate that phylogenetic signal is completely absent in trabecular bone structure in these taxa, the results strongly suggest that size-corrected variables are unlikely to contain a strong phylogenetic signal, and thus are acceptable for use in the multivariate analyses conducted in this study.

Discriminant Function Analyses

Discriminant function analyses were used to test the utility of the femoral and humeral head trabecular bone variables for differentiating anthropoid taxa into locomotor categories. Recent work on mammalian trabecular bone has demonstrated an allometric scaling effect on trabecular structural features [63]. To correct for the influence of body size, $\log_{10}$ transformed values for each trabecular bone variable were regressed against a $\log_{10}$ transformed estimate of body mass for each individual, using ordinary least squares linear regression. While using estimates of body mass based on regression equations introduces error, the non-isometric scaling of femoral head size with body size in *Homo sapiens* [64,65] precludes the use of femoral head breadth as a proxy for body mass in this sample. Body mass for each individual was estimated from femoral head dimensions using equations taken from the literature [66–68] and derived from analyses of the most appropriate taxonomic group (Table 1). Femoral head anteroposterior breadth, mediolateral breadth, and superoinferior height were measured to the nearest hundredth of a millimeter using digital calipers.

For all 115 individuals in the sample, unstandardized residuals calculated for the five trabecular bone variables were input into discriminant function analyses. Analyses were run separately for the humeral and femoral variables. To calculate structure matrices and locomotor group membership, unstandardized residuals were entered together and locomotor category was used as the grouping variable. To calculate the f-statistic for between locomotor group differences, discriminant analyses were re-run using a stepwise approach. All statistical analyses were performed in SPSS 18.0. For all statistical tests, null hypotheses were rejected for P-values less than 0.05.

Table 7. Pooled within-group correlations (r) between functions and variables.

Variable	Function 1	Function 2
Conn.D	0.423	0.351
SMI	−0.569	0.649
Tb.N	0.867	0.254
Tb.Th	−0.141	−0.061
DA	0.207	0.344

Results

The stepwise analysis of femoral head trabecular bone morphology for the complete sample generated two significant discriminant functions ($p<0.001$) that account for 68.5% and 23.1% of the variance, respectively (Figure 2). These functions correctly classify 85 of the 115 specimens (73.9%) into their assigned locomotor categories. The percentage of correct classifications varies by group (Table 3). Function 1 shows the strongest correlation with Tb.N and SMI, while Function 2 correlates most strongly with Tb.N and DA (Table 4). An F-test of among-group separations is highly significant ($P<0.001$, Table 5) for virtually all locomotor groups. The exception to this finding is the comparison of terrestrial versus arboreal quadrupeds and quadrumanous-climbers versus both arboreal quadruped-climbers and brachiators. This stepwise F-test initially included all five Tb variables.

Table 8. F-test results between groups (DF = 3, 106) for stepwise discriminant function analyses for locomotor group using five humeral head trabecular bone variables.

	Biped	Terrestrial quad	Arboreal quad	Arboreal quad-climber	Quadrumanous climber	Brachiator	Terrestrial quad-climber
Biped	X	<0.001	<0.001	<0.01	NS	<0.001	<0.001
Terrestrial quad	21.11	X	<0.001	<0.001	<0.001	<0.001	<0.001
Arboreal quad	12.06	5.68	X	<0.001	<0.01	<0.001	<0.001
Arboreal quad-climber	4.14	29.75	19.90	X	<0.05	<0.001	<0.001
Quadrumanous, climber	1.31	12.00	5.00	2.78	X	<0.01	<0.001
Brachiator	14.04	23.24	19.07	11.17	4.69	X	<0.001
Terrestrial quad- climber	28.94	5.88	10.55	28.92	12.67	20.69	X

Upper half of plot: p-values, lower half of plot: F-scores.
Stepwise analyses included DA, Tb.N. and ConnD in the final 'best fit' solution (thus excluding SMI and Tb.Th.), the results for which are presented here.

However, because SMI and Tb.Th were not included in the 'best fit' final solution, between group differences are based on three variables, DA, Tb.N and Conn.D.

Function 1 differentiates terrestrial quadrupedal-climbers (*Pan*) on one end of a continuum from bipeds (*Homo*) on the other. On this continuum, all remaining quadrupeds (*Alouatta, Macaca, Papio, Trachypithecus*) cluster together with quadrumanous climbers (*Pongo*) and brachiators (*Symphalangus*). Overlap exists between bipeds (*Homo*) and a few arboreally quadrupedal (*Macaca* and *Trachypithecus*) individuals. Function 2 separates brachiators (*Symphalangus*), arboreal quadrupedal-climbers (*Alouatta*) and, to a lesser degree, quadrumanous climbers (*Pongo*), from terrestrial quadrupeds (*Papio*). Arboreal quadrupeds (*Macaca, Trachypithecus*), bipeds (*Homo*) and terrestrial quadrupedal-climbers (*Pan*) fall in between these more extreme positions and overlap with all other groups.

The analysis of trabecular morphology of the proximal humerus also generated two significant discriminant functions ($p<0.001$) that accounted for 64.2% and 21.6% of the variance, respectively (Figure 3). These functions correctly classify 67 of the 115 specimens (58.3%) into their assigned locomotor groups, but the percentage of correct classifications varies by group (Table 6). Function 1 is strongly correlated with Tb.N and SMI, while Function 2 correlate with SMI and Conn.D (Table 7). Function 1 differentiates terrestrial quadrupeds and terrestrial quadrupedal-climbers (*Papio,* and *Pan*, respectively) from bipeds, quadrumanous climbers and arboreal quadrupedal-climbers (*Homo, Pongo, Alouatta*, respectively). Arboreal quadrupeds (*Macaca* and *Trachypithecus*) and brachiators (*Symphalangus*) overlap with all other groups. In contrast, for Function 2 brachiators (*Symphalangus*) are virtual outliers, separated from all other groups that are tightly clustered. Additionally, an F-test of between-group separations is significant among all locomotor groups ($p<0.001$, Table 8) other than bipeds and quadrumanous climbers. Similar to the outcome of the stepwise F-test conducted for femoral head trabecular analyses, the humeral head analysis initially included all five Tb variables. However, because SMI and Tb.Th are not included in the 'best fit' final solution, between group differences are based on only three variables, DA, Tb.N and Conn.D.

Discussion

Two hypotheses were tested in this study. Groups employing more distinct locomotor patterns were expected to have significantly divergent trabecular architecture, while groups with more similar locomotor patterns were expected to display more similar trabecular structure. The results reveal significant differences in trabecular architecture among locomotor categories. Nevertheless, overlap in trabecular morphology was found among individuals from both more (i.e. arboreal quadruped vs. arboreal quadruped-climber) and less distinct (i.e. brachiator vs. arboreal quadrupeds) locomotor behavioral groups. Because the forelimbs of primates generally experience lower vertical peak reaction forces during locomotion, it was hypothesized that humeral head trabecular structure would not distinguish locomotor groups as effectively as would trabecular structure from the femoral head. The results appear to support this hypothesis. Although significant differences exist among locomotor categories for both humeral and femoral head trabecular morphology, overlap among groups is more apparent in the proximal humerus.

The results of the current study suggest that when multiple trabecular bone variables are considered together as a functioning morphological suite, a locomotor signal may be detectable in the anthropoid femoral head, and less obviously in the humeral head. This finding may prove useful for reconstructions of locomotor behavior in the fossil record. Generally, the percentage of correct predictions derived from femoral head trabecular bone features (73.9%) indicates bone structural differences associated with generalized locomotor behaviors. Locomotor group predictions derived from the humeral head trabecular architecture were less accurate (58.3%).

The challenge stemming from the current study is to determine the mechanical and functional significance of the suite of morphological traits – Tb.N, Conn.D, DA, and SMI – that differentiates these locomotor groups. These features are intriguing due to their established relationships to the ultimate strength and elastic properties of trabecular bone [1–9]. The results from the current analysis suggest that multivariate analyses differentiate locomotor groups based on a combination of mechanically-relevant morphological features. This correspondence between a) variables that appear to delineate locomotor behavioral differences and, b) variables found to be significant in determining the mechanical behavior of trabecular bone (pre- and post-yield), suggests a locomotion-specific functional signal in the subarticular trabecular bone architecture of the femur and, less obviously, the humerus.

In spite of this apparent correspondence between the structural and mechanical properties of anthropoid trabecular bone, constructing direct links between trabecular bone variation and specific loading conditions for each locomotor mode is more problematic. It is apparent from these results that in the femoral

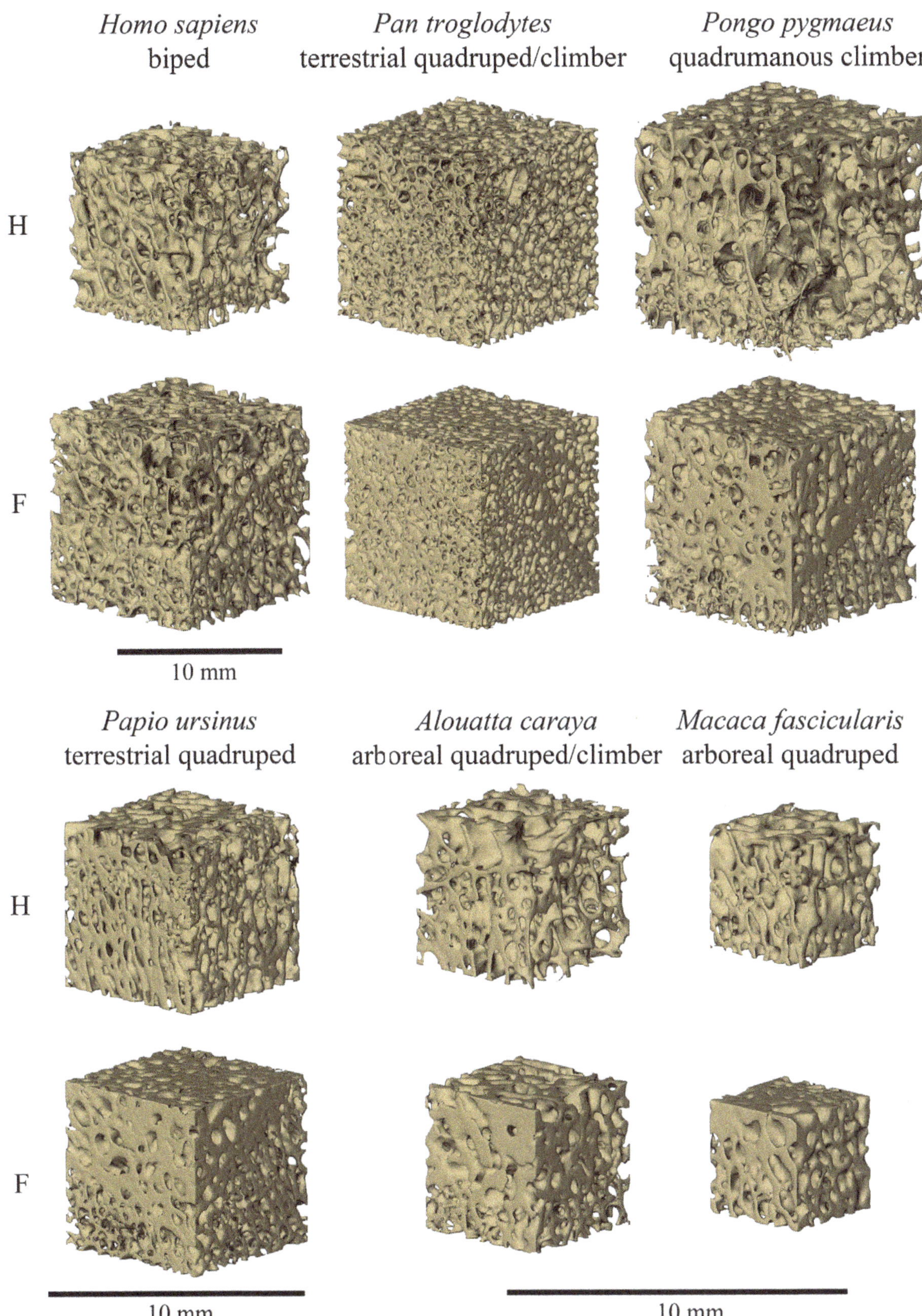

Figure 4. Three-dimensional reconstructions of cubic trabecular bone specimens from the humerus (top) and femur (bottom) from individuals used in the current study. Note variation in trabecular architecture between the femur and humerus, and among taxa.

head, bipeds (*Homo*) display unique trabecular bone characteristics that include a relatively low number of thin, concave plate-like, trabeculae that are highly anisotropic (Figure 4). This unique suite of traits sets them apart from almost all other taxa and, coupled with the low bone volume fraction [32], suggests relatively low tissue elasticity [1,3,4,6]. The asymmetric placement of trabecular bone in the femoral neck of humans, a phenomenon termed trabecular eccentricity, has been identified as a stress-reducing mechanism that reflects bone adaptation to applied loads [69]. Trabecular eccentricity and the femoral head bone architecture identified in this study suggest unique solutions to mechanical demands in the human proximal femur.

In direct contrast to the patterns seen in *Homo*, terrestrial quadruped-climbers (*Pan*) display relatively numerous, thick, highly concave trabeculae that form a dense, isotropic bone structure (Figure 4). These results suggest a fundamentally different trabecular bone architecture in the femur of Pan and, consequently, different mechanical properties. The femoral head trabecular structure of the remaining locomotor groups falls between the two ends of the continuum occupied by *Pan* and *Homo* (Figure 4). The terrestrial and arboreal quadrupedal specimens (*Papio* and *Macaca*, respectively) are associated with a more densely packed, concave, anisotropic trabecular bone structure. Brachiating (*Symphalangus*), quadrumanous climbing (*Pongo*), and arboreal quadruped-climbing (*Alouatta*) taxa have fewer, relatively isotropic trabeculae.

The microstructure of humeral head trabeculae presents a tripartite, though somewhat overlapping, separation of the locomotor groups. The brachiating locomotor pattern unique to *Symphalangus* corresponds with trabecular architecture that is relatively gracile, characterized by few, closed plate-like trabeculae that are loosely packed to form a relatively isotropic structure. In contrast, a more robust architecture is associated with the arboreal (*Macaca, Trachypithecus*) and terrestrial (*Papio*) quadrupedal and terrestrial quadrupedal-climbing (*Pan*) taxa, defined by numerous closed, concave trabeculae that form a densely packed relatively anisotropic structure (Figure 4). Finally, clustered tightly are the bipedal (*Homo*), quadrumanous climbing (*Pongo*), and arboreal quadruped-climbing (*Alouatta*) taxa, all of whom display a low number of trabeculae that are thickened and plate-like, and not highly connected. Along Function 1 *Homo, Pongo, Alouatta,* and *Symphalangus* overlap significantly, suggesting broadly similar bone structure, perhaps reflecting lower magnitude loading on the proximal humerus as compared to quadrupedal catarrhines.

Interestingly, bipeds and quadrumanous climbers present relatively similar humeral head trabecular bone morphology. The differences between the relative (un)loading of the forelimbs during terrestrial bipedal locomotion in *Homo* and forelimb loading during quadrumanous climbing in *Pongo* are presumably quite pronounced. The finding of microarchitectural similarities in the humeral head of these two taxa is therefore surprising. This result is interesting given the proposal that *Pongo*-like bipedal clambering may represent the primitive great ape locomotor pattern [70–72], but it is not immediately clear what drives these structural similarities.

Trabecular bone architecture is the product of both genetic and environmental influences [10,73,74,75]. The sensitivity of bone to mechanical signals, and the consequent functional importance of bone structural variation, is well established [76]. Environmental influences including locomotor, dietary, and manipulative behaviors can shape trabecular form throughout an individual's lifetime. Whether the interspecific differences in trabecular bone architecture described in this study are the result of selective or environmental forces, or a combination of both, remains unclear. While deciphering these influences is not the primary aim of this study, it is worth noting that the correspondence between trabecular architecture and distinct locomotor patterns in anthropoids may reflect selection over multiple generations and/or adaptation over the course of the lifetime of an individual.

One of the limitations of the present study is the use of relatively broad locomotor categories, each composed of a single taxon or a small number of taxa. As a result, structural differences across locomotor groups may reflect species-specific attributes rather than exclusively locomotor behavioral differences. Although it has been demonstrated that little or no phylogenetic signal exists in the morphological variables used in this study, phylogenetic heritage may nevertheless still be influencing the results. Given locomotor behavioral variation in extant primates, the number of potential species available for inclusion within certain locomotor categories is necessarily restricted (i.e. bipeds and quadrumanous climbers). Future studies that include a greater number of taxa within each locomotor category, where possible, will be better able to identify those characteristics of trabecular bone structural variation capable of differentiating among locomotor groups. It is also possible that the relatively coarse locomotor categories used in this study mask species-specific variation in locomotor behaviors. The ability to use trabecular bone architecture of the hip and shoulder joints to reconstruct locomotor behaviors in extinct primate taxa will depend on the continued refinement of the methods presented here and the determination of the relative importance of the phylogenetic, developmental, and functional components of bone architecture.

The challenge in future comparative trabecular bone analyses will be to elucidate further the nature of the behavior-specific osteological signal. Further analysis of ontogenetic changes in trabecular architecture will shed light on aspects of trabecular bone morphology that are mechanically mediated and functionally relevant [11,13,77]. Similarly, continued study of the interrelationships between trabecular bone architectural and mechanical variation will further delineate the functional significance of structural variation in the mammalian postcranial skeleton. Treating trabecular bone morphology as a suite of interrelated traits takes a step towards a Systems Biology approach, which considers complex interactions between components of a biological organism. Integrating trabecular bone architecture into analyses and models of whole bone structure and function will help define the interaction between the micro- and macro-scale structural adaptations of bone and how these interactions influence the function and behavior of the entire skeletal element.

Conclusions

By partitioning trabecular morphology into its component parts, previous studies may have inadvertently precluded identification of a more robust 'locomotor signal' in the primate locomotor skeleton. The findings of the present study suggest that morphological patterns reflective of adaptation to habitual locomotor mode may be identified in anthropoid primates through a combined analysis of multiple trabecular bone variables together. Applied to analyses of fossil primate skeletal remains, this approach might be a useful tool for inferring habitual locomotor patterns. Nevertheless, caution is advisable. While the eight taxa assessed here were reasonably successfully partitioned by general locomotor mode, such categorization does not encompass the variety of behaviors utilized by individuals or species as a whole. If a comparable approach were used to infer locomotor patterns from primate fossil remains, only general descriptions would be appropriate.

Acknowledgments

The authors thank Alan Walker for his support and helpful suggestions during the course of this project. The authors would also like to thank Darrin Lunde and Eileen Westwig at the American Museum of Natural History, Richard Thorington and Linda Gordon at the National Museum of Natural History, Smithsonian Institution, Judith Chupasko at the Museum of Comparative Zoology, Harvard University, George Milner at Pennsylvania State University, and Terrance Martin at the Illinois State Museum for their assistance with specimens and their willingness to loan specimens for scanning. Thanks to T. Stecko, A. Gordon, I. Carlson, M. Test, L. Souza, S. Kobos, A. Placke, S. Sukhdeo, and A. Swiatoniowski. Jim Gosman and two anonymous reviewers provided helpful feedback on this manuscript.

Author Contributions

Conceived and designed the experiments: TMR CNS. Performed the experiments: TMR CNS. Analyzed the data: TMR CNS. Wrote the paper: TMR CNS.

References

1. Kabel J, van Rietbergen B, Odgaard A, Huiskes R (1999) Constitutive relationships of fabric, density, and elastic properties in cancellous bone architecture. Bone 25: 481–486.
2. Mittra E, Rubin C, Qin Y-X (2005) Interrelationships of trabecular mechanical and microstructural properties in sheep trabecular bone. J Biomech 38: 1229–1237.
3. Odgaard A, Kabel J, van Rietbergen B, Dalstra M, Huiskes R (1997) Fabric and elastic principal directions of cancellous bone are closely related. J Biomech 30: 487–495.
4. Ulrich D, van Rietbergen B, Laib A, Rüegsegger P (1999) The ability of three-dimensional structural indices to reflect mechanical aspects of trabecular bone. Bone 25: 55–60.
5. van Rietbergen B, Odgaard A, Kabel J, Huiskes R (1996) Direct mechanics assessment of elastic symmetries and properties of trabecular bone architecture. J Biomech 29: 1653–1657.
6. van Rietbergen B, Odgaard A, Kabel J, Huiskes R (1998) Relationships between bone morphology and bone elastic properties can be accurately quantified using high-resolution computer reconstructions. J Orthop Res 16: 23–28.
7. Hodgskinson R, Currey JD (1990) The effect of variation in structure on the Young's modulus of cancellous bone: a comparison of human and non-human material. J Eng Med 204: 115–121.
8. Hodgskinson R, Currey JD (1990) Effects of structural variation on Young's modulus of non-human cancellous bone. J Eng Med 204: 43–52.
9. Turner CH, Cowin SC, Rho JY, Ashman RB, Rice JC (1990) The fabric dependence of the orthotropic elastic constants of cancellous bone. J Biomech 23: 549–561.
10. Barak MM, Lieberman DE, Hublin JJ (2011) A Wolff in sheep's clothing: Trabecular bone adaptation in response to changes in joint loading orientation. Bone 49: 1141–1151.
11. Gosman JH, Ketcham RA (2009) Patterns in ontogeny of human trabecular bone from SunWatch Village in the Prehistoric Ohio Valley: General features of microarchitectural change. Am J Phys Anthropol 138: 318–332.
12. Pontzer H, Lieberman DE, Momin E, Devlin MJ, Polk JD, et al. (2006) Trabecular bone in the bird knee responds with high sensitivity to changes in load orientation. J Exp Biol 209: 57–65.
13. Ryan TM, Krovitz GE (2006) Trabecular bone ontogeny in the human proximal femur. J Hum Evol 51: 591–602.
14. Fajardo RJ, MacLatchy LM, Müller R (2000) Analysis of femoral head trabecular architecture using mCT: evidence from some anthropoids and lorisoids. Am J Phys Anthropol S30: 147.
15. Fajardo RJ, Müller R (2001) Three-dimensional analysis of nonhuman primate trabecular architecture using micro-computed tomography. Am J Phys Anthropol 115: 327–336.
16. Fajardo RJ, Muller R, Ketcham RA, Colbert M (2007) Nonhuman anthropoid primate femoral neck trabecular architecture and its relationship to locomotor mode. Anat Rec 290: 422–436.
17. Ryan TM, Ketcham RA (2002) Femoral head trabecular bone structure in two omomyid primates. J Hum Evol 43: 241–263.
18. Ryan TM, Ketcham RA (2002) The three-dimensional structure of trabecular bone in the femoral head of strepsirrhine primates. J Hum Evol 43: 1–26.
19. Ryan TM, Ketcham RA (2005) The angular orientation of trabecular bone in the femoral head and its relationship to hip joint loads in leaping primates. J Morphol 265: 249–263.
20. Ryan TM, Walker A (2010) Trabecular bone structure in the humeral and femoral heads of anthropoid primates. Anat Rec 293: 719–729.
21. Saparin P, Scherf H, Hublin J, Fratzl P, Weinkamer R (2009) The trabecular bone architecture in proximal femora of primates with different locomotor preferences indicates different adaptation mechanisms. Bone 44: S63.
22. Cotter MM, Simpson SW, Latimer BM, Hernandez CJ (2009) Trabecular microarchitecture of hominoid thoracic vertebrae. Anat Rec 292: 1098–1106.
23. Scherf H (2007) Locomotion-related femoral trabecular architectures in Primates. Ph.D. Dissertation, Darmstadt University of Technology, Darmstadt, Germany.
24. Scherf H (2008) Locomotion-related femoral trabecular architectures in primates–high resolution computed tomographies and their implications for estimations of locomotor preferences of fossil primates. In: Endo H, Frey R, editors. Anatomical Imaging. Tokyo: Springer. 39–59.
25. Griffin NL (2008) Bone architecture of the hominin second proximal pedal phalanx: a preliminary investigation. J Hum Evol 54: 162–168.
26. MacLatchy L, Müller R (2002) A comparison of the femoral head and neck trabecular architecture of *Galago* and *Perodicticus* using micro-computed tomography (μCT). J Hum Evol 43: 89–105.
27. Maga M, Kappelman J, Ryan TM, Ketcham RA (2006) Preliminary observations on the calcaneal trabecular microarchitecture of extant large-bodied hominoids. Am J Phys Anthropol 129: 410–417.
28. Viola TB (2002) Locomotion dependent variation in the proximal femoral trabecular pattern in primates M.Sc. Thesis, University of Vienna, Vienna, Austria.
29. Griffin NL, D'Aout K, Ryan TM, Richmond BG, Ketcham RA, et al. (2010) Comparative forefoot trabecular bone architecture in extant hominids. J Hum Evol 59: 202–213.
30. Cotter MM, Loomis DA, Simpson SW, Latimer B, Hernandez CJ (2011) Human Evolution and Osteoporosis-Related Spinal Fractures. Plos One 6:(10): e26658.
31. Lazenby RA, Angus S, Cooper DML, Hallgrimsson B (2008) A three-dimensional microcomputed tomographic study of site-specific variation in trabecular microarchitecture in the human second metacarpal. J Anat 213: 698–705.
32. Shaw CN, Ryan TM (2012) Does skeletal anatomy reflect adaptation to locomotor patterns? Cortical and trabecular architecture in human and nonhuman anthropoids. Am J Phys Anthropol 147: 187–200.
33. Ruff CB (2002) Long bone articular and diaphyseal structure in old world monkeys and apes. I: Locomotor effects. Am J Phys Anthropol 119: 305–342.
34. Mittra E, Rubin C, Gruber B, Qin YX (2008) Evaluation of trabecular mechanical and microstructural properties in human calcaneal bone of advanced age using mechanical testing, microCT, and DXA. J Biomech 41: 368–375.
35. Shaw CN, Stock JT (2011) The influence of body proportions on femoral and tibial midshaft shape in hunter-gatherers. Am J Phys Anthropol 144: 22–29.
36. Shaw CN, Stock JT (2009) Habitual throwing and swimming correspond with upper limb diaphyseal strength and shape in modern human athletes. Am J Phys Anthropol 140: 160–172.
37. Shaw CN, Stock JT (2009) Intensity, repetitiveness, and directionality of habitual adolescent mobility patterns influence the tibial diaphysis morphology of athletes. Am J Phys Anthropol 140: 149–159.
38. Ruff CB (2008) Femoral/humeral strength in early African *Homo erectus*. J Hum Evol 54: 383–390.
39. Ruff CB (2009) Relative limb strength and locomotion in *Homo habilis*. Am J Phys Anthropol 138: 90–100.
40. Ruff CB (1987) Sexual dimorphism in human lower limb bone structure: relationships to subsistence strategy and sexual division of labour. J Hum Evol 16: 391–416.
41. Ruff C, Holt B, Trinkaus E (2006) Who's afraid of the big bad Wolff?:"Wolff's law" and bone functional adaptation. Am J Phys Anthropol 129: 484–498.
42. Smuts JC (1927) Holism and Evolution. London: MacMillan and Co. 368 p.
43. Ketcham RA, Ryan TM (2004) Quantification of anisotropy in trabecular bone. J Microsc 213: 158–171.
44. Harrigan TP, Jasty M, Mann RW, Harris WH (1988) Limitations of the continuum assumption in cancellous bone. J Biomech 21: 269–275.
45. Ridler TW, Calvard S (1978) Picture thresholding using an iterative selection method. IEEE Trans Sys Man Cyber SMC-8: 630–632.
46. Trussell HJ (1979) Comments on "Picture thresholding using an iterative selection method". IEEE Trans Sys Man Cyber SMC-9: 311.
47. Hildebrand T, Rüegsegger P (1997) A new method for the model-independent assessment of thickness in three-dimensional images. J Microsc 185: 67–75.
48. Hildebrand T, Rüegsegger P (1997) Quantification of bone microarchitecture with the structure model index. Comput Methods Biomech Biomed Eng 1: 15–23.
49. Odgaard A, Gundersen HJG (1993) Quantification of connectivity in cancellous bone, with special emphasis on 3-d reconstruction. Bone 14: 173–182.

50. Whitehouse WJ (1974) The quantitative morphology of anisotropic trabecular bone. J Microsc 101: 153–168.
51. Harrigan TP, Mann RW (1984) Characterization of microstructural anisotropy in orthtropic materials using a second rank tensor. J Mat Sci 19: 761–767.
52. Cowin SC (1986) Wolff's law of trabecular architecture at remodeling equilibrium. J Biomech Eng 108: 83–88.
53. Kim DG, Christopherson GT, Dong XN, Fyhrie DP, Yeni YN (2004) The effect of microcomputed tomography scanning and reconstruction voxel size on the accuracy of stereological measurements in human cancellous bone. Bone 35: 1375–1382.
54. O'Neill MC, Dobson SD (2008) The degree and pattern of phylogenetic signal in primate long-bone structure. J Hum Evol 54: 309–322.
55. Blomberg SP, Garland T, Ives AR (2003) Testing for phylogenetic signal in comparative data: Behavioral traits are more labile. Evolution 57: 717–745.
56. Garland T, Bennett AF, Rezende EL (2005) Phylogenetic approaches in comparative physiology. J Exp Biol 208: 3015–3035.
57. Eizirik E, Murphy WJ, Springer MS, O'Brien SJ, Ross CF, et al. (2004) Molecular phylogeny and dating of early primate divergences. Anthropoid Origins: New Visions. New York: Kluwer Academic. 45–61.
58. Porter CA, Page SL, Czelusniak J, Schneider H, Schneider MPC, et al. (1997) Phylogeny and evolution of selected primates as determined by sequences of the epsilon-globin locus and 5' flanking regions. Int J Primatol 18: 261–295.
59. Raaum RL, Sterner KN, Noviello CM, Stewart CB, Disotell TR (2005) Catarrhine primate divergence dates estimated from complete mitochondrial genomes: concordance with fossil and nuclear DNA evidence. J Hum Evol 48: 237–257.
60. Stauffer RL, Walker A, Ryder OA, Lyons-Weiler M, Hedges SB (2001) Human and ape molecular clocks and constraints on paleontological hypotheses. J Hered 92: 469–474.
61. Stewart CB, Disotell TR (1998) Primate evolution - in and out of Africa. Curr Biol 8: R582–R588.
62. Tosi AJ, Disotell TR, Morales JC, Melnick DJ (2003) Cercopithecine Y-chromosome data provide a test of competing morphological evolutionary hypotheses. Mol Phylogenet Evol 27: 510–521.
63. Doube M, Klosowski MM, Wiktorowicz-Conroy AM, Hutchinson JR, Shefelbine SJ (2011) Trabecular bone scales allometrically in mammals and birds. Proc R Soc Lond B Biol Sci 278: 3067–3073.
64. Jungers WL (1988) Relative joint size and hominoid locomotor adaptations with implications for the evolution of hominid bipedalism. J Hum Evol 17: 247–265.
65. Ruff C (1988) Hindlimb articular surface allometry in Hominoidea and *Macaca*, with comparisons to diaphyseal scaling. J Hum Evol 17: 687–714.
66. Payseur BA, Covert HH, Vinyard CJ, Dagosto M (1999) New body mass estimates for *Omomys carteri*, a Middle Eocene primate from North America. Am J Phys Anthropol 109: 41–52.
67. Ruff CB (2003) Long bone articular and diaphyseal structure in old world monkeys and apes. II: Estimation of body mass. Am J Phys Anthropol 120: 16–37.
68. Ruff CB, Scott WW, Liu AYC (1991) Articular and diaphyseal remodeling of the proximal femur with changes in body mass in adults. Am J Phys Anthropol 86: 397–413.
69. Fox JC, Keaveny TM (2001) Trabecular eccentricity and bone adaptation. J Theor Biol 212: 211–221.
70. Begun DR, Richmond BG, Strait DS (2007) Comment on "Origin of Human Bipedalism As an Adaptation for Locomotion on Flexible Branches". Science 318: 1066.
71. Crompton RH (2007) Locomotion and posture: from the common African ape ancestor to fully modern hominins. J Anat 210: 770.
72. Thorpe SKS, Holder RL, Crompton RH (2007) Origin of human bipedalism as an adaptation for locomotion on flexible branches. Science 316: 1328.
73. Havill LM, Allen MR, Bredbenner TL, Burr DB, Nicolella DP, et al. (2010) Heritability of lumbar trabecular bone mechanical properties in baboons. Bone 46: 835–840.
74. Judex S, Garman R, Squire M, Donahue LR, Rubin C (2004) Genetically based influences on the site-specific regulation of trabecular and cortical bone morphology. J Bone Miner Res 19: 600–606.
75. Wallace IJ, Middleton KM, Lublinsky S, Kelly SA, Judex S, et al. (2010) Functional significance of genetic variation underlying limb bone diaphyseal structure. Am J Phys Anthropol 143: 21–30.
76. Rubin J, Rubin C, Jacobs CR (2006) Molecular pathways mediating mechanical signaling in bone. Gene 367: 1–16.
77. Gosman JH, Stout SD, Larsen CS (2011) Skeletal biology over the life span: a view from the surfaces. Yearb Phys Anthropol 53: 86–98.

17

Torsion and Antero-Posterior Bending in the *In Vivo* Human Tibia Loading Regimes during Walking and Running

Peng-Fei Yang[1,2,3]*, Maximilian Sanno[3], Bergita Ganse[2], Timmo Koy[4], Gert-Peter Brüggemann[3], Lars Peter Müller[4], Jörn Rittweger[2,5]

1 Key Laboratory for Space Bioscience and Biotechnology, School of Life Sciences, Northwestern Polytechnical University, Xi'an, China, **2** Division of Space Physiology, Institute of Aerospace Medicine, German Aerospace Center, Cologne, Germany, **3** Institute of Biomechanics and Orthopaedics, German Sport University Cologne, Cologne, Germany, **4** Department of Orthopaedic and Trauma Surgery, University of Cologne, Cologne, Germany, **5** Institute for Biomedical Research into Human Movement and Health, Manchester Metropolitan University, Manchester, United Kingdom

Abstract

Bending, in addition to compression, is recognized to be a common loading pattern in long bones in animals. However, due to the technical difficulty of measuring bone deformation in humans, our current understanding of bone loading patterns in humans is very limited. In the present study, we hypothesized that bending and torsion are important loading regimes in the human tibia. *In vivo* tibia segment deformation in humans was assessed during walking and running utilizing a novel optical approach. Results suggest that the proximal tibia primarily bends to the posterior (bending angle: 0.15°–1.30°) and medial aspect (bending angle: 0.38°–0.90°) and that it twists externally (torsion angle: 0.67°–1.66°) in relation to the distal tibia during the stance phase of overground walking at a speed between 2.5 and 6.1 km/h. Peak posterior bending and peak torsion occurred during the first and second half of stance phase, respectively. The peak-to-peak antero-posterior (AP) bending angles increased linearly with vertical ground reaction force and speed. Similarly, peak-to-peak torsion angles increased with the vertical free moment in four of the five test subjects and with the speed in three of the test subjects. There was no correlation between peak-to-peak medio-lateral (ML) bending angles and ground reaction force or speed. On the treadmill, peak-to-peak AP bending angles increased with walking and running speed, but peak-to-peak torsion angles and peak-to-peak ML bending angles remained constant during walking. Peak-to-peak AP bending angle during treadmill running was speed-dependent and larger than that observed during walking. In contrast, peak-to-peak tibia torsion angle was smaller during treadmill running than during walking. To conclude, bending and torsion of substantial magnitude were observed in the human tibia during walking and running. A systematic distribution of peak amplitude was found during the first and second parts of the stance phase.

Editor: David Carrier, University of Utah, United States of America

Funding: No current external funding sources for this study.

Competing Interests: The authors have declared that no competing interests exist.

* E-mail: yangpf@nwpu.edu.cn

Introduction

Evidence suggests that both the geometry and thus the mechanical properties of long bones adapt to the mechanical load they are exposed to [1–3]. In the absence of an easy way to assess *in vivo* mechanical loads acting on bones, bone geometry, which is deemed to be causally related to its loading history, has been taken to predict the *in vivo* bone loading history [4,5]. For instance, by analyzing a stack of peripheral quantitative computed tomography (pQCT) images taken across the human tibia, it was concluded that the almost circular distal tibia seems to be adapted to compressive loading patterns, while the non-circular geometry of the proximal tibia is the result of increased torsion and bending [5]. However, there are several problems with this approach [6]. These include a lack of absolute values of cross-sectional geometric properties and a potential misalignment between the loading history and bone cross-sectional geometry [6]. It is obvious, and not only therefore, that accurate measurements of real-world *in vivo* bone loading patterns are needed.

Obtaining the information of the bone loading patterns is very important to better understand bone's mechano-adaptation, as bone responds differently to different deformation patterns, *e.g.* to torsion or compression [7]. Evidence also suggests that bone formation varies between anatomical sites due to the uneven local strain distribution and deformation patterns, as illustrated across the loaded ulna in rats [8]. Likewise, bending load, rather than local pressure, was capable of creating substantial periosteal mineral apposition in rats [9]. Moreover, understanding *in vivo* bone deformation is clinically relevant, in particular in relation to fatigue fracture. For example, *ex vivo* evidence suggests that mixed-mode loading is associated with greater bone fragility than uniaxial loading [10]. Similarly, changing the loading mode from pure compression to a combination of torsional and compressive loading facilitates propagation of microcracks within the bone

[11], and bones are relatively stronger when loaded by habitual load patterns than when exposed to novel loading regimes [12].

The *in vivo* bone deformation data currently available in literature mainly originates from studies that have used surgically implanted strain gauges. As noted previously, at least three strain gauges have to be attached around the long bone shaft to determine the neutral axis of bending and compute bending load or deformation. For most species, including humans, this operation is not feasible without affecting their regular muscle functions [6,13].

Harold Frost's mechanostat theory explains the functional adaptation capability of bone to mechanical stimulation [14]. However, it is still under debate which loading parameters in terms of deformation type, amplitude, repetition cycles and frequency, are most effective for bone adaptation [15]. Furthermore, the major sources of force, as well as the deformation modes required to effectively maintain or regulate bone structure and metabolism, remain unclear. Bending moments have been approximated in mammals, *e.g.* horse, dog and goat, using paired strains gauges from opposite surfaces of bones, in cases where limb motion is mainly in the parasagittal plane [7,16–18]. A series of classic studies on the bones of the lower extremities of animals in the 1980 s suggested that bending is occurring during different locomotor activities. This was demonstrated when strain gauge measurements showed that the anterior aspect of bone is under tension while the posterior aspect is under compression [16,17,19–21]. Recent studies in animal [18] and human models [22–24] suggest that bending is the primary component of long bone loading. The fact that most long bones are slightly curvatured also supports the idea that bending is notable, and that it may be enhanced by muscle contractions and the off-axis orientation of the bone to the center of body mass [25]. Furthermore, it has been speculated that the bone curvature is designed to improve the predictability of the bone load during different locomotor activities, since a curved bone is more likely to be bent than a straight bone [25]. Furthermore, studies have shown a shift of the bending neutral axis of long bones from the certroidal axis of the cross sectional area, indicating that long bones do indeed bend while experiencing axial loading [18,26]. In addition, it was shown that the bone loading pattern changes throughout the stance phase of the gait cycle and varies with speed [27–29]. The underlying cause will be that muscles attached to bone change their moment with joint movement. For example, most muscle groups in the human shank insert into the posterior aspect of tibia or fibula (Figure 1A). Although these muscles work against poor lever arms, they still generate very large flexion moments [30,31].

It is unclear in how far bending moments might be minimized by muscular contractions. Such contractions could protect the bone material and especially the long bones from bending stress accumulation, and therefore reduce fracture risks [32–35]. Muscle forces are thought by some to convert potential bending stress generated by reaction forces to compressive loading, which is less harmful for bone to tolerate [36]. An *in vivo* tibia strain study in humans seems to support the opinion. Milgrom *et al.* compared strain data in humans in fatigued and non-fatigued status [37]. The tensional strain of the antero-medial aspect of the tibia clearly increased when the gastrocnemius muscles were fatigue indicating that regular muscle activities might be crucial to maintain regular bone strains [37].

However, as noted above, one can apply paired or more gauges only where opposing sides of the bone are free of muscle insertions. Such an anatomical site is not available in any of large human long bones. To our knowledge, the *in vivo* bone loading patterns in humans during daily activities remains unknown.

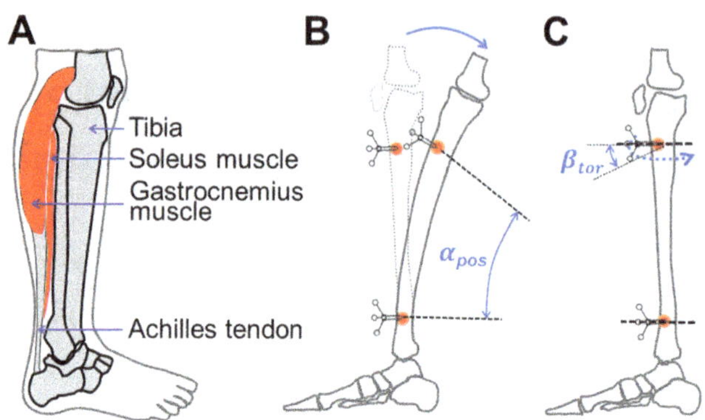

Figure 1. The demonstration of the human shank, the tibia posterior bending angle and torsion angle. A: anatomy of human shank. B: the demonstration of the posterior bending of the proximal tibia. α_{pos} indicates the posterior bending angle. C: tibia torsion deformation. β_{tor} indicates the internal torsion angle whist the tibia is twisted.

In comparison to bending, the role of torsion on bone mechanical adaptation has received little to no attention. Several classic studies have demonstrated that the strain gradient is highly correlated with periosteal bone formation on different sites [26,38]. If this holds true, then torsional loading would not be a crucial factor for periosteal bone formation, as torsional loading is only capable of generating relative small strain gradients for a near cylinder shaped long bone, compared to bending load. Contradictorily, some studies suggested that different constituents of the loading environment, namely axial loading and torsional loading, play a distinct role in regulating bone formation and structure [7,39]. These studies indicated that torsional loading might be one of the essential components of the entire bone loading regimes. Likewise, it was found that torsion dominates mechanical loading of the femur and tibiotarsus of the emu during running and gait [40]. Of note, torsion seems to be the main determinant of the design of long bones in birds [26,40–43]. To date, there is no salient evidence to suggest a strong role for torsion in the design of human long bones. One would intuitively assume that torsion is the driving loading pattern to maintain the almost circular cross-sectional geometry of long hollow bones [44], as torsion is capable of producing similar bone matrix deformation all along the circumference in different sites of the long bone. Results from an *in vivo* knee joint loading study indicated that the tibia-femur contact torsion moment was relatively small, with the normalized peak value (normalized by body weight times length) ranging from 0.53 to 1.1 [45]. However, considering the low capability of bone to resist torsional loading, we hypothesize that the human tibia may experience considerable torsional loading during walking and running.

Therefore, the goal of the present study was to use a novel optical segment tracking (OST) approach to investigate, for the first time, the *in vivo* human tibia loading regimes in terms of the tibia segment deformation regimes, including tibia antero-posterior (AP), medio-lateral bending angles (ML), torsion angles during most common locomotor activities for humans on the ground, *e.g.* walking and running. Furthermore, the relationship between the speed of walking and running, ground reaction force, moment and tibia deformation was assessed.

Material and Methods

Five healthy male subjects (26–50 years old) were recruited to participate in this study. They were free of any muscle or joint injuries and had not undergone orthopedic surgery in the lower extremities within twelve months prior to the study.

1.1 Ethics statement

Written and oral explanation of the purposes, benefits and risks of the study procedure were given to the subjects at least 3 days before they signed the consent forms. The subjects have given written informed consent, as outlined in the PLOS consent form, to the publication of their photograph. This study has been approved by the two relevant Ethics Committees, namely the ethical committee of the North-Rhine Medical Board in Düsseldorf and the ethical committee of the Faculty of Medicine in the University of Cologne. The operations and experiments were performed at the Department of Orthopedic and Trauma Surgery of the University Hospital of Cologne.

1.2 OST approach for tibia segment deformation measurements

A novel OST approach recently developed in our lab [46] has been adopted for tibia segment deformation recording in this study. Briefly, three mono-cortical bone screws were partially implanted into the anterior-medial aspect of the tibial cortex (Figure 2A–B). A marker cluster with a set of three non-collinear retro-reflective markers (Ø5 mm, Géodésie Maintenance Services, Nort Sur Erdre, France, Figure 2C) was mounted on each bone screw. The trajectories of the marker clusters were captured at 300 Hz by a Vicon MX optical motion capture system with eight Vicon F40 cameras (Vicon Motion System Ltd., LA, USA) (Figure 2A). In order to optimize resolution, accuracy and precision, the optical system used in this study included even more cameras than the previous validation study. The optical system was configured in line with our recent recommendations [46]. Specifications from our previous publication were followed, *i.e.*, positioning the cameras and adjusting the appropriate capture volume and the optimal distance between cameras and the tibia-affixed markers. It can therefore be taken as granted that the performance of the optical system was as good as in the mock-up study. This means that a resolution better than 20 µm within the capture volume of $400\times300\times300$ mm^3 was achieved. The maximal absolute error was 1.8 µm during displacements by 20 µm and repeatability was 2.5 µm. A detailed error analysis was performed in order to estimate absolute distance recording errors as a function of bending angle errors (see Discussion). Prior to the *in vivo* experiments, an *ex vivo* study on measuring tibia segment deformation under artificial loading in six cadaveric specimens has shown the fair repeatability and the feasibility of the OST approach (unpublished data). Briefly, the variance between the repeated tibia segment deformation measurements using the OST approach was assessed, whilst the cadaveric tibia was loaded by simulated muscle forces with a custom-made static loading device. Results suggested that the standard deviation of the mean bending and torsion deformation angles remains at a low level, from 0° to 0.04° for different loading conditions, indicating its potential to be applied *in vivo*. During the *in vivo* study, the stability of the bone screws in the tibial cortex was assessed by testing the resonance frequency of the screw-cluster structure and the relative position between the marker clusters prior to and after the exercises. It was shown to remain constant at ~260 Hz and ~380 Hz. The small location drift between the marker clusters during the course of the experimentation, which was maximally 0.06°, indicates that the implantation of the bone screws was extremely stable. The good toleration to the OST approach by the subjects also indicated its applicability for the *in vivo* measurements (See Results).

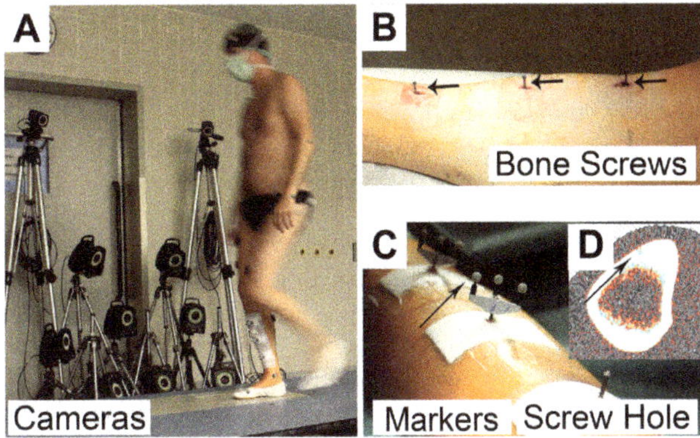

Figure 2. Illustration of the surgical details and the application of the OST approach in this study. A) The optical motion capture system with 8 high resolution cameras to track the retro-reflective markers affixed into tibial cortex, as well as two of the ten cameras for full body motion capturing; B) Implanted bone screws in the tibial cortex; C) Marker clusters were affixed to the endings of the bone screws; D) Cross-sectional pQCT image. The black arrow indicates the hole left behind after removal of the bone screw. OST: optical segment tracking.

In order to identify the tibia anatomical landmarks, general retro-reflective markers (Ø16 mm, Vicon Motion System Ltd., LA, USA) were attached on the skin over the medial and lateral malleolus, the tibia tuberosity and over the head of the fibula. Prior to each trial of the activities, the trajectories of skin-attached markers were recorded simultaneously with tibia-affixed markers for 1–2 seconds while the shank was in a static position and free of any loading. This static trial allowed the generation of the Shank Anatomical Coordinate System (SACS) required for data analysis. Tibia segment deformation was expressed as the relative movement between the tibia-affixed marker clusters in the SACS.

1.3 Surgical technique

Surgical implantation and explantation of the bone screws was performed under local anesthesia by injecting Xylocain 1% and Carbostesin 0.5% into the skin and the periosteum of the right shank of each subject. Prior to the operation, Ibuprofen (600 mg) and Cefuroxime (1500 mg) was administered to reduce pain perception and the risk of infection. The thickness of the tibial cortex was determined from transverse MRI (Magnetic Resonance Imaging, 1.5 T, Philips, Best, The Netherlands) images of the shank. To prevent intrusion into the bone marrow, the sites for screw implantation were selected so that the thickness of the tibial cortex was thicker than 4 mm. Thus, screws were implanted at approximately 10 cm below the tibia plateau, in the middle of the tibia diaphysis and at approximately 10 cm above the tibia medial malleolus.

Surgical incisions of approximately 1 cm length were made into the skin. A drill guide and a 2.1 mm diameter drill (Stryker Leibinger GmbH & Co. KG, Germany) were used to drill three holes into the tibial cortex to a depth of 2.5 mm. Bone screws (Asnis Micro cannulated titanium screws, Ø3 mm, 24/6 mm, Stryker Leibinger GmbH & Co. KG, Germany) were implanted with a dedicated screw driver. At the end of the experiment, *i.e.* between 6 and 8 hours later, bone screws were removed. Further details of the surgical procedure were described in another paper [47].

1.4 Investigated locomotor activities

All of the subjects wore gymnastic shoes during the experiments. Members of staff familiarized with the experimental procedure once a week during 6 months preceding the study, and study subjects underwent preparatory training during at least one day prior to the actual experiments in order to be fully acquainted with the protocol. During the practice training, the experimental protocol was followed closely to help the test subjects to be mentally well prepared for the *in vivo* experiments – the exception being that bone screws were installed into a shin pad above the shank instead of into the tibia. Testing included the most common locomotor activities during daily life: (1) walking on a walkway with a force plate embedded at self-selected slow, free and fast speed, respectively (Figure 2A); (2) walking at 2.5, 3.5, 4.5 and 5.5 km/h on a treadmill (Schiller MTM-1500 med, h/p/cosmos sports & medical GmbH, Germany); (3) running at 5.5 and 9 km/h on a treadmill (Two test subjects participated in the running test at 9 km/h). At least three repetitions have been performed at each speed of walking on the walkway, and a minimum of sixteen complete walking or running cycles were recorded on the treadmill, respectively.

1.5 Assessment of speed and ground reaction forces during walking

A second, independent motion capturing system with ten Bonita cameras (Vicon Motion System Ltd., LA, USA) was installed for the assessment of whole-body movement. Two general retro-reflective markers (Ø16 mm, Vicon Motion System Ltd., LA, USA) were attached to the skin of the left and right posterior superior iliac spine (PSIS). The trajectories of these two markers were sampled at 100 Hz for all subjects. Ground reaction forces during walking on the walkway were recorded at 1000 Hz with a force plate system (AMTI OR6-5, Watertown, MA, USA). The two motion capturing systems were synchronized by an external trigger.

1.6 Peripheral quantitative computed tomography (pQCT) imaging

Horizontal pQCT scans of the tibia on the sites of screw implantation were obtained one to three days after screw removal with a XCT3000 (Stratec Medizintechnik, Pforzheim, Germany) to document the screw holes and geometry of the tibia cross section area for further calculations (Figure 2D).

1.7 Data analysis

Raw marker trajectory data and ground reaction forces were further processed with custom-written MATLAB routines (The MathWorks, Inc. Version 7.9.0 R2009b). The raw marker trajectory data for tibia segment deformation recording was filtered using a 10-point moving average filter. Ground reaction force data was low-pass filtered using a 2nd order, zero lag Butterworth filter with cut-off frequency at 15 Hz.

1.7.1 Determination of SACS, tibia bending and torsion angles. For each subject, a randomly selected frame acquired during the static trial was utilized to determine an initial Cartesian SACS from the skin-attached tibia landmarks. In the SACS, X, Y and Z axes indicate the anterior-posterior, proximal-distal and medial-lateral direction, respectively [48]. The coordinates of the marker clusters implanted into the tibia were then subjected to coordinate transformation [49,50] to yield tibia segment deformation within the SACS. Differences between the relative position of each two sets of marker clusters in the SACS were then calculated and expressed as mean ± standard deviation (SD) of three Cardan/Euler angles and three translations along the axes of SACS, respectively. As the anterior-medial aspect of the tibia is free of muscle insertions, the effect of bone tissue inhomogeneity on anterior-medial tibia surface deformations was assumed to be negligible. AP bending angle, ML bending angle and inter-external torsion angle derived from Cardan/Euler angles were reported as tibia segment deformation. In the following, the relative movement of the proximal tibia-markers will be presented in relation to distal tibia-markers. Thus, AP bending (Figure 1B), ML bending and internal-external torsion (Figure 1C) always indicate the bending and torsion of the proximal tibia with respect to the distal tibia (Figure 1).

1.7.2 Calculation of the ground reaction force. Vertical ground reaction force (VGRF) during walking was derived from the filtered ground reaction force data. In general, there are two noticeable peaks for the VGRF during walking. These two peak values of VGRF were automatically identified and used for further analysis. Vertical Free moment (VFM) is the torque which acts about the vertical axis through the center of pressure of the ground reaction force. By subtracting the AP moment and the ML moment from the total transverse ground reaction moment, VFM about the vertical axis through the center of pressure of the force plate was determined. The details on the moment calculation can be referred to the 'Instruction Manual' of the AMTI Company [51]. VGRF was normalized to body weight (unit: N). VFM was normalized to the product of body weight (unit: N) and foot length (unit: m).

1.7.3 Calculation of walking speed on the walkway. During walking trials on the walkway, the coordinates of the mid-point of two PSIS markers in global transverse plane were extracted from the filtered total trajectories data. The average walking speed of the subjects was determined as the moving distance of the mid-point of two PSIS markers divided by time over the stance phase of the right leg on the force plate.

1.8 Statistics

Statistical analyses were performed using R statistic software (version 2.15.1, R Development Core Team, 2012). Least-squares linear regression was performed to determine the correlation between the tibia segment deformation angles and the moving speed, as well as VGRF or VFM for individual subjects. The 95% confidence interval for the slope was calculated. Furthermore, a one-way ANOVA linear model was employed to examine the main effects of subject, moving speed and the type of activity on the tibia segment deformation angles. Within-subject effects due to moving speed were assessed with the error analyses in an ANOVA linear model. Furthermore, considering that the sample size in the present study was limited, nonparametric tests were also adopted to assess the potential influence of small sample size on the statistical results. In particular, the correlation between tibia segment deformation angles, moving speed and VGRF or VFM for each individual subject was determined with Spearman's rank correlation rho (corresponding to Least-squares Linear regression in parametric tests). The effects of locomotor speed and the type of activity on tibia segment deformation angles during treadmill exercises were assessed with Friedman test or Wilcoxon Mann-Whitney test (corresponding to one-way ANOVA and t-test). Statistical significance was accepted at $p \leq 0.05$.

Results

Pain questionnaires (Visual analog scale form 0 to 10 indicating no pain to intolerable pain) were handed out during the *in vivo* experiments. All subjects report 0 during walking and running [47], indicating that the potential influence of pain caused by the bone screws and the wound on the motion is minimized. The bone screws were firmly inserted into the tibia until the end of the experiments. Statistical analysis suggested that there is no fundamental difference between parametric and nonparametric analysis. The details can be found in the following sections. The results in the corresponding figures were thus presented based on the parametric analysis.

1.1 Walking on the walkway with force plate embedded

A typical example of the tibia segment deformation angle during a stance phase of the gait cycle is presented in Figure 3. As the overground walking speed was not strictly controlled from subject to subject and computed after the experiments, the results in Figures 4–6 provide all data on an individual basis. During the stance phase, there were generally posterior bending, external torsion and medial bending of the proximal tibia relative to the distal tibia, with posterior bending being most pronounced during the first half, and torsion being predominant during the second half of the stance phase.

1.1.1 Tibia segment deformation versus walking speed. Statistical analysis yielded main effects of the test subject on the deformation angles ($p = 0.02$ and $r^2 = 0.57$ for tibia AP bending, $p<0.001$ and $r^2 = 0.09$ for tibia torsion, $p<0.001$ and $r^2 = 0.03$ for tibia ML bending). There were no significant within-subjects effects due to walking speed ($p = 0.36$ for tibia AP bending, $p = 0.07$ for tibia torsion, $p = 0.1$ for tibia ML bending). Therefore, the nonparametric and parametric statistic correlation analysis between deformation angles and walking speed was done separately for the individual test subjects (Figure 4). For all test subjects, the peak-to-peak AP bending angle linearly increased with walking speed. Peak-to-peak AP bending angles varied from 0.15° to 1.30° at the speed of 2.5 - 6.1 km/h. The slope of the regression line ranged from 0.17 to 0.32 with r-squared values between 0.70 and 0.96 (Figure 4A). Significant correlations between peak-to-peak tibia torsion angles and the speed were found in three out of five test subjects. The peak-to-peak tibia torsion angle varied between 0.67° and 1.66° at walking speed of 2.5–6.1 km/h (Figure 4B). By contrast, peak-to-peak ML bending angles were rather small, within 0.38°–0.90°, and were mostly unrelated to walking speed, except for test subject B (Figure 4C). The linear regression results are summarized in Table 1. Nonparametric statistical analysis (Spearman's rank correlation) yielded the similar correlation results to the parametric analysis between tibia bending angles and walking speed. The results were summarized in Table 2.

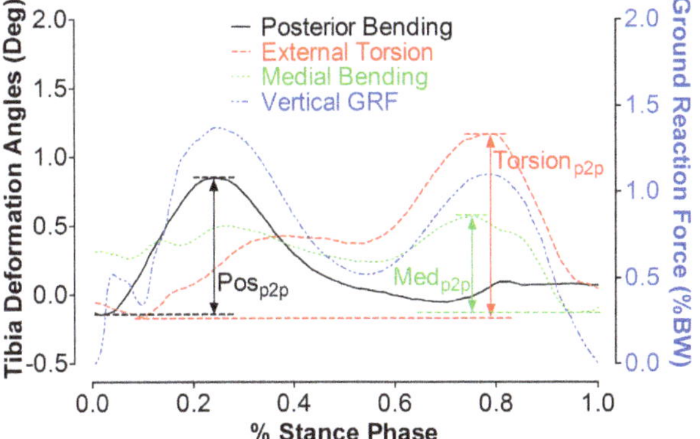

Figure 3. Illustration of the tibia segment deformation (example during the stance phase of an overground gait cycle). Solid black line: AP bending angle of the proximal tibia with respect to the distal tibia. Dashed red line: torsion angle, dotted green line: ML bending angle, dash-dot blue line: vertical ground reaction force. Pos_{p2p} refers to the peak-to-peak AP bending angle during the stance phase of the gait cycle. Med_{p2p} refers to the peak-to-peak ML bending angle of the proximal tibia. $Torsion_{p2p}$ refers to the peak-to-peak torsion angle. AP: antero-posterior, ML: medio-lateral. Pos: posterior, Med: medial, p2p: peak-to-peak.

1.1.2 Tibia segment deformation versus ground reaction force. Regression analysis suggests that the tibia peak-to-peak AP bending angle increased linearly ($p<0.001$) with the peak VGRF during the first half stance phase, with the slope of the regression line ranging between 1.99 degree*h/km and 2.56 degree*h/km (r^2: 0.77–0.97, Figure 5A). By contrast, there was no such relationship between peak-to-peak torsion angle and peak VGRF during the second half of the stance phase, except for subject C ($p<0.001$, $r^2 = 0.94$, Figure 5B).

VFM but not VGRF was correlated with peak-to-peak torsion angles in four test subjects, except subject A ($p = 0.056$, $r^2 = 0.22$, Figure 5C).

The linear regression results are summarized in Table 3. Similar correlation trends between the tibia bending angles and walking speed were found using nonparametric statistical analysis. The Spearman's rank correlation results are summarized in Table 4.

1.2 Walking and running on a treadmill

During treadmill walking, significant main effects of the test subjects on the AP bending angle ($p<0.001$, $r^2 = 0.89$), torsion angle ($p<0.001$, $r^2 = 0.85$) and ML bending angle ($p = 0.0046$, $r^2 = 0.62$) were found. Within-subjects effects of walking speed were not found ($p = 0.24$ for tibia AP bending, $p = 0.37$ for tibia torsion, $p = 0.16$ for tibia ML bending). Therefore, and as above, the deformation results are presented on the basis of the individual test subject (Figure 6). The AP bending angle increased with walking speed (posterior bending angles: from 0.23°±0.03° to 0.90°±0.22°, $p<0.001$) and running speed (posterior bending angles: from 1.07°±0.11° to 2.15°±0.27°, $p<0.001$). At the same speed, running induced a larger AP bending angle than walking (Figure 6A, $p<0.001$). No main effects of speed were found on tibia torsion during treadmill walking (external torsion angles: from 0.86°±0.10° to 1.85°±0.15 °, $p = 0.067$). Interestingly, for four test subjects, it seems that tibia torsion during running is lower than that during walking (Figure 6B, $p = 0.048$). During walking and running on the treadmill, ML bending, compared to bending deformation, occurred on somewhat low levels and was almost constant across speeds. One exception was that a larger ML bending angle was generated during running at 9 km/h than during running at 5.5 km/h and walking at different speeds (Figure 6C, $p<0.001$). Tibia torsion of two test subjects responded differently to the running speed. The tibia torsion angle significantly increased for test subject D ($p<0.001$), but decreased in test subject E (Figure 6B, $p = 0.0013$). The variation across the walking and running cycles was assessed by the standard deviation of the deformation angles, which was summarized in Table 5.

During treadmill walking, nonparametric analysis suggested a similar relationship between tibia deformation angles and moving speed as established during parametric analysis. More specifically, the AP bending angle increased with the walking speed ($p = 0.007$, except $p = 0.42$ for 2.5 km/h *v.s.* 3.5 km/h and $p = 0.22$ for 4.5 km/h *v.s.* 5.5 km/h comparisons). A larger AP bending angle

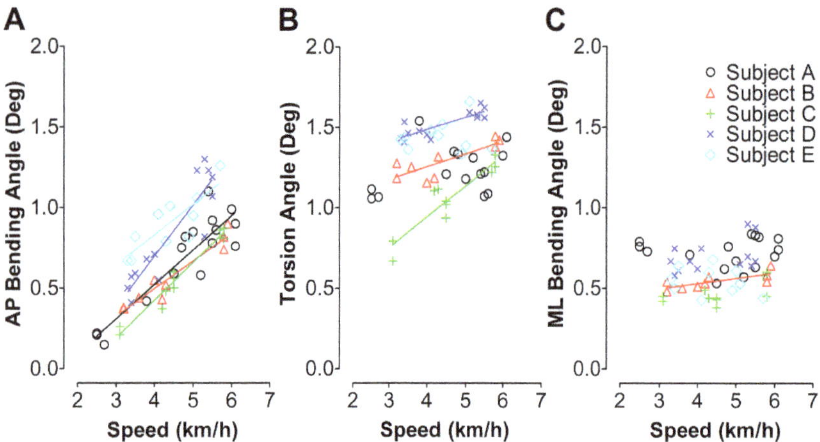

Figure 4. Illustration of individual tibia segment deformation during overground walking in relation to walking speed. The AP bending (A), torsion (B) and ML bending angle (C) indicate the extent of AP bending, external torsion and ML bending of the proximal tibia with respect to the distal tibia, respectively. The regression lines were given only when correlation between deformation angle and the walking speed was significant. It can be appreciated from these data that a high correlation exists between overground speed and bone deformation. This is despite the fact that locomotor patterns will contain elements that will not scale linearly with speed, which may underline the validity of the bone deformation measurements. AP: antero-posterior, ML: medio-lateral.

was induced by running than walking (walking at 5.5 km/h *v.s.* run at 9 km/h: $p = 0.03$). No significant effects of speed were found on tibia torsion during treadmill walking ($p = 0.22$) and running ($p = 0.08$). ML bending remained at a low level and nearly constant across speeds ($p = 0.45$) and types of locomotion ($p = 0.64$).

Discussion

In this paper, the *in vivo* tibia segment deformation regimes in humans, *e.g.* bending and torsion, during walking and running were investigated utilizing a novel optical segment tracking (OST) approach for the first time. Substantial effects of the walking and running speed, VGRF and VFM on the bending and torsion deformation angles of the human tibia were found. It should also be stated that these deformations were of surprisingly large magnitude during walking and running. In addition to the expected result that tibia segment deformation would generally increase with locomotor speed and with ground reaction forces, this study has yielded a number of novel and less obvious findings. Firstly, and most importantly, bone segment deformation, almost like a finger-print, contains highly specific personal information. In other words, very close relationships were found between *e.g.* ground reaction force and tibia segment deformation within each test subject, but the exact nature of these relationships varied between people. Secondly, anterior-posterior bending and torsion were the prevailing tibia loading regimes, whilst medio-lateral bending was much less pronounced. Thirdly, the different tibia deformation regimes did not scale uniformly with locomotor speed or ground reaction force. Each locomotor activity was rather characterized by a variable amount of bending and torsional deformation. Fourth, on the basis of many studies on the bone deformation amplitude in the past, this study provides rationale to

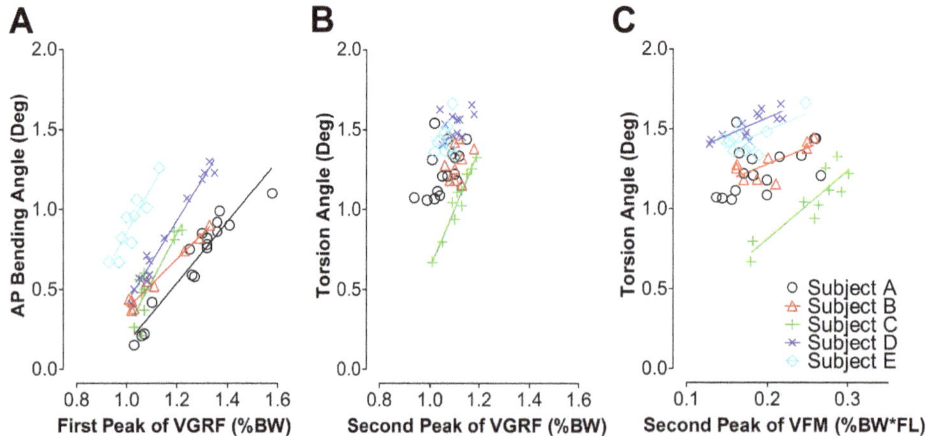

Figure 5. The relationship between the tibia segment deformation angles and the VGRF or VFM during walking. A: AP bending angles under different VGRF (the first peak value) during the first half stance phase of the gait cycle. B: Torsion angles under different VGRF (the second peak value) during the second half stance phase of the gait cycle. C: Torsion angles under different VFM during the second half stance phase of the gait cycle. The regression lines are displayed only where correlations between tibia deformation angles and the walking speed were significant. AP: antero-posterior, ML: medio-lateral. VGRF: vertical ground reaction force, VFM: vertical free moment.

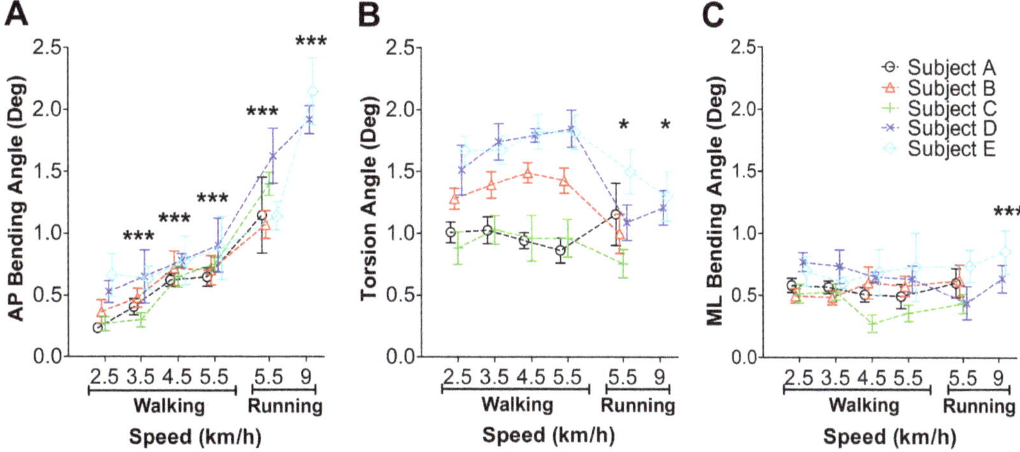

Figure 6. Tibia segment deformation angles during walking and running on a treadmill at different speed. A: tibia AP bending angles at different speed of walking and running. B: tibia torsion angle. C: tibia ML bending angle. *: $p<0.05$; ***: $p<0.001$. AP: antero-posterior, ML: medio-lateral.

revisit the potential importance of *in vivo* loading regimes and its features during common exercises, *e.g.* walking and running.

1.1 Analysis of recording errors

As with any new method, an assessment of limits arising from recording errors is vitally important. We see four major sources of error.

Firstly, the accuracy and the repeatability of the adopted optical system for recording minute marker movement in the targeted 3D volume have to be considered. As outlined above, the accuracy (absolute error) and the repeatability were very favorable within the volume of $400\times300\times300$ mm^3, namely maximum 1.8 µm and 2.5 µm, respectively, to assess displacements by 20 µm. The corresponding error can be translated in terms of angular deviation (α_{error} in Figure 7A) with the equations given as follows. The maximum between-marker distance within a marker cluster amounts to 25 mm, and we have to consider accuracy errors at both ends of the marker cluster. Thus, the total alignment error amounts to $2^{1/2} * 1.8 = 2.55$ µm, and the error for estimates of α_{error} would be $180°-2 * \arccos(2.55\ \mu m/25\ mm) = 0.012°$ (the calculations of arccos were based on angles, Figure 7A). The α_{error} value was smaller than reported deformation results by two orders of magnitude.

Secondly, there is an undeterminable source of error associated with longitudinal variation as per the biological experiment itself. Our experience from the afore-mentioned *ex vivo* study suggested a

Table 1. Least-squares linear regression statistics for tibia bending angles versus walking speed.

Subject	Deformation	b_1 (degree*h/km)	a_1 (degree)	r^2	*p* value	N
A	AP Bending	0.21***	−0.33	0.82	<0.001	16
	Torsion	0.05	1.02	0.16	0.12	
	ML Bending	7.57e-4	0.72	9.90e-05	0.97	
B	AP Bending	0.17***	−0.19	0.92	<0.001	9
	Torsion	0.08**	0.94	0.68	0.006	
	ML Bending	0.03*	0.40	0.56	0.02	
C	AP Bending	0.23***	−0.52	0.96	<0.001	10
	Torsion	0.19***	0.18	0.85	<0.001	
	ML Bending	0.04	0.28	0.36	0.07	
D	AP Bending	0.32***	−0.58	0.82	<0.001	13
	Torsion	0.08***	1.19	0.71	<0.001	
	ML Bending	0.05	0.49	0.19	0.14	
E	AP Bending	0.19**	0.07	0.70	0.0027	10
	Torsion	0.01	1.39	0.01	0.80	
	ML Bending	−0.03	0.67	0.07	0.46	

The linear model used in the statistics is: $y_1 = b_1 * x_1 + a_1$ (y_1 indicates the tibia bending angles, x_1 indicates walking speed, 95% Confident interval).
*: $p<0.05$,
**: $p<0.01$,
***: $p<0.001$.

Table 2. Nonparametric statistical analysis for tibia bending angles versus walking speed.

Subject	Deformation	r_s	*p* value	N
A	AP Bending	0.77***	<0.001	16
	Torsion	−0.38	0.14	
	ML Bending	−0.22	0.42	
B	AP Bending	0.88**	0.003	9
	Torsion	−0.73*	0.03	
	ML Bending	−0.76*	0.02	
C	AP Bending	0.98***	<0.001	10
	Torsion	−0.77**	0.0098	
	ML Bending	−0.41	0.24	
D	AP Bending	0.78**	0.002	13
	Torsion	−0.74**	0.004	
	ML Bending	−0.40	0.17	
E	AP Bending	0.82**	0.004	10
	Torsion	−0.006	1	
	ML Bending	0.15	0.68	

The coefficient of correlation (r_s) and level of significance (*p*) were yielded.
*: $p<0.05$,
**: $p<0.01$,
***: $p<0.001$.

reproducibility of approximately 0.04°. The value of 0.04° includes both measurement and experimental-longitudinal variation and is approximately twice as large as the measurement error only, but still substantially smaller than the reported results.

Thirdly, we have to consider that the bone screws could have loosened, *e.g.* due to the impact during the locomotor activities. However, the screws were deemed as stable upon removal after exercises were completed. Both orthopedic surgeons involved in the present study had performed hundreds of materials removals in their surgical practice. Moreover, the constant resonance frequency of the screw-cluster structure and the non-systematic

Table 3. Least-squares linear regression statistics for tibia deformation angles versus VGRF and VFM.

Subject	Deformation angles	b_3 (degree*h/km)	a_3 (degree)	r^2	*p* value	N
A	AP Bending *v.s.* VGRF	1.91***	−1.75	0.91	<0.001	16
	Torsion *v.s.* VGRF	1.34	−0.17	0.24	0.054	
	Torsion *v.s.* VFM	11.97	1.07	0.25	0.056	
B	AP Bending *v.s.* VGRF	1.56***	−1.18	0.97	<0.001	9
	Torsion *v.s.* VGRF	1.02	0.16	0.11	0.38	
	Torsion *v.s.* VFM	28.43*	0.60	0.51	0.046	
C	AP Bending *v.s.* VGRF	2.99***	−2.74	0.77	<0.001	10
	Torsion *v.s.* VGRF	3.67***	−3.03	0.94	<0.001	
	Torsion *v.s.* VFM	34.91**	0.33	0.66	0.008	
D	AP Bending *v.s.* VGRF	2.57***	−2.16	0.97	<0.001	13
	Torsion *v.s.* VGRF	0.85	0.59	0.21	0.11	
	Torsion *v.s.* VFM	10.71**	1.31	0.42	0.003	
E	AP Bending *v.s.* VGRF	2.90***	−2.04	0.84	<0.001	10
	Torsion *v.s.* VGRF	1.05	0.33	0.08	0.43	
	Torsion *v.s.* VFM	16.52*	1.10	0.47	0.04	

The linear model used in the statistics is: $y_3 = b_3 * x_3 + a_3$ (y_3 indicates the tibia deformation angles, x_3 indicates vertical ground reaction force or vertical free moment, 95% Confident interval).
*: $p<0.05$,
**: $p<0.01$,
***: $p<0.001$.

Table 4. Nonparametric statistical analysis for tibia bending angles versus VGRF and VFM.

Subject	Deformation angles	r_s	*p* value	N
A	AP Bending *v.s.* VGRF	0.96***	<0.001	16
	Torsion *v.s.* VGRF	−0.53*	0.04	
	Torsion *v.s.* VFM	−0.52*	0.04	
B	AP Bending *v.s.* VGRF	0.85**	0.003	9
	Torsion *v.s.* VGRF	−0.23	0.55	
	Torsion *v.s.* VFM	−0.89*	0.012	
C	AP Bending *v.s.* VGRF	0.78**	0.007	10
	Torsion *v.s.* VGRF	0.92***	<0.001	
	Torsion *v.s.* VFM	−0.81**	0.008	
D	AP Bending *v.s.* VGRF	0.96***	<0.001	13
	Torsion *v.s.* VGRF	−0.41	0.17	
	Torsion *v.s.* VFM	−0.78**	0.002	
E	AP Bending *v.s.* VGRF	0.91***	<0.001	10
	Torsion *v.s.* VGRF	−0.16	0.66	
	Torsion *v.s.* VFM	−0.42	0.27	

The coefficient of correlation (r_s) and level of significance (*p*) were yielded accordingly.
*: $p<0.05$,
**: $p<0.01$,
***: $p<0.001$.

and negligible drift between the marker clusters suggested firm fixation of the bone screws in the tibial cortex (unpublished data).

Fourthly, it is possible, in theory, that the marker cluster resonated during locomotor activities and thus produced artificial displacement. However, the vibration amplitude of the screw-cluster structure during the locomotor activities can be assessed with the known characteristics of the marker clusters and following equations, as illustrated in Figure 7B. The weight of the marker cluster is 5.6 grams. The most intense exercise, *i.e.* hopping, yielded acceleration of 3.5 times gravity, thus causing a force F of 0.19 N. The distance between the bone surface and the plane determined by three markers in the cluster is 26.6 mm (L), and the bending stiffness (flexural stiffness, *i.e.* the product of elastic modulus and area moment of inertia) of the bone screw shaft is 0.41 Nm^2 (elastic modulus of the screw material: $E = 110$ GPa, inner and outer diameters of 1.5 and 3 mm, respectively, and thus area moment of inertia $I = 3.73$ mm^4). Thus potential vibration amplitude of the markers induced by the acceleration of the marker cluster would be maximally [52]

$$d = F \times L^3/(3 \times E \times I) = 2.93\mu m$$

These results suggested that the amplitude of any vibration of the screw/cluster structure is relatively small, being certainly

Table 5. The variation across the walking and running cycles was assessed with the standard deviation (SD) of the deformation angles.

			SD (Deformation Angles, Degree)		
Subject	**Exercises**	**Cycles**	**AP Bending**	**Torsion**	**ML Bending**
A	walking	5–19	0.03–0.07	0.08–0.10	0.06–0.12
	running	22	0.31	0.25	0.12
B	walking	22–15	0.10–0.20	0.08–0.13	0.06–0.13
	running	41	0.11	0.16	0.13
C	walking	23–48	0.06–0.08	0.13–0.19	0.06–0.08
	running	30	0.09	0.11	0.08
D	walking	6–39	0.09–0.22	0.05–0.20	0.08–0.14
	running	39–53	0.11–0.22	0.14	0.11–0.13
E	walking	16–39	0.09–0.25	0.12–0.17	0.05–0.25
	running	18–28	0.12–0.27	0.18–0.20	0.13–0.18

SD: standard deviation.

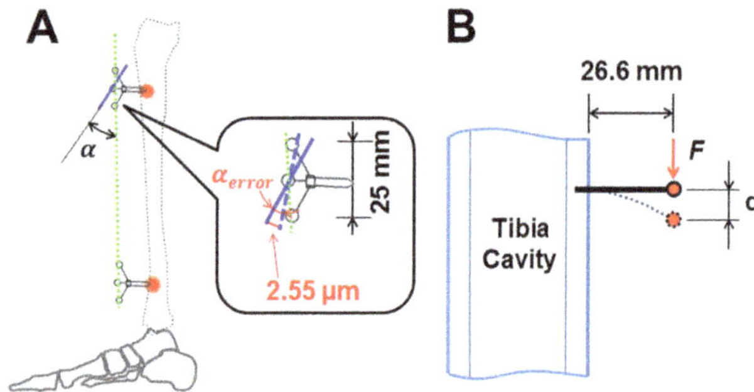

Figure 7. The recording error analysis of the OST approach. A: the deformation angle deviation α_{error} assumed from the absolute error of $2^{1/2}$ * 1.8 = 2.55 μm for both ends of the markers in the marker cluster. Bold black line referred to the plane determined by three markers in the marker cluster. 25 mm indicated the maximum distance between the markers in one marker cluster. α refers to the angle between the marker clusters. B: the potential marker displacement (d) due to the vibration induced by the acceleration force (*F*) of the screw/cluster structure. The bold black line refers to the bone screw. The red spot indicates the position of the plane determined by the markers in this cluster. 26.6 mm indicates the distance between the plane determined by three markers in one marker cluster and the bone surface. OST: optical segment tracking.

smaller than the resolution of the optical system, and probably negligible in comparison to the reported results.

1.2 Main findings on tibia segment deformation during walking on the walkway

Results from this study showed that the proximal tibia mainly twisted externally and bent to the posterior aspect, as well as to some extent to the medial aspect in relation to the distal tibia during the stance phase of walking and running. Previously, the tibia contact force and moment have been investigated with an instrumented knee implant [31,45]. These results are in accordance with our findings, especially regarding the occurrence of posterior and medial bending as well as torsion moments during the stance phase of level walking. In line with this, bending and torsion moments have been predicted to occur during walking in a musculoskeletal model calculation [30]. However, the results in our study disagree with previous reports of tibia bending assessed during running by inverse dynamics analysis, in which anterior, rather than posterior tibia bending moments were postulated during the stance phase of running [53]. The inconsistencies may relate to the inherent limitations of the inverse dynamics analysis approach, *e.g.* only joint reaction forces are calculated, which may derive unrealistic tibia load. In this context, the present results may provide further, indirect evidence to the view that the largest skeletal forces depend on muscle contractions, rather than simply arising from mass acceleration [54].

Another important finding is the non-uniform scaling of deformation regimes. As exemplified in Figure 3, there were generally two noticeable deformation peaks, one in antero-posterior bending that coincided with the heel-strike, and another one in torsion that coincided with toe lift-off. This pattern was also confirmed by statistical analyses, suggesting that the peak-to-peak antero-posterior bending angles are linearly correlated with the first peak of the vertical ground reaction force, while the peak-to-peak torsion angle is unrelated to the second peak of the VGRF, but correlates with the second peak of VFM during the second half of the stance phase. Considering the fact that the mechanical load on the tibia shaft is generally caused by body weight and muscle contractions, the plantar flexors are primarily active during the second half of the stance phase. It is therefore tempting to assume that the body weight primarily induces the posterior bending of the tibia, while torsion is mainly produced by the plantar flexors contraction. Certainly, further study into the relationship between the deformation angles and body weight or muscle activities is needed to draw a firm conclusion.

1.3 Effects of walking speed on tibia segment deformation

During walking on the walkway, tibia antero-posterior bending increased linearly with walking speed. This result is congruent with previous results of numerous animal experiments, *e.g.* dog tibia, dog radius, horse tibia, horse radius and goat tibia [21,55]. Similarly, for three test subjects, the torsion angles, but not the medio-lateral bending angles, slightly and linearly increased with walking speed. The medio-lateral bending angles remained rather constant with speed. Likewise, during treadmill walking, antero-posterior bending increased with speed. Interestingly, for three test subjects, tibia torsion angles increased linearly with walking speed during overground walking, but remained constant during treadmill walking, indicating that the tibia load might be different for these two cases. It has been shown that larger compression and tension strains on one site of bone were generated during the overground running than during the treadmill running [56]. The current results provide further evidence that the VGRF during the mid- and late-stance phase of treadmill walking differs from overground walking [57], which might be able to explain the deformation difference found in the present study.

1.4 Relationship between tibia segment deformation and ground reaction force or moment

The results from this study revealed a strong relationship between the VFM and the tibia torsion deformation for four of the test subjects. It is of interest in this context that VFM seems to be closely related to the loading history of the tibia [58]. Conversely, the results showed that tibia deformation or load could not be totally predicted from VGRF.

1.5 Tibia segment deformation during running on the treadmill

In general, running is a more demanding exercise than walking. The muscles in the lower extremities are generally more active during running than during walking. In addition, axial forces caused by mass acceleration are higher in running than in walking. Results from this study suggest that the antero-posterior bending angle during running is significantly larger than during walking, even at the same speed of locomotion (Figure 6). Despite the limited number of subjects ($n = 2$) participating in the jogging trials at 9 km/h, antero-posterior and medio-lateral bending were still significantly larger than at 5.5 km/h. Conversely, tibia torsion was profoundly decreased during jogging at 9 km/h, even below levels observed during walking. Previous strain gauge measurements generally found principal tibia strains to be larger during running than walking. However, no measurements in bending and torsion were available in these previous studies [59,60].

Taken all of the above together, results of the present study indicated that not only the amplitude, but the regimes of tibia load differ between running and walking. It has been well accepted that stress fractures in the anterior tibia shaft can occur among long distance runners [61]. Our experiment suggests that such stress fractures may be related to the high tension in the anterior aspect of tibia, whilst the posterior tibia was under even larger compression. Likewise, an inverse dynamics analysis study on runners indicated that the superposition of the joint reaction force and muscle force magnify the tibia posterior compression and attenuated the tibia shear force [62]. This might be one of the reasons why torsion angles from our measurements were lower during running than walking.

1.6 Limitations

Although new knowledge on human tibia segment deformation was contributed to understand the *in vivo* loading situations, the OST approach leaves some open questions. Firstly, unlike the strain gauge approaches, the local strain information of the tibia surface is not assessed in the proposed approach. Such a high-fidelity estimation or calculation should rely on an inversely-driven Finite Element Model (FEM), with anatomical tibia data – an approach that is by no means trivial but necessary to understand the strain distribution across the tibia. Secondly, the capture volume of the optical system was limited ($400\times300\times300$ mm^3 in this case) in order to maintain acceptable accuracy and repeatability during the deformation recording, meaning that tibia-affixed markers have to be in this volume during the recording trials of the exercises. As a consequence, the selection of exercises which can be performed, *e.g.* continuous recording of long term walking (Even for single gait cycle, the full swing phase is not always available due to the restriction of the capture volume) or running over ground, is limited. Thirdly, in the presented study, the comparatively small sample size ($n = 5$) raises the issue of interpretation of the parametric statistical analysis. Hence, nonparameteric statistics, which are conceived to be more robust for small sample size, were used in addition to parametric statistics to analyse the present results. No clear differences were found when comparing the two types of analyses, indicating that the small sample size in the present study is not likely to influence the conclusions we drew form the results. However, a larger sample size would still be appreciated in future studies. To summarize, it remains uncertain in how far the OST approach will be applied widely in future studies, due to its invasiveness. Understanding what can and what cannot be expected from the OST approach will guide the design of future studies, which firstly need to focus on improvement of the OST approach, and then further expand its application when justifiable.

Conclusions

In summary, taking together the tibia segment deformation results from this first application of the proposed OST approach in humans *in vivo*, we conclude that the human tibia experiences a considerable amount of bending and torsion loading during walking and running. The maximum peak-to-peak antero-posterior bending, torsion and medio-lateral bending angles reached up to 1.30°, 1.66° and 0.90° during walking, respectively. The tibia antero-posterior bending angles and torsion angles increased linearly with the walking speed and VGRF or VFM. More interestingly, a more or less fixed phase-relationship exists between different types of deformation during the stance phase of walking. Running generates larger antero-posterior bending angles, but smaller torsion angles than walking. These new findings on tibia segment deformation regimes during walking and running are therefore bound to change our understanding of long bone deformation in humans and provide more insights into the mechanical load distribution rather than mechanical load amplitude alone.

Acknowledgments

We would like to thank Peter Gauger, Wolfram Sies, Andreas Kriechbaumer and Jakob Kümmel for their kind help during data collection. We also would like to thank Hans-Martin Küsel-Feldker and Jürgen Geiermannat of the Institute of Biomechanics and Orthopaedics, German Sport University Cologne, Germany, for fine manufacturing the marker clusters. Special acknowledgements go to Alex Ireland for his kind language editing assistance. Peng-Fei Yang acknowledges Helmholtz Space Life Sciences Research School (SpaceLife) and his scholarship by the China Scholarship Council (CSC No.: 2009629013). Last but not least we are very grateful to our test subjects - without their selfless contribution, this work would not have been possible.

Author Contributions

Conceived and designed the experiments: PFY MS BG TK GPB LPM JR. Performed the experiments: PFY MS BG TK GPB LPM JR. Analyzed the data: PFY MS BG TK GPB LPM JR. Contributed reagents/materials/ analysis tools: PFY MS BG TK GPB LPM JR. Wrote the paper: PFY MS BG TK GPB LPM JR.

References

1. Main RP, Biewener AA (2004) Ontogenetic patterns of limb loading, *in vivo* bone strains and growth in the goat radius. J Exp Biol 207: 2577–2588.
2. Petit MA, Beck TJ, Lin HM, Bentley C, Legro RS, et al. (2004) Femoral bone structural geometry adapts to mechanical loading and is influenced by sex steroids: The Penn State Young Women's Health Study. Bone 35: 750–759.
3. Schulte FA, Ruffoni D, Lambers FM, Christen D, Webster DJ, et al. (2013) Local mechanical stimuli regulate bone formation and resorption in mice at the tissue level. PLoS ONE 8: e62172.
4. Augat P, Reeb H, Claes LE (1996) Prediction of fracture load at different skeletal sites by geometric properties of the cortical shell. J Bone Miner Res 11: 1356–1363.
5. Capozza RF, Feldman S, Mortarino P, Reina PS, Schiessl H, et al. (2010) Structural analysis of the human tibia by tomographic (pQCT) serial scans. J Anat 216: 470–481.
6. Lieberman DE, Polk JD, Demes B (2004) Predicting long bone loading from cross-sectional geometry. Am J Phys Anthropol 123: 156–171.
7. Rubin C, Gross T, Qin YX, Fritton S, Guilak F, et al. (1996) Differentiation of the bone-tissue remodeling response to axial and torsional loading in the turkey ulna. J Bone Joint Surg Am 78: 1523–1533.
8. Kotha SP, Hsieh YF, Strigel RM, Müller R, Silva MJ (2004) Experimental and finite element analysis of the rat ulnar loading model—correlations between strain and bone formation following fatigue loading. J Biomech 37: 541–548.
9. Raab-Cullen DM, Akhter MP, Kimmel DB, Recker RR (1994) Periosteal bone formation stimulated by externally induced bending strains. J Bone Miner Res 9: 1143–1152.
10. George WT, Vashishth D (2006) Susceptibility of aging human bone to mixed-mode fracture increases bone fragility. Bone 38: 105–111.
11. Wang XA, Niebur GL (2006) Microdamage propagation in trabecular bone due to changes in loading mode. J Biomech 39: 781–790.
12. Reilly GC, Currey JD (1999) The development of microcracking and failure in bone depends on the loading mode to which it is adapted. J Exp Biol 202: 543–552.
13. Yang PF, Bruggemann GP, Rittweger J (2011) What do we currently know from *in vivo* bone strain measurements in humans? J Musculoskelet Neuronal Interact 11: 8–20.
14. Frost HM (2000) The Utah paradigm of skeletal physiology: an overview of its insights for bone, cartilage and collagenous tissue organs. J Bone Miner Metab 18: 305–316.
15. Huiskes R, van Rietbergen B (2005) Biomechanics of bone. In: C. MV, R H, editors. Basic Orthopaedic Biomechanics & Mechano-biology. 3rd ed: Lippincott Williams & Wilkins. pp.123–180.
16. Biewener AA, Thomason JJ, Lanyon LE (1988) Mechanics of locomotion and jumping in the horse (Equus): *in vivo* stress in the tibia and metatarsus. J Zool 214: 547–565.
17. Biewener AA, Thomason J, Goodship A, Lanyon LE (1983) Bone stress in the horse forelimb during locomotion at different gaits - a comparison of 2 experimental methods. J Biomech 16: 565–576.
18. Gross TS, McLeod KJ, Rubin CT (1992) Characterizing bone strain distributions *in vivo* using three triple rosette strain gages. J Biomech 25: 1081–1087.
19. Biewener AA (1991) Musculoskeletal design in relation to body size. J Biomech 24 Suppl 1: 19–29.
20. Rubin CT, Lanyon LE (1984) Dynamic strain similarity in vertebrates; an alternative to allometric limb bone scaling. J Theor Biol 107: 321–327.

21. Rubin CT, Lanyon LE (1982) Limb mechanics as a function of speed and gait - a study of functional strains in the radius and tibia of horse and dog. J Exp Biol 101: 187–211.
22. Aamodt A, Lund-Larsen J, Eine J, Andersen E, Benum P, et al. (1997) *In vivo* measurements show tensile axial strain in the proximal lateral aspect of the human femur. J Orthop Res 15: 927–931.
23. Peterman MM, Hamel AJ, Cavanagh PR, Piazza SJ, Sharkey NA (2001) In vitro modeling of human tibial strains during exercise in micro-gravity. J Biomech 34: 693–698.
24. Macdonald HM, Cooper DML, McKay HA (2009) Anterior–posterior bending strength at the tibial shaft increases with physical activity in boys: evidence for non-uniform geometric adaptation. Osteopor Int 20: 61–70.
25. Bertram JE, Biewener AA (1988) Bone curvature: sacrificing strength for load predictability? J Theor Biol 131: 75–92.
26. Judex S, Gross TS, Zernicke RF (1997) Strain gradients correlate with sites of exercise-induced bone-forming surfaces in the adult skeleton. J Bone Miner Res 12: 1737–1745.
27. Szivek JA, Johnson EM, Magee FP (1992) *In vivo* strain analysis of the greyhound femoral diaphysis. J Invest Surg 5: 91–108.
28. Demes B, Stern JT Jr, Hausman MR, Larson SG, McLeod KJ, et al. (1998) Patterns of strain in the macaque ulna during functional activity. Am J Phys Anthropol 106: 87–100.
29. Demes B, Qin YX, Stern JT Jr, Larson SG, Rubin CT (2001) Patterns of strain in the macaque tibia during functional activity. Am J Phys Anthropol 116: 257–265.
30. Wehner T, Claes L, Simon U (2009) Internal loads in the human tibia during gait. Clin Biomech (Bristol, Avon) 24: 299–302.
31. Heinlein B, Kutzner I, Graichen F, Bender A, Rohlmann A, et al. (2009) ESB Clinical Biomechanics Award 2008: Complete data of total knee replacement loading for level walking and stair climbing measured *in vivo* with a follow-up of 6–10 months. Clin Biomech (Bristol, Avon) 24: 315–326.
32. Sverdlova NS, Witzel U (2010) Principles of determination and verification of muscle forces in the human musculoskeletal system: Muscle forces to minimise bending stress. J Biomech 43: 387–396.
33. Munih M, Kralj A (1997) Modelling muscle activity in standing with considerations for bone safety. J Biomech 30: 49–56.
34. Munih M, Kralj A, Bajd T (1992) Bending moments in lower-extremity bones for 2 standing postures. J Biom Eng 14: 293–302.
35. Pauwels F (1965) Gesammelte Abhandlungen zur funktionellen Anatomie des Be-wegungsapparates. Berlin Heidelberg New York: Springer.
36. Currey JD (2006) Bones: Structure and Mechanics: Princeton University Press; 1 edition. 297 p.
37. Milgrom C, Radeva-Petrova DR, Finestone A, Nyska M, Mendelson S, et al. (2007) The effect of muscle fatigue on *in vivo* tibial strains. J Biomech 40: 845–850.
38. Gross TS, Edwards JL, McLeod KJ, Rubin CT (1997) Strain gradients correlate with sites of periosteal bone formation. J Bone Miner Res 12: 982–988.
39. Guo XD, Cowin SC (1992) Periosteal and endosteal control of bone remodeling under torsional loading. J Biomech 25: 645–650.
40. Main RP, Biewener AA (2007) Skeletal strain patterns and growth in the emu hindlimb during ontogeny. J Exp Biol 210: 2676–2690.
41. De Margerie E, Sanchez S, Cubo J, Castanet J (2005) Torsional resistance as a principal component of the structural design of long bones: Comparative multivariate evidence in birds. Anat Rec 282A: 49–66.
42. Carrano MT, Biewener AA (1999) Experimental alteration of limb posture in the chicken (Gallus gallus) and its bearing on the use of birds as analogs for dinosaur locomotion. J Morphol 240: 237–249.
43. Swartz SM, Bennett MB, Carrier DR (1992) Wing bone stresses in free flying bats and the evolution of skeletal design for flight. Nature 359: 726–729.
44. Feldman S, Capozza RF, Mortarino PA, Reina PS, Ferretti JL, et al. (2012) Site and sex effects on tibia structure in distance runners and untrained people. Med Sci Sports Exerc 44: 1580–1588.
45. Kutzner I, Heinlein B, Graichen F, Bender A, Rohlmann A, et al. (2010) Loading of the knee joint during activities of daily living measured *in vivo* in five subjects. J Biomech 43: 2164–2173.
46. Yang PF, Sanno M, Bruggemann GP, Rittweger J (2012) Evaluation of the performance of a motion capture system for small displacement recording and a discussion for its application potential in bone deformation *in vivo* measurements. Proc Inst Mech Eng H 226: 838–847.
47. Ganse B, Yang PF, Bruggemann GP, Rittweger J, Mueller LP, et al. (2014) *In-vivo* measurements of human bone deformation using optical segment tracking: surgical approach and validation in a three-point bending test. J Musculoskelet Neuronal Interact: In press.
48. Grood ES, Suntay WJ (1983) A joint coordinate system for the clinical description of three-dimensional motions: application to the knee. J Biomech Eng 105: 136–144.
49. Soderkvist I, Wedin PA (1993) Determining the movements of the skeleton using well-configured markers. J Biomech 26: 1473–1477.
50. Lafortune MA, Cavanagh PR, Sommer HJ, 3rd, Kalenak A (1992) Three-dimensional kinematics of the human knee during walking. J Biomech 25: 347–357.
51. UO Motor Control and Cognition Lab website. Available: http://ganeshauoregonedu/images/c/c7/Force_Platform_Manual_20pdf. Accessed 2014 March 26.
52. Gere JM, Goodno BJ (2012) Machanics of Materials CL Engineering. 1152 p.
53. Haris Phuah A, Schache AG, Crossley KM, Wrigley TV, Creaby MW (2010) Sagittal plane bending moments acting on the lower leg during running. Gait Posture 31: 218–222.
54. Rittweger J (2007) Physiological targets of artificial gravity: adaptive processes in bone. In: Clement G, Bukley A, editors. Artificial Gravity.Berlin: Springer.pp. 191–231.
55. Biewener AA, Taylor CR (1986) Bone strain: a determinant of gait and speed? J Exp Biol 123: 383–400.
56. Milgrom C, Finestone A, Segev S, Olin C, Arndt T, et al. (2003) Are overground or treadmill runners more likely to sustain tibial stress fracture? Br J Sports Med 37: 160–163.
57. White SC, Yack HJ, Tucker CA, Lin HY (1998) Comparison of vertical ground reaction forces during overground and treadmill walking. Med Sci Sports Exerc 30: 1537–1542.
58. Milner CE, Davis IS, Hamill J (2006) Free moment as a predictor of tibial stress fracture in distance runners. J Biomech 39: 2819–2825.
59. Milgrom C, Finestone A, Levi Y, Simkin A, Ekenman I, et al. (2000) Do high impact exercises produce higher tibial strains than running? Br J Sports Med 34: 195–199.
60. Burr DB, Milgrom C, Fyhrie D, Forwood M, Nyska M, et al. (1996) *In vivo* measurement of human tibial strains during vigorous activity. Bone 18: 405–410.
61. Brubaker CE, James SL (1974) Injuries to runners. J Sports Med 2: 189–198.
62. Sasimontonkul S, Bay BK, Pavol MJ (2007) Bone contact forces on the distal tibia during the stance phase of running. J Biomech 40: 3503–3509.

18

Biomechanical Analysis of the Human Finger Extensor Mechanism during Isometric Pressing

Dan Hu[1,3], David Howard[2], Lei Ren[1]*

1 School of Mechanical, Aerospace and Civil Engineering, University of Manchester, Manchester, United Kingdom, 2 School of Computing, Science and Engineering, University of Salford, Manchester, United Kingdom, 3 State Key Laboratory of Automotive Simulation and Control, Jilin University, Changchun, P.R. China

Abstract

This study investigated the effects of the finger extensor mechanism on the bone-to-bone contact forces at the interphalangeal and metacarpal joints and also on the forces in the intrinsic and extrinsic muscles during finger pressing. This was done with finger postures ranging from very flexed to fully extended. The role of the finger extensor mechanism was investigated by using two alternative finger models, one which omitted the extensor mechanism and another which included it. A six-camera three-dimensional motion analysis system was used to capture the finger posture during maximum voluntary isometric pressing. The fingertip loads were recorded simultaneously using a force plate system. Two three-dimensional biomechanical finger models, a minimal model without extensor mechanism and a full model with extensor mechanism (tendon network), were used to calculate the joint bone-to-bone contact forces and the extrinsic and intrinsic muscle forces. If the full model is assumed to be realistic, then the results suggest some useful biomechanical advantages provided by the tendon network of the extensor mechanism. It was found that the forces in the intrinsic muscles (interosseus group and lumbrical) are significantly reduced by 22% to 61% due to the action of the extensor mechanism, with the greatest reductions in more flexed postures. The bone-to-bone contact force at the MCP joint is reduced by 10% to 41%. This suggests that the extensor mechanism may help to reduce the risk of injury at the finger joints and also to moderate the forces in intrinsic muscles. These apparent biomechanical advantages may be a result of the extensor mechanism's distinctive interconnected fibrous structure, through which the contraction of the intrinsic muscles as flexors of the MCP joint can generate extensions at the DIP and PIP joints.

Editor: Steve Milanese, University of South Australia, Australia

Funding: The China Scholarship Council (CSC) had partly supported the study design, data collection and analysis. The additional part of the funding of the study has been supported by the UK EPSRC from grant number EP/I033602/1. The funders had no role in study design, data collection and analysis, decision to publish, or preparation of the manuscript.

Competing Interests: The authors have declared that no competing interests exist.

* E-mail: lei.ren@manchester.ac.uk

Introduction

The structural and functional complexities of the human finger have long been recognised [1–5]. Effective function of the finger requires precise coordination of multiple muscles and the resulting finger motion is constrained by the forces exerted by the joint capsules, ligaments and joint articular surfaces. In manual activities, the highly complex musculoskeletal system of the hand and forearm is well coordinated to generate appropriate fingertip forces and finger postures. A good understanding of the biomechanical mechanisms of the finger would not only improve our knowledge of normal finger function and the etiology of hand diseases, but may also significantly improve prosthetic and biomimetic hand design.

However, finger mechanics is complicated by the finger extensor mechanism (also referred to as the extensor apparatus, extensor assembly or extensor expansion), which is a complex tendon network that brings together the forces of the lumbrical, interossei, and long extensor to produce precise functional movements of the phalanxes (see Figure 1). In recent decades, a number of studies have been conducted to investigate its anatomical structure [6–16] and the spatial relationships between its different components, to quantify its geometric configuration [17] and material properties [18]. In addition, recently there has been increasing use of extensor mechanism models for the biomechanical analysis of finger function [19–27]. However, despite this, little is known about how the extensor mechanism affects the mechanical loadings at finger joints and muscles.

Therefore, in this study, we aim to investigate the biomechanical effect of the extensor mechanism (tendon network) during isometric pressing using a combined experimental and modelling approach. Fingertip force and finger posture were recorded using a force plate and a three-dimensional (3D) motion analysis system. Force analysis was conducted using two different finger models, a minimal model excluding the extensor mechanism and a full model including the extensor mechanism. In this way, the effects of this complex tendon network on finger joint contact forces and extrinsic and intrinsic muscle forces were analysed. However, it should be noted that the conclusions drawn are based on interpreting the differences between the results generated by the two models and, as such, cannot be quoted with the confidence one would associate with wholly experimental results.

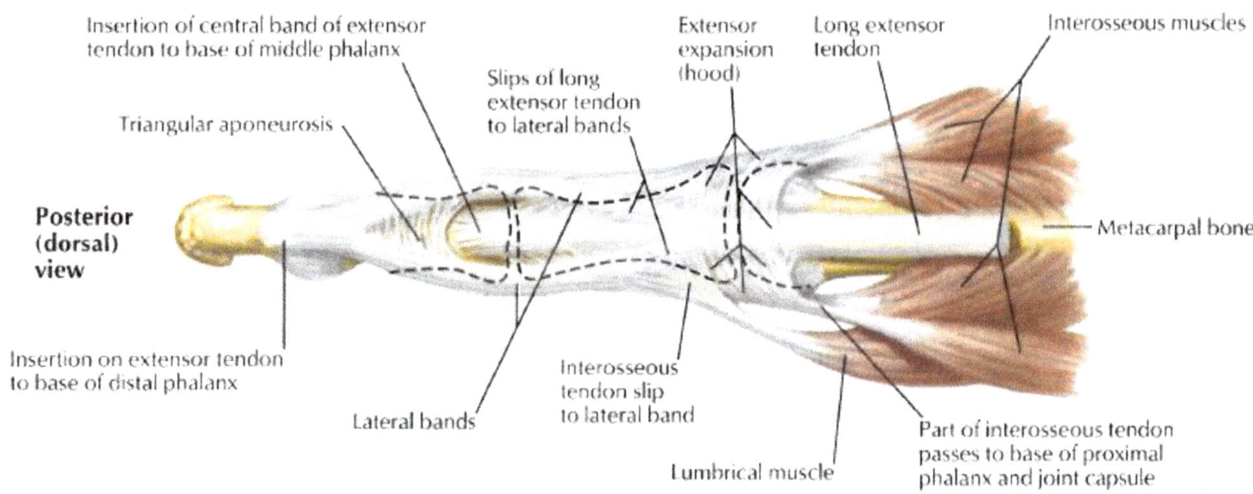

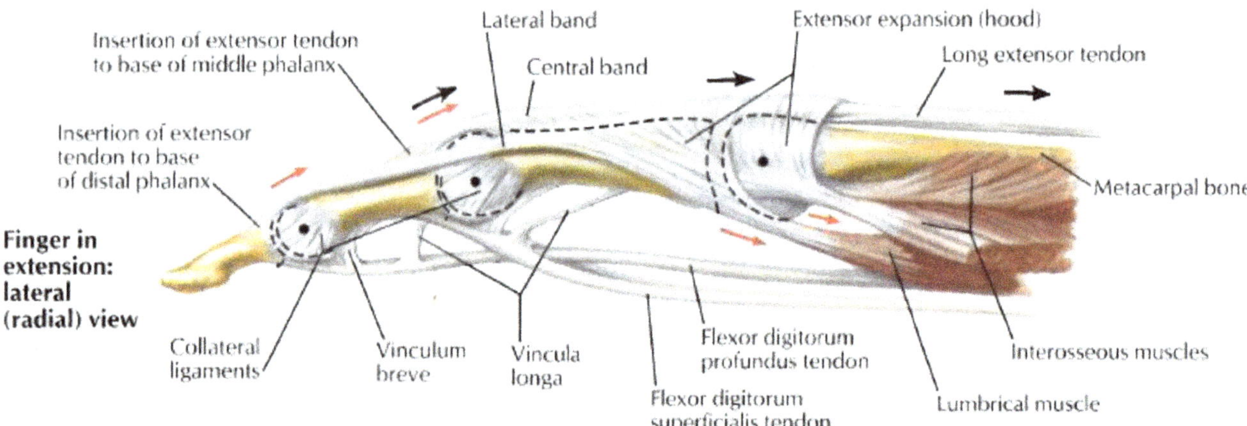

Figure 1. Musculotendonal structure of the human finger. The musculotendonal structure of the human finger from posterior (dorsal) and lateral (radial) views (from Netter, 2002)

Methods

Notation

PF: primary flexor

PE: primary extensor

FDP: flexor digitorum profundus

FDS: flexor digitorum superficials

TE: terminal extensor

ES: extensor slip

LE: long extensor

RI: radial interosseous

UI: ulnar interosseous

LU: lumbrical

RB: radial band

UB: ulnar band

DIP: distal interphalangeal

PIP: proximal interphalangeal

MCP: metacarpophalangeal

$a_{PF\_DIP\_FL}$, $a_{PF\_PIP\_FL}$, $a_{PF\_MCP\_FL}$: flexion/extension moment arm of *PF* around DIP, PIP and MCP joint

$a_{PE\_DIP\_FL}$, $a_{PE\_PIP\_FL}$, $a_{PE\_MCP\_FL}$: flexion/extension moment arm of *PE* around DIP, PIP and MCP joint

$a_{RI\_MCP\_FL}$, $a_{UI\_MCP\_FL}$: flexion/extension moment arm of *RI* and *UI* around MCP joint

$a_{RI\_MCP\_AD}$, $a_{UI\_MCP\_AD}$: adduction/abduction moment arm of *RI* and *UI* around MCP joint

$a_{TE\_DIP\_FL}$: flexion/extension moment arm of *TE* around DIP joint

$a_{FDP\_DIP\_FL}$, $a_{FDP\_PIP\_FL}$, $a_{FDP\_MCP\_FL}$: flexion/extension moment arm of *FDP* around DIP, PIP and MCP joint

$a_{ES\_PIP\_FL}$, $a_{UB\_PIP\_FL}$, $a_{RB\_PIP\_FL}$: flexion/extension moment arm of *ES*, *UB* and *RB* around PIP joint

$a_{LE\_MCP\_FL}$, $a_{RI\_MCP\_FL}$, $a_{UI\_MCP\_FL}$, $a_{LU\_MCP\_FL}$: flexion/extension moment arm of *LE*, *RI*, *UI* and *LU* around MCP joint

$a_{RI\_MCP\_AD}$, $a_{UI\_MCP\_AD}$, $a_{LU\_MCP\_AD}$: adduction/abduction moment arm of *RI*, *UI* and *LU* around MCP joint

$\theta_1,\theta_2,\theta_3,\theta_4$: angles between phalange segments and X axis of global coordinate system (which is horizontal)

θ_{PF_DIP}, θ_{PF_PIP}, θ_{PF_MCP}: angle between *PF* and X axis of global coordinate system at DIP,PIP and MCP joint

θ_{PE_DIP}, θ_{PE_PIP}, θ_{PE_MCP}: angle between *PE* and X axis of global coordinate system at DIP, PIP and MCP joint

$\theta_{x\_RI\_MCP}$, $\theta_{y\_RI\_MCP}$, $\theta_{z\_RI\_MCP}$: angles between *RI* and the X,Y,Z axes of the global coordinate system at MCP joint

$\theta_{x\_UI\_MCP}$, $\theta_{y\_UI\_MCP}$, $\theta_{z\_UI\_MCP}$: angles between *UI* and the X,Y,Z axes of the global coordinate system at MCP joint

θ_{FDP_DIP}, θ_{FDP_PIP}, θ_{FDP_MCP}: angle between *FDP* and X axis of global coordinate system at DIP, PIP and MCP joint

θ_{TE_DIP}: angle between *TE* and X axis of global coordinate system at DIP joint

θ_{ES_PIP}: angle between *ES* and X axis of global coordinate system at PIP joint

θ_{LE_MCP}: angle between *LE* and X axis of global coordinate system at MCP joint

$\theta_{x\_UB\_PIP}$, $\theta_{y\_UB\_PIP}$, $\theta_{z\_UB\_PIP}$: angles between *UB* and the X,Y,Z axes of the global coordinate system at PIP joint

$\theta_{x\_RB\_PIP}$, $\theta_{y\_RB\_PIP}$, $\theta_{z\_RB\_PIP}$: angles between *RB* and the X,Y,Z axes of the global coordinate system at PIP joint

$\theta_{x\_LU\_MCP}$, $\theta_{y\_LU\_MCP}$, $\theta_{z\_LU\_MCP}$: angles between *LU* and the X,Y,Z axes of the global coordinate system at MCP joint

l_1, l_2, l_3: phalangeal lengths

P_x, P_y, P_z: measured fingertip forces

Ethics Statement

This study was approved by Manchester University's Institutional Review Board, and the subjects provided written informed consent to participate in the experimental work.

Static pressing measurements

The experimental work involved six male subjects (age: 26±1years, weight: 75.8±8.1 kg, height: 174±4 cm) recruited from the University's population of postgraduate students. The subjects were instructed to press the force plate surface using their index finger for approximately 3 seconds using maximum voluntary isometric force (see Figure 2), while other parts of the body were not allowed to touch the force plate. Four different finger postures were adopted during static pressing, ranging from very flexed to fully extended (see Figure 3). Each experimental condition was measured ten times. Motion data were recorded at 200 Hz using a six-camera motion analysis system (Vicon, Oxford, UK) and the 3D external force acting on the fingertip was recorded at 1000 Hz using a force plate (Kistler, Switzerland). Referring to Figure 3, to capture finger motion, five semi-reflective markers of 8 mm diameter were attached to the distal phalange dorsal head (Marker01), middle phalange dorsal head (Marker02), proximal phalange dorsal head (Marker03), metacarpal bone dorsal head (Marker04), and metacarpal bone dorsal base (Marker05).

The raw marker data were processed using bespoke programs written in Matlab (Mathworks, MA, USA). All trials with more than 10 consecutive missing frames were discarded. After fill-gap processing, the data were filtered using a low-pass zero-lag fourth-order Butterworth digital filter with a cut-off frequency of 6.0 Hz. For both marker and force plate records, only the data in the middle of the trials was used when the subject had reached a steady isometric pressing condition. After data processing, the measured 3D external fingertip load P (P_x, P_y, P_z) and phalange angles (θ_1,θ_2,θ_3,θ_4) at a representative instant in time were used for the following biomechanical force analyses.

Minimal model without extensor mechanism

To represent the index finger musculoskeletal structure without the extensor mechanism, a simple 3D multi-segment model was constructed by scaling a standard finger model provided in the OpenSim biomechanical simulation environment [28]. The geometry of the digital bones was extracted from the OpenSim software and all other geometry (e.g. muscle insertion, origin positions etc.) was defined by referring to the Primal Pictures 3D anatomical software (Primal Picture Ltd., London, UK) and the literature [12]. The model consists of four segments, namely the distal, middle and proximal phalanxes, and the metacarpal bone, and three joints, namely the DIP, PIP and MCP. Both the DIP and PIP were modelled as hinge joints, each with 1 degree of freedom (DoF), and the MCP was modelled as a saddle joint with 2 DoF (see Figure 4). For this 4-DoF multi-segment system, a minimum of four muscles are needed to balance the external load during static pressing. Referring to Figure 4, a primary extensor (*PE*) was included to represent the combined action of the extensor muscles (mainly the long extensor) spanning the three joints. A primary flexor (*PF*) was used to represent the action of the flexor muscles (mainly the *FDP* and *FDS*). Two lateral muscles (*UI* and *RI*) are included on each side of the finger. This is analysed as a statically determinate system at equilibrium with the required minimum number of muscles. The force and moment equilibrium equations were derived as follows for each of the three joints (DIP, PIP and MCP respectively)

$$\begin{cases} F_{PE}\cos\theta_{PE\_DIP}+F_{PF}\cos\theta_{PF\_DIP}-F_{x\_DIP}+P_x=0 \\ F_{PE}\sin\theta_{PE\_DIP}+F_{PF}\sin\theta_{PF\_DIP}-F_{y\_DIP}+P_y=0 \\ -F_{z\_DIP}+P_z=0 \\ -F_{PE}a_{PE\_DIP\_FL}-P_yl_1\cos\theta_1+F_{PF}a_{PF\_DIP\_FL}+P_xl_1\sin\theta_1=0 \end{cases} \quad (1)$$

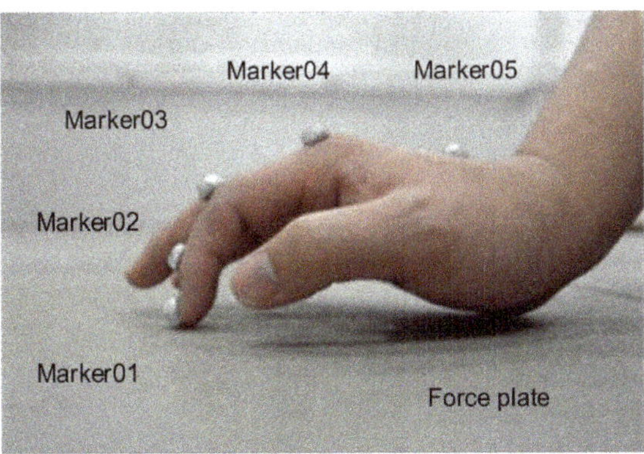

Lateral view

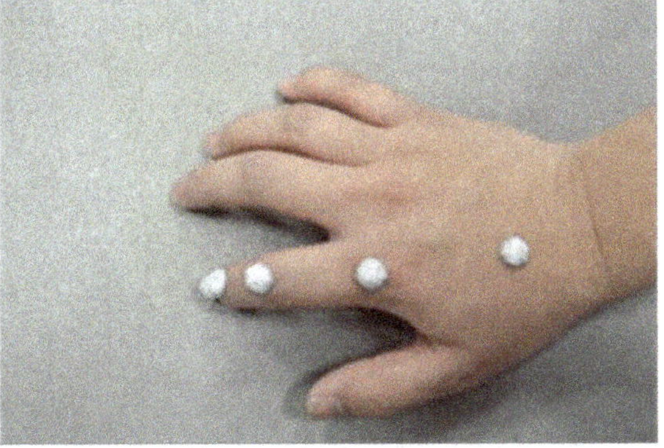

Superior view

Figure 2. Experimental setup. Experimental setup for the measurement of 3D fingertip force and finger posture during maximum voluntary isometric pressing. The subjects' wrists were not touching the surface of the force plate while measurements were being conducted.

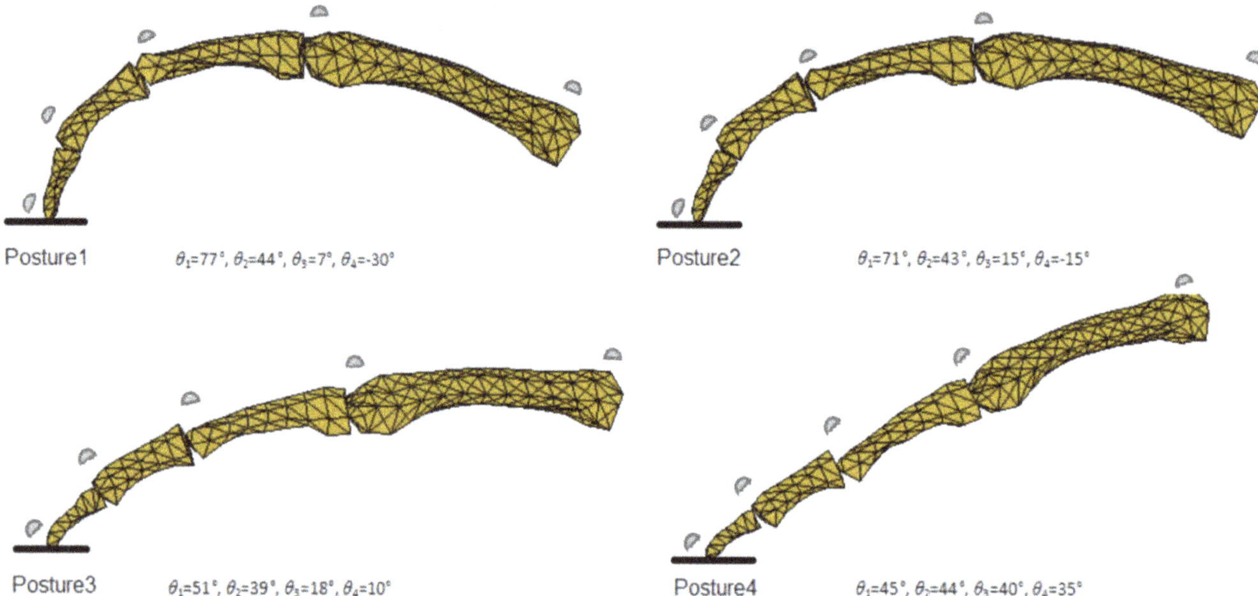

Figure 3. The four finger pressing postures. The four pressing postures, varying from flexed to fully extended, used in the experimental work. The segmental angles (θ_1, θ_2, θ_3, θ_4) are defined in Figure 4.

$$
\begin{cases}
F_{PE}\cos\theta_{PE\_PIP}+F_{PF}\cos\theta_{PF\_PIP}-F_{x\_PIP}+P_x=0\\
F_{PE}\sin\theta_{PE\_PIP}+F_{PF}\sin\theta_{PF\_PIP}-F_{y\_PIP}+P_y=0\\
-F_{z\_PIP}+P_z=0\\
-F_{PE}a_{PE\_PIP\_FL}-P_y(l_1\cos\theta_1+l_2\cos\theta_2)+F_{PF}a_{PF\_PIP\_FL}\\
+P_x(l_1\sin\theta_1+l_2\sin\theta_2)=0
\end{cases}
\tag{2}
$$

$$
\begin{cases}
F_{PE}\cos\theta_{PE\_MCP}+F_{PF}\cos\theta_{PF\_MCP}+F_{RI}\cos\theta_{x\_RI\_MCP}+\\
F_{UI}\cos\theta_{x\_UI\_MCP}-F_{x\_MCP}+P_x=0\\
F_{PE}\sin\theta_{PE\_MCP}+F_{PF}\sin\theta_{PF\_MCP}+F_{RI}\cos\theta_{y\_RI\_MCP}+\\
F_{UI}\cos\theta_{y\_UI\_MCP}-F_{y\_MCP}+P_y=0\\
F_{RI}\cos\theta_{z\_RI\_MCP}+F_{UI}\cos\theta_{z\_UI\_MCP}-F_{z\_MCP}+P_z=0\\
-F_{PE}a_{PE\_MCP\_FL}-P_y(l_1\cos\theta_1+l_2\cos\theta_2+l_3\cos\theta_3)+F_{PF}a_{PF\_MCP\_FL}\\
+F_{RI}a_{RI\_MCP\_FL}+F_{UI}a_{UI\_MCP\_FL}+\\
P_x(l_1\sin\theta_1+l_2\sin\theta_2+l_3\sin\theta_3)=0\\
F_{RI}a_{RI\_MCP\_AD}-F_{UI}a_{UI\_MCP\_AD}+P_z(l_1\cos\theta_1+l_2\cos\theta_2+l_3\cos\theta_3)=0
\end{cases}
\tag{3}
$$

Where the various muscle and tendon forces ($F_{\text{identifier}}$), moment arms ($a_{\text{identifier}}$), angles ($\theta_{\text{identifier}}$), and segment lengths ($l_{\text{identifier}}$) are defined in the notation list.

Equations 1 to 3 result in a total of 13 equilibrium equations with 13 unknowns (4 muscle forces and 9 bone-to-bone contact forces at the 3 joints). Therefore, the system is statically determinate and all of the unknowns can be determined from the measured finger posture and fingertip load during static pressing.

Full model with extensor mechanism

To investigate the effect of the extensor mechanism, a second multi-segment finger model was developed that represents the extensor apparatus as an interconnected tendon network (see Figure 5). The model shares the same segments, joint configurations, and bone geometry as the minimal model but with additional muscles and tendons. Referring to Figure 5, the five muscles included are the *LE*, *FDP*, *RI*, *UI* and *LU*. As the major extensor, *LE* has a similar function to that of the *PE* muscle in the minimal model. As the major flexor, *FDP* has a similar function to that of the *PF* muscle in the minimal model. In order to represent the key structural features of the extensor mechanism, another muscle (*LU*) is added to the full model on the radial side in addition to the *RI* and *UI* muscles. The force and moment equilibrium equations were derived as follows for each of the three joints (DIP, PIP and MCP respectively).

$$
\begin{cases}
F_{TE}\cos(\theta_{TE\_DIP})+F_{FDP}\cos(\theta_{FDP\_DIP})-F_{x\_DIP}+P_x=0\\
F_{TE}\sin(\theta_{TE\_DIP})+F_{FDP}\sin(\theta_{FDP\_DIP})-F_{y\_DIP}+P_y=0\\
-F_{z\_DIP}+P_z=0\\
-F_{TE}a_{TE\_DIP}+F_{FDP}a_{FDP\_DIP}+P_xl_1\sin\theta_1-P_yl_1\cos\theta_1=0
\end{cases}
\tag{4}
$$

$$
\begin{cases}
F_{ES}\cos(\theta_{ES\_PIP})+F_{FDP}\cos(\theta_{FDP\_PIP})+F_{UB}\cos(\theta_{x\_UB\_PIP})\\
+F_{RB}\cos(\theta_{x\_UB\_PIP})-F_{x\_PIP}+P_x=0\\
F_{ES}\sin(\theta_{ES\_PIP})+F_{FDP}\sin(\theta_{FDP\_PIP})+F_{UB}\cos(\theta_{y\_UB\_PIP})\\
+F_{RB}\cos(\theta_{y\_UB\_PIP})-F_{y\_PIP}+P_y=0\\
F_{UB}\cos(\theta_{z\_UB\_PIP})+F_{RB}\cos(\theta_{z\_RB\_PIP})-F_{z\_PIP}+P_z=0\\
F_{FDP}a_{FDP\_PIP\_FL}-F_{ES}a_{ES\_PIP\_FL}-F_{UB}a_{UB\_PIP\_FL}-F_{RB}a_{RB\_PIP\_FL}\\
+P_x(l_1\sin\theta_1+l_2\sin\theta_2)-P_y(l_1\cos\theta_1+l_2\cos\theta_2)=0
\end{cases}
\tag{5}
$$

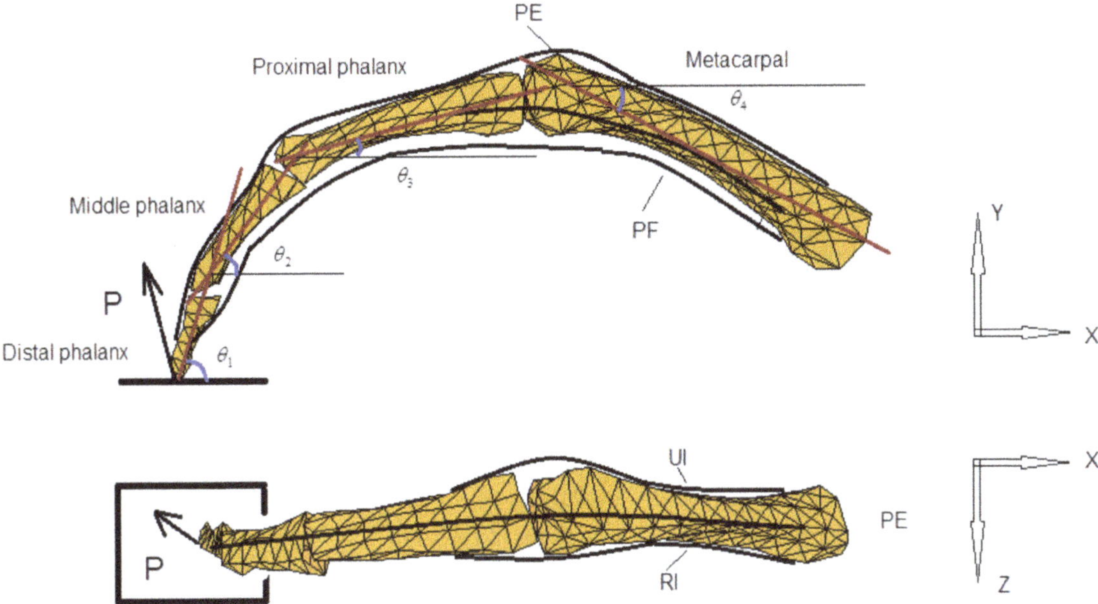

Figure 4. Minimal Model of the finger without extensor mechanism. Posterior (dorsal) and lateral (radial) views of the Minimal Model of the index finger without extensor mechanism. Four equivalent muscles (*PF, PE, UI, RI*) are considered to represent the actions of the finger flexor, extensor, lateral ulnar and lateral radial muscle groups respectively.

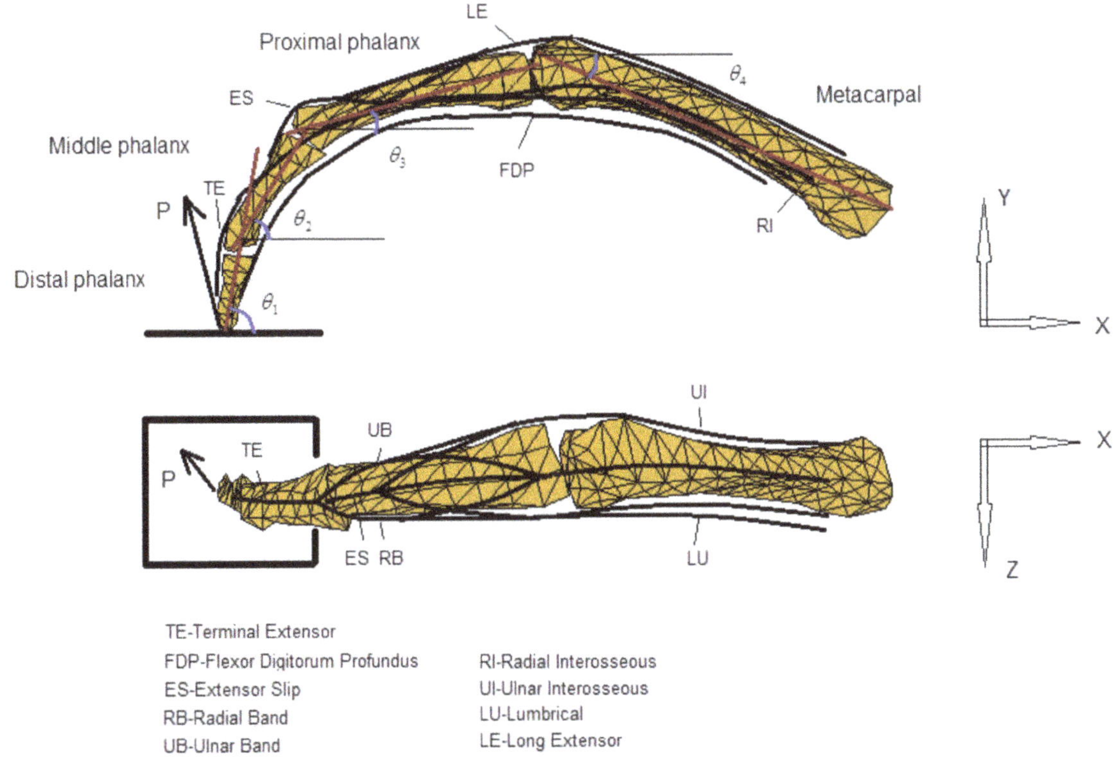

Figure 5. Full Model of the finger with extensor mechanism. Posterior (dorsal) and lateral (radial) views of the Full Model of the index finger with extensor mechanism (tendon network). In addition to the finger extensor muscle LE and flexor muscle FDP, the three major intrinsic muscles (*UI, RI* and *LU*) are included.

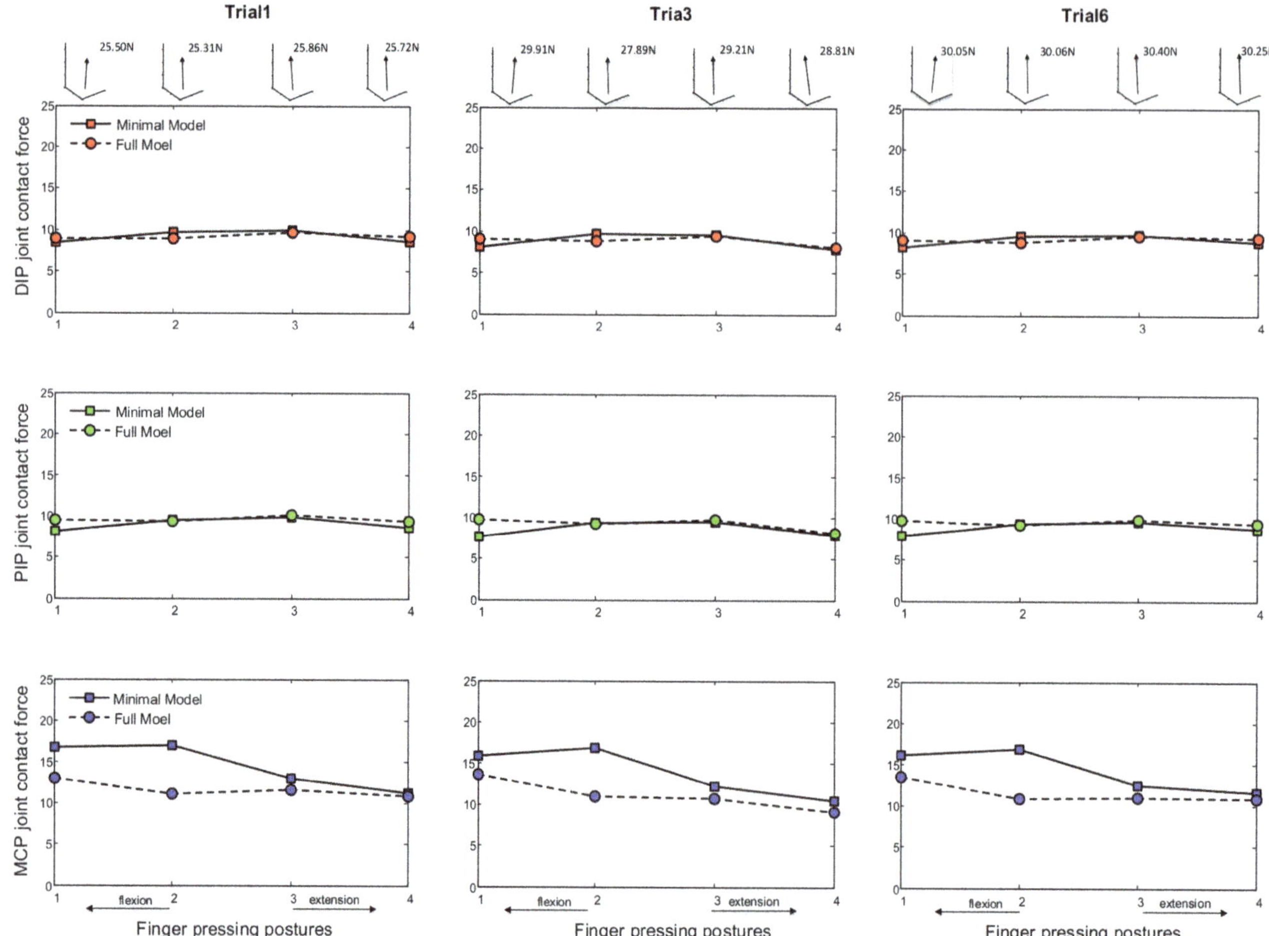

Figure 6. Bone-to-bone contact force calculation results. Calculated bone-to-bone contact forces (normalized by applied load) at the DIP, PIP and MCP joints obtained from both models for all finger postures. Based on measurement data from three typical trials (Trial 1, 3 and 6) for a representative subject (age: 25, weight: 75 kg, height: 1.72 m). The insets at the top show the measured 3D fingertip force vector for each posture.

$$\begin{cases} F_{LE}\cos(\theta_{LE\_MCP})+F_{FDP}\cos(\theta_{FDP\_MCP})+ \\ F_{RI}\cos(\theta_{x\_RI\_MCP})+F_{UI}\cos(\theta_{x\_UI\_MCP})+F_{LU}\cos(\theta_{x\_LU\_MCP})-F_{x\_MCP}+P_x=0 \\ F_{LE}\sin(\theta_{LE\_MCP})+F_{FDP}\sin(\theta_{FDP\_MCP})+ \\ F_{RI}\cos(\theta_{y\_RI\_MCP})+F_{UI}\cos(\theta_{y\_UI\_MCP})+F_{LU}\sin(\theta_{y\_LU\_MCP})-F_{y\_MCP}+P_y=0 \\ F_{RI}\cos(\theta_{z\_RI\_MCP})+F_{UI}\cos(\theta_{z\_UI\_MCP})+F_{LU}\cos(\theta_{z\_LU\_MCP})-F_{z\_MCP}+P_z=0 \\ F_{FDP}a_{FDP\_MCP\_FL}- \\ F_{LE}a_{LE\_MCP\_FL}+F_{RI}a_{RI\_MCP\_FL}+F_{UI}a_{UI\_MCP\_FL}+F_{LU}a_{LU\_MCP\_FL}+ \\ P_x(l_1\sin\theta_1+l_2\sin\theta_2+l_3\sin\theta_3)-P_y(l_1\cos\theta_1+l_2\cos\theta_2+l_3\cos\theta_3)=0 \\ F_{RI}a_{RI\_MCP\_AD}- \\ F_{UI}a_{UI\_MCP\_AD}+F_{LU}a_{LU\_MCP\_AD}+P_z(l_1\cos\theta_1+l_2\cos\theta_2+l_3\cos\theta_3)=0 \end{cases} \quad (6)$$

Where the various muscle and tendon forces ($F_{\text{identifier}}$), moment arms ($a_{\text{identifier}}$), angles ($\theta_{\text{identifier}}$), and segment lengths ($l_{\text{identifier}}$) are defined in the notation list.

Equations 4-6 define a statically indeterminate system at equilibrium with 13 equations and 18 unknowns. To resolve the static indeterminacy problem, the equations below are included, which are based on previous anatomical studies and cadaveric testing [29]. These equations describe the empirical distribution of forces between the muscles (F_{RI}, F_{UI}, F_{LU}, F_{LE}) and the tendon components (F_{RB}, F_{UB}, F_{TE}, F_{ES}) of the extensor mechanism [30,31].

$$F_{RB}=2/3F_{LU}+1/6F_{LE} \quad (7)$$

$$F_{UB}=1/3F_{UI}+1/6F_{LE} \quad (8)$$

$$F_{TE}=F_{RB}+F_{UB} \quad (9)$$

$$F_{ES}=1/3F_{RI}+1/3F_{UI}+1/3F_{LU}+1/6F_{LE} \quad (10)$$

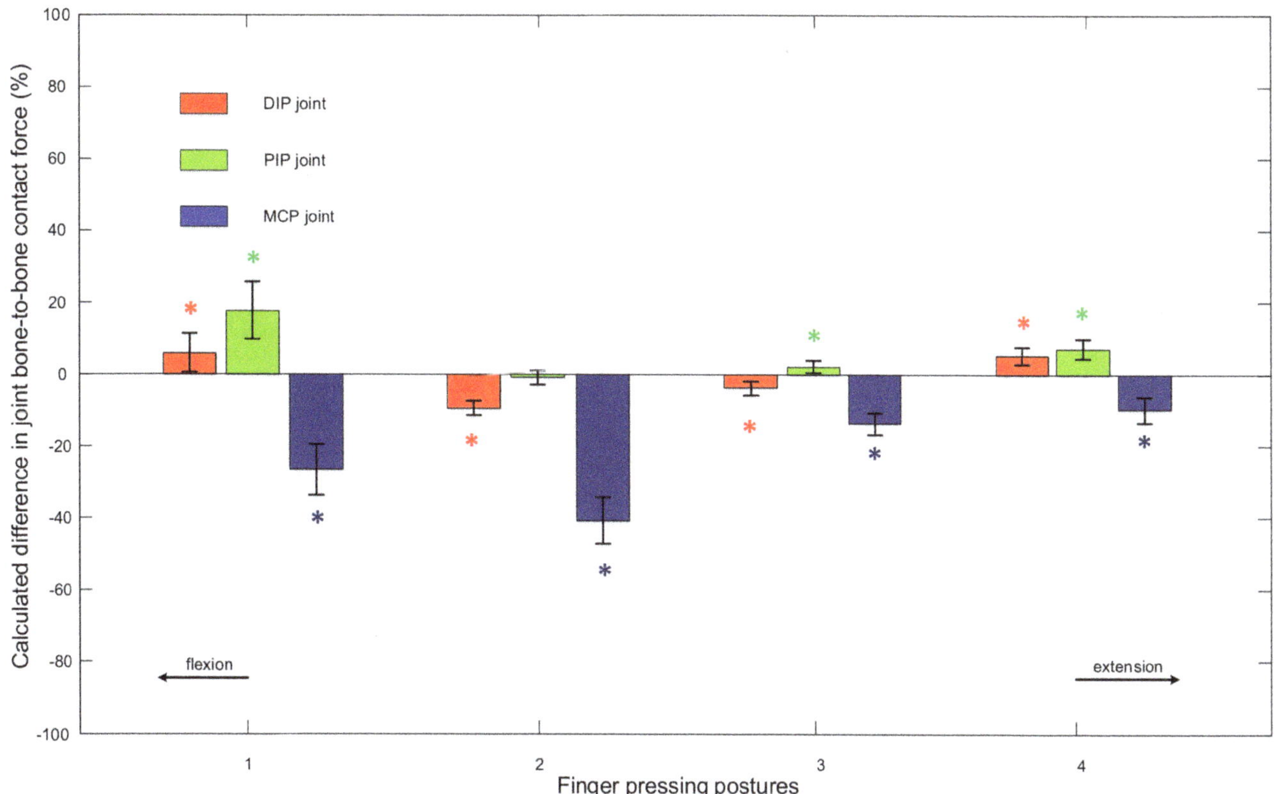

Figure 7. Percentage difference in bone-to-bone contact forces. The differences between the calculated bone-to-bone contact forces at the DIP, PIP and MCP joints obtained from the two models for all finger postures. The means and standard deviations were calculated across all trials and all subjects. A '*' indicates a significant difference between the results of the two models.

$$F_{LE} = F_{ES} \tag{11}$$

A more sophisticated optimisation based method could be employed to improve the solution of this statically indeterminate system [35–38]. However, finding an appropriate optimisation criterion may be challenging. Equations 4–11 can be used to solve for the bone-to-bone contact forces at all three joints and also the forces within the musculotendon network of the extensor mechanism for each measured finger posture and fingertip force.

Statistical analysis

All statistical analyses were conducted using SPSS 20.0 software (IBM, Armonk, NewYork, USA). The effects of finger model and posture on joint bone-to-bone contact forces and muscle forces were analysed using analysis of variance (ANOVA) with repeated measurements using a linear mixed model approach taking into account intra- and inter-subject variability. The different finger models and postures were the fixed effects, and subjects and trials were random effects. Differences between the two models and between each pair of postures were tested using Fisher's least significant difference (LSD) multiple comparison based on the least-squared means.

Table 1. Statistical analysis of results from the Minimal Model.

	Muscle forces				**Bone-to-bone contact forces**		
	F_{PE}	F_{PF}	F_{RI}	F_{UI}	F_{DIP}	F_{PIP}	F_{MCP}
Posture1	2.863 ± 0.571^a	5.150 ± 0.802^a	4.218 ± 0.892^a	4.121 ± 0.832^a	8.946 ± 0.998^a	8.641 ± 0.917^a	15.719 ± 1.921^a
Posture2	4.033 ± 1.110^b	8.293 ± 1.987^b	4.800 ± 1.378^b	7.437 ± 3.502^b	13.159 ± 2.562^b	12.879 ± 2.557^b	23.731 ± 6.568^b
Posture3	3.657 ± 1.024^c	8.817 ± 1.442^c	3.847 ± 1.156^c	7.059 ± 2.562^b	13.268 ± 1.777^b	13.032 ± 1.731^b	22.586 ± 4.840^b
Posture4	1.772 ± 0.613^d	7.565 ± 1.793^d	1.132 ± 0.259^d	2.375 ± 0.649^c	10.098 ± 2.164^c	10.092 ± 2.166^c	13.464 ± 2.797^c

Statistical analysis of the effect of finger posture on normalised muscle forces and joint bone-to-bone contact forces based on results from the Minimal Model. Values are means ± s.e.m. for all trials and all subjects. Identical letters indicate posture groups within a column do not differ significantly from each other ($p > 0.05$).

Table 2. Statistical analysis of results from the Full Model.

	Muscle forces				Bone-to-bone contact forces		
	F_{LE}	F_{FDP}	F_{RI}+F_{LU}	F_{UI}	F_{DIP}	F_{PIP}	F_{MCP}
Posture1	2.293±0.497[a]	4.992±0.932[a]	2.503±0.712[a]	2.287±0.788[a]	8.630±1.031[a]	9.028±1.348[a]	11.755±2.101[a]
Posture2	3.066±0.905[b]	7.999±2.308[b]	3.017±0.754[b]	3.066±1.598[b]	12.575±2.913[b]	13.693±3.502[b]	16.742±4.488[b]
Posture3	3.080±1.292[b]	8.671±1.498[c]	2.448±0.643[a]	3.075±1.287[b]	12.977±1.798[b]	14.025±2.173[b]	16.921±3.030[b]
Posture4	1.760±0.618[c]	7.446±1.728[d]	0.953±0.232[c]	1.294±0.446[c]	9.860±1.979[c]	10.064±2.041[c]	12.093±2.583[a]

Statistical analysis of the effect of finger posture on normalised muscle forces and joint bone-to-bone contact forces based on results from the Full Model. Values are means ± s.e.m. for all trials and all subjects. Identical letters indicate posture groups within a column do not differ significantly from each other (p>0.05).

Results

For all subjects, the measured finger joint angles (θ_1,θ_2,θ_3,θ_4) and fingertip forces (P_x, P_y, P_z) for each static pressing trial were used as inputs to both the minimal model and the full model. These models were implemented using bespoke programs written in Matlab (Mathworks, MA, USA). In this way, biomechanical analyses were conducted to assess the bone-to-bone contact forces at each joint and also the forces in the muscles and tendon components.

Figure 6 compares the calculated bone-to-bone contact forces at the DIP, PIP and MCP joints obtained from the two finger models, for all four pressing postures, using measurement data from three typical trials (Trial 1, 3, 6) for a representative subject (age: 25, weight: 75 kg, height: 1.72 m). The corresponding numerical data are presented in Tables S1 and S2. The DIP and

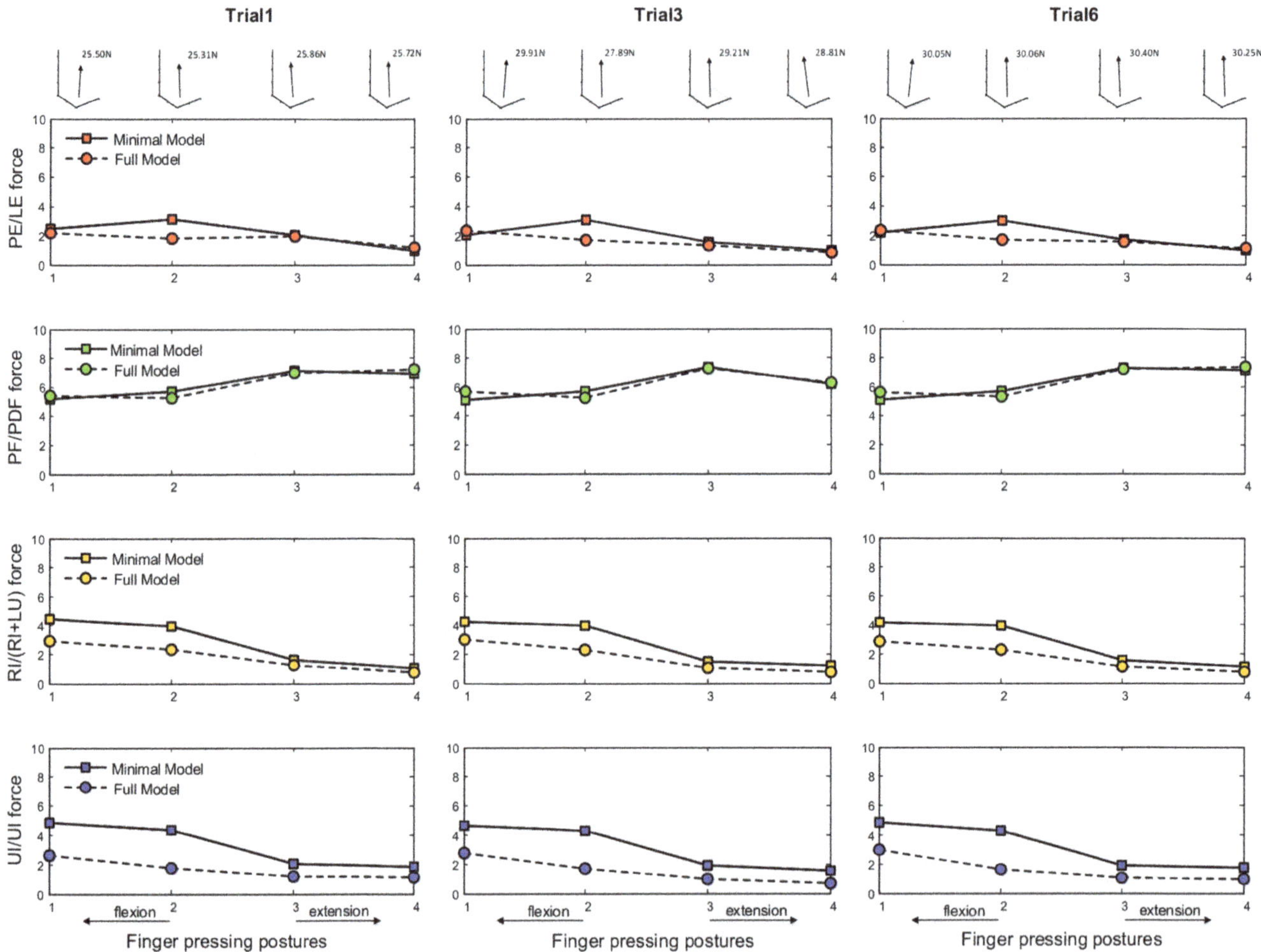

Figure 8. Muscle force calculation results. Calculated muscles forces (normalized by applied load) for the *PE* (*LE*), *PF* (*PDF*), *RI* (*RI+LU*) and *UI* muscles obtained from both models for all finger postures. Based on measurement data from three typical trials (Trial 1, 3 and 6) for a representative subject (age: 25, weight: 75 kg, height: 1.72 m). The insets at the top show the measured 3D fingertip force vector for each posture.

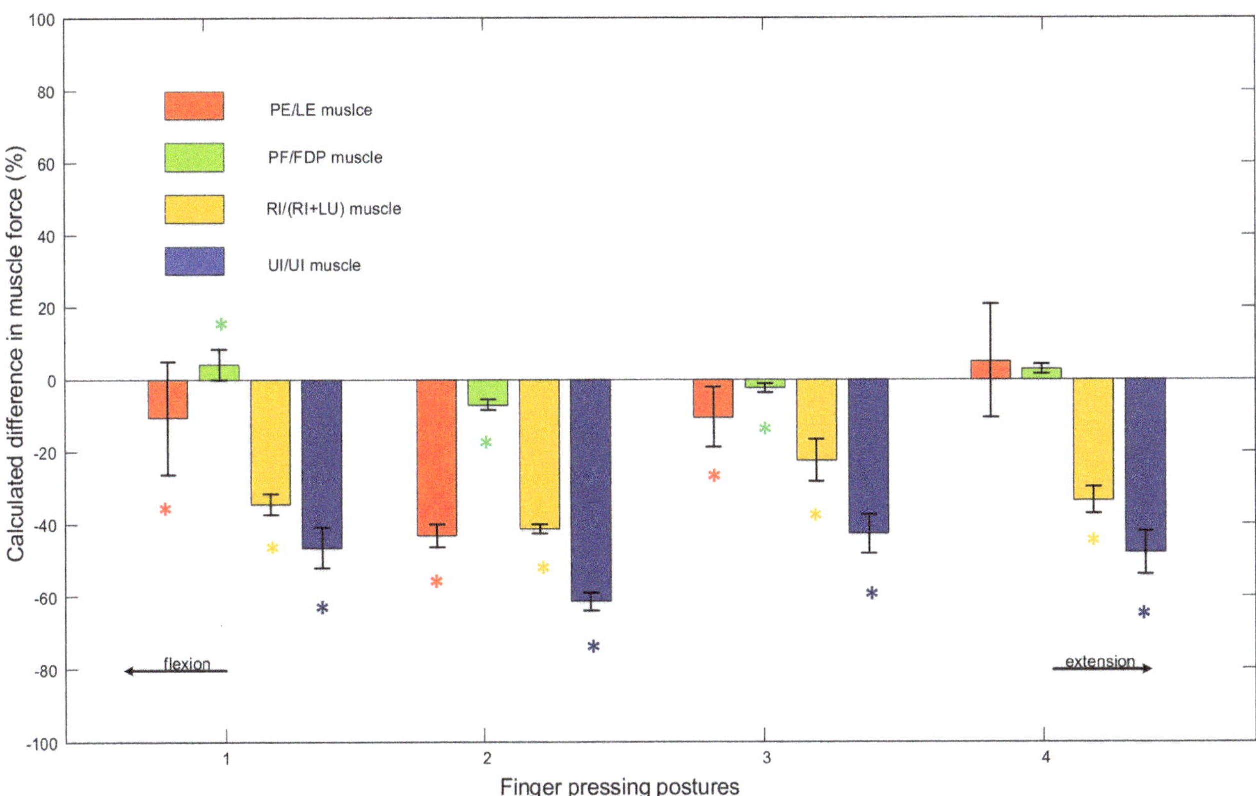

Figure 9. Percentage difference in muscle forces. The differences between the calculated muscle forces for the *PE* (*LE*), *PF* (*PDF*), *RI* (*RI+LU*) and UI muscles obtained from the two models for all finger postures. The means and standard deviations were calculated across all trials and all subjects. A '*' indicates a significant difference between the results of the two models.

PIP joint contact forces calculated by both models, normalized by the applied fingertip load, are in the range 7.7–9.8 for all finger postures. The MCP joint contact forces calculated by both models are in the range 10.5–17.0 times the applied fingertip load. This agrees well with the estimated contact force ranges for the index finger interphalangeal and metacarpal joints from previous studies for isometric key pinching [32]. However, it should be noted that, in this study, maximum voluntary isometric pressing was conducted on a large force plate surface, which differs slightly from key pinching. It can be seen from Figure 6 that both models show the MCP joint contact force increasing with more flexed postures. This is in general agreement with the posture-dependent pattern of MCP joint contact force reported by Harding et al. [21]. Comparing the joint contact forces generated by the minimal model and the full model in Figure 6, it appears that including the extensor mechanism does not have a significant effect on the calculated DIP and PIP joint contact forces. However, an appreciable effect can be observed on the calculated MCP joint contact force, where the full model predicts much lower values, especially in more flexed finger postures.

Figure 7 shows the percentage differences between the contact forces calculated by the full model and those calculated by the minimal model for each pressing posture (means and standard deviations across all trials and all subjects). This further supports the observation that including the extensor mechanism has a limited effect on the calculated DIP and PIP joint contact forces. With the exception of the PIP joint in the most flexed posture, the mean differences for the DIP and PIP joints are within ±9% and there is no consistent trend as the finger becomes more flexed or more extended. However, there is a consistent negative difference for the calculated MCP joint contact force across all finger postures (i.e. the full model produces lower force estimates). This difference becomes more pronounced when the finger becomes more flexed. For the two most flexed postures, mean decreases of 27% and 41% in estimated MCP contact force are obtained when the extensor mechanism is included. If the full model is assumed to be realistic, this suggests that the tendon network of the extensor mechanism might help to moderate the joint contact loads at the MCP during isometric pressing and hence may reduce the risk of injury or osteoarthritis [33,34].

In Figure 7, statistically significant differences ($p<0.05$) between models are labelled with a '*', which indicates that the mean bone-to-bone contact forces calculated by the two models differ significantly. With the exception of the PIP joint in posture 2, the differences between the results from the two models are all statistically significant (i.e. the calculated joint contact forces are significantly different when the extensor mechanism is included). Statistically significant differences between postures for both models are presented in Tables 1 and 2.

Figure 8 compares the calculated muscle forces obtained from the two finger models, for all four pressing postures, using measurement data from three typical trials (Trial 1, 3, 6) for a representative subject (age: 25, weight: 75 kg, height: 1.72 m). The corresponding numerical data are presented in Tables S1 and S2. The muscles from the two models are compared based on their anatomical functions, i.e. *PE* versus *LE* as extensors, *PF* versus *FDP* as flexors, *RI* versus *RI+LU* as lateral radial muscles and *UI* versus *UI* as lateral ulnar muscle. The range of muscle forces is approximately 1.2 to 7.0 times the applied fingertip load, which is in general agreement with the muscle force data reported in previous research on isometric pinching [30,32], which is similar to pressing on a flat surface. It can be seen from Figure 8 that posture-dependent trends are present for the *PF* or *FDP*, *RI* or *RI+LU* and *UI* muscles. The intrinsic muscle forces (*RI* or *RI+LU* and *UI*) increase with more flexed postures. However, the extrinsic flexor muscle (*PF* or *FDP*) shows decreasing force when the finger becomes more flexed. This is in a good agreement with the posture-dependent trends of the *FDP* muscle reported in the study by Weightman and Amis [20]. If the full model is assumed to be realistic, then the results from the two models suggest that the extensor mechanism may have a significant effect on the *RI+LU* and *UI* muscles for all finger postures. The full model, including the extensor mechanism, predicts much lower *RI+LU* and *UI* muscle forces than those predicted by the minimal model without the extensor mechanism.

Figure 9 shows the percentage differences between the muscle forces calculated by the full model and those calculated by the minimal model for each pressing posture (means and standard deviations across all trials and all subjects). It can be seen that the *RI+LU* and *UI* muscle forces are notably reduced when the extensor mechanism is included. The differences increase in magnitude with more flexed pressing postures, reaching 34% to 61% at the two most flexed postures. The differences are very small for the *PF* or *FDP* muscle forces. This agrees with the results obtained by Li et al. [23] who used simple 2D models without extensor forces to investigate the effect of fingertip load on flexor forces during isometric pressing with a fully extended finger. It can be seen from Figure 9 that mixed results are obtained for the *PE* or *LE* muscles. At postures 1, 3 and 4 the differences are small but at posture 2 there is a large negative difference (43%). In conclusion, if the full model is assumed to be realistic, the muscle force results suggest that the extensor mechanism helps to reduce the intrinsic muscle forces (*RI*, *LU* and *UI*), and this may also be the case for the extrinsic extensor muscles at moderately flexed postures.

In Figure 9, statistically significant differences ($p<0.05$) between models are labelled with a '*', which indicates that the mean muscle forces calculated by the two models differ significantly. With the exception of the *PE* (*LE*) and *PF* (*FDP*) in posture 4, the differences between the results from the two models are all statistically significant (i.e. the calculated muscle forces are significantly different when the extensor mechanism is included). Statistically significant differences between postures for both models are presented in Tables 1 and 2.

Discussion and Conclusion

By combining experimental measurement with biomechanical modelling, this study has investigated the calculated effects of the finger extensor mechanism on the contact forces at the interphalangeal and metacarpal joints and also on the forces exerted by the intrinsic and extrinsic muscles. If the full model is assumed to be realistic, then the results from the two models suggest some biomechanical advantages that may be provided by the tendon network of the extensor mechanism. The estimated forces in the intrinsic muscles (interosseus group and lumbrical) are significantly reduced by 22% to 61% when the extensor mechanism is included, especially in more flexed postures. The estimated contact force at the MCP joint is decreased by 10% to 41%, with larger reductions in more flexed postures, when the extensor mechanism is included. These effects may help to reduce the risk of injury at the finger joints and may also help to moderate the muscular effort required of the finger's intrinsic muscles.

The apparent biomechanical advantages provided by the finger extensor mechanism may be a result of its distinctive anatomical arrangement. The extensor apparatus surrounding the MCP joint receives muscle forces from the lumbricals (*LU*) and interossei (*RI* and *UI*). The contraction of these intrinsic muscles produces PIP and DIP extension by transmitting tension through the tendon network of the extensor mechanism (see Figures 1 and 5). The extensor slip (*ES*) attaches to the intermediate phalanx, where tension transmitted through the tendon network due to the intrinsic muscles extends the PIP joint. The lateral bands (radial band *RB* and ulnar band *UB*) on the dorsal side of the PIP joint merge over the dorsum of the intermediate phalanx, forming the terminal extensor (*TE*) slip, and insert into the distal phalanx, where the intrinsic muscle contraction leads to extension of the DIP joint. The tension generated by the contraction of the intrinsic muscles at the DIP and PIP joints tends to increase the force at the *FDP* muscle which further contributes to the flexion moment at the MCP joint, and thereby reduces the force demand imposed on the intrinsic muscles and hence moderates the bone-to-bone contact force at the MCP joint.

The biomechanical models used in this study have some limitations. The extensor apparatus is modelled as a tendon network with the individual tendon components represented by lines. However, in reality the finger extensor mechanism is a complex assembly of multi-directional fibres of varying viscoelastic properties. Three-dimensional solid mechanics models (e.g. based on the finite-element method) would be needed to better represent this interconnected fibrous structure in the future. To calculate the muscle and tendon forces in the full model, a set of empirical equations obtained from previous studies (Equations 7–11) was used to resolve the static indeterminacy problem. A more sophisticated optimisation based method could be employed to improve the solution of this statically indeterminate system of muscles and tendons [35–38]. However, finding an appropriate optimisation criterion may be challenging.

Supporting Information

Table S1 Calculation results from the Minimal Model. Force plate data and normalized calculation results from the Minimal Model for three typical trials (Trial 1, 3 and 6) with a representative subject (age: 25, weight: 75 kg, height: 1.72 m)

Table S2 Calculation results from the Full Model. Force plate data and normalized calculation results from the Full Model for three typical trials (Trial 1, 3 and 6) with a representative subject (age: 25, weight: 75 kg, height: 1.72 m)

Acknowledgments

Manxu Zheng's assistance with measurement data collection has been invaluable.

Author Contributions

Conceived and designed the experiments: LR D. Hu D. Howard. Performed the experiments: D. Hu LR. Analyzed the data: D. Hu. Contributed reagents/materials/analysis tools: D. Hu. Wrote the paper: D. Hu LR D. Howard.

References

1. Landsmeer JMF (1955) Anatomical and functional investigations on the articulation of the human fingers. Acta Anat Suppl 25: 1–69
2. Smith EM, Juvinall RC, Bender LF, Pearson JR (1964) Role of the finger flexors in Rheumatoid deformities of the metacarpophalangeal joints. Arthritis Rheum 7: 467–480
3. Cooney WP, Chao EY (1977) Biomechanical analysis of static forces in the thumb during hand function. J Bone Joint Surg 59: 27–36
4. Berme PW, Paul JP, Purves WK (1977) A biomechanical analysis of the metacarpophalangeal joint. J Biomech 10: 409–412
5. Fowler NK, Nicol AC (2000) Interphalangeal joint and tendon forces: normal model and biomechanical consequences of surgical reconstruction. J Biomech 33: 1055–1062
6. Eyler DL, Markee JE (1954) The anatomy and function of the intrinsic musculature of the fingers. J Bone Joint Surg (A) 36: 1–9
7. Landsmeer JMF (1961) Studies in the anatomy of articulation. 1. The equilibrium of the 'intercalated' bone. Acta Morph Neerl Scand 3: 287–303
8. Landsmeer JMF (1963) The coordination of finger-joint motions. J Bone Joint Surg 45: 1654–1662
9. Long C (1968) Intrinsic-extrinsic muscle control of the fingers. J Bone Joint Surg(A) 50: 973–984
10. Smith RJ (1974) Balance and kinetics of the finger under normal and pathological conditions. Clin Orthop Rel Res 104: 92–11
11. Ketchum LD, Thompson D, Pocock G, Wallingford D (1978) A clinical study of forces generated by the intrinsic muscles of the index finger and the extrinsic flexor and extensor muscles of the hand. J Hand Surg 3: 571–578
12. An KN, Chao EYS, Cooney WP, Linscheid RL (1979) Normative model of human hand for biomechanical analysis. J Biomech 12: 775–788
13. Darling WG, Cole KJ, Miller GF (1994) Coordination of index finger movements. J Biomech 12: 479–491
14. Dennerlein JT, Diao E, Mote CD, Rempel DM (1998) Tensions of the flexor digitorum superficialis are higher than a current model predicts. J Biomech 31: 295–301
15. Valero-Cuevas FJ, Zajac FE, Burgar CG (1998) Large index fingertip forces are produced by subject-independent patterns of muscle excitation. J Biomech 31: 693–703
16. Kursa K, Diao E, Lattanza L, Rempel D (2005) In vivo forces generated by finger flexor muscles do not depend on the rate of fingertip loading during an isometric task. J Biomech 38: 2288–2293
17. Garcia-Elias M, An KN, Berglund L, Linscheid RL, et al. (1991) Extensor mechanism of the fingers. I. A quantitative geometric study. J Hand Surg (A) 16: 1130–1136
18. Garcia-Elias M, An KN, Berglund L, Linscheid RL, et al. (1991) Extensor mechanism of the fingers. II. Tensile properties of components. J Hand Surg (A) 16: 1136–1140
19. Harris C, Rutledge AL (1972) The functional anatomy of the extensor mechanism of finger. J Bone Joint Surg (A) 54: 713–726
20. Weightman B, Amis AA (1982) Finger joint force predictions related to design of joint replacements. J Biomed Eng 4: 197–205
21. Harding DC, Brand KD, Hillberry BM (1993) Finger joint force minimization in pianists using optimization techniques. J Biomech 26: 1403–1412
22. Li ZM, Zatsiorsky VM, Latash ML (2000) Contribution of the extrinsic and intrinsic hand muscles to the moments in finger joints. Clin Biomech 15: 203–211
23. Li ZM, Zatsiorsky VM, Latash ML (2001) The effect of finger extensor mechanism on the flexor force during isometric tasks. J Biomech 34: 1097–1102
24. Lee SW, Chen H, Towles JD, Kamper DG (2008) Effect of finger posture on the tendon force distribution within the finger extensor mechanism. J Biomech Eng 130: 1–9
25. Vigouroux L, Quaine F, Labarre-Vila A, Amarantini D, Moutet F (2006) Estimation of finger muscle tendon tensions and pulley forces during specific sport-climbing grip techniques. J Biomech 39: 2583–2592
26. Valero-Cuevas FJ, Lipson H (2004) A computational Environment to simulate complex tendinous topologies. Proceedings of the 26th Annual International Conference of the IEEE EMBS, San Francisco, US
27. Valero-Cuevas FJ, Jae-Woong Y, Brown D, McNamara RV, Paul C (2007) The tendon network of the fingers performs anatomical computation at a macroscopic scale. IEEE Trans on Biomed Eng 54: 1161–1166
28. Scott LD, Frank CA, Allison SA, Peter L, Ayman H (2007) OpenSim: Open-source software to create and analyze dynamic simulations of movement. IEEE Trans Biomed Eng 54: 1940–1950
29. Chao EY, An KN (1978) Graphical interpretation of the solution to the redundant problem in biomechanics. J Biomech Eng 100: 159–167
30. Chao EY, Opgrance JD, Axmear FE (1976) Three-dimensional force analysis of finger joints in selected isometric hand functions. J Biomech 9: 387–396
31. Brook N, Mizrahi J, Shoham M, Dayan J (1995) A biomechanical model of index finger dynamics. Med Eng Phys 15: 54–63
32. An KN, Chao EYS, Cooney WP, Linscheid RL (1985) Forces in the normal and abnormal hand. J Orthop Res 3: 202–211
33. Kaab MJ, Ito K, Clark JM, Notzli HP (1998) Deformation of articular cartilage collagen structure under static and cyclic loading. J Orthop Res 16: 743–751
34. Arokoski JPA, Jurvelin JS, Vaatainen U, Helminen HJ (2000) Normal and pathological adaptions of articular cartilage to joint loading. Scand J Med Sci Sports 10: 186–198
35. Crowninshield RD, Brand RA (1981) A physiologically based criterion of muscle force prediction in locomotion. J Biomech 14:793–801
36. Sancho-Bru JL, Perez-Gonzalez A, Vergara-Monedero M, Giurintano D (2001) A 3-D dynamic model of human finger for studying free movements. J Biomech 34:1491–1500
37. Vigouroux L, Quaine F, Labarre-Vila A, Amarantini D, Moutet F (2007) Using EMG data to constrain optimization procedure improves finger tendon tension estimations during static fingertip force production. J Biomech 40:2846–2856
38. Fok KS, Chou SM (2010) Development of a finger biomechanical model and its considerations. J Biomech 43:701–713

19

Computed Tomographic Imaging of Subchondral Fatigue Cracks in the Distal End of the Third Metacarpal Bone in the Thoroughbred Racehorse Can Predict Crack Micromotion in an Ex-Vivo Model

Marie-Soleil Dubois[1], Samantha Morello[1], Kelsey Rayment[1], Mark D. Markel[1], Ray Vanderby Jr[2], Vicki L. Kalscheur[1], Zhengling Hao[1], Ronald P. McCabe[2], Patricia Marquis[1,3], Peter Muir[1]*

1 Comparative Orthopaedic Research Laboratory, School of Veterinary Medicine, University of Wisconsin-Madison, Madison, Wisconsin, United States of America, **2** Department of Orthopedics & Rehabilitation, School of Medicine & Public Health, University of Wisconsin-Madison, Madison, Wisconsin, United States of America, **3** Gulfstream Park, Hallandale Beach, Florida, United States of America

Abstract

Articular stress fracture arising from the distal end of the third metacarpal bone (MC3) is a common serious injury in Thoroughbred racehorses. Currently, there is no method for predicting fracture risk clinically. We describe an ex-vivo biomechanical model in which we measured subchondral crack micromotion under compressive loading that modeled high speed running. Using this model, we determined the relationship between subchondral crack dimensions measured using computed tomography (CT) and crack micromotion. Thoracic limbs from 40 Thoroughbred racehorses that had sustained a catastrophic injury were studied. Limbs were radiographed and examined using CT. Parasagittal subchondral fatigue crack dimensions were measured on CT images using image analysis software. MC3 bones with fatigue cracks were tested using five cycles of compressive loading at -7,500N (38 condyles, 18 horses). Crack motion was recorded using an extensometer. Mechanical testing was validated using bones with 3 mm and 5 mm deep parasagittal subchondral slots that modeled naturally occurring fatigue cracks. After testing, subchondral crack density was determined histologically. Creation of parasagittal subchondral slots induced significant micromotion during loading ($p<0.001$). In our biomechanical model, we found a significant positive correlation between extensometer micromotion and parasagittal crack area derived from reconstructed CT images ($S_R = 0.32$, $p<0.05$). Correlations with transverse and frontal plane crack lengths were not significant. Histologic fatigue damage was not significantly correlated with crack dimensions determined by CT or extensometer micromotion. Bones with parasagittal crack area measurements above 30 mm^2 may have a high risk of crack propagation and condylar fracture in vivo because of crack micromotion. In conclusion, our results suggest that CT could be used to quantify subchondral fatigue crack dimensions in racing Thoroughbred horses in-vivo to assess risk of condylar fracture. Horses with parasagittal crack arrays that exceed 30 mm^2 may have a high risk for development of condylar fracture.

Editor: Damian Christopher Genetos, University of California Davis, United States of America

Funding: This research [Project AOVET-12-05M] was supported by a grant from the AO Foundation. The funders had no role in study design, data collection and analysis, decision to publish, or preparation of the manuscript.

Competing Interests: Please note that although Patricia Marquis is affiliated with the Gulfstream Park company in Florida.

* Email: muirp@vetmed.wisc.edu

Introduction

Parasagittal fracture of the condyles of the third metacarpal/metatarsal bone (MC3/MT3), or condylar fracture, is common in Thoroughbred and Standardbred racehorses and is often identified as part of a syndrome of fetlock breakdown injury. Some of these injuries are catastrophic and require euthanasia of the horse [1,2]. In horses where surgical treatment is indicated, prognosis for return to athletic activity is not always favorable [2–4]. Risk of catastrophic injury may be as high as 2.17%, or 1 in every 46 race starts at some National Hunt racecourses in the United Kingdom [5]. Metacarpal fracture is the second most common cause of fatalities arising from a fracture in United States [6]. In the United Kingdom, condylar fractures are the most common type of fracture associated with racing and the most common reason for euthanasia of Thoroughbred racehorses with fracture [7].

Over the last 30 years, various etiologies for condylar fracture have been proposed. These theories fall into three main categories: first, accidental injury from mechanical overload [8]; second, pathological fracture associated with traumatic osteochondrosis [9–10]; and third, failure of functional adaptation and development of stress fracture [11–14]. Functional adaptation is a process by which bone remodels in response to mechanical loading. Bones are typically adapted to normal loads, but may be poorly designed to resist propagation of macroscopic fatigue cracks [15]. Although research data are primarily associative, it is now widely accepted that condylar fractures are site-specific articular stress fractures that essentially represent failure of functional adaptation to protect the subchondral bone plate of affected joints from cumulative fatigue injury [11–16]. Functional strains normally range from −1,500 to −3,000 microstrain in cursorial mammals [17]. However, in-vivo strains of more than −5,000 microstrain have been recorded in the MC3 mid-diaphysis of Thoroughbreds during galloping [18].

Functional adaptation is readily detectable by 4 months of race training [19]. Contact stresses on the palmar or plantar regions of the distal end of the MC3/MT3 bones from the proximal sesamoid bones are more than twice the stresses imposed on the dorsal region at the canter; this is a result of more load being shifted to the suspensory apparatus during increased fetlock joint extension [20]. As training increases, adaptation in the subchondral plate leads to sclerosis of the trabecular bone in the palmar/plantar aspect of the condyles, endochondral ossification of the joint surface, and advancement of the tidemark to the articular surface [11,14]. These changes are associated with site-specific microdamage accumulation in calcified cartilage and the underlying subchondral bone of the parasagittal condylar grooves [11,12,14]. Microcrack initiation occurs in the calcified cartilage layer [14] and stimulates a targeted remodeling response that results in the formation of resorption spaces containing activated osteoclasts in the damaged bone [14]. This reparative response is associated with an increase in bone porosity, and may make horses more vulnerable to stress fracture if athletic activity is ongoing [14]. Accumulation and coalescence of these microcracks leads to development of macroscopic crack arrays in the subchondral bone of the condylar grooves [11,12,14]. Crack propagation through porous bone compromises the overlying cortical shell at the distal end of the MC3/MT3 bone [15,21]. Once the cortical shell of the distal end of the MC3/MT3 bone is mechanically compromised, crack propagation proximally along trabecular planes can easily develop, thereby rendering the horse at high risk of developing condylar stress fracture [15,21].

Currently, there are differing opinions in the field regarding the etiology of fetlock breakdown injury in the racing Thoroughbred. The causative mechanism is likely complex and involves all of the joint structures, the third metacarpal or metatarsal, the proximal sesamoids, and the proximal phalanx. Very little is known about the mechanical stability of the fatigue cracks in the subchondral bone plate that precede development of a condylar stress fracture. It is likely that condylar stress fracture is preceded by cracks in the subchondral plate that become sufficiently severe to permit development of micromotion at the high joint loads associated with training or racing. Therefore, knowledge of the relationship between crack dimensions determined by cross-sectional imaging and crack micromotion at high load may facilitate early identification of horses that are at high risk of condylar stress fracture. Ultimately, this knowledge could help reduce the incidence of serious or catastrophic injuries at the racetrack.

Multiple imaging methods relevant to the distal limb are available to the equine clinician. Radiography is inferior to computed tomography (CT) and magnetic resonance imaging (MRI) for identification of pathologic features in subchondral bone and articular cartilage, such as fatigue cracks in the subchondral bone plate [22,23]. In addition to increased sensitivity for identifying pathologic changes in the articular surface of the fetlock joint, CT allows for multi-planar analysis of cross-sectional images of bone, facilitating a more accurate determination of size or extent of specific structures, such as subchondral fatigue cracks.

The objective of the present study was to develop an ex-vivo biomechanical model in which subchondral crack micromotion at high loads could be measured in distal MC3. We then used this model to determine the relationship between subchondral crack dimensions measured using CT and crack micromotion. We hypothesized that subchondral crack micromotion would be commonly detectable in the distal end of the MC3 bone in Thoroughbred racehorses at joint loads that model racing activity. Such a result would suggest that athletic Thoroughbred horses commonly train and race with incipient condylar stress fracture and are vulnerable to fracture propagation during athletic activity. A secondary objective was to study detection of fetlock joint abnormalities by CT imaging.

Materials and Methods

Thoroughbred racehorses

Thirty-six pairs of entire distal forelimbs and 4 individual limbs from 40 Thoroughbred racehorses that died or were euthanatized for reasons unrelated to the present study were given for use in this work (**Fig. 1**). Horses were euthanatized humanely by a veterinarian at the racetrack using an intravenous anesthetic overdose. Euthanasia was performed for clinical reasons because of serious injury during racing. Only thoracic limbs were used for this study. Condylar fractures most commonly affect the thoracic limbs [2,3,24,25]. Limbs were transected at the level of the carpus, sealed in plastic bags, and stored at -20C until needed. The age, gender, and racing history were collected from the Jockey Club Information Systems, Inc. Thoroughbred racehorse database (www.equineline.com) for horses with parasagittal subchondral cracks that were tested mechanically.

Digital radiography (DR)

DR radiographs of the metacarpophalangeal joint of each limb specimen were made using a single dorsopalmar radiographic view (70 kVp, 0.08 Ms, EDR3-MFA, Sound-Eklin, Carlsbad, CA) to determine whether fractures of the MC3 bone, proximal sesamoid bones or proximal phalanx were present. Limbs were excluded if a fracture of the MC3 bone was present.

Computed tomography (CT)

CT imaging was performed at high-resolution using 0.625 mm contiguous slices (64 slices GE Discovery CT750 HD, GE Healthcare Technologies, Waukesha, WI, USA). CT images were reconstructed in the sagittal, transverse, and frontal planes using a 64-bit Dicom viewer (OsiriX, Pixmeo SARL, Bernex, Switzerland). CT images were examined for evidence of pathological changes, including the presence of subchondral sclerosis, fractures, defects in the joint surface, and parasagittal fatigue cracks within the condylar grooves. The presence of palmar osteochondral disease (POD), initially referred to in the literature as traumatic osteochondrosis [26,27], was defined by the presence of subchondral bone lysis in the palmar condyle area [22]. The dimensions of subchondral cracks were measured radiographically on transverse and reconstructed frontal plane CT images (**Fig. 2**). In addition, crack area was measured in the parasagittal plane using image analysis (Image J, NIH) (**Fig. 2**). Using commercially available software (Mimics 13.1 Materialise, Ann Arbor, Michigan), the distal end of each MC3 bone with a parasagittal condylar groove lesion was segmented manually. A 3D volumetric model of the subchondral crack lesion was then created from the segmented images on a voxel-by-voxel basis to yield measurements of subchondral crack volume and the surface area of the subchondral crack volume.

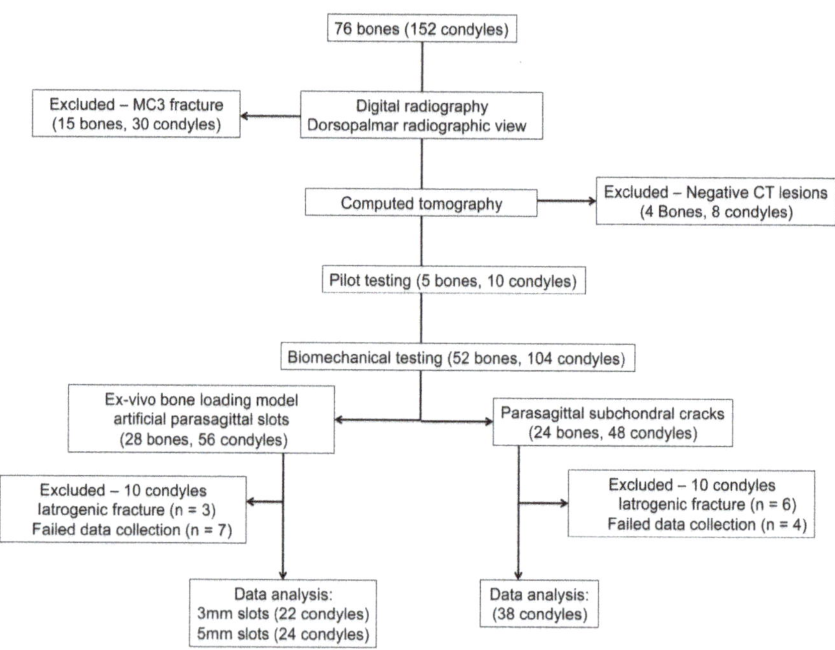

Figure 1. Flow diagram for limb inclusion and exclusion. Of the 152 condyles from 76 limbs horses initially screened, 38 condyles with naturally occurring subchondral fatigue cracks were ultimately studied in detail.

Visual examination and photography

After CT imaging, all soft tissue was removed from each MC3 bone. The shaft was cut with a band saw in the mid-diaphysis, 12 cm proximal to the dorsal articular margin of the distal end of the bone. The second and fourth metacarpal bones were removed. The articular surface at the distal end of the bone was photographed and the articular cartilage and remaining soft tissues were then digested using 0.15–0.2 M sodium hydroxide at 37°C. The solution was changed as needed every 1 to 3 days. Once the soft tissues were removed, bones were fixed in 70% ethanol and additional photographs of the distal articular surface were made. Severity of the parasagittal crack arrays was graded using a visual analogue scale as previously described [12]. The articular surface was also evaluated for any other pathology before and after digestion. The presence of POD was considered positive if there was discoloration of the cartilage or subchondral bone of the palmar condyle, ulceration/collapse of the cartilage, or presence of subchondral defect in the palmar region of the condyle [26,27]. Severity of POD was also graded using a visual analogue scale [12].

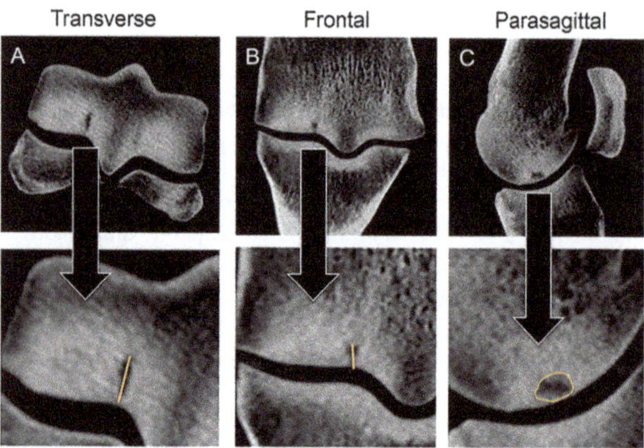

Figure 2. Subchondral fatigue crack dimensions were measured in transverse (**A**) and reconstructed frontal plane (**B**) computed tomography (CT) images. In addition, the area of the crack array was measured in the parasagittal plane (**C**).

Ex-vivo bone loading model

To study subchondral crack micromotion at high loads associated with athletic performance, we developed a non-destructive MC3 bone-loading model. An isolated single bone model was chosen for this work because of the high compressive load used for mechanical testing. Each bone was potted in an aluminum cylinder that was 10 cm long using epoxy (Evercoat 100156 Lite Weight Autobody Filler, Fiber Glass-Evercoat, Cincinnati, OH, USA). An 8 mm hole was drilled in the proximal end of the potted bone and the surrounding cylinder approximately 2 cm from the end of the cylinder, perpendicular to the long axis of the bone and the joint surface, and a stainless steel pin was inserted for additional stability.

Bone specimens without detectable CT lesions in the condylar grooves were used to validate the biomechanical model. Holes, 1.25 mm in diameter, were drilled at the distal palmar aspect of the sagittal ridge and 1 mm abaxial to the condylar groove in the same oblique frontal plate to span the region-of-interest. The potted bone specimen was then positioned in a custom jig (**Fig. 3**). The bones were oriented obliquely in the jig with the palmar-odistal aspect facing up in order to mimic compressive loading by the proximal sesamoid bones from weight-bearing. Hypodermic needles (18 gauge) were placed in the drill holes and connected to an extensometer (MTS Systems Corp., Model 632-120-20, Eden Prairie, MN). Lateral and medial condyles of each bone were tested separately. As the bones were not tested destructively each specimen acted as it's own control. Each intact condyle was tested once, in order to obtain a baseline extensometer measurement

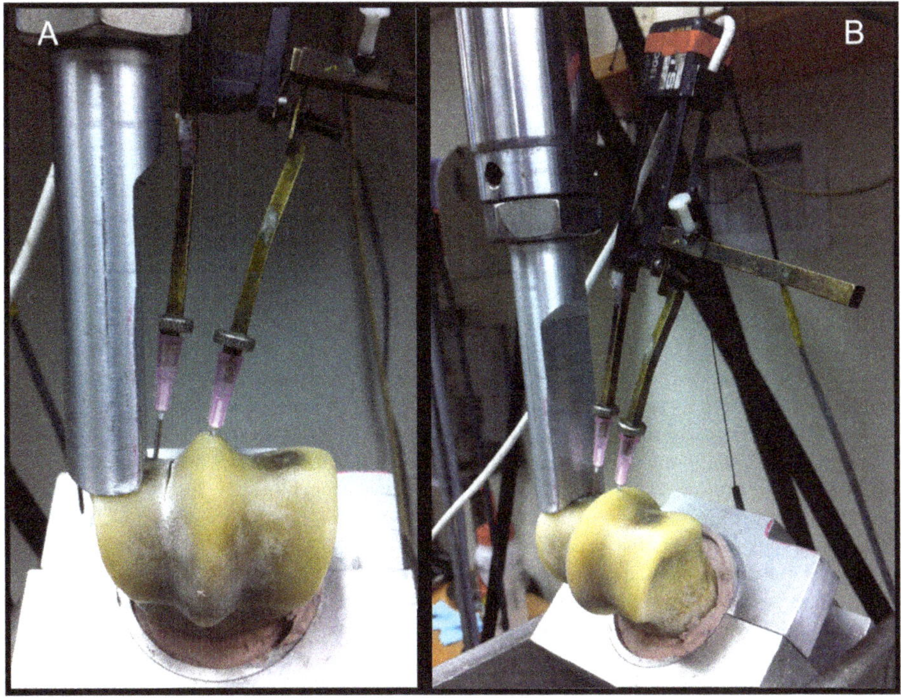

Figure 3. Photograph illustrating the custom-made jig that secures the distal end of the MC3 bone to the platen of a materials testing machine (MTS 858, Minneapolis, MN). (**A**) Drill holes 1.25 mm in diameter were made on the lateral and medial side of the artificial slot or crack array in the parasagittal condylar groove. (B) Hypodermic needles (18 g) were then placed in the drill holes and attached to an extensometer to measure motion across the slot or crack. The actuator consisted of a metal rod that was contoured to conform to the curved surface of the condyle.

before creation of an artificial subchondral slot to model an in-vivo fatigue crack.

Crack micromotion was measured using a materials testing system (modified MTS Bionics 858 hydraulic test machine; MTS Systems Corp, Eden Prairie, Minneapolis, MN) under load control. Before the mechanical test, each bone was pre-loaded at 100 N. Five cycles of compressive load of 7,500 N were then applied to the condyle abaxial to the extensometer at 0.1 Hz. This load was selected based on biomechanical modeling of fetlock joint loading [20]. Data were collected at 30 Hz for all channels (load, displacement and extensometer motion) and stored on a computer in a data file for future analysis. Mean micromotion for each test was determined by peak-to-peak measurements for the five load cycles. It has been previously estimated that the peak compressive load on the palmar surface of the distal end of the MC3 bone exerted by each proximal sesamoid bone on its respective condyle is at least 7,500 N for a 500 kg horse at the canter, giving rise to a peak stress of 23.9 MNm^{-2} [20].

After an initial baseline testing, an artificial slot was created in the palmar region of the condylar groove using a high-speed rotary tool with a circular diamond wheel, 0.6 mm thick (Dremel 545, Racine, WI) to model a naturally occurring parasagittal array of fatigue cracks. Lateral and medial condyles were randomly assigned to slots that were either 3 mm or 5 mm deep and approximately 18 mm long in a dorsopalmar direction. Mechanical testing was then repeated.

Mechanical testing of parasagittal subchondral fatigue cracks

Bone specimens that were found to have macroscopic parasagittal crack arrays in the condylar groove after cartilage digestion and corresponding lesions detectable on CT cross-sectional images were also tested biomechanically. In order to separate pre-existing fatigue cracking from artifactual damage induced by mechanical testing, a bulk-staining method was used [28]. The entire distal end of the MC3 bone was bulk-stained in 1% basic fuchsin for three days, changing the solution daily. The bones were then placed in 100% ethyl alcohol for 20 minutes before being incrementally rehydrated and then placed in 0.9% saline. The bones were mounted and tested as described above. Movement during loading of the condyle was detected by placement of the extensometer across the array of cracks in the condylar groove. Lateral and medial condyles were again tested separately, but testing was not repeated.

Bone morphometry

After mechanical testing, 1.1 mm thick oblique frontal sections of the distal end of each MC3 bone were prepared using a diamond saw. Sections were cut in a proximodorsal distopalmar plane to pass through the palmar crack array in the condylar groove [12]. Microradiographs (Faxitron, Wheeling, IL, USA) of each section were made for comparison with equivalent frontal plane CT images.

Bone sections were examined for condylar groove cracking [14]. Subchondral cracks that were stained with basic fuchsin were counted within the condylar groove region and normalized to the length of the regional bone boundary to give a crack boundary density (N.Cr/B.Bd, #/mm) by a single observer (KR) [14]. Sections were also examined for unstained artifactual subchondral cracks associated with mechanical testing and bone sectioning. In addition, stained subchondral cracks were examined for evidence of crack extension during mechanical testing.

Statistical analysis

The Shapiro-Wilk test was used to determine whether data approximated a normal distribution. To validate the ex-vivo bone-loading model, baseline extensometer motion was subtracted from extensometer motion recorded after slot creation. Because data did not approximate a normal distribution, the Wilcoxon Signed Rank test was used to determine whether data for each slot group differed from a theoretical median of zero (no extensometer displacement). Distribution of condyles between groups was examined using the Chi-squared test. The Wilcoxon Signed Rank test or the Student's t test for paired data, as appropriate, were used to analyze pathological change in the lateral and medial joint regions. The correlative relationships between measurements of fatigue crack dimensions on CT images and extensometer micromotion and subjective and objective measures of pathologic change in the joint surface were examined using the Spearman Rank test. Baseline micromotion for bones with naturally occurring fatigue cracks was determined from extensometer measurements of all condyles without fatigue cracks evident on CT examination (n = 14 condyles). A mean baseline extensometer reading was subtracted from the mean micromotion value for each bone before analysis. The Spearman Rank test was also used to determine whether a correlative relationship existed between athletic history (horse age, number of race starts, number of career wins, and racing surface [turf or dirt]) and fatigue crack dimensions measured by CT. A similar analysis was performed for crack micromotion measured by mechanical testing, and subjective and objective measurement of pathologic change.

The relationship between fatigue crack micromotion from mechanical testing and crack dimensions was also examined using logistic regression. Extensometer micromotion was coded as 1 – motion is >15% above baseline, or 0 – ≤15% above baseline for condyles without CT evidence of subchondral fatigue cracks from the pool of bones with naturally occurring fatigue crack arrays. 15% above baseline was arbitrarily chosen to create a conservative assessment of crack micromotion within the statistical model. Horse identity and the presence or absence of a proximal sesamoid bone fracture were included as variables in the logistic regression model. For crack measurement methods with significant results in the logistic regression model, postestimation was used to determine probability of a positive outcome for each CT measurement. Results were considered significant at $p<0.05$. Fatigue cracks with a probability estimate >0.8 for micromotion 15% above baseline were considered clinically relevant.

Results

Digital radiography

DR radiographs were made of 76 forelimbs (**Fig. 1**). Fifteen limbs (20%) revealed a fracture of MC3. Eleven limbs (14%) had a condylar fracture (9 lateral and 2 medial). A comminuted diaphyseal fracture was seen in 4 limbs (5%). These limbs were excluded from further analysis (**Fig. 1**). Lesions other than a fracture were identified in distal MC3 bone in 2 of 76 limbs. In one limb, a small radiolucency in the lateral condylar groove was seen, which, subsequently, was associated with a fatigue crack in the subchondral plate identified using CT. Severe POD of both condyles characterized by a subchondral bone defect and associated radiolucency adjacent to the joint surface was seen in another limb. These changes were also visible on CT. Biaxial proximal sesamoid fracture was seen in 12 of 76 limbs (16%) and uniaxial proximal sesamoid fracture was seen in 6 of 76 limbs (8%). Condylar fracture was seen concurrently in three limbs with proximal sesamoid fracture.

Metacarpophalangeal joint osteoarthritis was seen in three limbs, and evidence of rupture of the intersesamoidian ligament (abnormal distance between both proximal sesamoid bones) was seen in one limb. Lateral condylar fracture was also seen concurrently with a comminuted fracture of the proximal phalanx in one limb.

Computed tomography

Sixty-one bones were examined via CT imaging (see Fig. 1 for exclusions). Palmar subchondral bone sclerosis was identified in all condyles studied. Parasagittal crack arrays in the palmar subchondral plate of the distal end of the MC3 bone were identified in 42 of 122 condyles (34%), or 27 of 61 limbs (44%) (Table 1). Of those, 24 were located in a lateral condyle, and 18 in a medial. Fifteen limbs had cracks in both the medial and lateral grooves. The appearance of these subchondral lesions within the condylar grooves varied tremendously in shape and density, ranging from a faint lucency to a distinctive crack in the subchondral plate (Figs. 4, 5). POD was found in 46 of 122 condyles (38%), or 28 of 61 limbs (46%) (Fig. 6). In addition, several other fetlock joint abnormalities were identified, including fractures of the proximal sesamoid bone (15 limbs), osteoarthritis (10 limbs), dorsoproximal proximal phalanx fracture (7 limbs), irregularities on the dorsoproximal aspect of the proximal phalanx (5 limbs), irregularities of the distal mid-sagittal ridge (3 limbs), enthesophytosis of the proximal sesamoid bone (2 limbs), and frontal proximal phalanx fracture (1 limb). Fractures of 26 proximal sesamoid bones were seen. Of the 26 fractures, 12 were comminuted, 7 were mid-body, 5 were basilar, and 2 were apical. Four limbs were not studied further because of the absence of CT lesions (Fig. 1).

Visual examination and photography

The distal end of the MC3 bone was examined in 57 limbs, after exclusion for MC3 fracture (15 limbs) and absence of CT lesions (4 limbs) (**Fig. 1**). On gross examination of the joints before digestion of articular cartilage, multiple different pathologies were identified (**Table 1**).

Wear lines. Wear lines were identified on the cartilage of the distal end of 24 MC3 bones (42%).

Parasagittal subchondral crack arrays. Results are summarized in **Table 2**. Focal or linear cartilage defects were present in the condylar grooves of 58 of 114 condyles (51%). Of these 58 condyles, parasagittal subchondral crack arrays were identified in 33 (57%) after articular cartilage digestion (**Figs. 4, 5**). No cracks in the subchondral plate were seen in the other 25 condyles. After cartilage digestion, subchondral bone crack arrays were identified in 51 of 114 condyles (45%), of which 33 were also identified before cartilage digestion. Of those 51 condyles with visible cracks after removal of the articular cartilage, 28 were evident with CT imaging (55%). Subchondral cracking identified in 11 condyles using CT imaging had no visible lesions in the joint surface of the condylar grooves. Median (range) severity scores for lateral and medial parasagittal linear cartilage defects were 8 (0,48) and 10 (0,42) respectively; severity of disease was not significantly different between lateral and medial condyles. Median (range) severity scores for lateral and medial parasagittal fatigue crack arrays in the subchondral plate were 21.5 (0,92) and 1 (0,90) respectively. Severity of subchondral fatigue damage was increased in the lateral condyle, compared with the medial condyle ($p<0.05$). Severity of subchondral fatigue damage assessed by subjective scoring was not significantly correlated with crack dimensions measured on reconstructed CT images or extensometer micromotion during mechanical testing.

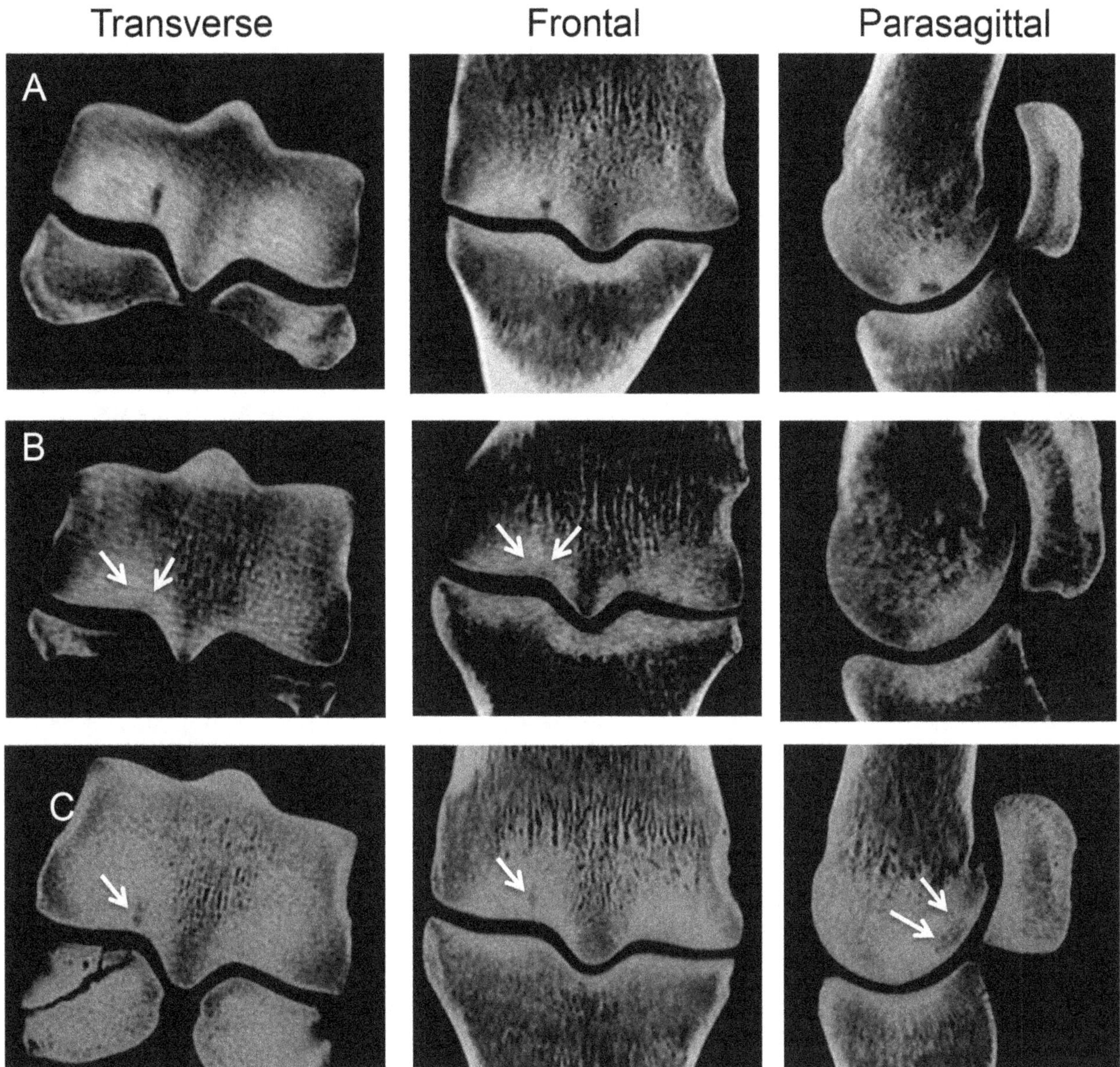

Figure 4. Representative computed tomography images of the distal end of the third metacarpal bone illustrating variation in appearance of parasagittal subchondral crack arrays in the condylar grooves of racing Thoroughbreds. (**A**) A large subchondral crack is evident within the lateral condylar groove. The crack is evident in all three planes. (**B**) In this horse, a small radiolucency is evident in the subchondral plate in the condylar groove (arrows) associated with the presence of a smaller array of fatigue cracks in the transverse and frontal plane images (arrows). (**C**) In this horse, a small well-defined crack is present in the subchondral bone of the medial condylar groove (arrow), which was associated with a large parasagittal crack area that exceeded 30 mm^2. Fracture of the adjacent proximal sesamoid is also evident.

Palmar osteochondral disease. POD was identified in 67 of 114 condyles (59%) after cartilage digestion. Abnormality in the cartilage overlying the subchondral bone lesion was evident in 50 (75%) of these condyles (**Fig. 6, 7**). Of the 67 condyles in which POD was identified after removal of the articular cartilage, 39 were evident with CT imaging (58%). Median (range) severity scores for lateral and medial parasagittal fatigue crack arrays in the subchondral plate were 5 (0,54) and 8 (0,48) respectively. Severity of POD was increased in the medial condyle, compared with the lateral condyle ($p<0.05$).

Ex-Vivo Bone Loading Model

In the 3 mm slot group, there were 22 condyles (14 medial and 8 lateral) analyzed from 19 MC3 bones. In the 5 mm slot group, there were 24 condyles (11 medial and 13 lateral) analyzed from 20 MC3 bones. Three condyles did not yield interpretable data and were excluded due to fracture of the bone during biomechanical testing. Six other condyles were excluded because of failure of extensometer data collection (**Fig. 1**).

There was no significant difference in the distribution of medial to lateral condyles in both groups. In both the 3 mm and 5 mm groups, significant micromotion was detected with compressive

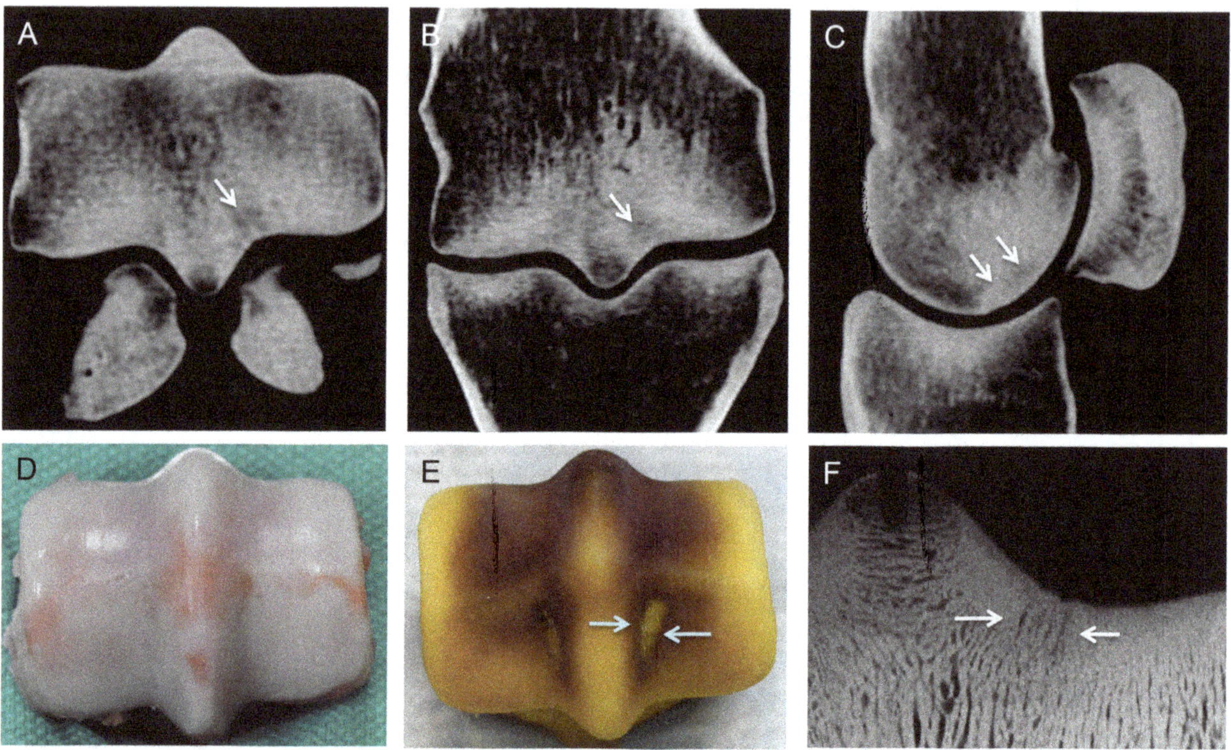

Figure 5. Representative images of the distal end of the third metacarpal bone illustrating the appearance of a large parasagittal subchondral crack array in the lateral condylar groove of the joint surface (arrows) evident on transverse (**A**), frontal (**B**), and parasagittal reconstructed computed tomography images (**C**). A large array of subchondral cracks is present in the subchondral bone of lateral condylar groove (arrows) with relatively little change in the overlying cartilage (**D, E**). An array of fatigue cracks that extend into the proximal part of the subchondral plate is also evident (arrows) on a microradiograph of an oblique frontal bone section (**F**).

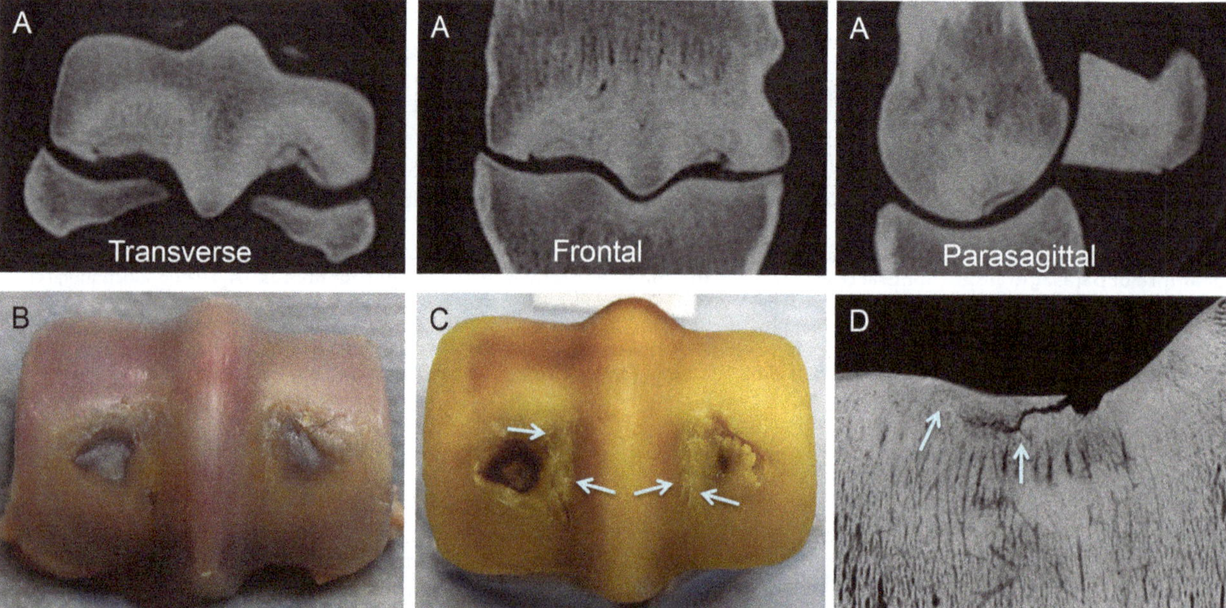

Figure 6. Representative images of the distal end of the third metacarpal bone illustrating articular saucer stress fracture formation in a racing Thoroughbred horse with severe palmar osteochondral disease. (**A**) In reconstructed computed tomography images, a circular articular saucer fracture is present in both condyles. A halo of reduced bone density adjacent to the saucer fracture is caused by the reparative remodeling response in the subchondral plate. Extensive adaptive subchondral sclerosis is also evident. (**B**) Hyaline cartilage overlying the stress fracture has been replaced by fibrocartilage. (**C**) Extensive fatigue damage to the underlying subchondral plate is also evident, including parasagittal cracks in the condylar grooves (arrows). (**D**) Propagation of the fracture line at the interface of the vascular remodeling response to the fatigue injury in the subchondral plate is evident (arrows) on a microradiograph of an oblique frontal bone section.

Table 1. Distribution of fetlock joint abnormalities in Thoroughbred racehorses identified by radiographic imaging and direct observation.

	Digital radiography	Computed tomography	Observation of articular cartilage	Observation of the subchondral plate
	Wear lines			
Horses (n = 38)	n/a	n/a	20 (53%)	n/a
Bones (n = 57)	n/a	n/a	24 (42%)	n/a
Condyles (n = 114)	n/a	n/a	46 (40%)	n/a
	Parasagittal subchondral crack array			
Horses (n = 38)	1 (3%)	21 (55%)	23 (61%)	25 (66%)
Bones (n = 57)	1 (2%)	27 (47%)	31 (54%)	31 (54%)
Condyles (n = 114)	1 (1%)	42 (37%)	58 (51%)	51 (45%)
	Palmar osteochondral disease			
Horses (n = 38)	1 (3%)	19 (50%)	23 (61%)	29 (76%)
Bones (n = 57)	1 (2%)	27 (47%)	32 (56%)	41 (72%)
Condyles (n = 114)	2 (2%)	42 (37%)	53 (46%)	67 (59%)
	Proximal sesamoid fracture			
Horses (n = 38)	15 (39%)	15 (39%)	n/a	n/a
Bones (n = 57)	15 (26%)	15 (26%)	n/a	n/a
Condyles (n = 114)	27 (24%)	27 (24%)	n/a	n/a

Note: One hundred fourteen condyles from 57 MC3 bones from 38 horses were dissected and digested to evaluate the articular surface (see also Fig. 1). Subchondral plate observations were made after cartilage digestion.

loading, ($p<0.001$), with median values of 0.008 mm and 0.038 mm, respectively. Micromotion was significantly increased in the 5 mm slot group when compared with the 3 mm slot group ($p<0.001$) (**Fig. 8**).

Relationship between crack micromotion and crack dimensions derived from computed tomographic imaging

MC3 bones from 24 limbs were used for mechanical testing. Of the 48 condyles, 6 did not yield interpretable data and were excluded because the bone sustained a fracture during mechanical testing. Iatrogenic fractures did not propagate from the condylar groove, and affected either the potted region of the bone shaft (n = 2) or the region of the condyle in direct contact with the actuator (n = 4). Four other condyles were excluded because of failure of extensometer data collection. Mechanical data were acquired for the remaining 38 condyles (**Fig. 1**). These condyles were derived from 21 bones from 18 Thoroughbred horses.

Micromotion 15% above baseline was detected in 18 of 38 condyles (47%) (**Fig. 9**). Median micromotion corrected for the baseline value was 0.007 mm, with a maximum value of 0.103 mm. There was a significant positive correlation between extensometer micromotion and parasagittal crack area measured from reconstructed CT images ($S_R = 0.32$, $p<0.05$). Correlations with transverse and frontal plane crack lengths were not significant. Similarly, correlations with volumetric and surface measurements on 3D reconstructed images were not significant. All CT measurements were significantly correlated with each other ($S_R>0.74$, $p<0.001$). When extensometer motion data were transformed into a binary format, we found a significant relationship between crack dimensions on CT and the presence of fatigue crack micromotion ($p<0.05$ for frontal plane crack length, parasagittal crack area, crack volume, and crack surface area, when data were corrected for motion 15% above baseline (**Table 3**); significance was greatest for parasagittal crack area. For parasagittal crack area, a similar result was obtained with a simple baseline correction ($p = 0.06$). Comparisons of other CT measurements with baseline-corrected crack micromotion were not significant. The presence of a proximal sesamoid fracture was not significantly correlated with subchondral crack micromotion and was not a significant factor in the logistic regression model.

Table 2. Identification of parasagittal subchondral crack arrays in the distal end of the third metacarpal bone of Thoroughbred racehorses by computed tomography and direct observation.

	Computed tomography	Observation of articular cartilage	Observation of the subchondral plate
Computed tomography	42 (37%)		
Observation of articular cartilage	30 (26%)	58 (51%)	
Observation of the subchondral plate	28 (25%)	33 (29%)	51 (45%)

Note: One hundred fourteen condyles from 57 MC3 bones from 38 different horses were dissected and digested to evaluate the articular surface (see also Fig. 1). Data represent number of condyles. Percentages represent proportion of total (114 condyles).

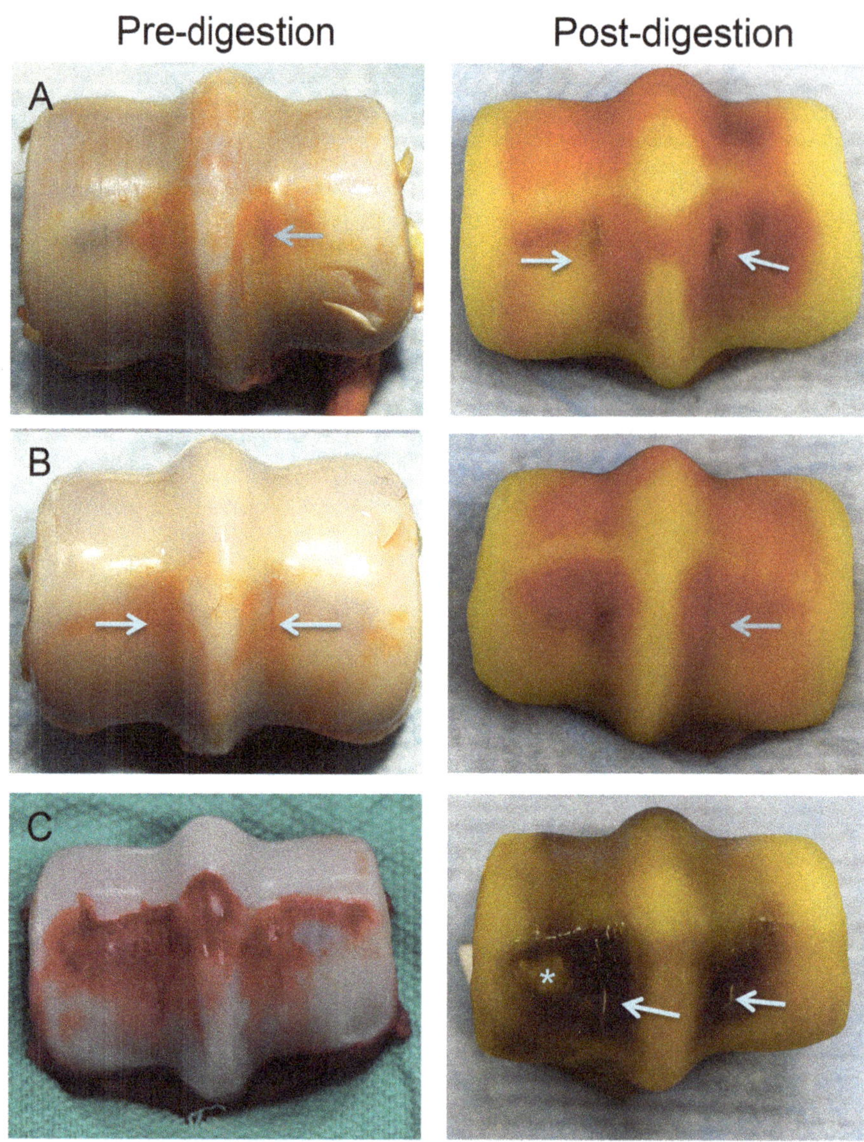

Figure 7. Representative images of the distal end of the third metacarpal bone before and after cartilage digestion illustrating fetlock abnormalities commonly associated with the presence of subchondral fatigue crack arrays. Extensive wear lines in hyaline cartilage (**A**), subchondral bruising (**A–C**) and flattening of the palmar region of the condyles (**C**) were commonly found. In some horses parasagittal defects in the hyaline articular cartilage of the condylar grooves were of mild severity and associated with varying degrees of fatigue cracking of the underlying subchondral plate (arrows) (**A–C**). Palmar osteochondral disease was commonly associated with condylar groove fatigue cracks (* in **C**). Images obtained from the same horses as Figure 4.

In the logistic regression model, 3 of 38 condyles (7.9%) in the limbs of three different horses had parasagittal fatigue cracks in the condylar groove with a parasagittal crack area measurement that exceeded 30 mm^2. Specimens with parasagittal crack area measurements above this value had a probability of >0.8 that crack micromotion in our biomechanical model would exceed baseline +15% and be deemed clinically significant (**Figs. 4,5,7**).

Subchondral fatigue crack histomorphometry

Mean ± standard deviation N.Cr/B.Bd was 0.62±0.34 and 0.55±0.32 respectively for the lateral and medial condyles; severity of histologic fatigue damage was not significantly different between lateral and medial condyles. Severity of histologic fatigue damage was not significantly correlated with crack dimensions measured on reconstructed CT images or extensometer micromotion during mechanical testing. Examination of the oblique frontal bone sections after mechanical loading did not reveal any evidence of crack extension from mechanical testing. One or two unstained cracks were identified in the articular surface of the condylar groove in 6 of 38 condyles after mechanical testing.

Relationship between athletic history and severity of subchondral fatigue damage

Mechanical data were obtained for 38 condyles from 22 limbs of 18 horses. Of these 18 Thoroughbreds, a racing history was available for 15 animals. The study group was comprised of 7 females and 8 males consisting of 5 stallions and 3 geldings. The median age was 4 years old (range of 2 to 8). Median number of career starts was 12 (range of 0 to 46). Seven horses were racing on

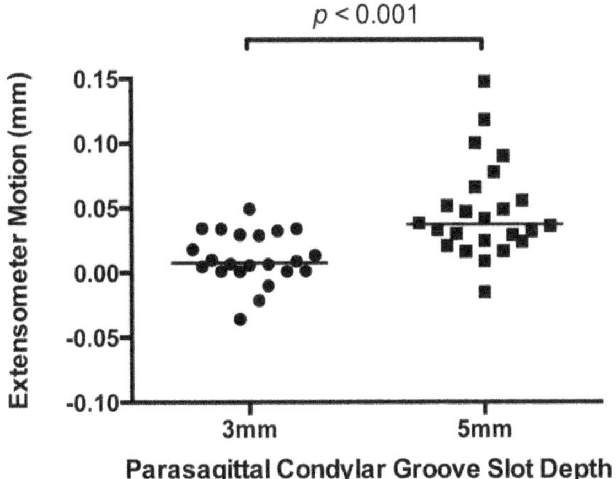

Figure 8. In our ex-vivo biomechanical model, extensometer micromotion associated with creation of shallow parasagittal slots in the palmar region of the condylar groove was used to model naturally occurring arrays of fatigue cracks. In both the 3 mm and 5 mm groups, baseline-corrected extensometer motion was significantly different from zero (no motion) ($p<0.001$). Increased slot depth was associated with increased micromotion. In our model, the condyle was loaded at −7,500 N in compression. In the scatterplot, the horizontal bar represents the median value for each group.

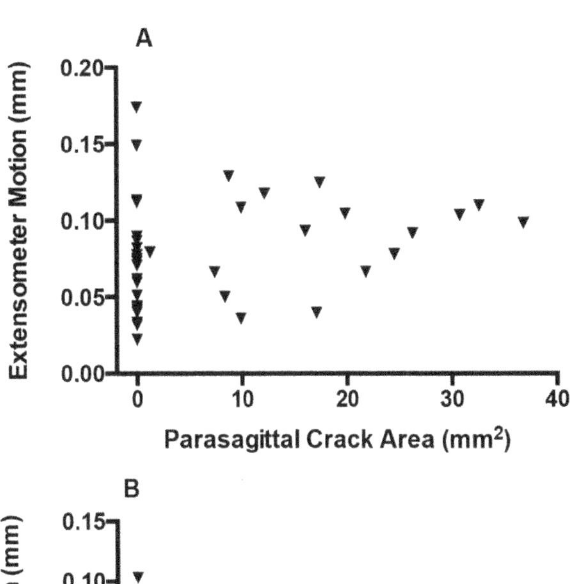

Figure 9. In our ex-vivo biomechanical model, extensometer micromotion associated with naturally occurring parasagittal fatigue cracks in the palmar region of the condylar groove was also determined. (**A**) There was a significant correlation between extensometer motion and parasagittal crack area measured from reconstructed computed tomographic images ($S_R=0.32$, $p<0.05$). (**B**) Extensometer motion corrected for baseline. Micromotion 15% above baseline was detected in 18 of 38 condyles (47%).

dirt and 4 on turf. One horse never raced. Athletic history was not available for the other three horses. There were no significant correlations between athletic history and the magnitude of parasagittal fatigue crack dimensions from CT imaging of the distal end of the MC3 bone. Similarly, there were no significant correlations between athletic history and detection of crack micromotion. Subjective scoring and histomorphometric assessment of parasagittal subchondral fatigue damage, but not severity of POD, was significantly correlated with horse age and athletic activity (**Table 4**). Significant correlations between severity of subchondral fatigue damage and racing surface were not detected.

Discussion

Collectively, past observations suggest that condylar stress fractures arise from site-specific accumulation of fatigue damage in the subchondral plate of the distal end of the MC3/MT3 bone [12–16]. However, the mechanism by which fatigue damage ultimately precipitates structural failure of the MC3/MT3 bone during athletic activity is poorly understood and little investigated. Results from our ex-vivo model suggest that it is likely that some degree of fatigue crack micromotion is present in a large proportion of Thoroughbred racehorses during training and racing. Although subchondral crack micromotion may not be the only determinant of a stress fracture, microcrack propagation, as opposed to initiation, is likely an important component of stress fracture development [29]. Microstructural features of the subchondral plate, such as resorption spaces, may also have an important role in crack propagation [14,29]. Our results suggest that CT imaging could be used to quantify subchondral fatigue crack dimensions in racing Thoroughbred horses and assess risk of condylar fracture in clinical longitudinal studies. Horses with parasagittal crack arrays that exceed 30 mm^2 may have a high risk for development of condylar fracture; based on our results it is likely that fatigue crack arrays exceeding these dimensions are exposed to micromotion during high speed running and are, therefore, vulnerable to catastrophic crack propagation [14,15].

During initial screening with DR, we found that condylar fracture was present in 14% of limbs of the Thoroughbred horses in this study. This observation is similar to other epidemiological studies that suggest that condylar stress fracture is commonly associated with catastrophic injuring in racing Thoroughbreds [5–7]. Fractures of the proximal sesamoid bones were also commonly detected using DR and CT imaging in the Thoroughbred horses of the present study. The majority of these were comminuted. Similar observations have been made in clinical studies in Thoroughbred racehorses with catastrophic injuries [6,7].

The lesions we identified on examination of the articular surface before and after cartilage digestion were similar to earlier studies [11,12,23,30] and support the concept that pathological changes to the fetlock joint are common in racing Thoroughbreds, including young horses at the beginning of their racing career.

Previous work from our laboratory suggests that cross-sectional imaging, particularly with CT, is superior to digital radiography for lesion identification in the fetlock joint of racing Thoroughbreds [22,23]. This observation was reaffirmed in the present study. However, CT imaging was only able to identify 55% of condyles with visible subchondral cracking after cartilage digestion. This might be explained by the fact that some visible crack arrays are small and only affect the subchondral bone plate superficially, thus preventing identification on CT examination. Histologic examination of the distal joint surface of the MC3 bone

Table 3. Relationship between computed tomography measurement of parasagittal fatigue crack dimensions and detection of crack micromotion during mechanical loading.

	Statistical Model	Odds ratio	95% Confidence Interval	Likelihood Ratio Chi-square	Significance
Crack length in the transverse plane	Crack length + horse			5.57	0.06
	Crack length				0.41
Crack length in the frontal plane	Crack length + horse			7.79	0.02
	Crack length				0.1
Parasagittal crack area	Crack area + horse			9.53	0.01
	Crack area	1.08	1.00–1.16		0.05
Crack volume	Crack volume + horse			6.90	0.03
	Crack volume				0.17
Crack surface	Crack surface + horse			7.43	0.02
	Crack surface				0.13

Note: A logistic regression model was used to determine whether there was a significant relationship between fatigue crack dimensions determined by measurement from computed tomography images and crack micromotion under clinically relevant joint loads in an ex-vivo model (micromotion corrected to 15% above baseline) (n = 38 condyles from 21 bones from 18 horses). Within the multivariate models of CT measurement parameter and horse identity, parasagittal crack area was the only CT measurement that yielded a significant result.

from racing Thoroughbreds suggests that fatigue injury is initiated in the calcified cartilage of the joint surface [14]. However, in the present study, we found that subchondral cracking identified in 11 condyles on CT imaging had no visible lesions in the joint surface of the condylar grooves after cartilage digestion. This may suggest site-specific remodeling in the subchondral plate proximal to the articular surface is also an early event in the disease mechanism. Alternatively, crack initiation may occur deeper within the subchondral plate in some horses. It should be noted that our evaluation of these condyles occurred at a specific point in time, and cannot consider how adaptive remodeling may lead to changes in pathological features within the subchondral plate over time. Therefore, it is possible that some of these lesions represent the early phase of the damage process before development of a more extensive crack array in the subchondral plate, or alternatively the beginning of a healing process.

The appearance of parasagittal subchondral crack arrays in the condylar grooves of the MC3 joint surface was quite variable using CT imaging. Subchondral cracks surrounded by radiolucency may have a greater area or volume than cracks with more clearly defined margins. This is likely important, as stressed volume is thought to be an important factor in the pathogenesis of stress fracture [31]. Our regression analyses suggested that measurement of parasagittal crack area, as opposed to transverse or frontal plane measurements of crack length, yielded the best predictor of crack micromotion. Detection of radiolucency in the parasagittal condylar groove on CT may suggest that the array of interconnected fatigue cracks occupies a larger volume in the subchondral plate. This concept could be examined by more detailed histomorphometric examination of fatigue-damaged bone with this CT abnormality. In the present study, we did not identify a significant correlation between crack array dimensions on CT and

Table 4. Relationship between athletic history and severity of pathologic change observed in the joint surface of the distal end of the third metacarpal of racing Thoroughbreds.

Parameter	S_R	Significance
Horse age		
Condylar groove cartilage defect severity score	−0.25	NS
Condylar groove subchondral bone damage severity score	0.61	$p<0.001$
N.Cr/B.Bd, #/mm	0.57	$p<0.001$
Number of race starts		
Condylar groove cartilage defect severity score	−0.38	$p<0.05$
Condylar groove subchondral bone damage severity score	0.50	$p<0.005$
N.Cr/B.Bd, #/mm	0.37	$p<0.05$
Number of career wins		
Condylar groove cartilage defect severity score	−0.30	NS ($p=0.09$)
Condylar groove subchondral bone damage severity score	0.35	$p=0.05$
N.Cr/B.Bd, #/mm	0.37	$p<0.05$

Note: Correlations with severity scoring of palmar osteochondral disease were not significant for any athletic history parameter (n = 32 condyles).

objective measurement of histologic fatigue damage or subjective grading of joint pathology. Even though CT imaging was performed at high resolution, precise determination of crack margins was not always straightforward. Improvements in image resolution may help to identify horses with more subtle fatigue damage in the subchondral plate of the distal end of the MC3/MT3 bone.

CT imaging was also able to identify POD in a large proportion of the condyles studied. However, not all POD lesions seen on examination of the subchondral plate after cartilage digestion were evident with CT imaging. The main reason for this discrepancy is that those POD lesions not identified on CT imaging were mostly a discoloration of the palmar condyle area, and not a bony defect. Ten of 24 limbs in the naturally occurring crack group were affected by POD, potentially complicating measurement of subchondral crack motion during mechanical testing. In specimens with this lesion, care was taken to place the extensometer needle axial to the POD lesion. By doing so, any POD-associated micromotion should not be included in the motion measured by the extensometer. Although subchondral bone cracks and POD are different clinical entities, they have a similar etiology and both represent fatigue injury to the joint surface [16]. They are a consequence of repetitive stresses from strenuous exercise [12–14,16,26,27], which predisposes them to occurring simultaneously in the same condyle. It is unclear why some horses develop POD instead of parasagittal subchondral fatigue cracks, or vice versa.

To validate our ex-vivo model, we measured micromotion before and after creation of parasagittal slots of two different depths in the palmar region of the condylar groove. Data from this initial experiment supported the validity of our biomechanical model and yielded micromotion values that approximated the values obtained from bones with naturally occurring fatigue crack arrays. Loading conditions for the model were based on earlier studies [20]. Although removal of the articular cartilage may have influenced load distribution during testing, cartilage removal was necessary to observe parasagittal subchondral crack arrays, if present.

We found evidence of fatigue crack micromotion in 47% of condyles, suggesting that a large proportion of racing Thoroughbreds may experience some degree of crack micromotion in vivo. This is an important observation, since it is unlikely that articular fatigue damage will heal well clinically in the face of ongoing instability from habitual training and racing. Horses with parasagittal crack areas that exceed 30 mm^2 are likely to experience substantial crack micromotion under high joint loads, based on our regression analysis. This result was identified in 7.9% of horses, suggesting that a large number of Thoroughbreds racing in the United States are vulnerable to condylar stress fracture during racing.

In this experiment, extensometer motion was detected in condyles without detectable subchondral crack arrays. This is likely a consequence of the large compressive load that was applied to the joint surface during testing to model weight-bearing during high-speed running. Rotational motion and creep of some of the bones inside the potting cylinder was noticed during the mechanical testing and there was a tendency for some degree of extensometer drift during the five loading cycles of each test. To account for this limitation, mechanical data were baseline-corrected before statistical analysis. Further, we chose to only consider crack micromotion as relevant when it increased $\geq$15% above baseline. As there is no established model to determine what amount of motion is truly relevant, this value was chosen arbitrarily as a conservative approach to data interpretation. Development of an improved method for measurement of crack motion during mechanical testing may be help improve precision of mechanical testing in future work.

Histomorphometric quantification and severity scoring of subchondral cracking were significantly correlated with horse age and number of race starts, suggesting that accumulation of MC3 subchondral fatigue injury is related to habitual athletic activity. Cumulative cyclic loading of the fetlock is influenced by accumulation of racing starts as well as high-speed timed workout. Another important component of fetlock loading history is the frequency of these events, which can significantly influence risk of a catastrophic musculoskeletal injury [32]. Severity of the defect in the condylar groove cartilage was significantly and inversely related to number of race starts suggesting that cartilage damage is an early feature of joint injury from habitual athleticism. We did not identify any significant correlation between the cumulative racing history and the magnitude of parasagittal fatigue crack dimensions from CT imaging of the distal end of the MC3 bone, or detection of crack micromotion. However, data were only collected from a limited number of horses, so this finding should be interpreted with caution in the absence of relevant data describing the training activity, as the amount and intensity of workout sessions is likely important to accumulation of subchondral fatigue damage over time. More work is needed to comprehensively understand the relationship between athletic history and subchondral fatigue injury. Clinically, condylar fractures are more common in younger horses that may not have an extensive racing history [1,3,25].

A limitation of this project in accurately modeling an *in vivo* scenario was our use of frozen limbs collected from catastrophically injured racing Thoroughbreds. Limbs were thawed for DR and CT imaging and then refrozen until further dissection, digestion, and basic fuchsin staining. It is possible that post-mortem change and freeze-thaw effects could have influenced our results. Such effects are likely relatively small in a high load biomechanical model. Furthermore, all specimens tested were treated in a similar manner. Removal of the articular cartilage was necessary to appreciate the subchondral crack array in the condylar grooves. Another limitation is that we studied an isolated single bone model with our mechanical testing. Therefore, our study does not address the role of the first phalanx in loading of the distal MC3 bone. It is likely that the articulation between the proximal phalanx and the metacarpus and the loading pattern resulting from this is of importance in the pathogenesis of condylar fracture. Although currently unknown, this interaction, as well as the forces placed on the condyles by the adjacent soft tissues structures (collateral ligaments) probably plays a role in the formation and propagation of these fractures. Our goal was to isolate one portion of the bone that is of known importance in condylar fractures to estimate crack micromotion during direct loading via the articulation between the condyle and the sesamoid. While of great importance, addressing the roles of other anatomical structures is outside the scope of this study, but relevant to future work. The presence of a proximal sesamoid fracture was not significantly related to detection of crack micromotion in our model. Although actuator placement modeled the position of the proximal sesamoid during mechanical testing, in-vivo loading of the distal MC3 bone by the proximal sesamoid may be different. This may explain the iatrogenic fracture that occurred in some bones during testing. Finally, athletic history was obtained from a relatively limited number of horses. Additional epidemiological work is needed to comprehensively understand the relationship between habitual athleticism and fetlock injuries, such as accumulation of MC3 subchondral fatigue damage.

The current design of equine CT scanners requires general anesthesia, which limits the use of CT as a diagnostic modality for equine athletes in race training. However, CT scanning of the foot in the standing horse using a gantry in a horizontal orientation has been performed [33]. Results of the present study suggest that this approach to equine CT imaging needs to be expanded to include the fetlock. With cross-sectional imaging of the fetlock, particularly if available as a standing modality, longitudinal screening of a population of Thoroughbred racehorses in training or racing could improve our ability to recognize and monitor the progression of specific pathologic features in vivo. This would be extremely informative to understanding and treatment of distal MC3/MT3 injury or disease. While reduction in joint loading may contribute to bone healing, it is unknown whether healing of condylar groove subchondral cracks occurs if habitual athletic activity is withdrawn.

In conclusion, condylar stress fractures are common in Thoroughbred racehorses. Parasagittal arrays of fatigue cracks in the subchondral plate of the condylar grooves of the distal end of the MC3 bone are readily detectable by CT. Our results suggest that measurement of crack area on reconstructed parasagittal CT images is a predictive marker for crack micromotion at joint loads associated with high-speed running. Consequently, this parameter may prove to be a useful predictive marker for condylar fracture risk in longitudinal in-vivo studies of Thoroughbred racehorses. Improved determination of fracture risk promises reduction in serious injuries during racing and better clinical management of horses with incipient condylar fracture. Furthermore, such knowledge promises improved understanding of the epidemiological relationship between habitual athletic activity and fetlock breakdown injury.

Acknowledgements

The authors gratefully acknowledge the help of all the Comparative Orthopaedic Research Laboratory students who contributed to this project. Molly VanBommel provided assistance with bone sectioning.

Author Contributions

Conceived and designed the experiments: P. Muir MDM RV RPM. Performed the experiments: MSD SM KR VK ZH RPM P. Muir. Analyzed the data: MSD P. Muir. Wrote the paper: MSD SM P. Muir. Contributed limb specimens for analysis: P. Marquis.

References

1. Richardson DW (1984) Medial condylar fractures of the third metatarsal bone in horses. J Am Vet Med Assoc 185: 761–765.
2. Bassage LH, Richardson DW (1998) Longitudinal fractures of the condyles of the third metacarpal and metatarsal bones in racehorses: 224 cases (1986–1995). J Am Vet Med Assoc 212: 1757–1764.
3. Ellis DR (1994) Some observations on condylar fractures of the third metacarpus and third metatarsus in young Thoroughbreds. Equine Vet J 26: 178–183.
4. Zekas LJ, Bramlage LR, Embertson RM, Hance SR (1999) Results of treatment of 145 fractures of the third metacarpal/metatarsal condyles in 135 horses (1986–1994). Equine Vet J 31: 309–313.
5. McKee SL (1995) An update on racing fatalities in the UK. Equine Vet Educ 7: 202–204.
6. Stover SM, Murray A (2008) The California Postmortem Program: Leading the Way. Vet Clin North Am Equine Pract 24: 21–36.
7. Clegg PD (2011) Musculoskeletal disease and injury, now and the future. Part 1: Fractures and fatalities. Equine Vet J 43: 643–649.
8. Rooney JR (1974) Distal condylar fractures of the cannon bone in the horse. Mod Vet Pract 55: 113–114.
9. Kaneko M, Oikawa M, Yoshihara T (1993) Pathological analysis of bone fractures in racehorses. J Vet Med Sci 55: 181–183.
10. Krook L, Maylin G (1988) Fractures in Thoroughbred racehorses. Cornell Vet 78: 7–133.
11. Riggs CM, Whitehouse GH, Boyde A (1999) Pathology of the distal condyles of the third metacarpal and third metatarsal bone of the horse. Equine Vet J 31: 140–148.
12. Radtke CL, Danova NA, Scollay MC, Santschi EM, Markel MD, et al. (2003) Macroscopic changes in the distal ends of the condyles of the third metacarpal and third metatarsal bone in Thoroughbred racehorses with condylar fracture. Am J Vet Res 64: 1110–1116.
13. Stepnik MW, Radtke CL, Scollay MC, Oshel PE, Albrecht RM, et al. (2004) Scanning electron microscopic examination of third metacarpal/third metatarsal bone failure surfaces in Thoroughbred racehorses with condylar fracture. Vet Surg 33: 2–10.
14. Muir P, McCarthy J, Radtke CL, Markel MD, Santschi EM, et al. (2006) Role of endochondral ossification of articular cartilage and functional adaptation of the subchondral plate in the development of fatigue microcracking of joints. Bone 38: 342–349.
15. Currey JD (2003) How well are bones designed to resist fracture? J Bone Miner Res 18: 591–598,
16. Muir P, Peterson AL, Sample SJ, Scollay MC, Markel MD, et al. (2008) Exercise-induced metacarpophalangeal joint adaptation in the Thoroughbred racehorse. J Anat 213: 706–717.
17. Rubin CT, Lanyon LE (1982) Limb mechanics as a function of speed and gait: A study of function strains in the radius and tibia of the horse and dog. J Exp Biol 101: 187–211.
18. Nunamaker DM, Butterweck DM, Provost MT (1990) Fatigue fractures in Thoroughbred racehorses: Relationships with age, peak bone strain, and training. J Orthop Res 8: 604–611.
19. Reilly GC, Currey JD, Goodship AE (1997) Exercise of young Thoroughbred horses increases impact strength of the third metacarpal bone. J Orthop Res 15: 862–868.
20. Riggs CM, Whitehouse GH, Boyde A (1999) Structural variation of the distal condyles of the third metacarpal bone and third metatarsal bone in the horse. Equine Vet J 31: 130–139.
21. Boyde A, Haroon Y, Jones SJ, Riggs CM (1999) Three dimensional structure of the distal condyles of the third metacarpal bone of the horse. Equine Vet J 31: 122–129.
22. Morgan JW, Santschi EM, Zekas LJ, Scollay-Ward MC, Markel MD, et al. (2006) Comparison of radiography and computed tomography to evaluate metacarpo/metatarsophalangeal joint pathology of paired limbs of Thoroughbred racehorses with severe condylar fracture. Vet Surg 35: 611–617.
23. O'Brien T, Baker TA, Brounts SH, Sample SJ, Markel MD, et al. (2011) Detection of articular pathology of the distal aspect of the third metacarpal bone in Thoroughbred racehorses: Comparison of radiography, computed tomography, and magnetic resonance imaging. Vet Surg 40: 942–951.
24. Zekas LJ, Bramlage LR, Embertson RM, Hance SR (1999) Characterization of the type and location of fractures of the third metacarpal/metatarsal condyles in 135 horses in central Kentucky (1986–1994). Equine Vet J 31: 304–308.
25. Jacklin BD, Wright IM (2012) Frequency distributions of 174 fractures of the distal condyles of the third metacarpal and metatarsal bones in 167 Thoroughbred racehorses (1999–2009). Equine Vet J 44: 707–713.
26. Hornof WJ, O'Brien TR, Pool RR (1981) Osteochondritis dissecans of the distal metacarpus in the adult racing Thoroughbred horse. Vet Radiol 22:98–106.
27. Pool RR (1996) Pathologic manifestations of joint disease in the athletic horse. In: McIlwraith CW, Trotter GW, editors. Joint Disease in the Horse. Philadelphia: W.B Saunders. pp 87–104.
28. Burr DB, Hooser M (1995) Alterations to the en bloc basic fuchsin staining protocol for the demonstration of microdamage produced in vivo. Bone 17: 431–433.
29. Taylor D, O'Reilly P, Vallet L, Lee TC (2003) The fatigue strength of compact bone in torsion. J Biomech 36:1103–1109.
30. Barr ED, Pinchbeck GL, Clegg PD, Boyde A, Riggs CM (2009) *Post mortem* evaluation of palmar osteochondral disease (traumatic osteochondrosis) of the metacarpo/metatarsophalangeal joint in Thoroughbred racehorses. Equine Vet J 41:366–371.
31. Taylor D (1998) Fatigue of bone and bones: An analysis based on stress volume. J Orthop Res 16:163–169.
32. Estberg L, Gardner IA, Stover SM, Johnson BJ (1998) A case-crossover study of intensive racing and training schedules and risk of catastrophic musculoskeletal injury and lay-up in California Thoroughbred racehorses. Prev Vet Med 33:159–170.
33. Desbrosse FG, Vandeweerd JMEF, Perrin RAR, Clegg PD, Launois MT, et al (2008) A technique for computed tomography (CT) of the foot in the standing horse. Equine Vet Educ 20:93–98.

20

Genes Involved in the Osteoarthritis Process Identified through Genome Wide Expression Analysis in Articular Cartilage; the RAAK Study

Yolande F. M. Ramos[1,2*❦], Wouter den Hollander[1❦], Judith V. M. G. Bovée[3], Nils Bomer[1], Ruud van der Breggen[1], Nico Lakenberg[1], J. Christiaan Keurentjes[4], Jelle J. Goeman[5], P. Eline Slagboom[1,2], Rob G. H. H. Nelissen[4], Steffan D. Bos[1,2¶], Ingrid Meulenbelt[1,2¶]

1 Department of Molecular Epidemiology, Leiden University Medical Center, Leiden, The Netherlands, **2** The Netherlands Genomics Initiative, sponsored by the NCHA, Leiden-Rotterdam, The Netherlands, **3** Department of Pathology, Leiden University Medical Center, Leiden, The Netherlands, **4** Department of Orthopeadics, Leiden University Medical Center, Leiden, The Netherlands, **5** Department of Biostatistics and Bioinformatics, Leiden University Medical Center, Leiden, The Netherlands

Abstract

Objective: Identify gene expression profiles associated with OA processes in articular cartilage and determine pathways changing during the disease process.

Methods: Genome wide gene expression was determined in paired samples of OA affected and preserved cartilage of the same joint using microarray analysis for 33 patients of the RAAK study. Results were replicated in independent samples by RT-qPCR and immunohistochemistry. Profiles were analyzed with the online analysis tools DAVID and STRING to identify enrichment for specific pathways and protein-protein interactions.

Results: Among the 1717 genes that were significantly differently expressed between OA affected and preserved cartilage we found significant enrichment for genes involved in skeletal development (e.g. *TNFRSF11B* and *FRZB*). Also several inflammatory genes such as *CD55*, *PTGES* and *TNFAIP6*, previously identified in within-joint analyses as well as in analyses comparing preserved cartilage from OA affected joints versus healthy cartilage were among the top genes. Of note was the high up-regulation of *NGF* in OA cartilage. RT-qPCR confirmed differential expression for 18 out of 19 genes with expression changes of 2-fold or higher, and immunohistochemistry of selected genes showed a concordant change in protein expression. Most of these changes associated with OA severity (Mankin score) but were independent of joint-site or sex.

Conclusion: We provide further insights into the ongoing OA pathophysiological processes in cartilage, in particular into differences in macroscopically intact cartilage compared to OA affected cartilage, which seem relatively consistent and independent of sex or joint. We advocate that development of treatment could benefit by focusing on these similarities in gene expression changes and/or pathways.

Editor: Joseph Najbauer, University of Pécs Medical School, Hungary

Funding: This study was supported by the Leiden University Medical Center, the Dutch Arthritis Association, the Centre of Medical System Biology and the Netherlands Consortium for Healthy Ageing both in the framework of the Netherlands Genomics Initiative (NGI). The authors also acknowledge support by TreatOA which is funded by the European Commission framework 7 program (PF7/2007) under grant agreement no. 200800, and the European Union's Seventh Framework Program (FP7/2007-2011) under grant agreement n° 259679. The funders had no role in study design, data collection and analysis, decision to publish, or preparation of the manuscript.

Competing Interests: The authors have declared that no competing interests exist.

* Email: y.f.m.ramos@lumc.nl

❦ These authors contributed equally to this work.

¶ Shared last author position.

Introduction

Osteoarthritis (OA) is a degenerative disease of the joints causing pain and disability for an increasing proportion of the population thereby imposing a large patient and socio-economic burden [1,2]. Risk factors for OA include age, sex, joint injury, obesity, and mechanical stresses. In addition, predisposition to OA has a considerable genetic component and it has been proposed that OA can be viewed as a continuum resulting from the interaction between genetics affecting cartilage extracellular matrix composition and joint shape and sensitivity to the other factors mentioned [3,4]. Major efforts are made to identify loci associated with OA susceptibility to elucidate underlying mechanisms [5]. Treatment options to slow down or reverse the OA process are still very limited and at the time of diagnosis the damage is already irreversible. Together, this emphasizes the importance to increase insight into the disease process and to identify genes and pathways involved in development of OA. A way to achieve this is by investigating the pathophysiological processes in articular cartilage by means of gene expression analyses.

Initially, expression profiles were established for cartilage from knee OA joints in comparison to healthy joints using only a limited number of genes [6]. More recently, exploratory genome wide expression profiling has been performed for the intact cartilage of hip and knee OA joints of patients undergoing joint replacement surgery compared to non-OA joints either derived from autopsies or from neck of femur fractures [7,8]. These studies showed that many genes involved in extracellular matrix (ECM) production as well as genes involved in ECM degradation or in inflammation were changed. Together, this resulted in significant enrichment for genes involved in skeletal development and response to external stimuli. Although studies that compare healthy cartilage with the preserved cartilage of joints from OA patients are very useful to acquire insight into the pathogenetic differences, the findings are likely biased by confounding factors such as innate differences, age, and stratification by joint. Moreover, due to the study design distinction between age-related changes and early or late changes of OA pathophysiology is hampered.

One of the characteristics of OA is focal loss of articular cartilage, resulting in areas of degradation as well as areas with a relative preservation of cartilage thickness and appearance in the joint. Insight into gene expression specific for the focal areas of cartilage degradation compared to those in preserved areas can provide clues towards dynamic changes of genes and pathways involved in OA pathophysiology independent of confounding factors such as age. Gene expression profiles of cartilage from OA affected and macroscopically preserved areas of the same joint have been determined before, however, in most of these studies limited numbers of donors (4–5 knee joints) were included [9–11].

As part of the ongoing Research Arthritis and Articular Cartilage (RAAK) study we set out to perform genome wide analysis of differential gene expression by comparing 33 pairs of matched OA affected and preserved cartilage samples, originating from the same joint of patients that underwent total joint replacement of either hip or knee. Results provide further insights in the ongoing OA disease processes in cartilage, in particular into differences in macroscopically intact cartilage compared to OA affected cartilage.

Materials and Methods

Ethics statement

Participants of the RAAK study provided written informed consent. The ongoing RAAK study and its consent procedure is approved by the institutional ethics review committee (Commissie Medische Ethiek of the Leiden University Medical Center; protocol no. P08.239).

Discovery cohort

The RAAK study is aimed at the biobanking of joint materials as well as mesenchymal stem cells and primary chondrocytes from patients and controls in the Leiden University Medical Center and collaborating outpatient clinics in the Leiden area. In the current study we used paired preserved and OA affected cartilage samples for 33 donors undergoing joint replacement surgery for primary OA (22 hips, 11 knees). Characteristics of the donors are shown in Table S1.

At the moment of collection (within 2 hours following surgery) tissue was washed extensively with phosphate buffered saline (PBS) to decrease the risk of contamination by blood. Cartilage was classified macroscopically and collected separately from OA affected and preserved regions around the weight-bearing area of the joint (Figure S1). Classification was done based on predefined features of OA related damage as described previously [9,10]: color/whiteness of the cartilage, surface integrity as determined by visible fibrillation/crack formation, and depth and hardness of the cartilage upon sampling with a scalpel. Care was taken to avoid contamination with bone or synovium. Collected cartilage was snap frozen in liquid nitrogen and stored at −80°C prior to RNA extraction.

Validation and replication cohort

Validation was performed by RT-qPCR in 8 sample pairs of the discovery cohort (3 knee and 5 hip) and for replication of the results we included 28 additional matched sample pairs (20 knee, 8 hip) of similar mean age (shown in Table S1). Sampling procedures were according to the discovery cohort.

RNA isolation

Cartilage samples were pulverized using a Retsch MM200 under cryogenic conditions. On average 150 mg of pulverized cartilage was dissolved in 1 ml of Trizol reagent, and mixed vigorously. After addition of 200 µl of chloroform the sample was mixed and centrifuged for 15 minutes (16,000 g). The clear aqueous layer was transferred to a new vial and 1 volume of 70% ethanol/DEPC-treated water was added to precipitate RNA. RNA was collected using Qiagen mini columns according to the manufacturers protocol and quality was assessed using a Bioanalyzer lab-on-a-chip. RNA integrity numbers above 8 were considered suitable for microarray analysis.

Microarrays

After *in vitro* transcription, amplification, and labeling with biotin-labeled nucleotides (Illumina TotalPrep RNA Amplification Kit) Illumina HumanHT-12 v3 microarrays were hybridized. Sample pairs were randomly dispersed over the microarrays, however each pair was measured on a single chip. Microarrays were read using an Illumina Beadarray 500GX scanner and after basic quality checks using Beadstudio software data were analyzed in R statistical programming language. Intensity values were normalized using the "rsn" option in the Lumi-package and absence of large scale between-chip effects was confirmed using the Globaltest-package in which the individual chip numbers were tested for association to the raw data [12]. After removal of probes that were not reliably detected (detection $P>0.05$ in more than 50% of the samples) a paired t-test was performed for the remaining 13277 probes comprising 11421 unique genes on all sample pairs while adjusting for chip (to adjust for possible batch effects) and using multiple testing correction as implemented in the "BH" (Benjamini and Hochberg) option in the Limma-package. Analyses for differential expression between OA and healthy and between preserved and healthy cartilage was performed likewise, adjusting in addition for sex and for age.

Gene expression profiles of the samples have been deposited in NCBI's Gene Expression Omnibus [13] and are accessible through GEO Series accession number GSE57218.

Quantitative reverse transcription PCR (RT-qPCR)

0.5 µg of total RNA was processed with the First Strand cDNA Synthesis Kit according to the manufacturer's protocol (Roche Applied Science) and RT-qPCR was performed for the 19 genes showing at least 2-fold expression differences in the microarray analysis (Taqman gene expression assays used are listed in Table S2) using the Biomark 96.96 Dynamic Arrays Fluidigm RT-qPCR platform [14]. Relative gene expressions were calculated with the

$2^{-\Delta\Delta Ct}$ method [15], using household gene Beta Actin (*ACTB*) expression as internal standard.

Immunohistochemistry and staining analysis

For histological examination, joints were fixed using a 4% formaldehyde solution. Subsequently, samples were decalcified using a 10% EDTA solution and embedded in paraffin. Sections (5 µm) adjacent to the collected area were stained using hematoxilin and eosin (H&E) and toluidine blue. Immunohistochemistry was performed for SERPINE1 (mouse monoclonal antibody from American Diagnostica Inc.) without antigen retrieval and for CD55 (rabbit polyclonal antibody from Santa Cruz Biotechnology Inc.) with heat antigen retrieval (0,01 M Citratebuffer pH = 6.0) as described previously [16].

Quantification of OA related cartilage damage was scored by 2 observers (JVMGB and YFMR) according to Mankin *et al* [17]. Quantification of SERPINE1 expression was performed by scoring staining of chondrocytes in the superficial, middle, and deep cartilage layer with a score of 0 (no staining), 1 (moderate staining), or 2 (strong staining). Using Generalized Estimating Equations, scores were summed and used as a predictor variable with Mankin score as outcome whilst correcting for sex and age of each donor.

Pathway analysis and protein-protein interaction

Gene enrichment among the 1717 genes showing significant differential expression was performed with the Database for Annotation, Visualization and Integrated Discovery (DAVID) tool [18] selecting for biological processes identified in the Gene Ontology database (GOTERM_BP_FAT in the options menu implemented in DAVID), selecting for cell compartment (GOTERM_CC_FAT), or selecting for molecular function (GOTERM_MF_FAT) and using the microarray background (HumanHT-12_V3_0_R2_11283641_A). Pathways with $P \leq 0.05$ after correction for multiple testing according to Bonferroni were considered significant (Bonferroni corrections were performed by multiplying the raw P-values with the number of genes included in the analysis).

Enrichment in protein-protein interactions among the significant genes was analyzed with the Search Tool for the Retrieval of Interacting Genes/Proteins (STRING) 9.0 [19] available online.

Literature based candidate genes

Based on selected publications of genome wide association study meta-analyses [20–29] we investigated our expression dataset for evidence of differential gene expression of the reported significant candidate genes.

Results

Differential expression between preserved and OA affected cartilage

To identify genes with changed expression in response to ongoing OA processes genome wide expression profiles were generated for preserved and OA affected cartilage of the same joint of 33 donors. Characteristics of the donors are shown in Table S1. Males (N = 13) and females (N = 20) included in the study were aged between 54 and 80 years (mean age: 66.2). In total, 22 patients received a hip replacement and 11 patients underwent total knee replacement. Among all OA joints included in this study (61 in total), 28 pairs were randomly selected to assess the Mankin scores of preserved and affected areas. Mankin scores were significantly higher in the samples macroscopically designated as 'OA affected' as compared to sections distinguished as 'preserved' (mean Mankin score 7.8 vs. 4.7, respectively, $P = 4 \times 10^{-4}$, paired t-test) and as a result gene expression differences can be directly linked to these differences in Mankin scores.

After normalization and correction for multiple testing, significant differential expression between the OA affected and preserved cartilage was identified for 1893 probes, representing 1717 unique genes (Table S3). Among the 1717 unique genes 19 were differently expressed with fold-changes of 2 and higher (Table 1). Notably, 14 of these were up-regulated in OA as compared to preserved cartilage and only 5 were down-regulated. Overall, 748 (44%) of the differentially expressed genes were up-regulated. Larger fold changes were observed in expression of genes well known for their association with OA cartilage such as tumor necrosis factor alpha-induced protein 6 (*TNFAIP6* also known as *TSG-6*, 2.9-fold up in OA cartilage; $P = 4.4 \times 10^{-8}$), cytokine receptor-like factor 1 (*CRLF1*, 3-fold up in OA cartilage; $P = 4.4 \times 10^{-8}$), and *Wnt*-inhibitor frizzled related protein beta (*FRZB*, 2.5-fold down in OA cartilage; $P = 1.3 \times 10^{-6}$). A notable gene highly up-regulated in OA cartilage was neuronal growth factor (*NGF*, 2.3-fold up; $P = 3.4 \times 10^{-7}$).

Validation of the 19 genes with fold-changes of 2 or higher in 8 sample pairs used in the microarray analyses by means of RT-qPCR showed similar effect sizes and directions as those found in the microarray analysis (Table S5). Replication performed in an additional set of 28 independent preserved and affected cartilage sample pairs also showed comparable effect sizes and directions and, except for cysteine-rich secretory protein LCCL domain-containing 1 precursor (*CRISPLD1*), all genes were significantly different expressed (Table 1). Individual expression boxplots of the replicated genes are shown in Figure S2.

Expression profiles of genes with fold-changes of 2 and higher were analyzed for association with Mankin score as a grade of disease severity (Table 2). Almost all genes associated with Mankin score, except for *COL9A1*, *HBA2* and *HBB*. To further characterize expression of the 19 genes with highest fold changes in OA affected cartilage, we investigated whether the observed changes were either joint or sex specific. As shown in Table 2, for most of the genes fold changes of the (joint or sex) stratified analyses were highly comparable and not statistically different from those of the discovery analysis. However, increased expression of pregnancy-associated plasma protein A (*PAPPA*) was significantly less pronounced in knee OA (1.3-fold increase) than in hip OA (2.6-fold increase).

In addition to the gene expression profiles of preserved and OA affected cartilage, gene expression profiles were also generated for 7 healthy cartilage (characteristics of the donors are shown in Table S1) and explored for the 19 genes. For most of these 19 genes we did not find significant differences between healthy and preserved cartilage. However, when analyzing the trend of the differences between healthy, preserved and OA affected cartilage we did find a significant linear effect on the expression of most genes. In contrast, expression changes of *CRISPLD1* and *COL9A1* in healthy versus preserved cartilage were not significant and appeared to be increased while the expression in preserved versus OA affected cartilage was found to be decreased (Figure S3).

Functional annotation of genes differently expressed in OA affected cartilage

To investigate whether the genes differently expressed between preserved and OA affected cartilage belonged to specific pathways, we used the online functional annotation tool DAVID. Seven GO-terms referring to 6 independent pathways were identified

Table 1. Genes significantly differently expressed in OA affected cartilage.

Gene symbol	Function	Discovery FC	Discovery Dir.	Discovery Pval	Replication FC	Replication Dir.	Replication Pval
TNFAIP6	cartilage development	2.90	Up	4.40×10^{-8}	4.01	Up	3.61×10^{-4}
CRLF1	immune response	2.97	Up	4.40×10^{-8}	4.01	Up	8.09×10^{-6}
LEPREL1	cartilage development	2.37	Up	4.40×10^{-8}	2.88	Up	9.49×10^{-4}
CD55	complement cascade	2.39	Up	4.40×10^{-8}	3.00	Up	5.18×10^{-5}
RARRES2	immune response	2.26	Down	6.06×10^{-8}	3.32	Down	1.23×10^{-4}
NGF	neurogenesis	2.26	Up	3.36×10^{-7}	4.54	Up	2.50×10^{-5}
FRZB	bone development	2.54	Down	1.28×10^{-6}	3.04	Down	4.39×10^{-4}
SERPINE1	complement cascade	2.40	Up	1.30×10^{-6}	3.13	Up	1.54×10^{-4}
PTGES	immune response	2.34	Up	1.46×10^{-6}	3.29	Up	1.76×10^{-5}
SPP1	ECM-receptor interaction	2.53	Up	3.40×10^{-6}	2.56	Up	7.05×10^{-3}
CXCL14	immune response	2.16	Up	3.54×10^{-6}	4.97	Up	1.01×10^{-4}
TNFRSF11B	bone development	2.10	Up	4.23×10^{-6}	2.69	Up	6.58×10^{-4}
FN1	ECM-receptor interaction	2.31	Up	1.13×10^{-5}	1.52	Up	3.28×10^{-2}
HBA2	oxygen transport	2.26	Up	2.02×10^{-5}	2.97	Up	6.15×10^{-3}
HBB	oxygen transport	2.00	Up	6.97×10^{-5}	2.50	Up	1.69×10^{-2}
PAPPA	wound healing	2.08	Up	7.69×10^{-5}	2.25	Up	4.05×10^{-3}
CRISPLD1	–	2.50	Down	1.42×10^{-4}	1.05	–	7.54×10^{-1}
COL9A1	cartilage development	2.18	Down	2.67×10^{-4}	3.14	Down	2.27×10^{-4}
CHRDL2	cartilage development	2.39	Down	3.55×10^{-4}	5.33	Down	5.71×10^{-4}

Shown are results of the microarray analysis (Discovery) and the replication for genes with at least 2-fold change (Dir.: direction of effects relative to OA; FC: fold change; Pval: P-value).

Table 2. Characteristics of the replicated genes.

		Hip		Knee	Male		Female		
Gene symbol	**pVal$_{Mankin}$**	**FC**	**pVal**	**FC**	**pVal**	**FC**	**pVal**	**FC**	**pVal**
TNFAIP6	1.E-05	2.80	3.89E-05	3.10	6.19E-03	3.09	7.88E-04	2.78	2.11E-04
CRLF1	3.E-07	2.93	1.49E-04	3.06	1.47E-03	3.51	1.22E-03	2.67	2.34E-04
LEPREL1	5.E-15	2.50	3.85E-05	2.12	1.67E-02	2.90	7.88E-04	2.07	2.52E-04
CD55	8.E-11	2.67	3.85E-05	1.92	6.86E-03	2.63	1.53E-03	2.25	2.34E-04
RARRES2	6.E-08	0.42	3.85E-05	0.48	3.18E-02	0.44	5.51E-03	0.44	2.11E-04
NGF	2.E-09	2.39	1.49E-04	2.03	7.26E-03	2.68	5.48E-03	2.02	2.69E-04
FRZB	1.E-05	0.35	1.30E-04	0.50	3.67E-02	0.36	3.20E-03	0.41	1.95E-03
SERPINE1	1.E-03	2.40	6.10E-04	2.41	6.19E-03	2.64	8.36E-03	2.26	1.15E-03
PTGES	5.E-05	2.40	3.54E-04	2.21	1.70E-02	2.81	5.05E-03	2.07	1.84E-03
SPP1	3.E-05	2.56	1.94E-04	2.46	5.87E-02	2.64	9.09E-03	2.45	2.36E-03
CXCL14	2.E-04	2.49	1.87E-04	1.63	3.16E-02	2.73	9.09E-03	1.85	1.29E-03
TNFRSF11B	1.E-05	2.27	1.87E-04	1.80	8.65E-02	2.63	8.10E-03	1.82	2.71E-03
FN1	9.E-05	2.64	1.49E-04	1.83	1.40E-01	2.89	9.35E-03	2.00	4.48E-03
HBA2	1.E-01	2.46	1.01E-03	1.91	5.04E-02	1.96	2.46E-02	2.49	2.87E-03
HBB	2.E-01	2.17	1.50E-03	1.70	1.30E-01	1.72	2.86E-02	2.21	5.56E-03
PAPPA	2.E-05	2.59	4.68E-04	1.34	1.98E-01	2.22	4.79E-02	1.99	6.10E-03
CRISPLD1	6.E-02	0.38	5.98E-03	0.44	4.28E-02	0.36	2.56E-03	0.43	3.47E-02
COL9A1	6.E-01	0.42	6.24E-03	0.54	6.46E-02	0.42	4.95E-03	0.49	4.52E-02
CHRDL2	3.E-04	0.37	3.56E-03	0.52	2.09E-01	0.34	2.70E-02	0.48	3.50E-02

Results of the analysis for association of the genes with Mankin score and for joint- and sex-stratified analyses.

(Table 3). The most significant GO-term was observed for "skeletal system development". This term captured several of the genes with fold-changes of 2 or higher (e.g. *FRZB* and *TNFRSF11B*). Furthermore, of note was the GO-term referring to "extracellular matrix organization" including decorin (*DCN*) and several collagens (e.g. *COL1A2*, *COL2A1*, *COL3A1*). When analyzing for enrichment using the cellular compartment option, most significant GO-term was "extracellular matrix", and analyzing for molecular function showed genes involved in "copper ion binding" and "glycosaminoglycan binding" to be significantly enriched (Table 3).

Among the 19 genes that were highly changed in OA affected cartilage (at least 2-fold), 3 pathways were significantly enriched with lowest P-value for GO-term "response to wounding" (Table 4), which included the genes *TNFAIP6*, *SERPINE2*, and *CD55*. When analyzing for interaction among proteins encoded by these genes using STRING, we found significant enrichment for protein-protein interactions ($P = 4.7 \times 10^{-10}$) in which fibronectin-1 (*FN1*) seemed to play a central role considering that 6 of the 19 proteins were found to relate to *FN1* (Figure 1).

Immunohistochemical assessment of proteins encoded by genes identified in the microarray analysis

In addition to differential expression of proteins encoded by genes found in the microarray analysis, immunohistochemical (IHC) staining provides insight in expression pattern and localization of differentially expressed genes in the different cartilage layers. Therefore, as a proof of principal, IHC was performed for SERPINE1 and CD55. Figure 2 shows representative sections for the staining of preserved (P) versus OA affected cartilage, with Figure 2A and B showing an example of the H&E and Toluidine blue staining respectively (upper panel: 4x magnification, lower panel 20x magnification).

Immunohistochemistry for SERPINE1 showed that the protein is expressed in chondrocytes and differential expression between OA and preserved cartilage at the protein level was very pronounced (Figure 2C). In OA affected cartilage, SERPINE1 was not only expressed in the superficial layer, but also in the middle layer. In the most affected parts, we even observed SERPINE1 protein expression in chondrocytes residing in the deep zone. In addition, increasing matrix staining of SERPINE1 was observed with increasing OA affection state. We performed a quantification of the staining as described in Materials and Methods, and statistical analysis showed a significant difference between protein abundance in OA and preserved cartilage ($P = 2.4 \times 10^{-4}$). The expression difference seemed to correlate mostly with toluidine blue staining, and thus with the level of proteoglycan constituents of chondromucin aggregates in the samples ($P = 2.9 \times 10^{-9}$).

CD55 protein expression was most pronounced in the superficial layer, with higher levels in the more OA affected zones of the cartilage, while hardly any CD55 positive cells were detected in the deep layer (Figure 2D). The differences, however, were more subtle than for SERPINE1 and the range in the quantification did not allow for statistical analysis.

Prioritization of genes residing in compelling genome wide association signals

In order to explore whether genes identified by genome wide association studies are active in cartilage and/or change in response to the OA process, we screened for differential expression of genes originating from recently published large scale meta analyses on OA (Table 5). Sixteen of the 29 genes selected were well detected in the microarray ($P_{detection} \leq 0.05$) and from these, 8 were significantly different between OA and preserved cartilage. Most genes showed only modest expression changes. Of note was differential expression of the HMG-box transcription factor 1 (*HBP1*) gene, identified in the Rotterdam study [24], which showed 1.1-fold up-regulation in OA cartilage ($P = 2.0 \times 10^{-3}$).

Discussion

As part of the RAAK study we compared genome wide expression levels between preserved and OA affected cartilage of the same joint from 33 donors. Such a paired study design allows the detection of genes specifically involved in the OA pathophysiological process, independent of inter-individual or age-related confounding factors as also reflected by the highly comparable differential gene expression patterns when stratifying according to joint and sex. After correction for multiple testing 1717 unique genes showed significant differential expression, of which 19 genes had a fold-change of 2 or higher. In an independent paired cartilage sample set, differential expression was confirmed for 18 genes by RT-qPCR. For most of these genes, except *HBA2*, *HBB*, and *COL9A1*, expression associated with disease severity as determined by scoring according to Mankin [17], and OA-associated increase in protein expression for 2 genes (*CD55* and *SERPINE1*) was demonstrated by immunohistochemistry.

We confirmed several genes previously identified in within-joint analyses for OA affected versus preserved cartilage as well as analyses comparing preserved cartilage from OA affected joints versus healthy cartilage such as the inflammatory genes *CD55* [8], *PTGES* and *TNFAIP6* [11]. This overlap is noteworthy since in our analysis considerably more samples were included. A large sample size increases power to detect replicable findings and allows detection of differences that were previously missed or more subtle. Our data thus indicate that at least a number of genes are consistently involved in the OA disease process despite the appreciated heterogeneous pathophysiology. Another gene present among the top genes and highly up-regulated in OA affected cartilage was the tumor necrosis factor receptor superfamily 11b (*TNFRSF11B*) gene encoding osteoprotegerin. Very recently we reported in this protein on a gain of function mutation likely causal in a family with early onset OA with chondrocalcinosis [30]. In this respect, the up-regulated expression, could contribute to respective mineralization of the cartilage and eventually formation of bone, a major hallmark of the ongoing osteoarthritis disease process.

Studies comparing intact cartilage with OA affected cartilage of the same joint allow detection of gene expression changes specific to the ongoing OA pathophysiological processes independent of confounding factors such as sex and age and joint as was also demonstrated by the highly comparable results of our stratified analysis. Identification of such genes commonly changing during OA independent of joint site or sex could be very useful with respect to drug development. On the other hand, differences identified between the intact cartilage derived from patients undergoing joint replacement surgery and healthy cartilage of independent joints are of a cross-sectional nature and provide information on innate differences among OA patients as well as genes changing during OA. Therefore, genes overlapping among the different studies may be of interest to better understand dynamic changes during onset and ongoing OA. A notable example was the expression of the *COL9A1* gene that was higher in preserved as compared to healthy cartilage (3.6-fold), but was subsequently decreased in the OA affected cartilage (Figure S3).

Table 3. Gene enrichment analysis in OA affected versus preserved cartilage.

Analysis option:	GO-Term	Count	Pct.	Enr.	Pval	$Pval_{adj}$	FDR
Biological Processes	GO:0001501~skeletal system development	59	3.86	2.12	5.21×10^{-8}	7.97×10^{-5}	9.53×10^{-5}
Biological Processes	GO:0007167~enzyme linked receptor protein signaling pathway	56	3.66	1.88	5.74×10^{-6}	8.78×10^{-3}	1.05×10^{-2}
Biological Processes	GO:0008285~negative regulation of cell proliferation	57	3.73	1.81	1.52×10^{-5}	2.32×10^{-2}	2.77×10^{-2}
Biological Processes	GO:0005996~monosaccharide metabolic process	40	2.61	2.07	1.64×10^{-5}	2.51×10^{-2}	3.00×10^{-2}
Biological Processes	GO:0030198~extracellular matrix organization	24	1.57	2.67	2.10×10^{-5}	3.22×10^{-2}	3.85×10^{-2}
Biological Processes	GO:0007155~cell adhesion	93	6.08	1.53	3.11×10^{-5}	4.76×10^{-2}	5.69×10^{-2}
Biological Processes	GO:0022610~biological adhesion	93	6.08	1.53	3.30×10^{-5}	5.06×10^{-2}	6.04×10^{-2}
Cellular Compartment	GO:0031012~extracellular matrix	69	4.51	2.26	1.49E-10	2.29E-07	2.19E-07
Cellular Compartment	GO:0005578~proteinaceous extracellular matrix	65	4.25	2.03	2.63E-10	4.02E-07	3.86E-07
Cellular Compartment	GO:0044421~extracellular region part	133	8.69	1.56	1.10E-07	1.68E-04	1.61E-04
Cellular Compartment	GO:0044420~extracellular matrix part	30	1.96	2.90	2.16E-07	3.31E-04	3.17E-04
Cellular Compartment	GO:0005581~collagen	14	0.92	4.45	5.20E-06	7.95E-03	7.62E-03
Molecular Function	GO:0005507~copper ion binding	19	1.24	3.36	6.69E-06	1.02E-02	1.08E-02
Molecular Function	GO:0005539~glycosaminoglycan binding	29	1.90	2.40	1.99E-05	3.04E-02	3.20E-02
Molecular Function	GO:0005198~structural molecule activity	84	5.49	1.58	2.52E-05	3.85E-02	4.06E-02

Analysis considering the biological processes option in DAVID (GOTERM_BP_FAT), the cellular compartment option (GOTERM_CC_FAT), or the molecular function option (GOTERM_MF_FAT) as indicated in the first column, using medium classification stringency for all genes significantly differently expressed between OA affected and preserved cartilage (GO-Term: GO-terms within the different clusters; Count: number of genes identified for the respective GO-term; Pct: percentage of genes from total number of genes tested; Enr.: fold enrichment of indicated pathway; Pval: P-value; $Pval_{adj}$: adjusted P-value; FDR: false discovery rate).

Table 4. Gene enrichment analysis.

Term	Count	Pct	Enr.	Pval	$Pval_{adj}$	FDR
GO:0009611~response to wounding	6	31.58	8.87	2.96E-04	5.63E-03	3.94E-01
GO:0001501~skeletal system development	5	26.32	12.10	4.95E-04	9.40E-03	6.58E-01
GO:0006954~inflammatory response	5	26.32	12.06	5.01E-04	9.51E-03	6.65E-01

Pathway analysis considering the biological processes option in DAVID (GOTERM_BP_FAT) using the genes from Table 1 with at least 2-fold expression difference between OA affected and preserved cartilage (GO-Term: GO-terms within the different clusters; Count: number of genes identified for the respective GO-term; Pct: percentage of genes from total number of genes tested; Enr.: fold enrichment of indicated pathway; Pval: P-value; $Pval_{adj}$: adjusted P-value; FDR: false discovery rate).

Although we acknowledge the fact that the included 7 healthy cartilage samples had a large age-range, our results are in line with the findings of Karlsson *et al* [8] and Xu *et al* [7] showing increased expression of *COL9A1* in cartilage from patients undergoing joint replacement surgery in comparison to healthy cartilage. This altered direction of effect in ongoing OA may explain the fact that *COL9A1* was found not to be associated with Mankin score and suggests that it is mainly involved in the initial response of the chondrocyte to cartilage damage. Gene enrichment analyses performed with all significant genes showed especially that genes involved in the skeletal development were changed in OA affected as compared to preserved cartilage. Notably, this is in accordance with observations from Xu *et al* [7] who found enrichment of genes involved in skeletal development by comparing healthy cartilage versus cartilage of OA affected joints, suggesting that this is a pathway commonly affected in OA cartilage, both in the initiation phases as well as in ongoing OA. The fact that genes involved in skeletal development (e.g. *FRZB* and *TNFRSF11B*, but also *OSTF1*, *FGFR3*, and *IGFBP3*; Table S3) change during ongoing OA processes confirms the hypothesis that OA chondrocytes lose their maturational arrested phenotype, specific for articular cartilage, towards their end-stage differentiation, resembling growth plate during skeletal development [3].

As reviewed by Barter and Young [31], gene expression differences in OA affected tissues may originate from changes in epigenetic control mechanisms. More recently, a comparison between the methylome of hip OA cartilage with cartilage of non-OA hips indeed showed more than 5000 differentially methylated loci whereas the annotated genes were mainly involved in pathways related to skeletal development [32] similar to the current and previous transcriptomic analyses [7]. Although direct association between such changes in DNA methylation and respective gene expression remains to be demonstrated, the skeletal developmental processes appear to consistently mark ongoing OA pathophysiology.

Recently, a GWAS for hand OA identified a locus in the aldehyde dehydrogenase 1 family, member A2 (*ALDH1A2*) gene [33]. Expression of *ALDH1A2* was shown to be allele dependent and with decreased expression in OA affected cartilage. Despite this and other recent successes of genome wide association studies [24,28] a variety of the identified signals indicate chromosomal regions without obvious OA candidate genes or regions of high linkage disequilibrium with many relative unknown genes [24,28].

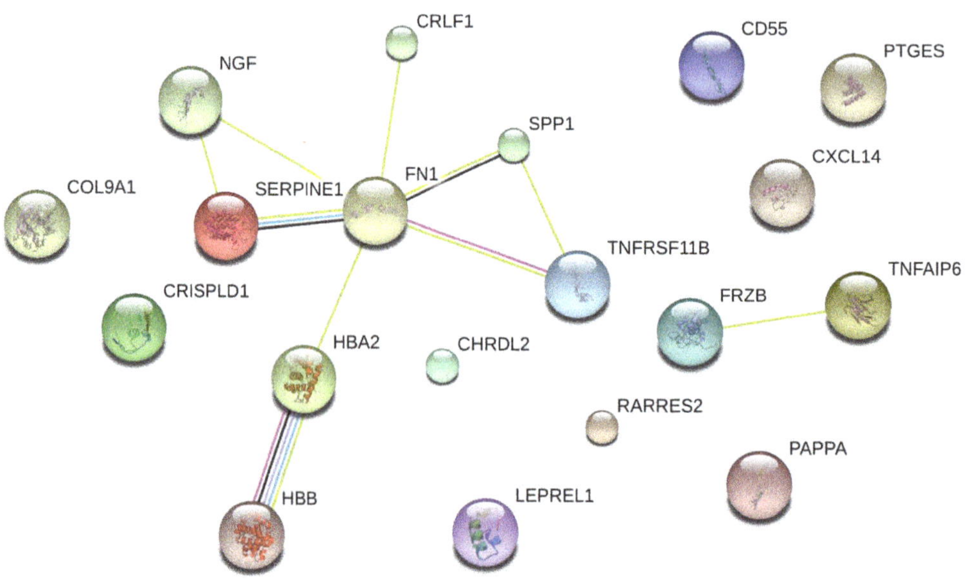

Figure 1. Protein-protein interaction between the genes with expression changes of at least 2-fold (Table 1) as determined with STRING.

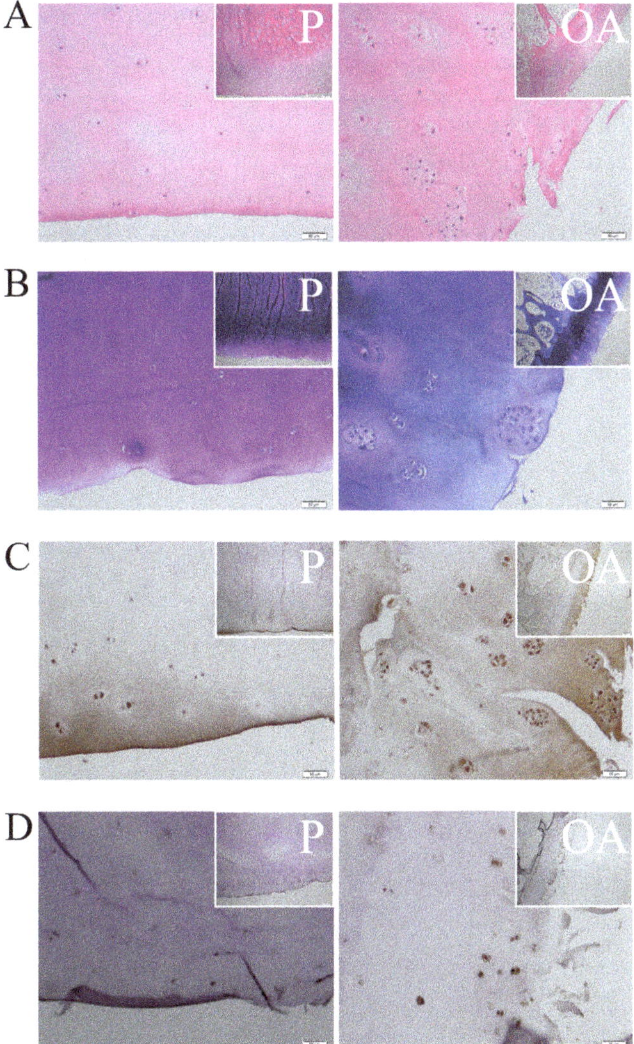

Figure 2. Representative slides of immunohistochemical staining. A) H&E staining. B) Toluidine blue staining. C) SERPINE1. D) CD55 (magnification 20x; insets show larger overview at magnification 4x; white scale bars indicate 50 μm and 200 μm, respectively). The left panels show preserved cartilage area (P) and the right panels show the OA affected cartilage area (OA).

Here, we provide a means of exploring the overall expression and behavior during disease in cartilage. Although OA should be considered a 'whole joint disease' [2] and expression profiles of other OA affected joint tissues such as those performed recently in subchondral bone [34] are highly valuable, expression profiles in OA cartilage could serve as one of the selection criteria to prioritize genes for functional follow-up studies and research directed at understanding pathophysiological mechanisms of OA and drug design. In our cartilage dataset, we found differential expression for several of the genes, among which *PAPPA* was most significant ($P = 1.1 \times 10^{-6}$), positionally localized in close neighborhood of one the arcOGEN genome wide hits: rs4836732 within the *ASTN2* gene. The exact linkage disequilibrium across this locus needs to be further explored. We also found *HBP1*, at the chr7q22 locus, to be differently expressed, although with small effect size in the OA versus preserved comparison (1.1-fold higher in OA affected cartilage). When comparing diseased cartilage (OA affected as well as macroscopically intact cartilage) with healthy cartilage we observed a much stronger and opposite direction of effects: healthy versus OA and healthy versus preserved both showed 1.4-fold lower expression (Table S4) in accordance with a previous study by Raine *et al.* showing increased expression of *HBP1* in OA affected cartilage [35]. Given that *HBP1* resides in the 7q22 gene cluster [24] results mark this gene as most likely candidate for further functional follow-up investigations.

Although *MCF2L* (MCF.2 cell line derived transforming sequence-like), a gene previously identified in GWA as an OA susceptibility gene [22], was not well-detected in the microarray analysis, the significant increased expression of neuronal growth factor (*NGF*) is worth mentioning in this respect. Neurotrophin-3 (NT3), another member of the NGF-family of proteins, enhances migration of premyelinating Schwann cells via Dbs/MCF2L [36], possibly implicating nociception in OA. Interestingly, antibodies generated against NGF or its receptor have been used successfully to treat OA patients and effectively reduced their pain [37]. The fact that *NGF* was not identified previously by comparing healthy with OA affected cartilage [7,8] suggests that *NGF* may be more specific for the "late" OA process. Alternatively, selection of druggable targets from early-responsive genes that start changing

Table 5. Genes identified in robust genome wide approaches with fold-changes and P-values for OA versus preserved cartilage (OA vs P).

			OA vs P	
Gene	**Ref**	**Joint published**	**FC**	**Pval**
ASTN2	[28]	Hip&Knee	–	–
BCAP29	[24]	Knee	1.1	1.7×10^{-2}
BTNL2	[26]	Knee	–	–
C6ORF130	[27]	Hip&Knee	0.88	1.6×10^{-3}
CDC5L	[28]	Hip&Knee	–	–
CHST11	[28]	Hip&Knee	–	–
COG5	[24]	Knee	0.98	2.1×10^{-1}
COL11A1	[27]	Hip&Knee	0.94	4.5×10^{-1}
DOT1L	[20]	Hip	–	–
DUS4L	[24]	Knee	–	–
DVWA	[25]	Knee	–	–
FILIP1	[28]	Hip&Knee	–	–
FTO	[28]	Hip&Knee	1.0	8.5×10^{-1}
GDF5	[21]	Hip&Knee	1.1	4.3×10^{-2}
GLT8D1	[28]	Hip&Knee	1.0	3.0×10^{-1}
GNL3	[28]	Hip&Knee	1.1	4.6×10^{-2}
GPR22	[24]	Knee	–	–
HBP1	[24]	Knee	1.1	2.0×10^{-3}
HLA-DQB1	[26]	Knee	–	–
KLHDC5	[28]	Hip&Knee	1.0	4.8×10^{-1}
MCF2L	[22]	Hip&Knee	–	–
MICAL3	[27]	Hip&Knee	–	–
NCOA3	[23]	Hip	0.93	7.9×10^{-3}
PAPPA	[28]	Hip&Knee	2.1	1.1×10^{-6}
PRKAR2B	[24]	Knee	1.0	9.9×10^{-1}
PTHLH	[28]	Hip&Knee	1.4	1.8×10^{-3}
SENP6	[28]	Hip&Knee	1.1	3.3×10^{-1}
SUPT3H	[28]	Hip&Knee	1.0	6.1×10^{-1}
TP63	[28]	Hip&Knee	–	–
VEGF	[29]	Hip	1.0	4.5×10^{-1}

(Ref: reference, where indicated gene was published as OA susceptibility gene; Pval: nominal P-value; FC: fold change; –: not detected on microarray).

before damage is irreversible could be more eligible to effectively slow-down or stop the OA process.

The sample collection is performed by well-trained lab personnel, however, we cannot exclude the possibility of minor contamination with bone tissue. In this respect, it is of note that several cartilage-specific genes (e.g. decorin or *DCN*, collagen type 2 A1 (*COL2A1*), cartilage intermediate layer protein (*CILP*), and cartilage oligomeric matrix protein (*COMP*) were amongst the 100 genes with highest levels of expression in the dataset while no bone-specific genes (e.g. *COL1A1, COL1A2, TNFRSF11B*, and bone sialoprotein II or *IBSP*) were identified here.

In conclusion, our results add to the insight into the ongoing pathological processes in OA cartilage by the identification of different gene expression patterns depending on OA severity as determined by Mankin score. This large scale analysis of joint-matched OA affected and preserved cartilage seems to hint at relatively consistent changes in gene expression during OA development. We think research and development of OA treatment could benefit by focusing on these similarities in gene expression changes and/or pathways.

Supporting Information

Figure S1 Typical example of hip (A) and knee (B) joint with areas of macroscopically preserved (arrow head) and OA affected cartilage (arrow; white scale bars indicate 500 mm). Insets show detail of preserved (right) and OA affected area (left), in A separated by a dashed line (scale bar inset in B: 250 mm).

Figure S2 Individual box plots per status for genes validated by RT-qPCR.

Figure S3 Relative changes in gene expression levels in preserved and OA affected cartilage relative to healthy

cartilage for the 19 genes with at least 2-fold difference in the OA versus preserved analysis (note that the line does not imply continues changes given the fact that the healthy cartilage was derived from independent donors).

Table S1 Characteristics of OA donors included in the microarray analyses (discovery) and in the replication and characteristics of the healthy donors included in the microarray analysis.

Table S2 Taqman probes used in the fluidigm RT-qPCR experiment.

Table S3 Genes significantly differently expressed between OA and preserved cartilage in microarray analysis of 33 paired OA affected and preserved samples (FC: fold change; Pval: P-value; highlighted in yellow the genes that are also significantly different in the healthy versus preserved cartilage comparison).

Table S4 Genes significantly differently expressed between preserved and healthy cartilage (FC: fold change; Pval: P-value).

Table S5 Results of the validation of the genes with at least 2-fold significant differential expression between OA affected and preserved cartilage in the microarray analyses (Dir: direction of effects; FC: fold change; Pval: P-value).

Acknowledgments

We thank I. Briaire-de Bruin for expert technical assistance with the immunohistochemistry.

Author Contributions

Conceived and designed the experiments: YR PS SB IM. Performed the experiments: YR WH RB NL NB SB. Analyzed the data: YR WH SB JG JB IM. Contributed reagents/materials/analysis tools: YR WH NB RB NL JCK JG RN SB. Wrote the paper: YR WH SB IM. Critical reviewing and approval of the manuscript: YR WH JB NB RB NL JCK JG PS RN SB IM.

References

1. Goldring MB, Marcu KB (2009) Cartilage homeostasis in health and rheumatic diseases. Arthritis Res Ther 11: 224.
2. Loeser RF, Goldring SR, Scanzello CR, Goldring MB (2012) Osteoarthritis: a disease of the joint as an organ. Arthritis Rheum 64: 1697–1707.
3. Bos SD, Slagboom PE, Meulenbelt I (2008) New insights into osteoarthritis: early developmental features of an ageing-related disease. Curr Opin Rheumatol 20: 553–559.
4. Sandell LJ (2012) Etiology of osteoarthritis: genetics and synovial joint development. Nat Rev Rheumatol 8: 77–89.
5. Gonzalez A (2013) Osteoarthritis year 2013 in review: genetics and genomics. Osteoarthritis Cartilage 21: 1443–1451.
6. Aigner T, Fundel K, Saas J, Gebhard PM, Haag J, et al. (2006) Large-scale gene expression profiling reveals major pathogenetic pathways of cartilage degeneration in osteoarthritis. Arthritis Rheum 54: 3533–3544.
7. Xu Y, Barter MJ, Swan DC, Rankin KS, Rowan AD, et al. (2012) Identification of the pathogenic pathways in osteoarthritic hip cartilage: commonality and discord between hip and knee OA. Osteoarthritis Cartilage 20: 1029–1038.
8. Karlsson C, Dehne T, Lindahl A, Brittberg M, Pruss A, et al. (2010) Genome-wide expression profiling reveals new candidate genes associated with osteoarthritis. Osteoarthritis Cartilage 18: 581–592.
9. Geyer M, Grassel S, Straub RH, Schett G, Dinser R, et al. (2009) Differential transcriptome analysis of intraarticular lesional vs intact cartilage reveals new candidate genes in osteoarthritis pathophysiology. Osteoarthritis Cartilage 17: 328–335.
10. Tsuritani K, Takeda J, Sakagami J, Ishii A, Eriksson T, et al. (2010) Cytokine receptor-like factor 1 is highly expressed in damaged human knee osteoarthritic cartilage and involved in osteoarthritis downstream of TGF-beta. Calcif Tissue Int 86: 47–57.
11. Sato T, Konomi K, Yamasaki S, Aratani S, Tsuchimochi K, et al. (2006) Comparative analysis of gene expression profiles in intact and damaged regions of human osteoarthritic cartilage. Arthritis Rheum 54: 808–817.
12. Goeman JJ, van de Geer SA, de KF, van Houwelingen HC (2004) A global test for groups of genes: testing association with a clinical outcome. Bioinformatics 20: 93–99.
13. Edgar R, Domrachev M, Lash AE (2002) Gene Expression Omnibus: NCBI gene expression and hybridization array data repository. Nucleic Acids Res 30: 207–210.
14. Citri A, Pang ZP, Sudhof TC, Wernig M, Malenka RC (2012) Comprehensive qPCR profiling of gene expression in single neuronal cells. Nat Protoc 7: 118–127.
15. Livak KJ, Schmittgen TD (2001) Analysis of relative gene expression data using real-time quantitative PCR and the 2(-Delta Delta C(T)) Method. Methods 25: 402–408.
16. Bos SD, Bovee JV, Duijnisveld BJ, Raine EV, van Dalen WJ, et al. (2012) Increased type II deiodinase protein in OA-affected cartilage and allelic imbalance of OA risk polymorphism rs225014 at DIO2 in human OA joint tissues. Ann Rheum Dis 71: 1254–1258.
17. Mankin HJ, Dorfman H, Lippiello L, Zarins A (1971) Biochemical and metabolic abnormalities in articular cartilage from osteo-arthritic human hips. II. Correlation of morphology with biochemical and metabolic data. J Bone Joint Surg Am 53: 523–537.
18. Huang DW, Sherman BT, Lempicki RA (2009) Systematic and integrative analysis of large gene lists using DAVID bioinformatics resources. Nat Protoc 4: 44–57.
19. Szklarczyk D, Franceschini A, Kuhn M, Simonovic M, Roth A, et al. (2011) The STRING database in 2011: functional interaction networks of proteins, globally integrated and scored. Nucleic Acids Res 39: D561–D568.
20. Castano Betancourt MC, Cailotto F, Kerkhof HJ, Cornelis FM, Doherty SA, et al. (2012) Genome-wide association and functional studies identify the DOT1L gene to be involved in cartilage thickness and hip osteoarthritis. Proc Natl Acad Sci U S A 109: 8218–8223.
21. Chapman K, Takahashi A, Meulenbelt I, Watson C, Rodriguez-Lopez J, et al. (2008) A meta-analysis of European and Asian cohorts reveals a global role of a functional SNP in the 5′ UTR of GDF5 with osteoarthritis susceptibility. Hum Mol Genet 17: 1497–1504.
22. Day-Williams AG, Southam L, Panoutsopoulou K, Rayner NW, Esko T, et al. (2011) A Variant in MCF2L Is Associated with Osteoarthritis. Am J Hum Genet 89: 446–450.
23. Evangelou E, Kerkhof HJ, Styrkarsdottir U, Ntzani EE, Bos SD, et al. (2013) A meta-analysis of genome-wide association studies identifies novel variants associated with osteoarthritis of the hip. Ann Rheum Dis, doi: 10.1136/annrheumdis-2012-203114.
24. Kerkhof HJ, Lories RJ, Meulenbelt I, Jonsdottir I, Valdes AM, et al. (2010) A genome-wide association study identifies an osteoarthritis susceptibility locus on chromosome 7q22. Arthritis Rheum 62: 499–510.
25. Miyamoto Y, Shi D, Nakajima M, Ozaki K, Sudo A, et al. (2008) Common variants in DVWA on chromosome 3p24.3 are associated with susceptibility to knee osteoarthritis. Nat Genet 40: 994–998.
26. Nakajima M, Takahashi A, Kou I, Rodriguez-Fontenla C, Gomez-Reino JJ, et al. (2010) New sequence variants in HLA class II/III region associated with susceptibility to knee osteoarthritis identified by genome-wide association study. PLoS One 5: e9723.
27. Panoutsopoulou K, Southam L, Elliott KS, Wrayner N, Zhai G, et al. (2011) Insights into the genetic architecture of osteoarthritis from stage 1 of the arcOGEN study. Ann Rheum Dis 70: 864–867.
28. Zeggini E, Panoutsopoulou K, Southam L, Rayner NW, Day-Williams AG, et al. (2012) Identification of new susceptibility loci for osteoarthritis (arcOGEN): a genome-wide association study. Lancet 380: 815–823.
29. Rodriguez-Fontenla C, Calaza M, Evangelou E, Valdes AM, Arden N, et al. (2013) Assessment of osteoarthritis candidate genes in a meta-analysis of 9 genome-wide association studies. Arthritis Rheum 66: 940–949.
30. Ramos YF, Bos SD, van der Breggen R, Kloppenburg M, Ye K, et al. (2014) A gain of function mutation in TNFRSF11B encoding osteoprotegerin causes osteoarthritis with chondrocalcinosis. Ann Rheum Dis, doi: 10.1136/annrheumdis-2013-205149.
31. Barter MJ, Young DA (2013) Epigenetic mechanisms and non-coding RNAs in osteoarthritis. Curr Rheumatol Rep 15: 353.
32. Rushton MD, Reynard LN, Barter MJ, Refaie R, Rankin KS, et al. (2014) Characterization of the cartilage DNA methylome in knee and hip osteoarthritis. Arthritis Rheumatol, doi: 10.1002/art.38713.

33. Styrkarsdottir U, Thorleifsson G, Helgadottir HT, Bomer N, Metrustry S, et al. (2014) Severe osteoarthritis of the hand associates with common variants within the ALDH1A2 gene and with rare variants at 1p31. Nat Genet 46: 498–502.
34. Chou CH, Wu CC, Song IW, Chuang HP, Lu LS, et al. (2013) Genome-wide expression profiles of subchondral bone in osteoarthritis. Arthritis Res Ther 15: R190; doi: 10.1186/ar4380.
35. Raine EV, Wreglesworth N, Dodd AW, Reynard LN, Loughlin J (2012) Gene expression analysis reveals HBP1 as a key target for the osteoarthritis susceptibility locus that maps to chromosome 7q22. Ann Rheum Dis 71: 2020–2027.
36. Yamauchi J, Chan JR, Miyamoto Y, Tsujimoto G, Shooter EM (2005) The neurotrophin-3 receptor TrkC directly phosphorylates and activates the nucleotide exchange factor Dbs to enhance Schwann cell migration. Proc Natl Acad Sci U S A 102: 5198–5203.
37. Seidel MF, Lane NE (2012) Control of arthritis pain with anti-nerve-growth factor: risk and benefit. Curr Rheumatol Rep 14: 583–588.

21

Moderate-Intensity Rotating Magnetic Fields Do Not Affect Bone Quality and Bone Remodeling in Hindlimb Suspended Rats

Da Jing[1]‡, Jing Cai[2]‡, Yan Wu[3]‡, Guanghao Shen[1], Mingming Zhai[1], Shichao Tong[1], Qiaoling Xu[4], Kangning Xie[1], Xiaoming Wu[1], Chi Tang[1], Xinmin Xu[5], Juan Liu[1], Wei Guo[1], Maogang Jiang[1], Erping Luo[1]*

1 Department of Biomedical Engineering, Fourth Military Medical University, Xi'an, China, **2** Department of Endocrinology, Xijing hospital, Fourth Military Medical University, Xi'an, China, **3** Institute of Orthopaedics, Xijing hospital, Fourth Military Medical University, Xi'an, China, **4** Department of Nursing, Fourth Military Medical University, Xi'an, China, **5** Department of Medical Engineering, PLA No. 323 Hospital, Xi'an, China

Abstract

Abundant evidence has substantiated the positive effects of pulsed electromagnetic fields (PEMF) and static magnetic fields (SMF) on inhibiting osteopenia and promoting fracture healing. However, the osteogenic potential of rotating magnetic fields (RMF), another common electromagnetic application modality, remains poorly characterized thus far, although numerous commercial RMF treatment devices have been available on the market. Herein the impacts of RMF on osteoporotic bone microarchitecture, bone strength and bone metabolism were systematically investigated in hindlimb-unloaded (HU) rats. Thirty two 3-month-old male Sprague-Dawley rats were randomly assigned to the Control ($n = 10$), HU ($n = 10$) and HU with RMF exposure (HU+RMF, $n = 12$) groups. Rats in the HU+RMF group were subjected to daily 2-hour exposure to moderate-intensity RMF (ranging from 0.60 T to 0.38 T) at 7 Hz for 4 weeks. HU caused significant decreases in body mass and soleus muscle mass of rats, which were not obviously altered by RMF. Three-point bending test showed that the mechanical properties of femurs in HU rats, including maximum load, stiffness, energy absorption and elastic modulus were not markedly affected by RMF. µCT analysis demonstrated that 4-week RMF did not significantly prevent HU-induced deterioration of femoral trabecular and cortical bone microarchitecture. Serum biochemical analysis showed that RMF did not significantly change HU-induced decrease in serum bone formation markers and increase in bone resorption markers. Bone histomorphometric analysis further confirmed that RMF showed no impacts on bone remodeling in HU rats, as evidenced by unchanged mineral apposition rate, bone formation rate, osteoblast numbers and osteoclast numbers in cancellous bone. Together, our findings reveal that RMF do not significantly affect bone microstructure, bone mechanical strength and bone remodeling in HU-induced disuse osteoporotic rats. Our study indicates potentially obvious waveform-dependent effects of electromagnetic fields-stimulated osteogenesis, suggesting that RMF, at least in the present form, might not be an optimal modality for inhibiting disuse osteopenia/osteoporosis.

Editor: Robert Lafrenie, Sudbury Regional Hospital, Canada

Funding: The authors acknowledge support from the National Natural Science Foundation of China (No. 51077128 and 31270889), Shaanxi Provincial Natural Science Foundation (No. 2014JQ4139), and the Doctoral Thesis Foundation of the Fourth Military Medical University (No. 2012D01). The funders had no role in study design, data collection and analysis, decision to publish, or preparation of the manuscript.

Competing Interests: The authors have declared that no competing interests exist.

* Email: luoerping@fmmu.edu.cn

‡ These authors contributed equally to this work.

Introduction

Osteoporosis, a progressive 'silent bone disease' caused by age, disuse or disease, is characterized by loss of bone mass and deterioration of bone microarchitecture, resulting in pain and deformity and increased risk of bone fracture [1,2]. Bone loss due to the removal of weight-bearing physical activities, which occurs during therapeutic bed rest, limb immobilization and spaceflight, has become a non-negligible health concern in clinics and space medicine. Mechanical unloading induces negative skeletal calcium homeostasis, uncoupling of osteoclast and osteoblast activities, and resultant bone mineral loss [3]. Studies have shown that astronauts experienced loss of bone mineral density (BMD) with approximately 1.5% per month during spaceflight, equaling to that for postmenopausal women in 1 year [4,5,6]. It has been proved that individuals subjected to long-term bed rest or immobilization exhibited dramatic bone mass loss, deterioration of cancellous and cortical bone microarchitecture, and increased risk of falls and bone fracture [7,8]. In view of the side effects or high cost of anti-osteoporosis drugs (e.g., bisphosphonates, calcitonin and hormones) [9,10,11], safe and noninvasive biophysical stimuli for the prevention and treatment of disuse osteoporosis might be more promising in clinical application, and especially favorable for the use of spaceflight.

Our growing understanding of the intricate piezoelectric and electromagnetic properties of bone tissues raised the possibility that exogenous electric or magnetic stimulation might regulate the activities and functions of bone cells. Since the 1970s when Bassett et al. for the first time promoted fracture healing in clinics using pulsed electromagnetic fields (PEMF) [12], abundant evidence has substantiated that electromagnetic fields (EMF) therapy was capable of producing satisfying therapeutic effects in a diverse range of bone diseases in the past four decades [13,14]. The EMF has been approved by the FDA as a safe noninvasive treatment method in 1979. Basically, the three most common EMF application modalities well documented thus far include PEMF, static magnetic fields (SMF) and rotating magnetic fields (RMF). A large body of evidence has shown that PEMF displayed strong osteogenic potential both experimentally and clinically [15,16,17,18], which was primarily associated with the induction of electric currents in tissues to initiate a battery of biological cascades. Several investigators also reported that SMF exposure was able to stimulate *in vivo* skeletal anabolic responses and increase BMD [19,20]. Unlike PEMF, SMF induced no remarkable electrical potential in tissues and might directly affect bone cells through magnetic actions [20]. In recent years, several commercial therapeutic devices with RMF exposure are available on the market. Several previous studies have reported the beneficial effects of RMF on the musculoskeletal system [21,22]. Zhang and colleagues found that 0.4 T RMF increase BMD and serum calcium and phosphatase (ALP) in ovariectomized (OVX) rats [21]. Pan et al. reported that 0.4 T RMF exposure mitigated hyperlipidaemia and steroid-induced necrosis of femoral head in rabbits [22]. However, to date the possible impacts of RMF on disuse-induced osteopenia/osteoporosis remain unknown. Thus, systemic assessment of the regulatory effects of RMF exposure on bone mass, bone microarchitecture, bone strength and bone metabolism in animal models of disuse-induced osteopenia is of great significance for the scientific application of RMF.

One of the best-recognized animal models to study disuse osteoporosis is the hindlimb unloading (HU) model via tail suspension [23,24], which could induce decreased bone formation and increased bone resorption, and thus lead to the loss of bone mass and reduction of bone mechanical strength [25,26]. Therefore, in the present investigation, the efficiency of RMF exposure on disuse-induced bone loss was systematically evaluated via analyses for serum biochemical, bone biomechanical, μCT and histomorphometric parameters in rats subjected to tail suspension.

Materials and Methods

Animals and experimental design

Thirty two mature 3-month-old male Sprague-Dawley rats (276.8±13.5 g, Vital River Laboratory Animal Technology, Beijing, China) were used in the present study. All procedures in the experiment were in strict accordance with the guiding principles of Institutional Animal Ethical Committee (IAEC), Committee for the Purpose of Control and Supervision of Experiments on Animals (CPCSEA), and the Guide for the Care and Use of Laboratory Animals published by the National Institutes of Health [NIH Publication.85–23]. The animal protocol was approved by the Institutional Animal Care and Use Committee of Fourth Military Medical University. All efforts were made to minimize the number of animals used. Animals were housed at 23±1°C temperature, 50%–60% relative humidity, 12:12 h light-dark cycle. Rats were randomly assigned to the Control ($n = 10$), HU ($n = 10$) and HU with RMF exposure (HU+RMF, $n = 12$) groups. The disuse of rat hindlimbs was induced by the tail-suspension technique according to the previously described protocol [27,28]. Briefly, the tail after cleaned with 70% ethanol, was coated with a thin layer of liquid-like benzoin and resin dissolved in 99% ethanol. Then, a strip of adhesive tape was firmly attached laterally along the proximal portion of the tail and allowed thorough air dry, forming a loop close to the end of the tail. The adhesive tape was subsequently secured by three tape strips in its perpendicular direction. A plastic paperclip was employed to attach the loop of the surgical tape to a swivel hoop mounted at the top of a custom-designed plexiglass cage (length = 35 cm, width = 30 cm, height = 45 cm). The rat was maintained in an approximately 30° head-down-tilt position with its hindlimbs unloaded. Rats were caged individually and allowed free access to tap water and chow. The rats in the HU+RMF group were exposed to daily 2 h/day whole-body RMF for 4 weeks. Animals were intramuscularly injected with 25 mg/kg tetracycline (Sigma-Aldrich, Louis, MO, USA) at 14 and 13 days and 5 mg/kg calcein (Sigma-Aldrich) at 4 and 3 days before sacrifice, respectively. Rats were euthanatized with an overdose of chloral hydrate at the end of 4-week experiment. Serum samples were obtained via abdominal aorta puncture, centrifuged for 20 min and stored at −70°C for biochemical analysis. Bilateral femora were harvested, wrapped in saline-soaked gauze and stored at −70°C, which were used for mechanical testing and μCT analysis, respectively. Right tibiae were also harvested for bone histomorphometric analysis.

RMF treatment

As shown in **Fig. 1**, a commercial treatment system with RMF exposure (CRSMART-C, Chaoruishi Medical Supplies Co., Ltd, Zibo, China) was used in the present study. The therapeutic device mainly consisted of a treatment table, two opposite anti-parallel arrays of NdFeB permanent magnets, and a signal display and control module. Each magnet array comprised a total of 20 disc-shaped NdFeB magnets. The maximum magnetic flux density for each magnet was 400 mT. The network topology of the lower NdFeB permanent magnet array is shown in **Fig. 1B**. The lower magnet array was rotated at 7 Hz driven by a high-power spinning motor. The upper magnet array was also rotated accordingly at the same frequency driven by the upper motor. The rotation of both magnet arrays generated non-uniform RMF in the space between the arrays. The cage was placed coaxially with the upper and lower magnet arrays. A Gaussmeter (Model 455, Lake Shore Cryotronics, Westerville, OH, USA) with a transversal Hall Probe (HMFT-3E03-VF) was used to determine the spatial distribution of the magnetic field intensity. The determined magnetic flux density distribution in the position of the cage region ranged from 0.60 T to 0.38 T. The measured environmental background electromagnetic field was 0.5±0.02 Gs.

Serum biochemical analysis

Commercial ELISA kits were employed for quantifying serum biochemical markers, including bone formation-associated osteocalcin (OC) and N-terminal propeptide of type 1 procollagen (P1NP), bone resorption-related tartrate-resistant acid phosphatase (TRAcP5b) and C-terminal cross-linked telopeptides of type I collagen (CTX-I) (Biomedical Technologies, Stoughton, MA, USA). ELISA kits were also used to determine the serum concentrations of two essential osteogenesis-associated cytokines, including prostaglandin E_2 (PGE_2) and transforming growth factor-β1 (TGF-β1) (JRDUN Biotechnology Co., Ltd., Shanghai, China). Assays were performed according to the manufacturers' instructions.

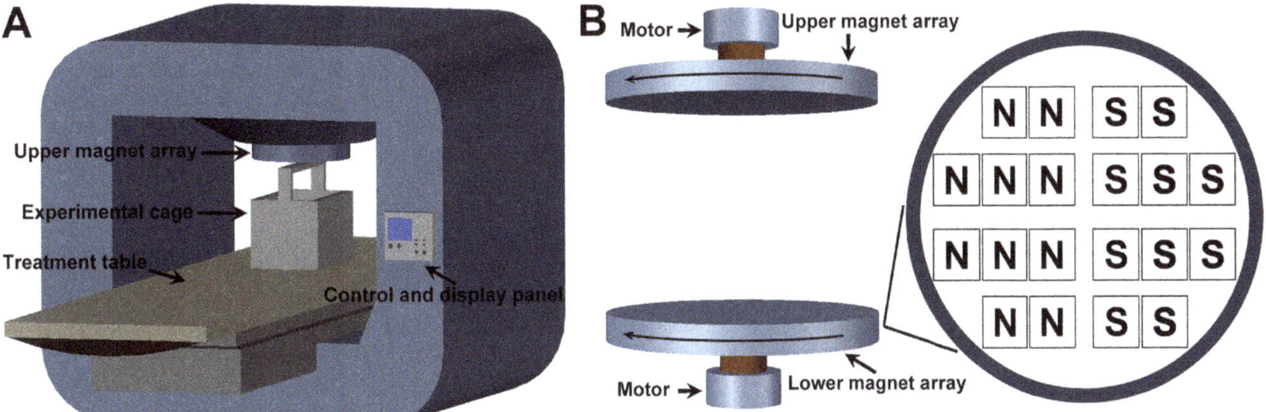

Figure 1. Schematic representation of the treatment device with RMF exposure used in the present study. (**A**) The therapeutic device mainly consists of a treatment table, two opposite anti-parallel arrays of NdFeB permanent magnets, and a signal display and control module. (**B**) Each magnet array comprises a total of 20 disc-shaped NdFeB magnets. The maximum magnetic flux density for each magnet is 400 mT. The right panel in (**B**) shows the network topology of the lower NdFeB permanent magnet array (**N** and **S** in the figure indicate the north pole and south pole of the magnet, respectively). The lower magnet array is rotated at 7 Hz driven by a high-power spinning motor, and thus driving the rotation of the upper magnet array. The rotation of both magnet arrays generates non-uniform RMF in the space between the arrays. The cage is placed coaxially with the upper and lower magnet arrays. The magnetic flux density distribution in the position of the cage region was determined to be 0.60–0.38 T.

Biomechanical examination

The left femora after thawing in phosphate buffer solution (PBS) at room temperature were used for three-point bending test. The mechanical properties were evaluated at the femoral mid-diaphysis using a commercial mechanical testing system (*AGS-10 kNG, Shimadzu*, Kyoto, Japan). The femur with its physiological curvature facing up was stabilized on a supporter with two fixed loading points with 20-mm distance. A stabilizing preload with 2 N was applied on the femoral medial surface using a steel cross-bar plate, which was oriented perpendicularly to the long axis of the sample and at the midpoint between the lower loading points. The bending load was applied at a constant displacement rate of 2 mm/min until fracture occurred. Then, the internal and external major axis and minor axis lengths of the femur at the fracture point were immediately measured using a vernier caliper. The following indices were determined from the load-deformation curve: maximum load (the maximum tensile load that the femur can sustain before failure), stiffness (slope of the linear part of the curve representing elastic deformation), and energy absorption (area under the load-deformation curve). Elastic modulus was calculated according to the formula: $E = FL^3/48dI$, where F is the maximum load, L is the distance between supporting points, d is the displacement, I is the moment of inertia of the cross-section in relation to the horizontal axis.

μCT analysis

The right femora of rats were scanned at a spatial resolution of 16 μm/slice using a high-resolution μCT system (GE healthcare, Madison, WI, USA). The femoral samples were placed in a 20-mm-diameter tube perpendicularly to the scanning axis with a total of 12-mm reconstruction height. After scanning, the 2-D image sequences were transferred to a workstation and 3-D images were reconstructed. For analyses of trabecular bone microarchitecture, a volume of interest (VOI) with 2.0-mm height was selected. The VOI started at a distance of 0.4 mm from the lowest end of the growth plate of the distal femur and extended to the proximal end with a distance of 2.0 mm, which excluded all the primary spongiosa and only contained the second spongiosa. The trabecular bone parameters, including trabecular BMD, trabecular number (Tb.N), trabecular thickness (Tb.Th), trabecular separation (Tb.Sp), bone volume per tissue volume (BV/TV), and structure model index (SMI) were automatically quantified using the MicroView program (GE healthcare, Madison, WI, USA). Moreover, the mid-diaphyseal cortical bone was manually traced by another VOI. The cortical bone parameters, including cortical thickness (Ct.Th) and cortical area (Ct.Ar) were also determined.

Histology and histomorphometry

Right tibiae were immediately cut longitudinally into two pieces along the sagittal plane after animal dissection. One piece was fixed in 4% paraformaldehyde (PFA), decalcified in 10% ethylenediaminetetraacetic acid (EDTA), and embedded in paraffin. Five-μm-thick sections were stained with toluidine blue to visualize osteoblasts, and stained with tartrate resistant acid phosphatase (TRAP) to label osteoclasts. Static bone histomorphometric parameters, including osteoblast numbers per millimeter of trabecular bone surface (N.Ob/BS) and osteoclast numbers per millimeter of trabecular bone surface (N.Oc/BS) were quantified. The other piece was fixed in 80% ethanol for 24 h, and then embedded in methylmethacrylate. Eighty-μm-thick unstained sections were imaged with fluorescence microscope (LEICA DM LA, Leica Microsystems, Heidelberg, Germany) to observe and calculate the distance between the tetracycline and calcein labels divided by the labeling intervals of 10 days. Then, the dynamic bone histomorphometric parameters were quantified, including mineral apposition rate (MAR) and bone formation rate per bone surface (BFR/BS).

Statistical analysis

All data presented in this study were expressed as the mean ± standard deviation (S.D.). Statistical analyses were performed using SPSS version 13.0 for Windows software (SPSS, Chicago, IL, USA). One-way analysis of variance (ANOVA) was employed for evaluating the existence of differences among the three groups and once a significant difference was detected, Bonferroni's post hoc analysis was used to determine the significance between every two groups. The significance level was set at 0.05.

Results

Effects of RMF on body mass and soleus muscle mass in HU rats

The results of body mass and soleus muscle mass of rats before and after RMF exposure are shown in **Table 1**. No significant difference in body mass was observed between the Control, HU and HU+RMF groups before RMF exposure ($P>0.05$). HU for 4 weeks induced dramatic loss in body mass ($P<0.01$), soleus muscle mass ($P<0.01$) and soleus muscle mass normalized with body mass ($P<0.01$) as compared with the Control group; nevertheless, 4-week RMF exposure did not significantly alter the body mass, soleus muscle mass, or normalized soleus muscle mass in HU rats ($P>0.05$).

Effects of RMF on serum biochemical indices in HU rats

As shown in **Fig. 2**, bone formation markers, including serum OC and PINP in the HU group were significantly lower than those in the Control group ($P<0.01$). Serum TRAcP5 b and CTX-I, two serum markers for bone resorption, were remarkably higher in the HU group than those in the Control group ($P<0.01$). However, no significant difference in serum OC, PINP, TRAcP5 b or CTX-I levels was found between the HU and HU+RMF groups ($P>0.05$). Moreover, serum levels of PGE_2 and TGF-β1 in the HU group were lower than those in the Control group ($P<0.05$), whereas RMF did not significantly increase serum PGE_2 or TGF-β1 concentrations ($P>0.05$).

Effects of RMF on the biomechanical properties of bone in HU rats

The results of biomechanical testing of three-point bending are shown in **Fig. 3**. HU resulted in prominent decreases in the biomechanical properties of femora, including maximum load, stiffness, energy absorption and elastic modulus ($P<0.01$), whereas RMF exposure for 4 weeks exerted no significant impacts on maximum load, stiffness, energy absorption or elastic modulus in HU rats ($P>0.05$).

Effects of RMF on bone microarchitecture in HU rats

Representative 3-D and 2-D μCT images in the Control, HU and HU+RMF groups are shown in **Fig. 4**. The rat femur in the HU group exhibited notable reductions in the trabecular number, trabecular area and cortical thickness as compared with that in the Control group. RMF exposure did not exhibit remarkable effects on trabecular bone microarchitecture and cortical bone thickness in HU rats. The statistical results for the μCT analysis of trabecular and cortical bone structure in rat femora are shown in **Fig. 5**. Four-week skeletal disuse by HU caused significant decreases in trabecular BMD, Tb.N, Tb.Th and BV/TV ($P<0.01$), and increase in Tb.Sp and SMI ($P<0.01$). Moreover, HU induced significant deterioration in cortical bone structure of rat femora, as evidenced by decreased Ct.Ar and Ct.Th ($P<0.01$). However, no significant difference was observed in any trabecular or cortical bone parameter between the HU and HU+RMF groups, including BMD, Tb.N, Tb.Th, Tb.Sp, BV/TV, SMI, Ct.Ar or Ct.Th ($P>0.05$).

Effects of RMF on bone remodeling in HU rats

As shown in **Fig. 6**, the HU rats exhibited significant decrease in N.Ob/BS ($P<0.01$) and increase in N.Oc/BS ($P<0.01$) comparing to those in the Control group; nevertheless, RMF exposure did not alter N.Ob/BS or N.Oc/BS in HU rats. Furthermore, HU for 4 weeks also led to significant decreases in MAR and BFR/BS ($P<0.01$). However, no significant difference in MAR or BFR/BS was found between the HU and HU+RMF groups ($P>0.05$).

Effects of RMF on bone microstructure and bone turnover in normal rats

The descriptions for the methods for evaluating the effects of RMF on bone microstructure and bone turnover in normal rats are shown in File S1. As shown in **Fig. S1 in File S1**, RMF exposure did not significantly affect the parameters of bone microstructure in normal rats, including trabecular BMD, trabecular BV/TV or Cr.Ar ($P>0.05$). Moreover, no significant difference was observed in serum OC (the bone formation marker), and serum TRAcP5b (the bone resorption marker) between the Control and RMF groups ($P>0.05$).

Discussion

Accumulating evidence has demonstrated the promotional effects of PEMF and SMF on osteogenesis both *in vivo and in vitro*, whereas few studies have reported the efficiency of RMF in the musculoskeletal system. A previous study has demonstrated that moderate-intensity RMF was able to increase BMD and regulate bone metabolism in OVX rats [21]. However, the impacts of RMF on disuse-induced osteopenia/osteoporosis have never been previously investigated. Therefore, in the present study, we systematically evaluated the effects of RMF on HU-induced bone loss in rats subjected to tail suspension. Our findings clearly demonstrated that 4-week RMF exposure did not obviously affect soleus muscle mass, bone mass, bone microarchitecture, bone mechanical strength or bone remodeling in HU rats.

In the present study, soleus muscle atrophy and deceased body mass in rats were induced by 4-week HU. Disturbed balance between protein synthesis and protein degradation are regarded to

Table 1. Comparisons of body mass and soleus muscle mass of rats in the three experimental groups.

	Control ($n=10$)	HU ($n=10$)	HU+RMF ($n=12$)
Body Mass Day 0 (g)	275.6±12.9	275.6±12.6	279.4±16.4
Body Mass Day 29 (g)	354.3±20.9	293.6±16.7*	291.4±14.4*
Body Mass Change (g)	78.6±14.5	18.0±12.5*	12.0±17.6*
Soleus Mass (mg)	174.9±15.7	79.0±13.3*	89.8±13.5*
Soleus Mass/Body Mass (μg/g)	494.3±42.7	270.4±51.1*	308.6±48.3*

Values are expressed as mean ± S.D.
*Significant difference from Control group with $P<0.05$.

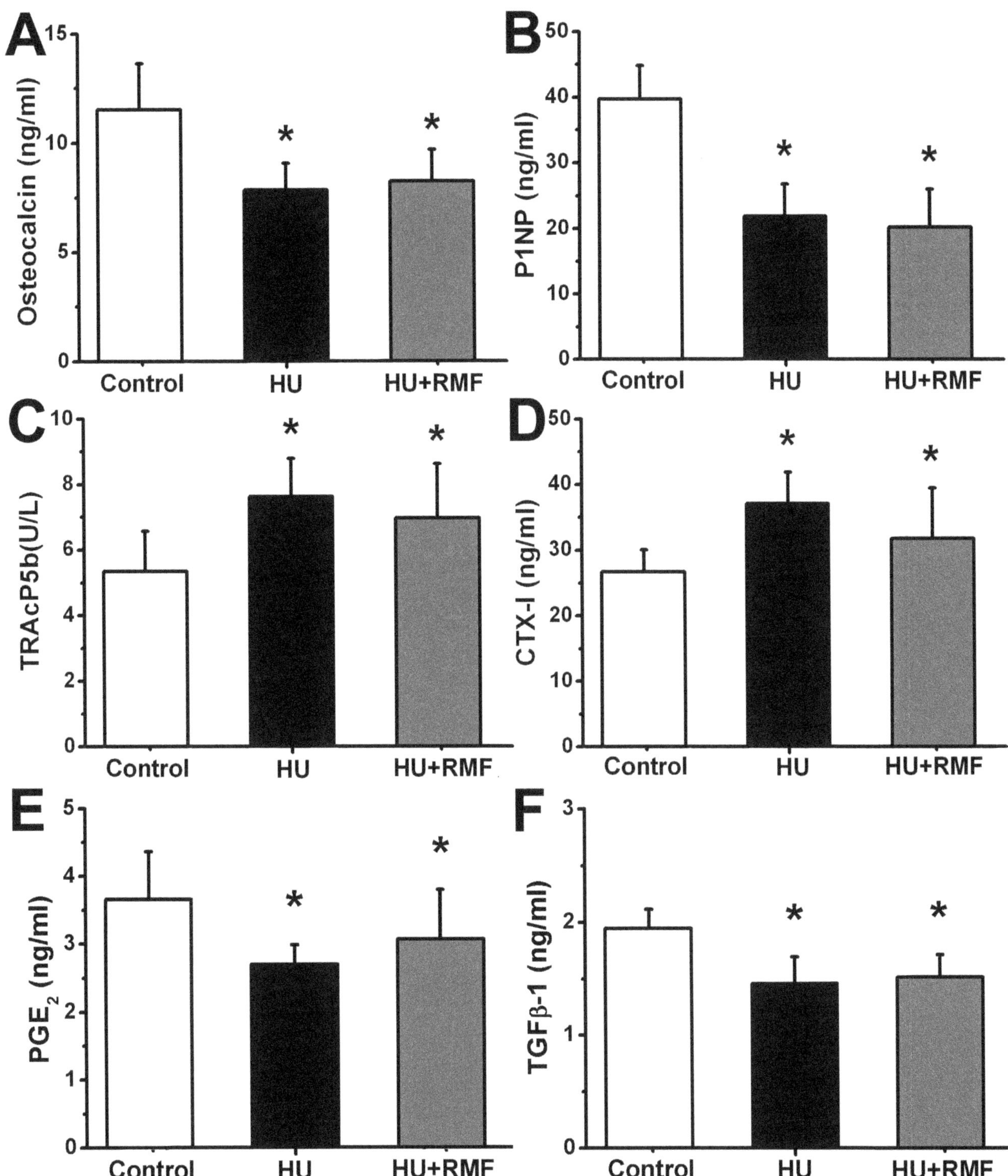

Figure 2. Effects of 4-week RMF exposure on serum biochemical indices (bone turnover markers and osteogenesis-associated cytokines) in HU rats, including bone formation markers (A) serum osteocalcin (OC) and (B) serum N-terminal propeptide of type 1 procollagen (P1NP), bone resorption markers (C) serum tartrate-resistant acid phosphatase (TRAcP5b) and (D) serum C-terminal cross-linked telopeptides of type I collagen (CTX-I), (E) prostaglandin E_2 (PGE_2), and (F) transforming growth factor-β1 (TGF-β1). Control, the control group ($n = 10$); HU, the hindlimb unloading group ($n = 10$); HU+RMF, the hindlimb unloading with RMF exposure group ($n = 12$). Values are all expressed as mean ± S.D. *Significant difference from the Control group with $P<0.05$.

be the major mechanism of HU-induced muscle atrophy [29], although the exact signaling pathways and molecular mechanisms remain elusive. Previous investigation has demonstrated that pulsed electrical stimulation with 20 Hz has the potency to inhibit

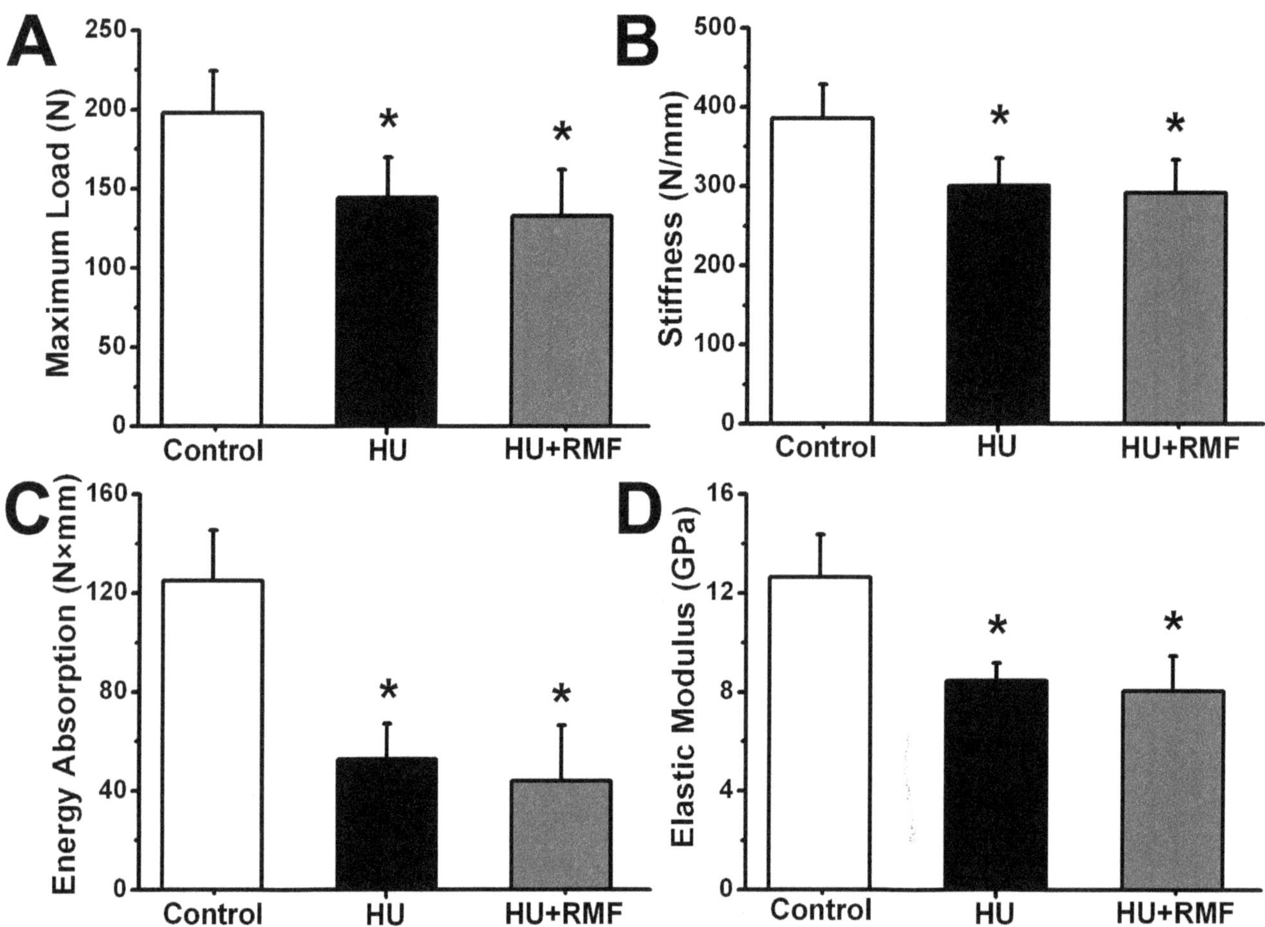

Figure 3. Effects of 4-week RMF exposure on femoral biomechanical parameters in HU rats, including (A) maximum load (B) stiffness (C) energy absorption and (D) elastic modulus. Control, the control group ($n = 10$); HU, the hindlimb unloading group ($n = 10$); HU+RMF, the hindlimb unloading with RMF exposure group ($n = 12$). Values are all expressed as mean ± S.D. *Significant difference from the Control group with $P<0.05$.

muscle atrophy by rescuing myonuclei and satellite cells [30]. It has also been shown that SMF exposure contributed significantly to the promotion of myogenic differentiation and myoblast alignment [31]. However, no obvious attenuation of soleus muscle atrophy in HU rats was observed after 4-week exposure to RMF in the present study.

The skeleton is a highly mechanoadaptive system, and insufficient mechanical stimuli to weight-bearing regions of the skeleton lead to bone mass loss [32,33]. In line with previous studies [34,35], HU resulted in marked deterioration in trabecular bone microarchitecture, as evidenced by decreased trabecular BMD, Tb.N, Tb.Th and BV/TV, and increased Tb.Sp. More importantly, increased trabecular SMI was also observed in HU rats, revealing a potentially dramatic reduction of trabeculae with plate-like structures [36]. Moreover, in accordance with previous findings [35], skeletal disuse by HU caused lower cortical bone thickness in the present study. Further observations by mechanical testing demonstrated that the skeletal extrinsic mechanical properties (maximum load, stiffness and energy absorption) and intrinsic mechanical properties (elastic modulus) were decreased in HU rats, implying the impaired mechanical integrity and declining capacity of fracture toughness [37]. However, RMF exposure did not obviously contribute to the improvement of trabecular bone microarchitecture, cortical bone thickness or bone mechanical strength.

To further evaluate whether RMF regulated osteoblastic and osteoclastic activities in HU rats, systemic analyses of serum biomarkers and bone histomorphometry for bone remodeling were performed. Similar with previous investigations [33], dramatically reduced bone formation was observed in HU rats, as evidenced by decreased serum markers (OC and P1NP) and histomorphometric parameters in trabecular bones (MAR, BFR/BS and N.Ob/BS). Our results also showed elevated serum TRAcP5b, serum CTX-I and N.Oc/BS in trabecular bones, revealing remarkably enhanced bone resorption induced by HU. However, we found no obvious regulatory effects of RMF on either serum markers or bone histomorphometric parameters for bone turnover, implying no direct impacts of RMF on skeletal anabolic or catabolic activities in HU rats. Moreover, many cytokines have proven to play essential roles in regulating the process of bone remodeling, such as PGE_2 and TGF-β1. PGE_2 is the most extensively produced prostanoid and has the capacity of stimulating bone formation and promoting fracture healing [38,39]. Chang et al. showed that PEMF inhibited osteopenia in OVX rats and stimulated serum PGE_2 secretions [40]. Significant evidence has demonstrated that TGF-β1 was able to regulate osteoblastic and osteoclastic functions [41]. More importantly,

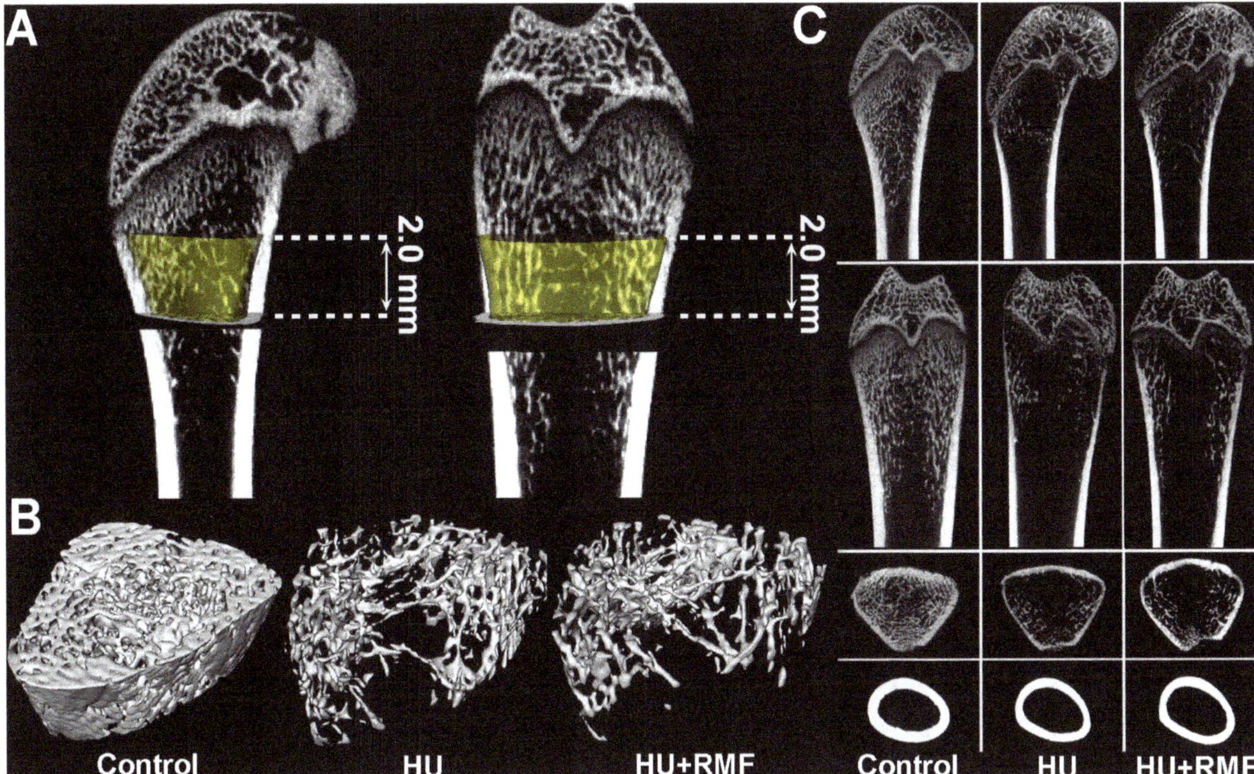

Figure 4. Effects of 4-week RMF exposure on trabecular bone microarchitecture in the distal femora and cortical bone thickness in the mid-diaphyseal femora. (**A**) The selected trabecular volume of interest (VOI) with yellow color in 2.0 mm height, which is represented with yellow color and only contains the secondary spongiosa. (**B**) 3-D μCT images of trabecular bone microarchitecture determined by the VOI. (**C**) 2-D μCT images of trabecular bone microarchitecture from the axial, coronal and sagittal plane observation in the distal femora, and cortical bone images in the femoral mid-diaphysis. The rat femur in the HU group exhibited significant decrease in the trabecular number, trabecular area and cortical thickness as compared with that in the Control group, whereas RMF exposure did not exhibit remarkable effects on trabecular bone microarchitecture and cortical bone thickness in HU rats.

TGF-β1 has also proven to be an essential mediator for the coupling of dynamic bone resorption and bone formation [42,43]. Our present study showed that serum PGE_2 and TGF-β1 secretions were decreased in the absence of regular mechanical stimulation. However, 4-week RMF exposure did not significantly change the concentrations of serum PGE_2 or TGF-β1.

The discovery of the skeletal piezoelectric effect by Fukada et al. in 1957 raised the possibility of the application of exogenous electrical stimulus on bone repair [44]. Subsequent studies have confirmed the osteogenic effects of electrical stimulation [45,46]. Bassett et al. for the first time found that PEMF treatment, a more accessible and affordable non-contact modality, was able to dramatically accelerate fracture healing in patients [12]. Numerous studies have further proved that PEMF could promote potently osteogenesis and enhance bone mineralization both *in vivo* and *in vitro* [15,16,47]. Clinical investigations revealed that PEMF produced satisfying therapeutic effects on fresh and nonunion fractures and osteoporosis [14,17]. It should be noted that the positive effects derived from PEMF stimulation revealed by Bassett et al. and other investigators were based on low-intensity and low-frequency non-thermal exposure levels, which were anticipated to primarily induce weak low-frequency electric current inside bone tissues. Moreover, these PEMF waveforms previously used were unidirectional single pulse or pulse burst. Several previous studies demonstrated that time-varying electromagnetic fields, e.g., sinusoidal wave, led to marked decreases of BMD and mechanical strength in rats [48]. Zhang et al. also demonstrated that sinusoidal EMF treatment decreased the osteoblasts proliferation and suppressed mineralized nodules formation, which exhibited opposite effects by unidirectional PEMF stimulation [47]. In the present study, moderate-intensity RMF we used could also induce spatial time-varying bidirectional electric fields in body tissues. However, different exposure waveforms, intensities and directionalities may contribute to the dramatically distinct effects between PEMF and RMF on the skeleton.

The beneficial effects of moderate-intensity and high-intensity SMF on osteogenesis have also been well documented thus far. Previous investigation has demonstrated that SMF promoted the differentiation and activation of osteoblasts *in vitro* [49]. It has been shown that SMF have the potency to enhance the local BMD in osteoporotic rats and accelerate fracture healing [19,50,51]. More interestingly, Kotani et al. found that high-intensity SMF exposure stimulated skeletal anabolic responses, and the orientation of bone formation and osteoblast growth was parallel to the magnetic field both *in vivo* and *in vitro* [20]. Thus, SMF may only induce a direct magnetic field to regulate osteoblast orientation, proliferation, differentiation, and bone formation, which shows distinct osteogenic mechanism with PEMF. However, unlike SMF with constant magnetic field direction, time-varying spatial magnetic fields generated by RMF we used in the present study might not facilitate the orientation of bone cells and

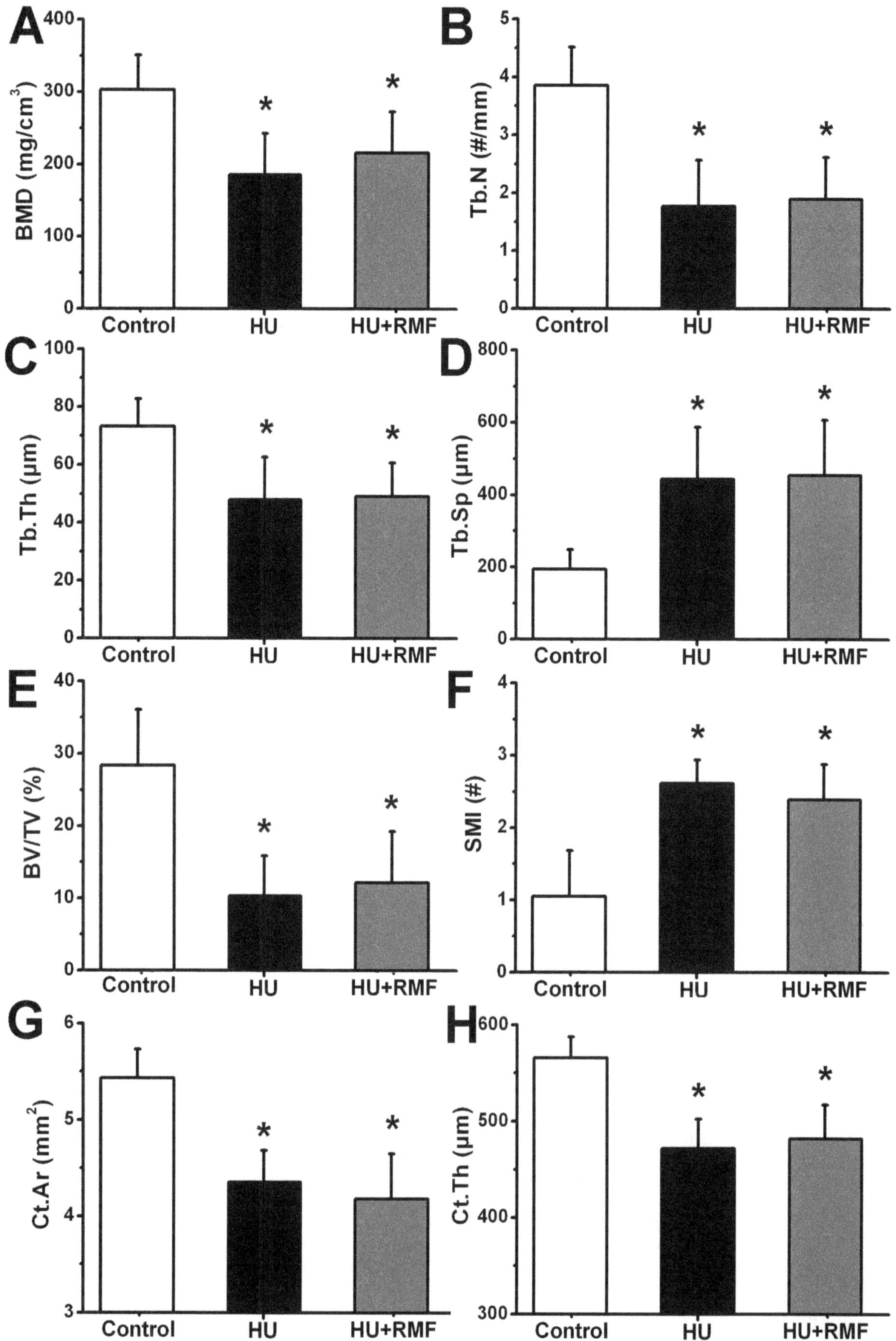
A
BMD (mg/cm^3)
400
300
200
100
0
Control
HU
HU+RMF
B
Tb.N (#/mm)
5
4
3
2
1
0
Control
HU
HU+RMF
C
Tb.Th (μm)
100
80
60
40
20
0
Control
HU
HU+RMF
D
Tb.Sp (μm)
800
600
400
200
0
Control
HU
HU+RMF
E
BV/TV (%)
40
30
20
10
0
Control
HU
HU+RMF
F
SMI (#)
4
3
2
1
0
Control
HU
HU+RMF
G
Ct.Ar (mm^2)
6
5
4
3
Control
HU
HU+RMF
H
Ct.Th (μm)
600
500
400
300
Control
HU
HU+RMF

Figure 5. Effects of 4-week RMF exposure on μCT indices of femoral trabecular and cortical bone microstructure in HU rats, including (A) trabecular bone mineral density (BMD), (B) trabecular number (Tb.N), (C) trabecular thickness (Tb.Th), (D) trabecular separation (Tb.Sp), (E) bone volume per tissue volume (BV/TV), (F) structure model index (SMI), (G) cortical area (Ct.Ar) and (H) cortical thickness (Ct.Th). Control, the control group ($n = 10$); HU, the hindlimb unloading group ($n = 10$); HU+RMF, the hindlimb unloading with RMF exposure group ($n = 12$). Values are all expressed as mean ± S.D. *Significant difference from the Control group with $P<0.05$.

their cytoskeletons, and thus might not facilitate stimulating bone formation in one particular direction. This might be one of the possible reasons for the minor impacts of RMF on bone quality and bone metabolism in HU rats in the present study.

Another interesting aspect for helping decipher the mechanism of RMF on the tissues is the quantification of the electromagnetic energy absorbed by the tissues and the heat effect because of the energy absorption. According to the previous description, the Specific Absorption Rate (SAR) of the tissue is calculated in the following equation [52]: $SAR = \sigma \cdot E^2/\rho$, where σ is the conductivity of the tissue, ρ is the tissue mass, and E is the electric field intensity inside the tissue. The temperature alterations due to the energy absorption are able to be numerically quantified by analyzing the bioheat transfer equation based on the obtained SAR value [53]. A systematic numerical calculation based on finite element analysis will be performed in our following studies to obtain comprehensive understanding for the electromagnetic energy absorption in the tissues.

In conclusion, the present study demonstrated that exposure with moderate-intensity RMF at 7 Hz did not affect bone mass, bone microstructure, bone mechanical strength and bone remodeling in HU-induced osteoporotic rats, as evidenced by systemic evaluation for the serum biochemical, bone biomechanical, μCT and histomorphometric analyses. Although RMF stimulation may yield both a time-varying magnetic field and an electric current inside tissues, the RMF exposure was indeed not an optimal modality for regulating bone quality and bone remodeling, at least in its present form. It is regarded that treatment with EMF on various disorders probably exists "biological windows" of stimulus parameters. Thus, further investigations for the regulatory effects of high-intensity and low-intensity RMF on bone loss in HU rats are necessary to obtain a more comprehensive understanding for

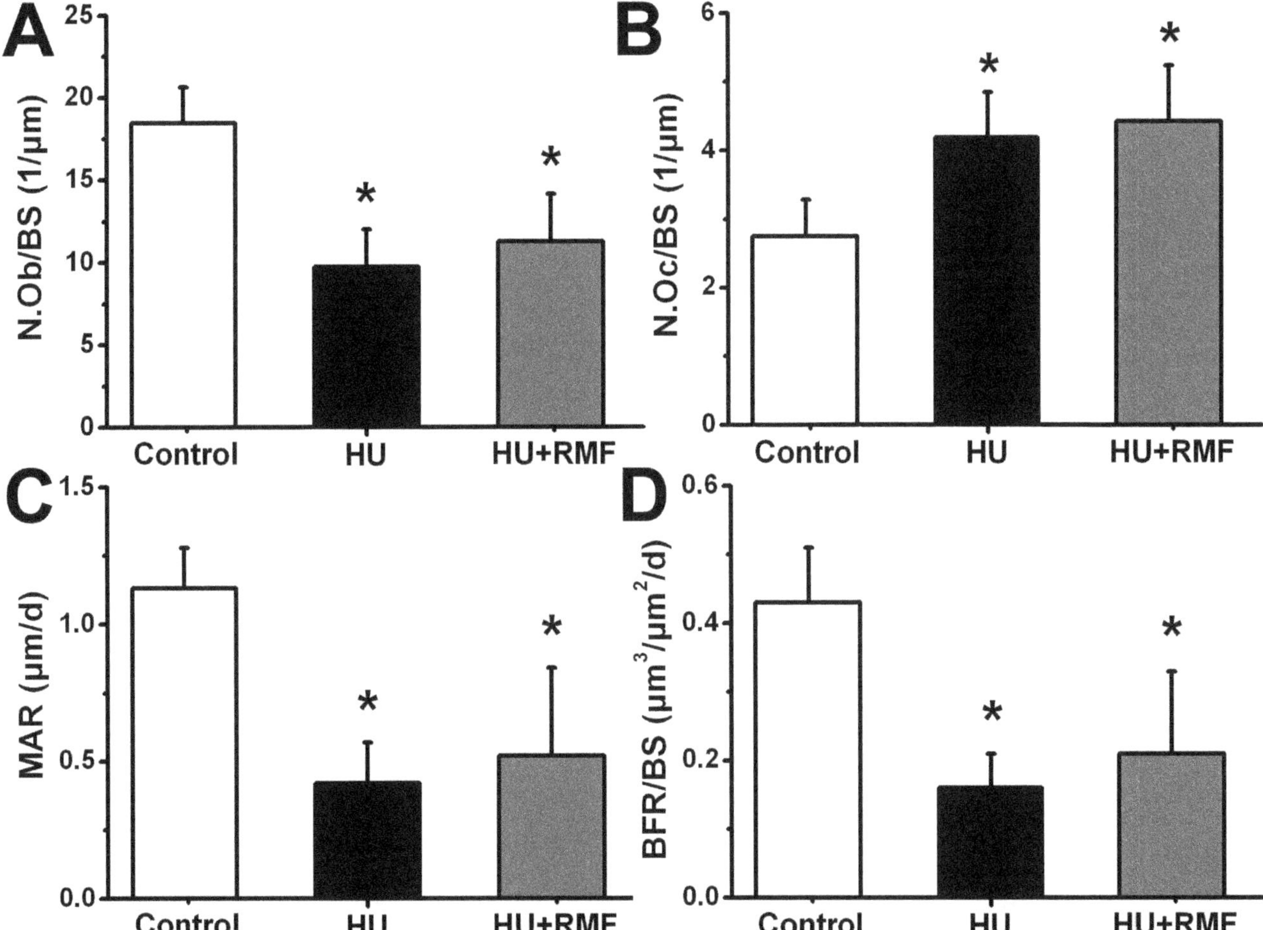

Figure 6. Effects of 4-week RMF exposure on tibial static and dynamic bone histomorphometric parameters in HU rats, including (A) osteoblast numbers per millimeter of trabecular bone surface (N.Ob/BS), (B) osteoclast numbers per millimeter of trabecular bone surface (N.Oc/BS), (C) mineral apposition rate (MAR) and (D) bone formation rate per bone surface (BFR/BS). Control, the control group ($n = 10$); HU, the hindlimb unloading group ($n = 10$); HU+RMF, the hindlimb unloading with RMF exposure group ($n = 12$). Values are all expressed as mean ± S.D. *Significant difference from the Control group with $P<0.05$.

the osteogenic effects of RMF, which may be helpful for more scientific evaluation of RMF stimulation on osteopenia/osteoporosis in clinics.

Supporting Information

File S1 Combined file containing supporting materials and methods and Figure S1. Figure S1: Effects of 4-week RMF exposure on femoral trabecular and cortical bone microarchitecture and serum markers for bone turnover in normal rats, including **(A)** trabecular bone mineral density (BMD), **(B)** trabecular bone volume per tissue volume (BV/TV), **(C)** cortical area (Ct.Ar), the bone formation marker **(D)** serum osteocalcin (OC), and bone resorption marker **(E)** serum tartrate-resistant acid phosphatase (TRAcP5b). Control, the control group; RMF, the RMF exposure group. Values are all expressed as mean ± S.D. ($n = 8$).

Acknowledgments

The authors sincerely thank Dr. Yaochun Wang (Department of Aerospace Biodynamics, Fourth Military Medical University, Xi'an, China) for his assistance in the establishment of animal model.

Author Contributions

Conceived and designed the experiments: DJ EL JC. Performed the experiments: DJ JC YW ST. Analyzed the data: DJ JC YW GS QX KX XW MJ. Contributed reagents/materials/analysis tools: MZ CT XX JL WG. Wrote the paper: DJ.

References

1. Heaney RP, Abrams S, Dawson-Hughes B, Looker A, Marcus R, et al. (2000) Peak bone mass. Osteoporos Int 11: 985–1009.
2. McCombs JS, Thiebaud P, McLaughlin-Miley C, Shi J (2004) Compliance with drug therapies for the treatment and prevention of osteoporosis. Maturitas 48: 271–287.
3. Takata S, Yasui N (2001) Disuse osteoporosis. J Med Invest 48: 147–156.
4. LeBlanc A, Schneider V, Shackelford L, West S, Oganov V, et al. (2000) Bone mineral and lean tissue loss after long duration space flight. J Musculoskelet Neuronal Interact 1: 157–160.
5. Lang TF, Leblanc AD, Evans HJ, Lu Y (2006) Adaptation of the proximal femur to skeletal reloading after long-duration spaceflight. J Bone Miner Res 21: 1224–1230.
6. Riggs BL, Khosla S, Melton LJ 3rd (1998) A unitary model for involutional osteoporosis: estrogen deficiency causes both type I and type II osteoporosis in postmenopausal women and contributes to bone loss in aging men. J Bone Miner Res 13: 763–773.
7. Thomsen JS, Morukov BV, Vico L, Alexandre C, Saparin PI, et al. (2005) Cancellous bone structure of iliac crest biopsies following 370 days of head-down bed rest. Aviat Space Environ Med 76: 915–922.
8. Lazo MG, Shirazi P, Sam M, Giobbie-Hurder A, Blacconiere MJ, et al. (2001) Osteoporosis and risk of fracture in men with spinal cord injury. Spinal Cord 39: 208–214.
9. Mahavni V, Sood AK (2001) Hormone replacement therapy and cancer risk. Curr Opin Oncol 13: 384–389.
10. Musette P, Brandi ML, Cacoub P, Kaufman JM, Rizzoli R, et al. (2010) Treatment of osteoporosis: recognizing and managing cutaneous adverse reactions and drug-induced hypersensitivity. Osteoporos Int 21: 723–732.
11. Rizzoli R, Reginster JY, Boonen S, Breart G, Diez-Perez A, et al. (2011) Adverse reactions and drug-drug interactions in the management of women with postmenopausal osteoporosis. Calcif Tissue Int 89: 91–104.
12. Bassett CA, Pawluk RJ, Pilla AA (1974) Augmentation of bone repair by inductively coupled electromagnetic fields. Science 184: 575–577.
13. Bassett CA, Mitchell SN, Gaston SR (1982) Pulsing electromagnetic field treatment in ununited fractures and failed arthrodeses. JAMA 247: 623–628.
14. Assiotis A, Sachinis NP, Chalidis BE (2012) Pulsed electromagnetic fields for the treatment of tibial delayed unions and nonunions. A prospective clinical study and review of the literature. J Orthop Surg Res 7: 24.
15. Jing D, Cai J, Shen G, Huang J, Li F, et al. (2011) The preventive effects of pulsed electromagnetic fields on diabetic bone loss in streptozotocin-treated rats. Osteoporos Int 22: 1885–1895.
16. Rubin CT, McLeod KJ, Lanyon LE (1989) Prevention of osteoporosis by pulsed electromagnetic fields. J Bone Joint Surg Am 71: 411–417.
17. Tabrah F, Hoffmeier M, Gilbert F Jr, Batkin S, Bassett CA (1990) Bone density changes in osteoporosis-prone women exposed to pulsed electromagnetic fields (PEMFs). J Bone Miner Res 5: 437–442.
18. Jing D, Cai J, Wu Y, Shen G, Li F, et al. (2014) Pulsed Electromagnetic Fields Partially Preserve Bone Mass, Microarchitecture, and Strength by Promoting Bone Formation in Hindlimb-Suspended Rats. J Bone Miner Res. doi:10.1002/jbmr.2260.
19. Yan QC, Tomita N, Ikada Y (1998) Effects of static magnetic field on bone formation of rat femurs. Med Eng Phys 20: 397–402.
20. Kotani H, Kawaguchi H, Shimoaka T, Iwasaka M, Ueno S, et al. (2002) Strong static magnetic field stimulates bone formation to a definite orientation in vitro and in vivo. J Bone Miner Res 17: 1814–1821.
21. Zhang XY, Xue Y, Zhang Y (2006) Effects of 0.4 T rotating magnetic field exposure on density, strength, calcium and metabolism of rat thigh bones. Bioelectromagnetics 27: 1–9.
22. Pan X, Xiao D, Zhang X, Huang Y, Lin B (2009) Study of rotating permanent magnetic field to treat steroid-induced osteonecrosis of femoral head. Int Orthop 33: 617–623.
23. Morey-Holton ER, Globus RK (1998) Hindlimb unloading of growing rats: a model for predicting skeletal changes during space flight. Bone 22: 83S–88S.
24. Swift JM, Nilsson MI, Hogan HA, Sumner LR, Bloomfield SA (2010) Simulated resistance training during hindlimb unloading abolishes disuse bone loss and maintains muscle strength. J Bone Miner Res 25: 564–574.
25. Halloran BP, Bikle DD, Wronski TJ, Globus RK, Levens MJ, et al. (1986) The role of 1, 25-dihydroxyvitamin D in the inhibition of bone formation induced by skeletal unloading. Endocrinology 118: 948–954.
26. Machwate M, Zerath E, Holy X, Hott M, Godet D, et al. (1995) Systemic administration of transforming growth factor-beta 2 prevents the impaired bone formation and osteopenia induced by unloading in rats. J Clin Invest 96: 1245–1253.
27. Morey-Holton ER, Globus RK (2002) Hindlimb unloading rodent model: technical aspects. J Appl Physiol 92: 1367–1377.
28. Zhang LN, Zhang LF, Ma J (2001) Simulated microgravity enhances vasoconstrictor responsiveness of rat basilar artery. J Appl Physiol 90: 2296–2305.
29. Fitts RH, Riley DR, Widrick JJ (2000) Physiology of a microgravity environment invited review: microgravity and skeletal muscle. J Appl Physiol (1985) 89: 823–839.
30. Guo BS, Cheung KK, Yeung SS, Zhang BT, Yeung EW (2012) Electrical stimulation influences satellite cell proliferation and apoptosis in unloading-induced muscle atrophy in mice. PLoS One 7: e30348.
31. Coletti D, Teodori L, Albertini MC, Rocchi M, Pristera A, et al. (2007) Static magnetic fields enhance skeletal muscle differentiation in vitro by improving myoblast alignment. Cytometry A 71: 846–856.
32. Kazakia GJ, Tjong W, Nirody JA, Burghardt AJ, Carballido-Gamio J, et al. (2014) The influence of disuse on bone microstructure and mechanics assessed by HR-pQCT. Bone.
33. Spatz JM, Ellman R, Cloutier AM, Louis L, van Vliet M, et al. (2013) Sclerostin antibody inhibits skeletal deterioration due to reduced mechanical loading. J Bone Miner Res 28: 865–874.
34. Hu M, Cheng J, Qin YX (2012) Dynamic hydraulic flow stimulation on mitigation of trabecular bone loss in a rat functional disuse model. Bone 51: 819–825.
35. Lloyd SA, Bandstra ER, Willey JS, Riffle SE, Tirado-Lee L, et al. (2012) Effect of proton irradiation followed by hindlimb unloading on bone in mature mice: a model of long-duration spaceflight. Bone 51: 756–764.
36. Parkinson IH, Badiei A, Stauber M, Codrington J, Muller R, et al. (2012) Vertebral body bone strength: the contribution of individual trabecular element morphology. Osteoporos Int 23: 1957–1965.
37. Sun Y, Shuang F, Chen DM, Zhou RB (2013) Treatment of hydrogen molecule abates oxidative stress and alleviates bone loss induced by modeled microgravity in rats. Osteoporos Int 24: 969–978.
38. Li M, Thompson DD, Paralkar VM (2007) Prostaglandin E(2) receptors in bone formation. Int Orthop 31: 767–772.
39. Keila S, Kelner A, Weinreb M (2001) Systemic prostaglandin E2 increases cancellous bone formation and mass in aging rats and stimulates their bone marrow osteogenic capacity in vivo and in vitro. J Endocrinol 168: 131–139.
40. Chang K, Chang WH (2003) Pulsed electromagnetic fields prevent osteoporosis in an ovariectomized female rat model: a prostaglandin E2-associated process. Bioelectromagnetics 24: 189–198.
41. Janssens K, ten Dijke P, Janssens S, Van Hul W (2005) Transforming growth factor-beta1 to the bone. Endocr Rev 26: 743–774.
42. Tang Y, Wu X, Lei W, Pang L, Wan C, et al. (2009) TGF-beta1-induced migration of bone mesenchymal stem cells couples bone resorption with formation. Nat Med 15: 757–765.
43. Buijs JT, Stayrook KR, Guise TA (2012) The role of TGF-beta in bone metastasis: novel therapeutic perspectives. Bonekey Rep 1: 96.
44. Fukada E, Yasuda I (1957) On the Piezoelectric Effect of Bone. J Phys Soc Jpn 12: 1158–1162.

45. O'Connor BT, Charlton HM, Currey JD, Kirby DR, Woods C (1969) Effects of electric current on bone in vivo. Nature 222: 162–163.
46. McElhaney JH, Stalnaker R, Bullard R (1968) Electric fields and bone loss of disuse. J Biomech 1: 47–52.
47. Zhang X, Zhang J, Qu X, Wen J (2007) Effects of different extremely low-frequency electromagnetic fields on osteoblasts. Electromagn Biol Med 26: 167–177.
48. Gurgul S, Erdal N, Yilmaz SN, Yildiz A, Ankarali H (2008) Deterioration of bone quality by long-term magnetic field with extremely low frequency in rats. Bone 42: 74–80.
49. Yamamoto Y, Ohsaki Y, Goto T, Nakasima A, Iijima T (2003) Effects of static magnetic fields on bone formation in rat osteoblast cultures. J Dent Res 82: 962–966.
50. Xu S, Okano H, Tomita N, Ikada Y (2011) Recovery Effects of a 180 mT Static Magnetic Field on Bone Mineral Density of Osteoporotic Lumbar Vertebrae in Ovariectomized Rats. Evid Based Complement Alternat Med 2011.
51. Puricelli E, Ulbrich LM, Ponzoni D, Filho JJ (2006) Histological analysis of the effects of a static magnetic field on bone healing process in rat femurs. Head Face Med 2: 43.
52. Shiba K, Nukaya M, Tsuji T, Koshiji K (2008) Analysis of current density and specific absorption rate in biological tissue surrounding transcutaneous transformer for an artificial heart. IEEE Trans Biomed Eng 55: 205–213.
53. Pennes HH (1998) Analysis of tissue and arterial blood temperatures in the resting human forearm. 1948. J Appl Physiol (1985) 85: 5–34.

22

Inactivation of Factor VIIa by Antithrombin *In Vitro, Ex Vivo* and *In Vivo:* Role of Tissue Factor and Endothelial Cell Protein C Receptor

Rit Vatsyayan[1], Hema Kothari[1], Nigel Mackman[2], Usha R. Pendurthi[1], L. Vijaya Mohan Rao[1]*

1 Department of Cellular and Molecular Biology, The University of Texas Health Science Center at Tyler, Tyler, Texas, United States of America, **2** Division of Hematology and Oncology, McAllister Heart Institute, Department of Medicine, University of North Carolina at Chapel Hill, Chapel Hill, North Carolina, United States of America

Abstract

Recent studies have suggested that antithrombin (AT) could act as a significant physiologic regulator of FVIIa. However, *in vitro* studies showed that AT could inhibit FVIIa effectively only when it was bound to tissue factor (TF). Circulating blood is known to contain only traces of TF, at best. FVIIa also binds endothelial cell protein C receptor (EPCR), but the role of EPCR on FVIIa inactivation by AT is unknown. The present study was designed to investigate the role of TF and EPCR in inactivation of FVIIa by AT *in vivo*. Low human TF mice (low TF, ~1% expression of the mouse TF level) and high human TF mice (HTF, ~100% of the mouse TF level) were injected with human rFVIIa (120 $\mu g\ kg^{-1}$ body weight) via the tail vein. At varying time intervals following rFVIIa administration, blood was collected to measure FVIIa-AT complex and rFVIIa antigen levels in the plasma. Despite the large difference in TF expression in the mice, HTF mice generated only 40–50% more of FVIIa-AT complex as compared to low TF mice. Increasing the concentration of TF *in vivo* in HTF mice by LPS injection increased the levels of FVIIa-AT complexes by about 25%. No significant differences were found in FVIIa-AT levels among wild-type, EPCR-deficient, and EPCR-overexpressing mice. The levels of FVIIa-AT complex formed *in vitro* and *ex vivo* were much lower than that was found *in vivo*. In summary, our results suggest that traces of TF that may be present in circulating blood or extravascular TF that is transiently exposed during normal vessel damage contributes to inactivation of FVIIa by AT in circulation. However, TF's role in AT inactivation of FVIIa appears to be minor and other factor(s) present in plasma, on blood cells or vascular endothelium may play a predominant role in this process.

Editor: Toshiyuki Miyata, National Cerebral and Cardiovascular Center, Japan

Funding: The work was supported by National Institutes of Health grant HL107483. The funders had no role in study design, data collection and analysis, decision to publish, or preparation of the manuscript.

Competing Interests: The authors have declared that no competing interests exist.

* Email: Vijay.rao@uthct.edu

Introduction

Tissue factor pathway inhibitor (TFPI) is the primary physiological regulator of factor VIIa (FVIIa)-tissue factor (TF)-induced blood coagulation [1,2]. Although antithrombin III (AT) was shown to inhibit FVIIa [3–6], the physiological significance of this inhibition was debatable [7,8]. AT could effectively inhibit FVIIa only when it was bound to TF and not free FVIIa [3,4]. Still, compared to TFPI, AT was a poor inhibitor of FVIIa-TF [5,8,9]. Interestingly, Smith et al. [10] showed that levels of FVIIa-AT complex were surprisingly abundant in plasma (2% of plasma FVII antigen), and suggested that AT could be a significant regulator of FVIIa function and turnover in plasma. Recently, Agerso et al. [11] showed that rFVIIa-AT complex formation was responsible for 65% of the total rFVIIa clotting activity clearance following intravenous administration of rFVIIa in hemophilia patients. This is somewhat surprising as *in vitro* studies showed little inhibition of FVIIa by AT in the absence of TF, even in the presence of saturating concentrations of heparin [3,4]. Furthermore, circulating blood contains either no detectable TF, or at best, traces of TF [12–14]. The above studies raise an interesting question that whether TF, either circulating or intravascular, or some other factors in blood are responsible for relatively rapid inactivation of FVIIa by AT *in vivo*.

Since AT preferentially inhibits FVIIa bound to TF, and FVIIa-AT complex rapidly disassociates from TF [9], the circulating levels of FVIIa-AT complex is thought to be an important indirect indicator of intravascular TF exposure *in vivo* [10]. Therefore, a number of recent studies measured plasma FVIIa-AT levels in various patient groups to investigate whether FVIIa-AT levels in plasma could predict hypercoagulable state and thrombotic risk [15–18]. Although these studies indicate that the FVIIa-AT levels may be useful in identifying hypercoagulable state in specific patient groups, they strongly suggest that large prospective cohort studies were needed to consider the clinical application of FVIIa-AT complex determination [17]. More importantly, to date, there is no empirical data in the literature showing that exposure of blood to intravascular TF is primarily responsible for the generation of FVIIa-AT complex *in vivo*.

Studies from our laboratory [19] and others [20,21] have established that FVIIa binds endothelial protein C receptor (EPCR) in a true ligand manner. The interaction between FVIIa and EPCR is capable of not only eliciting protease activated receptor-1 (PAR1)-mediated barrier protective signaling [22,23], but also promotes internalization of the receptor–ligand complex [24]. At present, it is unknown whether FVIIa binding to EPCR influences AT inactivation of FVIIa. Recently, we have shown that rFVIIa administered to mice intravenously (i.v) associates with EPCR, and EPCR facilitates the entry of FVIIa from circulation into perivascular tissues [25]. Once entered into perivascular tissues, FVIIa was retained there in functionally active state for extended time periods (24 h to 7 days) [25], which sharply contrasts to the short circulating half-life (<30 min) of FVIIa [26]. Since EPCR is present primarily on the endothelium whereas TF is mainly localized in extravascular cells, it raises the possibility that TF may be involved in FVIIa retention in extravascular tissues.

Development of transgenic mice that express either low levels of human TF (low TF) or high levels of human TF (HTF) in place of murine TF were useful in obtaining valuable insights into TF's role in hemostasis, thrombosis and vascular development [27,28]. Compared to wild-type TF, low TF mice express ~1% of TF [29] whereas HTF mice express ~100% of TF, except in the heart [30]. Similarly, development of EPCR-deficient and EPCR-overexpressing mice helped in elucidating the role of EPCR in hemostasis and inflammation [31,32]. In the present study, we used the above mice to investigate the role of TF and EPCR in generation of FVIIa-AT complex *in vivo*. In order to compare the rates of AT inactivation of FVIIa *in vitro, ex vivo* and *in vivo,* human rFVIIa was administered to mice, or added to whole blood or plasma. Evaluation of the role of TF and EPCR in AT inactivation of exogenously administered rFVIIa is clinically relevant as AT was believed to be primarily responsible for rapid inactivation of therapeutically administered rFVIIa to hemophilic patients [11]. In addition, we also measured endogenous levels of FVIIa-AT complex in wild-type, TF and EPCR transgenic mice.

Materials and Methods

Ethics statement

Human participants: Blood from healthy donors was obtained following a written consent. Human subject research was approved by the Institutional Review Board at The University of Texas Health Science Center at Tyler.

Animals: All studies involving animals were conducted in accordance with the animal welfare guidelines set forth in the Guide for the Care and Use of Laboratory Animals and Department of Health and Human Services, and approved by the Institutional Animal Use and Care Committee of The University of Texas Health Science Center at Tyler, Tyler, TX (Animal Welfare Assurance Number A3589-01; Protocol Number: 530).

Reagents

Human rFVIIa was obtained from Novo Nordisk A/S (Maaloev, Denmark). Mouse rFVIIa was provided by Mirella Ezban/Lars Petersen, Novo Nordisk (Denmark). Affinity purified polyclonal antibodies against human FVIIa were provided by the late Walter Kisiel (University of New Mexico, Albuquerque, NM, USA). Murine FVIIa antibodies were raised in-house by immunizing rabbits with recombinant mouse FVIIa. Antithrombin and sheep anti-AT antibodies, for both human and murine, were purchased from Haematologic Technologies, Inc (Essex Junction VT, USA). Human factor X was from Enzyme Research Laboratories (South Bend, IN, USA). Chromogenic substrate Chromogenix S-2765 was from DiaPharma (West Chester, OH, USA). Rat anti-mouse TF mAb (1H1) antibodies were provided by Daniel Kirchhofer, Genentech, CA, USA. Donkey anti-sheep biotinylated IgG was obtained from Thermo Scientific (Rockford, IL, USA). Lipopolysaccharide (LPS) from *Escherichia coli* 0111:B4 were from Sigma (St. Louis. MO, USA). Streptavidin alkaline phosphatase (ALP) and BluePhos microwell phosphatase substrate system were from KPL (Gaithersburg, MD, USA).

Cells

Primary human umbilical vein endothelial cells (HUVEC), EBM-2 basal medium, and growth supplements were purchased from Lonza (Walkersville, MD, USA). Endothelial cells were cultured in EBM-2 basal medium supplemented with growth supplements, 1% penicillin/streptomycin, and 2% fetal bovine serum.

Mice

The generation of low TF and HTF mice was described earlier [29,30]. Breeding pairs of EPCR-deficient (EPCR-def) and EPCR-overexpressing (EPCR-OE) mice were obtained from Chuck Esmon (Oklahoma Medical Research Foundation, Oklahoma City, OK, USA), and their generation was described in earlier reports [31,32]. Where available, littermate controls were used as wild-type mice. Otherwise, wild-type mice were obtained from Jackson Laboratory (Bar Harbor, ME, USA) or in-house breeding program. All mice were in C57BL/6J genetic background.

Administration of rFVIIa to mice, collection of blood and tissues

Human rFVIIa was administered to mice via the tail vein at a dose of 120 μg kg^{-1} body weight in 100 μL of Tris-buffered saline (TBS, 50 mM Tris–HCl, 0.15 M NaCl, pH 7.5). At various time intervals, ranging from 5 min to 7 days after rFVIIa administration, blood was collected either via submandibular vein or by cardiac puncture at right ventricle if it was a terminal time point. Only two or three blood samples were obtained from each mouse. Blood was collected into 1/10 volume of 0.13 M sodium citrate anticoagulant unless otherwise specified. Mice were subsequently exsanguinated by severing the renal artery and perfused by flushing ice-cold saline containing 5 mM $CaCl_2$+1 mM $MgCl_2$ through the heart. Knee bone joints were excised, rinsed briefly with ice-cold saline containing 5 mM $CaCl_2$+1 mM $MgCl_2$, and then processed for measuring FVIIa activity and antigen levels. Briefly, excised knee bone joints were cut into fine pieces with a sharp razor blade, and added to TBS buffer containing EDTA (20 mM) (0.5 mL buffer per 100 mg tissue), freeze-thawed, vortexed, and centrifuged to obtain clear supernatant for measuring FVIIa antigen or activity levels.

Ex vivo studies were conducted using blood drawn into factor Xa inhibitor, rivaroxaban (100 μg/ml blood) as an anticoagulant. Plasma was separated by centrifugation at 6, 000×g for 15 min.

Isolation of microparticles (MPs) from plasma, and TF activity assay

Microparticles from mouse plasma were isolated essentially as described earlier [33]. TF activity in MPs was measured by adding either mouse (in wild-type mice) or human FVIIa (in low TF and HTF mice) (10 nM), and human FX (175 nM), and measuring the amount of FXa generated at the end of 1 or 2 h activation period in a chromogenic assay. In some experiments, TF activity was measured both in the presence and absence of neutralizing TF antibodies to determine TF-specific coagulant activity.

Generation and isolation of cell-derived microparticles

Confluent monolayers of HUVEC cultured in 100 mm dish were infected with control and TF adenovirus [34] (10 moi/cell). Two days post-infection, cells were washed with buffer A (10 mM Hepes, 0.15 M NaCl, 4 mM KCl, 11 mM glucose, pH 7.5), and then treated with calcium ionomycin (10 μM) in buffer B (buffer A containing 5 mM $CaCl_2$ and 1 mg/ml bovine serum albumin) for 20 min at 37°C. Supernatant was collected and centrifuged first at 200×g for 5 min to remove any cell debris, and then centrifuged for 1 h at 20,000×g at 4°C to sediment microparticles. Microparticle pellet was washed once with buffer A, resuspended in 100 μl of buffer A, and stored at 4°C until used. Characterization of microparticles derived from endothelial cells transfected with control adenovirus (TF^- microparticles) and TF adenovirus (TF^+ microparticles) in prothrombin activation assay revealed that their prothrombin activation potential was essentially equal, indicating that both TF^- and TF^+ MPs express equal amounts of phosphatidylserine. As expected, TF^+ microparticles and not TF^- microparticles effectively activated FX. TF concentration in TF^+ microparticles was estimated in factor X activation assay using known concentrations of relipidated TF as a standard.

FVIIa antigen and activity assays

rFVIIa antigen levels were determined by ELISA using rabbit anti-human FVIIa as the capture antibody and biotinylated rabbit anti-human FVIIa as the detecting antibody. FVIIa clotting activity was measured in a FVIIa-specific clotting assay as described previously [25] using STart coagulation analyzer (Diagnostica Stago, Parsippany, NJ, USA). Briefly, 50 μl of sample was incubated with 50 μl of 100 nM soluble TF in 1 mM phospholipids (40% phosphatidyl choline/25% phosphatidyl serine/35% phosphatidyl ethanolamine) and 100 μl of FVII-deficient plasma (George King Biomedical Inc., Overland Park, KS, USA) for 3 min at 37°C, and clotting was initiated by the addition of 100 μl of 25 mM $CaCl_2$. Varying known concentrations of rFVIIa (0.5 ng to 30 ng/ml for the ELISA; 0.25 to 50 ng/ml for the activity assay) were used to construct a standard curve.

Measurement of FVIIa-AT complexes

Majority of experiments described in this study required the measurement of human rFVIIa-mouse AT complex. The amount of rFVIIa-AT complex generated in our experimental system was determined by using an in-house developed ELISA, which is specific to measure the complex between human rFVIIa and mouse AT. Briefly, rabbit anti-human FVIIa antibodies (5 μg/ml) were coated onto 96-well ELISA plate for overnight at 4°C. After blocking the wells with 0.1% gelatin, diluted samples were added to the wells to capture rFVIIa. After 1 h incubation at room temperature, unbound material was removed, wells were washed 4 times, and then sheep anti–mouse AT antibody (5 μg/ml) was added to the wells for 1 h, followed by donkey anti-sheep biotinylated IgG (1:500), and streptavidin ALP (1:200 dilution) for 1 h each with ample washings of the wells prior to the addition of each reagent. Color was developed by using BluePhos microwell phosphatase substrate system, and measured at 650 nm. A background reading obtained in a zero min time point sample was subtracted from the readings of other time points. To generate rFVIIa-AT standard, a known concentration of rFVIIa (100 nM, 5 μg/ml) was incubated with soluble TF (200 nM), mouse AT (1 μM), and heparin (10 U/ml) overnight at 37°C, and the samples were subjected to non-reducing SDS-PAGE followed by immunoblot analysis to evaluate the extent of FVIIa-AT complex formation. The concentration of rFVIIa-AT in the standard was determined by the relative band intensities of rFVIIa-AT and free rFVIIa. Typically, more than 80% of FVIIa was in complex with AT. Varying concentrations of rFVIIa-AT complex (0.325 to 80 ng/ml, FVIIa-AT concentration depicts ng FVIIa in complex with AT) were used to generate a standard curve. The lower detection limit of the assay was between 0.25 to 0.5 ng ml^{-1} rFVIIa-AT complexes. The assay was specific to detect human FVIIa-mouse AT complex (substitution of free human FVIIa, mouse FVIIa, mouse AT or mouse control plasma in place of human FVIIa-mouse AT complex gave a reading similar to that of the blank (buffer), OD<0.1).

A similar procedure was used for measuring mouse FVIIa-mouse AT complexes or human FVIIa-human AT complexes. For this, ELISA plates were coated with either rabbit anti-mouse FVIIa antibodies or anti-human FVIIa antibodies to capture FVII/FVIIa from that particular species. The species-specific FVIIa-AT complexes were detected using either sheep anti-mouse AT or anti-human AT. It may be pertinent to note here that anti-mouse FVIIa antibodies do not cross react with human FVIIa and *vice versa*. Mouse FVIIa-AT standard was made by complexing recombinant mouse rFVIIa with mouse AT, and human FVIIa-AT standard was made by incubating human rFVIIa with human AT as described in the above paragraph.

Statistics

All *in vitro* and *ex vivo* experiments were repeated three or more times. For *in vivo* studies, 3 to 9 mice were used for each group. Analysis of a data set using statistical software (GraphPad, Prism vs. 4.03, La Jolla, CA, USA) where n was 8 or more passed the normality test (D'Agostino and Pearson omni bus normality test). The data were shown as the mean ± SEM. Statistical significance between the two experimental groups was determined by Students t-test. One-way analysis of variance was used to determine statistical significance among three groups.

Results

Formation of FVIIa-AT complex in buffer, plasma and blood

First, we compared the rate of rFVIIa-AT complex formation in buffer, plasma, and blood in the absence of exogenously added heparin or TF. We included the plasma concentration of AT in a buffer system, and rFVIIa (1 μg/ml) was added to all three systems. As shown in Fig. 1A, increasing amounts of rFVIIa-AT complex was formed with increase in times under all experimental conditions. However, only less than 1% of FVIIa was found to be in complex with AT in a buffer system at the end of 1 h incubation with AT (Fig. 1A). The rate of rFVIIa-AT complex formation was significantly higher in plasma compared in buffer (about 4-fold). The rate of rFVIIa-AT complex formation was 2-fold higher in blood, compared in plasma.

It is possible that increased levels of rFVIIa-AT generated in plasma and blood, compared to a buffer system, may be due to the presence of traces of TF in plasma and blood. To investigate this possibility, we first attempted to measure TF antigen levels in mouse plasma. However, the sensitivity of TF ELISA assay was not suitable for detecting picograms of TF that may be present in plasma. Next, we measured MP-associated TF activity in plasma in factor X activation assay, using known concentrations of relipidated TF as the standard. This assay revealed that plasma of wild-type mice contains ~2 pg/ml TF (data not shown). Actual concentration of TF in plasma may be slightly higher since this assay does not take into account soluble TF and TF that may not associate with MPs. To determine the role of trace amounts of TF in plasma in rFVIIa inactivation by AT, first we attempted to

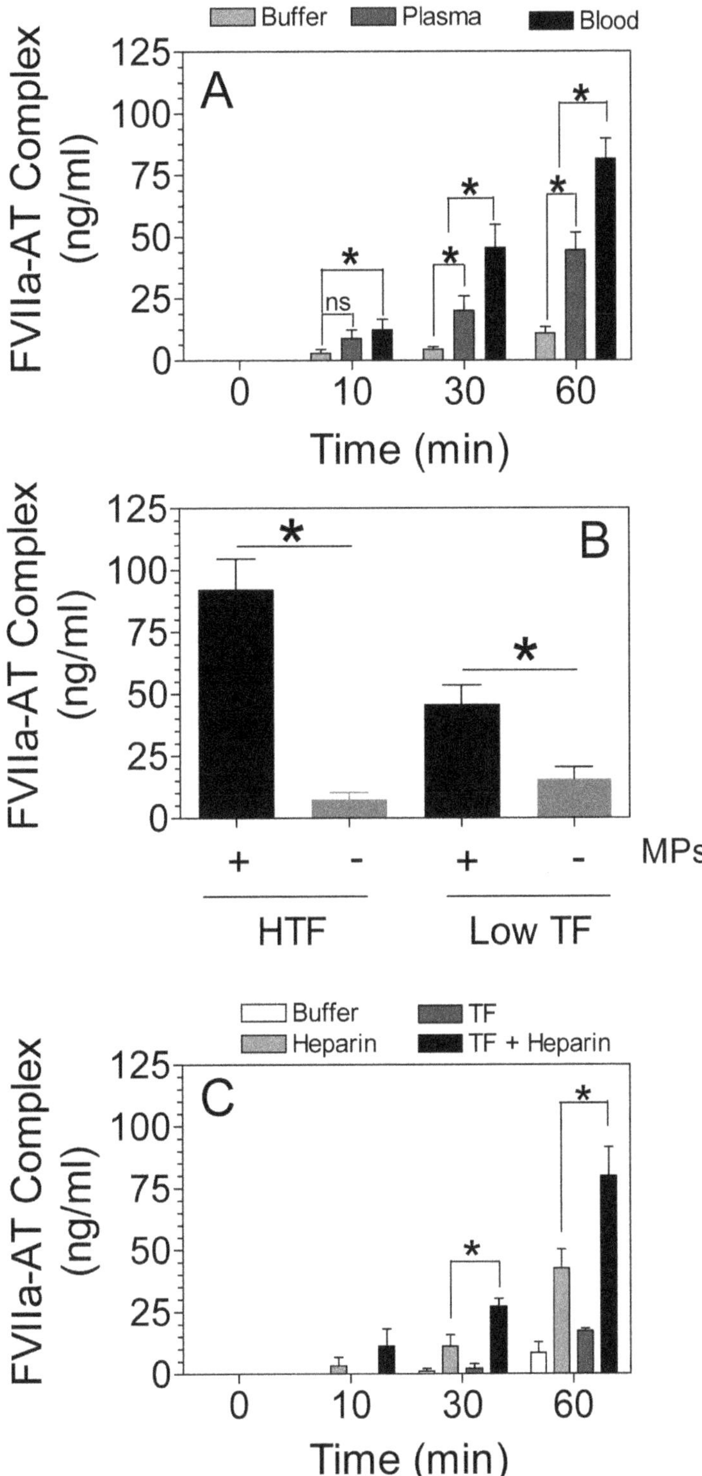

Figure 1. Comparison of FVIIa-AT complex formation *in vitro* and *ex vivo* conditions. (A) Blood from wild-type mice was drawn into rivaroxaban as an anticoagulant. Plasma was separated by centrifugation at 6,000×g for 5 min. To a reaction system not containing plasma or blood, a plasma concentration of AT (125 μg/ml) was added to Tris-buffered saline (TBS) containing 1 mg/ml bovine serum albumin (BSA), 5 mM $CaCl_2$ and 1 mM $MgCl_2$. rFVIIa was added to all three reaction systems (buffer, plasma and blood) to a final concentration of 1 μg/ml. At various time points, an aliquot was removed from the reaction mixtures and diluted 1:10 in TBS/BSA containing 10 mM EDTA, and frozen immediately until they were used for the assay. Levels of FVIIa-AT complex was measured in an ELISA as described in Methods (n = 6 to 9). (B) Plasma obtained from HTF and low TF mice was divided into two equal aliquots, and one of the aliquots was subjected to centrifugation 20,000×g for 1 h at 4°C to remove microparticles. rFVIIa (1 μg/ml) was added to both the plasmas, and FVIIa-AT complex generated at 60 min was determined. (C) rFVIIa (1 μg/ml) was incubated for varying times with AT (125 μg/ml) in TBS/BSA buffer containing 5 mM $CaCl_2$+1 mM $MgCl_2$ in the presence or absence of heparin (1 U/ml) and relipidated TF (100 pg/ml). FVIIa-AT levels were determined in an ELISA (n = 4). The concentration of FVIIa-AT (ng/ml) reflects ng of FVIIa complexed with AT. *Indicates that the compared values differ in statistically significant manner ($P<0.05$).

inhibit plasma TF activity by using TF neutralizing antibodies. However, both TF antibodies and control IgG interfered in measuring FVIIa-AT complex levels in an ELISA. Therefore, next we compared the generation of rFVIIa-AT complexes in plasma of low TF and HTF mice. As shown in Fig. 1B, the formation of rFVIIa-AT complex in plasma of HTF mice was significantly higher than in plasma of low TF mice. Furthermore, removal of MPs from the plasma by centrifugation significantly reduced the levels of rFVIIa-AT formation in plasma. These data indicate that traces of TF in plasma significantly accelerate inactivation of FVIIa by AT.

The effect of low concentrations of TF on FVIIa-AT complex formation was examined further in a buffer system where rFVIIa was incubated with AT ± heparin (1 U/mL) in the presence or absence of relipidated TF (100 pg/ml). As shown in Fig. 1C, a low concentration of TF substantially enhanced the formation of FVIIa-AT complex both in the absence and presence of heparin. In the presence of both TF and heparin, we observed ~10-fold increase in the rate of FVIIa-AT generation in comparison to a buffer system containing AT alone. However, even in the presence of heparin and TF, only less than 10% of rFVIIa was found to be in complex with AT at the end of 60 min incubation time (Fig. 1C).

In additional studies, to examine the role of MPs on FVIIa-AT complex formation in plasma, endothelial cell-derived MPs bearing TF or lacking TF were added to human plasma or whole blood supplemented with rFVIIa (1 μg/ml), and the levels of FVIIa-AT formed at the end of 1 h was measured. The concentration of MP TF chosen for this study was 30 pg/ml, an outer limit of MP-TF concentration that could possibly be present in patients with high thrombotic risk (see rev [35] for references). Although we found a modest, 20 and 50%, increase in FVIIa-AT levels in plasma supplemented with TF^- and TF^+ MPs, respectively, over the control plasma, this increase was not statistically significant (FVIIa-AT levels, ng/ml : no MPs, 6.14±1.45; TF^- MPs, 8.23±2.84; TF^+ MPs, 11.13±5.9; n = 6). Heparin (1 U/ml) increased FVIIa-AT levels in plasma by 4-fold, but the presence of TF^- or TF^+ MPs had no measurable influence on AT inactivation of FVIIa. Similarly, no differences were found in FVIIa-AT levels in whole blood in the presence or absence of MPs (data not shown).

Role of TF in generation of FVIIa-AT complex *in vivo*

First to determine the extent of FVIIa-AT complex formed *in vivo* in mice under basal conditions and the role of TF in generation of FVIIa-AT, we measured mouse FVIIa-AT complexes in plasma obtained from wild-type, HTF and low TF mice. Both wild-type and HTF mice contained similar levels of mouse FVIIa-AT complex (wild-type, 6.93±2.47 ng/ml, n = 6; HTF, 7.66±2.40 ng/ml, n = 8) whereas FVIIa-AT levels were substantially low in low TF mice (1.21±0.19 ng/ml, n = 12).

Next to compare the rate of AT inactivation of FVIIa *in vivo* vs. *in vitro* or *ex vivo*, and to determine the role of TF or other *in vivo* parameters in influencing AT inactivation of therapeutic concentrations of rFVIIa, low TF and HTF mice were administered with human rFVIIa (120 μg kg^{-1} body weight). Blood was collected at various time intervals following rFVIIa administration, and rFVIIa-AT complex and rFVIIa antigen levels in plasma were measured. As shown in Fig. 2A, rFVIIa complex formation with AT was evident as early as 1 min following rFVIIa administration in both the genotypes. rFVIIa-AT levels peaked at 60 min, and start to decline thereafter. At 24 h following rFVIIa administration, rFVIIa-AT complexes were barely detectable in plasma. The levels of rFVIIa-AT complex were significantly higher in HTF mice as compared with low TF mice at 30 and 60 min following rFVIIa administration (Fig. 2A). It may be pertinent to note here that measurement of TAT at these points showed no significant differences between HTF and low TF mice (TAT levels ng/ml at 30 min: low TF, 19.69±4.38; HTF 14.30±2.7; at 60 min: low TF, 24.27±9.78; HTF 18.93±4.7, n = 6).

We also measured rFVIIa antigen levels in the plasma of HTF and low TF mice to investigate whether TF influences pharmacokinetics of rFVIIa, which in turn could influence the formation of rFVIIa-AT complex *in vivo*. As shown in Fig. 2B, no significant differences were found in rFVIIa antigen levels in the HTF and low TF mice, indicating that differences in rFVIIa-AT complex levels in these mice at 30 and 60 min is not due to the difference in the plasma rFVIIa antigen levels in these mice.

The comparison of rFVIIa antigen and rFVIIa-AT complex levels, particularly in samples obtained at 60 min or later following rFVIIa administration, suggests that rFVIIa antigen assay does not fully recognize rFVIIa in rFVIIa-AT complex. Thus, rFVIIa antigen levels were substantially lower than rFVIIa-AT complex levels at these later time points, and also lower than predicted rFVIIa antigens levels based on our earlier FVIIa clearance studies utilizing ^{125}I-labeled rFVIIa. Here, it may be pertinent to note that we evaluated several other FVIIa antibodies, both prepared in-house and obtained commercially or from other investigators, and none of the antibodies recognized rFVIIa in complex with AT to the same extent as of free rFVIIa.

Role of EPCR in generation of FVIIa-AT complex *in vivo*

Recently, we have shown that FVIIa binds EPCR both *in vitro* and *in vivo* [19,36]. Therefore, we investigated here whether FVIIa binding to EPCR influences FVIIa-AT complex formation *in vivo*. Human rFVIIa was injected into wild-type, EPCR over-expressing (EPCR-OE), and EPCR-deficient mice (EPCR-def) and the levels of rFVIIa-AT complex were measured. As shown in Fig. 3A, there were no significant differences in the levels of rFVIIa-AT complex generated among the wild-type, EPCR-def and EPCR-OE mice. We also measured endogenous FVIIa-AT levels in the above groups of mice (no rFVIIa was administered). These data also showed no significant differences in FVIIa-AT levels among the three groups (Fig. 3B). It may pertinent to note here that while human FVIIa binds murine EPCR, murine FVIIa does not bind murine EPCR in any significant manner [36].

Effect of enhanced TF expression on FVIIa-AT complex formation *in vivo*

If traces of TF contribute to the generation of FVIIa-AT complex formation *in vivo,* then pathological conditions (e.g., sepsis, atherosclerosis etc.), where TF expression is upregulated in cells that come in contact with blood, may accelerate FVIIa-AT complex formation. Wang et al. [33] showed that TF MP levels were increased several fold in endotoxemic mice. To test the effect of increased expression of TF *in vivo* on FVIIa-AT generation, wild-type mice were injected with saline or LPS (5 mg/kg body weight), and 5 h after LPS administration blood was collected from these mice by cardiac puncture, and plasma was processed for measuring MPs procoagulant activity and mouse FVIIa-AT complexes. As shown in Fig. 4A, LPS administration markedly increased the procoagulant activity of plasma MPs. The increased procoagulant activity was due to the generation of TF^+ MPs since the incubation of MPs with mouse TF mAb blocked the increased procoagulant activity. LPS administration increased the levels of FVIIa-AT complexes in plasma by about 50% compared to the saline control, but the difference is not statistically significant, probably due to a wider variation in FVIIa-AT levels in these

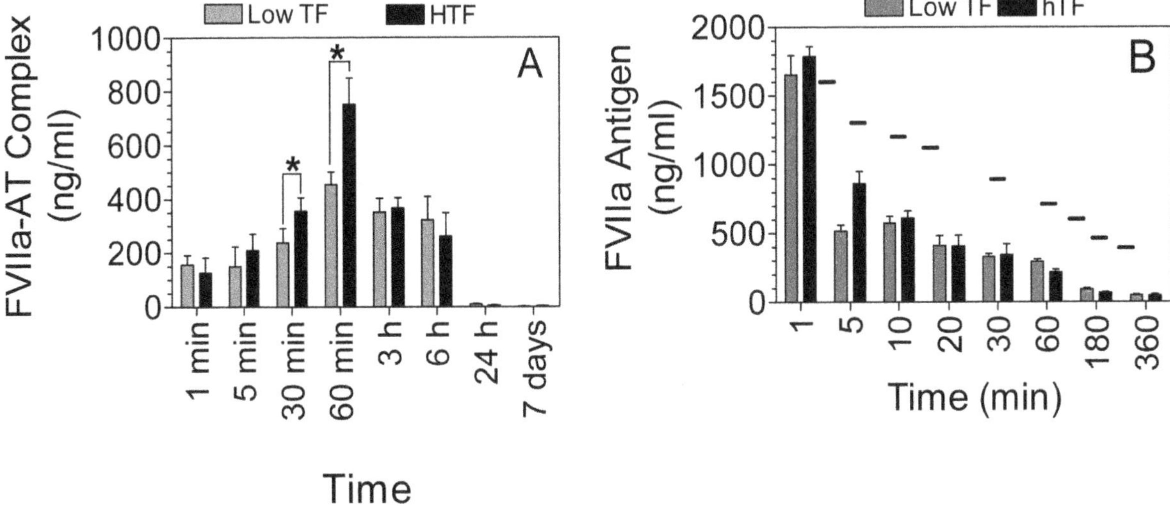

Figure 2. Levels of FVIIa-AT generated *in vivo* in HTF and low TF mice following administration of rFVIIa. HTF and low TF mice were injected with rFVIIa (120 μg/kg body weight) intravenously via the tail vein. FVIIa-AT complex (A) and FVIIa antigen (B) levels were determined in plasma obtained from these mice at various time points following rFVIIa administration (n = 4 or more). The small bar (–) in the figure represents expected FVIIa antigen levels, based on our previous study of rFVIIa clearance in wild-type mice using ^{125}I-rFVIIa as a tracer [26], at 3, 5, 15, 30, 60, 120, 180, and 240 min following rFVIIa administration. The concentration of FVIIa-AT (ng/ml) reflects ng of FVIIa complexed with AT. *Indicates the value differs in statistically significant manner (*P<0.05*) between HTF and low TF mice at the given time point.

mice. It may be important to note here that measuring endogenous murine FVIIa-AT complexes in LPS administered mice may not provide a complete picture of the role of TF on AT inactivation of FVIIa since FVIIa-AT complex formation is limited by the availability of FVIIa. LPS administration may not significantly increase FVIIa levels *in vivo* [37].

Therefore, to investigate the effect of enhanced *in vivo* TF on AT inactivation of FVIIa more accurately, HTF mice were injected with LPS (5 mg/kg body weight), and after 5 h, human rFVIIa was given to these mice via tail vein injection, and the amount of rFVIIa-AT complex generated in plasma was measured. As shown in Fig. 5A, MP TF activity was increased by 6-fold in HTF mice administered with LPS compared to control HTF mice. Measurement of rFVIIa-AT complex in these mice showed a slight but statistically significant increase in rFVIIa-AT levels in LPS-challenged mice compared to control mice

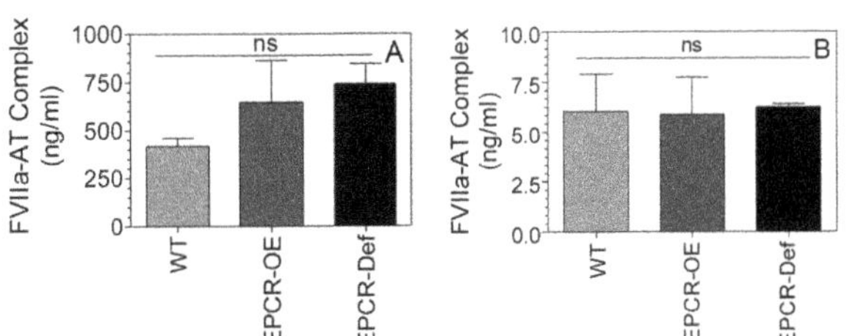

Figure 3. Levels of FVIIa-AT generated *in vivo* in wild-type, EPCR-overexpressing (EPCR-OE), and EPCR-deficient (EPCR-def) mice. (A) Wild-type, EPCR-OE and EPCR-def mice were injected with rFVIIa (120 μg/kg body weight) intravenously via the tail vein. FVIIa-AT levels in plasma obtained from these mice at 60 min post-rFVIIa administration was measured in an ELISA assay (n = 3–4). (B) Endogenous FVIIa-AT levels. Plasma obtained from wild-type, EPCR-OE and EPCR-def mice that were not subjected to any treatment were used to measure endogenous FVIIa-AT levels. The concentration of FVIIa-AT (ng/ml) reflects ng of FVIIa complexed with AT. ns, not statistically significant as determined in one-way analysis of variance.

(Fig. 5B). We also measured the levels of endogenous mouse FVIIa-AT complexes generated in the above experimental system. LPS treatment increased the levels of endogenous mouse FVIIa-AT in these mice by 40% (data not shown).

Role of TF in retention of rFVIIa activity and antigen *in vivo*

Recently, we have shown that rFVIIa entered into extravascular tissues via EPCR-dependent mechanism is retained in tissues for extended time periods [25]. It has been thought that TF present on extravascular cells may play a role in retention of FVIIa in tissues [25]. Our earlier analysis of TF expression by immunohis-

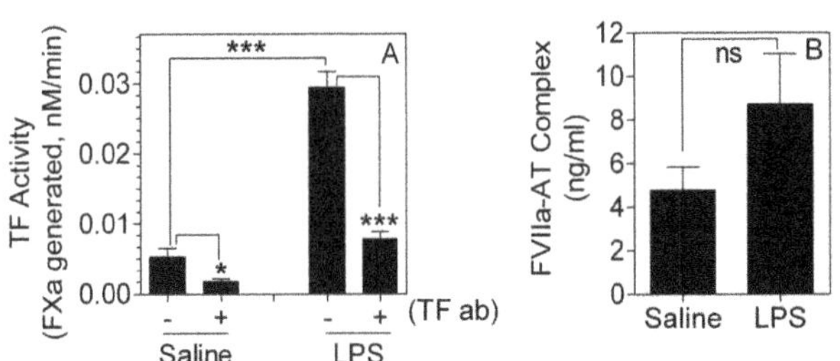

Figure 4. Measurement of microparticle TF procoagulant activity and FVIIa-AT levels in plasma following LPS administration in wild-type mice. Wild-type mice (C57BL/6J) were injected with saline or LPS (5 mg/kg body weight) intraperitoneally. 5 h after saline or LPS administration, blood was obtained from these mice by cardiac puncture, and plasma samples were processed for isolation of microparticles to measure TF procoagulant activity (A) or for determination of FVIIa-AT levels (B). Procoagulant activity measured in factor Xa generation assay in the absence or presence of mouse TF mAb (10 μg/ml, preincubated for 30 min) (n = 5). *Indicates the values differ in statistically significant manner between the control and LPS-treated mice. The concentration of FVIIa-AT (ng/ml) reflects ng of FVIIa complexed with AT. *, *P<0.05*; ***, *P<0.001*; ns, not statistically significant.

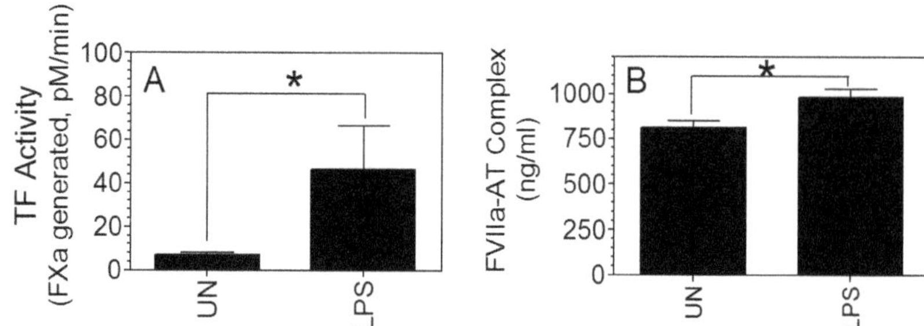

Figure 5. Effect of increased TF expression on formation of FVIIa-AT complex in HTF mice administered with therapeutic concentrations of rFVIIa. HTF mice were injected with LPS (5 mg/kg body weight) intraperitoneally. 5 h after LPS administration, rFVIIa (120 µg/kg body weight) was injected into these mice as well as unchallenged mice. 1 h following rFVIIa administration, blood was drawn from these mice by cardiac puncture, and plasma samples were processed for isolation of TF microparticles or determination of FVIIa-AT levels. (A) Microparticle TF activity; (B) FVIIa-AT levels (n = 4). The concentration of FVIIa-AT (ng/ml) reflects ng of FVIIa complexed with AT. *Indicates the values differ in statistically significant manner between the control and LPS-treated mice.

tochemistry in various tissues of wild-type mice revealed the presence of TF in bone joints in the zone of calcified cartilage in the growth plate region and the mineralized bone [38]. To investigate the effect of TF in retaining FVIIa in bone joints, rFVIIa was administered to low TF and HTF mice, and seven days after rFVIIa administration, bone joints from these mice were collected, and rFVIIa antigen and activity levels in bone joints were measured. As shown in Fig. 6A, rFVIIa antigen levels were significantly higher in the bone joints of HTF mice as compared with low TF mice. Measurement of FVIIa activity in these samples showed that rFVIIa in the bone joint of HTF is functionally active. As with rFVIIa antigen level, FVIIa activity level was substantially higher in bone joints of HTF as compared to low TF mice (Fig. 6B).

Discussion

The present study carried out with low TF mice expressing ~1% of wild-type TF and HTF mice expressing ~100% of wild-type TF indicates that TF contributes to the formation of FVIIa-AT complex *in vivo*. Increased levels of FVIIa-AT complex were found in plasma of HTF mice compared to low TF mice endogenously as well as after administration of a therapeutic concentration of rFVIIa. Further, the observation that increased intravascular exposure of TF by LPS administration to HTF mice moderately, but statistically significant fashion, increased FVIIa-AT levels in the plasma confirms that increased FVIIa-AT levels in plasma may reflect exposure of blood to increased levels of intravascular TF. Nonetheless, our data also indicate that the effect of TF on AT inactivation of FVIIa appears to be modest, and therefore, measurement of FVIIa-AT levels in plasma may not be a very sensitive indicator of intravascular TF exposure, and may lack robustness in accurately predicting hypercoagulable state. For example, despite a ~100-fold difference in TF expression between HTF and low TF mice, differences in FVIIa-AT levels between the two genotypes following rFVIIa administration was less than 2-fold, that too only at 30 and 60 min following rFVIIa administration but not at later time points. Similarly, LPS administration increased MP-associated TF activity in plasma of HTF mice by more than 600% whereas it only led to a small increase (~25%) in FVIIa-AT levels in plasma.

Recent studies of pharmacokinetics of rFVIIa in hemophilia patients or animals showed that the majority of rFVIIa clotting activity following rFVIIa intravenous administration was inhibited by AT by forming rFVIIa-AT complexes [11,39,40]. These results suggest that AT inhibition of rFVIIa controls drug duration in hemophilia treatment with rFVIIa. Furthermore, these data also showed that the rate of inhibition of rFVIIa by AT is significantly higher *in vivo* than *in vitro* [40]. Consistent with these data, we found that most of rFVIIa in circulation was in complex with AT at 60 min following rFVIIa administration as the levels of FVIIa-AT complex measured at this time were very similar to total FVIIa antigen levels in the circulation (compare Fig. 2A and 2B). Although TF contributes to the formation of rFVIIa-AT complex *in vivo*, it does not appear to influence the overall pharmacokinetics of rFVIIa as rFVIIa was cleared in a similar fashion in low TF and HTF mice. These data were also consistent with the earlier observation that showed clearance of FVIIa was unaffected

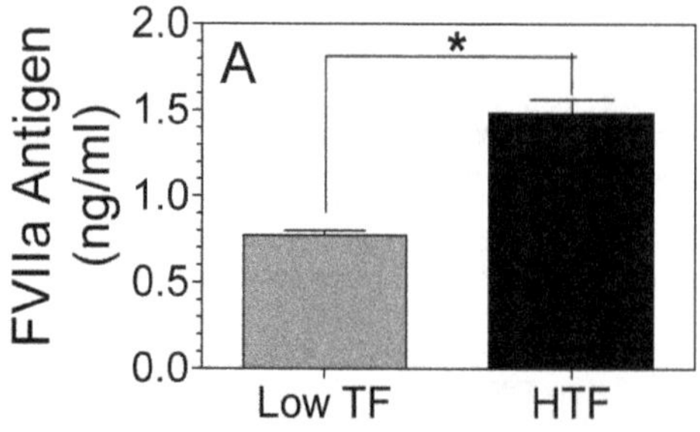

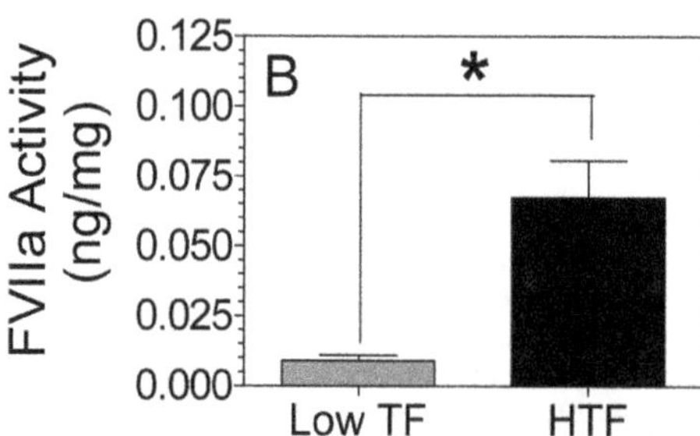

Figure 6. Higher levels of FVIIa retained in bone joints of HTF compared to low TF mice. HTF and low TF mice were injected intravenously via the tail vein with rFVIIa (120 µg/kg body weight). Seven days later, bone joints were collected, bone joint fluids were eluted, and assayed for FVIIa antigen (A) and FVIIa activity (B) levels (n = 3). *Indicates the value differs in statistically significant manner *(P<0.05)* between HTF and low TF mice.

by its inactivation with AT [41]. The observation that rFVIIa-AT complex formation was impeded, but not markedly impaired in low TF mice indicates that TF plays probably a minor role in FVIIa inactivation by AT *in vivo*. Overall, our data suggest that although TF contributes to FVIIa-AT generation *in vivo*, it may not be the principle player that regulate rFVIIa inactivation by AT *in vivo*.

Comparison of rFVIIa-AT complex formation *in vitro, ex vivo* and *in vivo* conditions show that only traces of rFVIIa was complexed with AT *in vitro* (in buffer) in the absence of heparin. Although rFVIIa-AT complex formation was higher in plasma and blood, relative to that in buffer, still only less than 10% of rFVIIa formed complex with AT even after 1 h of incubation time. A significantly higher level of rFVIIa-AT formation in blood, compared to plasma, indicates that blood cells may promote rFVIIa inactivation by AT. At present, blood cell types that are responsible for this are unknown. Addition of heparin and a low concentration of relipidated TF increased FVIIa-AT formation in a buffer system, reaching to comparable level obtained in the blood in *ex vivo* condition. At present, it is unclear whether heparin-like proteoglycans and/or TF on blood cells is responsible for increasing FVIIa-AT complex formation in blood. It may be pertinent to add here that exogenous addition of TF^{+} MPs to human slightly increased AT inactivation of FVIIa in *ex vivo*, but this increase was not statistically significant. It is possible that other clotting factors in blood or other components of blood may contribute for the increased FVIIa-AT generation in blood. Here, one should note that both clotting factors IX and X were shown to enhance the inhibition of FVIIa-TF by AT on a human bladder carcinoma cell line [42]. In contrast to *in vitro* and *ex vivo*, rFVIIa complex formation with AT was relatively rapid *in vivo*. Within one minute following rFVIIa administration, the formation of rFVIIa-AT complex was evident, and most of rFVIIa present in circulation at 60 min following rFVIIa administration was in complex with AT. It is unclear at present the exact mechanism(s) by which FVIIa was rapidly inactivated by AT *in vivo*.

Recently, we have shown that rFVIIa administered to mice rapidly associates with EPCR on vascular endothelium *in vivo* [25,26,36]. Therefore, it is entirely possible that FVIIa binding to EPCR could facilitate FVIIa inactivation by AT. However, studies conducted herein with EPCR-deficient mice and EPCR overexpressing mice (at least 8- or more fold higher EPCR expression over the wild-type [32]) clearly show that EPCR does not play a role in FVIIa-AT complex formation *in vivo* as we observed similar levels of rFVIIa-AT complex in these mice following rFVIIa administration.

Our recent studies showed that although most of the rFVIIa administered to mice was cleared rapidly from circulation with a half-life of less than 30 min, a small amount of rFVIIa enters into extravascular tissues, and this FVIIa was retained for extended time periods in tissues [25,26,38,43]. Since most of the extravascular cells express TF, and FVIIa binds to TF with a high affinity, it had been thought that TF may be playing a role in retaining FVIIa entered into extravasculature [25]. Our present observation of increased levels of rFVIIa activity and antigen in bone joints of HTF mice compared to low TF mice even 7 days after rFVIIa administration clearly supports the above hypothesis that FVIIa entered into extravasculature associates with TF, and this association could retain FVIIa for extended time periods in extravascular tissues. The potential significance of this finding to hemostasis and hemophilia therapy with rFVIIa had been discussed earlier [25].

In summary, data presented in the manuscript show that TF contributes to FVIIa-AT complex formation *in vivo*. However, presence of traces of intravascular TF alone cannot explain the generation of high levels of FVIIa-AT complex rapidly *in vivo* following rFVIIa administration. EPCR does not influence FVIIa-AT complex formation *in vivo*. Finally, our data also show that TF plays a role in retaining FVIIa entered into extravasculature.

Acknowledgments

The authors are thankful to Charles T. Esmon, Oklahoma Medical Research Foundation, Oklahoma City, OK for providing EPCR-deficient and EPCR-overexpressing mice breeding pairs, and Jagan Sundaram, The University of Texas Health Science Center, Tyler, TX for breeding these mice. We thank Curtis Clark, The University of Texas Health Science Center, Tyler, TX, for his technical assistance in tail vein injections in initial experiments. We thank the late Walter Kisiel, University of New Mexico, Albuquerque, NM for providing affinity purified antibodies against human FVIIa; Mirella Ezban and Lars Peterson, Novo Nordisk, Denmark, for providing mouse FVIIa; and Daniel Kirchhofer, Genentech, CA, USA for providing rat anti-mouse TF mAb.

Author Contributions

Conceived and designed the experiments: RV URP LVMR. Performed the experiments: RV HK URP. Analyzed the data: RV HK LVMR. Contributed reagents/materials/analysis tools: NM LVMR. Wrote the paper: RV LVMR. Reviewed and edited the manuscript, and provided important suggestions: HK NM URP. Approved the final version of the manuscript: RV HK NM URP LVMR.

References

1. Rapaport SI, Rao LVM (1992) Initiation and regulation of tissue factor-dependent blood coagulation. Arterioscler Thromb 12: 1111–1121.
2. Broze Jr. GJ (1995) Tissue factor pathway inhibitor and the current concept of blood coagulation. Blood Coagul Fibrinolysis 6: S7–S13.
3. Lawson JH, Butenas S, Ribarik N, Mann KG (1993) Complex-dependent inhibition of factor VIIa by antithrombin III and heparin. J Biol Chem 268: 767–770.
4. Rao LVM, Rapaport SI, Hoang AD (1993) Binding of factor VIIa to tissue factor permits rapid antithrombin III/heparin inhibition of factor VIIa. Blood 81: 2600–2607.
5. Hamamoto T, Yamamoto M, Nordfang O, Petersen JGL, Foster DC, et al. (1993) Inhibitory properties of full-length and truncated recombinant tissue factor pathway inhibitor (TFPI). Evidence that the third kunitz-type domain of TFPI is not essential for the inhibition of factor VIIa-tissue factor complexes on cell surfaces. J Biol Chem 268: 8704–8710.
6. Shigematsu Y, Miyata T, Higashi S, Miki T, Sadler JE, et al. (1992) Expression of human soluble tissue factor in yeast and enzymatic properties of its complex with factor VIIa. J Biol Chem 267: 21329–21337.
7. Rapaport SI, Rao LVM (1995) The tissue factor pathway: How it has become a "prima ballerina". Thromb Haemost 74: 7–17.
8. Broze GJ Jr., Likert K, Higuchi D (1993) Inhibition of factor VIIa/tissue factor by antithrombin III and tissue factor pathway inhibitor. Blood 82: 1679–1680.
9. Rao LVM, Nordfang O, Hoang AD, Pendurthi UR (1995) Mechanism of antithrombin III inhibition of VIIa/tissue factor activity on cell surfaces. Comparison with tissue factor pathway inhibitor/factor Xa induced inhibition of factor VIIa/tissue factor activity. Blood 85: 121–129.
10. Smith SA, Antonaci FC, Woodhams BJ, Morrissey JH (2007) Factor VIIa-antithrombin complexes in human plasma. J Thromb Haemost 5: O-S-040 (abstract).
11. Agerso H, Brophy DF, Pelzer H, Martin EJ, Carr M, et al. (2011) Recombinant human factor VIIa (rFVIIa) cleared principally by antithrombin following intravenous administration in hemophilia patients. J Thromb Haemost 9: 330–338.
12. Butenas S, Bouchard BA, Brummel-Ziedins KE, Parhami-Seren B, Mann KG (2005) Tissue factor activity in whole blood. Blood 105: 2764–2770.
13. Giesen P, Rauch U, Bohrmann B, Kling D, Roque M, et al. (1999) Blood-borne tissue factor: another view of thrombosis. Proc Natl Acad Sci USA 96: 2311–2315.

14. Takahashi H, Satoh N, Wada K, Takakuwa E, Seki Y, et al. (1994) Tissue factor in plasma of patients with disseminated intravascular coagulation. Am J Hematol 46: 333–337.
15. Spiezia L, Rossetto V, Campello E, Gavasso S, Woodhams B, et al. (2010) Factor VIIa-antithrombin complexes in patients with arterial and venous thrombosis. Thromb Haemost 103: 1188–1192.
16. Spiezia L, Campello E, Gentilomo C, Gavasso S, Woodhams B, et al. (2011) Factor VIIa-antithrombin complexes in children with ischemic stroke. Thromb Res 128: 303–304.
17. Simioni P, Spiezia L (2011) Factor VIIa-AT complex plasma levels and arterial thrombosis. Thromb Res 128: 507.
18. Silveira A, Scanavini D, Boquist S, Ericsson CG, Hellenius ML, et al. (2012) Relationships of plasma factor VIIa-antithrombin complexes to manifest and future cardiovascular disease. Thromb Res 130: 221–225.
19. Ghosh S, Pendurthi UR, Steinoe A, Esmon CT, Rao LV (2007) Endothelial cell protein C receptor acts as a cellular receptor for factor VIIa on endothelium. J Biol Chem 282: 11849–11857.
20. Preston RJ, Ajzner E, Razzari C, Karageorgi S, Dua S, et al. (2006) Multifunctional specificity of the protein C/activated protein C Gla domain. J Biol Chem 281: 28850–28857.
21. Lopez-Sagaseta J, Montes R, Puy C, Diez N, Fukudome K, et al. (2007) Binding of factor VIIa to the endothelial cell protein C receptor reduces its coagulant activity. J Thromb Haemost 5: 1817–1824.
22. Sen P, Gopalakrishan R, Kothari H, Keshava S, Clark C, et al. (2011) Factor VIIa bound to endothelial cell protein C receptor activates protease activated receptor-1 and mediates cell signaling and barrier protection. Blood 117: 3199–3208.
23. Sundaram J, Keshava S, Gopalakrishan R, Esmon CT, Pendurthi UR, et al. (2014) Factor VIIa binding to endothelial cell protein C receptor protects vascular barrier integrity *in vivo*. J Thromb Haemost 12: 690–700.
24. Nayak RC, Sen P, Ghosh S, Gopalakrishnan R, Esmon CT, et al. (2009) Endothelial cell protein C receptor cellular localization and trafficking. Blood 114: 1974–1986.
25. Clark CA, Vatsyayan R, Hedner U, Esmon CT, Pendurthi UR, et al. (2012) Endothelial cell protein C receptor-mediated redistribution and tissue-level accumulation of factor VIIa. J Thromb Haemost 10: 2383–2391.
26. Gopalakrishnan R, Pendurthi UR, Hedner U, Agerso H, Esmon CT, et al. (2012) Influence of endothelial cell protein C receptor on plasma clearance of factor VIIa. J Thromb Haemost 10: 971–973.
27. Mackman N (2004) Role of tissue factor in hemostasis, thrombosis, and vascular development. Arterioscler Thromb Vasc Biol 24: 1015–1022.
28. Mackman N (2008) Tissue-specific hemostasis: role of tissue factor. J Thromb Haemost 6: 303–305.
29. Parry GC, Erlich JH, Carmeliet P, Luther T, Mackman N (1998) Low levels of tissue factor are compatible with development and hemostasis in mice. J Clin Invest 101: 560–569.
30. Pawlinski R, Tencati M, Holscher T, Pedersen B, Voet T, et al. (2007) Role of cardiac myocyte tissue factor in heart hemostasis. J Thromb Haemost 5: 1693–1700.
31. Li W, Zheng X, Gu JM, Ferrell GL, Brady M, et al. (2005) Extraembryonic expression of EPCR is essential for embryonic viability. Blood 106: 2716–2722.
32. Li W, Zheng X, Gu J, Hunter J, Ferrell GL, et al. (2005) Overexpressing endothelial cell protein C receptor alters the hemostatic balance and protects mice from endotoxin. J Thromb Haemost 3: 1351–1359.
33. Wang JG, Manly D, Kirchhofer D, Pawlinski R, Mackman N (2009) Levels of microparticle tissue factor activity correlate with coagulation activation in endotoxemic mice. J Thromb Haemost 7: 1092–1098.
34. Kothari H, Nayak RC, Rao LV, Pendurthi UR (2010) Cystine186-cystine 209 disulfide bond is not essential for the procoagulant activity of tissue factor or for its de-encryption. Blood 115: 4273–4283.
35. Geddings JE, Mackman N (2013) Tumor-derived tissue factor-positive microparticles and venous thrombosis in cancer patients. Blood 122: 1873–1880.
36. Sen P, Clark CA, Gopalakrishnan R, Hedner U, Esmon CT, et al. (2012) Factor VIIa binding to endothelial cell protien C receptor: Differences between mouse and human systems. Thromb Haemost 107: 951–961.
37. Warr TA, Rao LVM, Rapaport SI (1990) Disseminated intravascular coagulation in rabbits induced by administration of endotoxin or tissue factor: effect of anti-tissue factor antibodies and measurement of plasma extrinsic pathway inhibitor activity. Blood 75: 1481–1489.
38. Gopalakrishnan R, Hedner U, Ghosh S, Nayak R, Allen TC, et al. (2010) Biodistribution of pharmacologically administered rFVIIa. J Thromb Haemost 8: 301–310.
39. Agerso H, Kristensen NR, Ostergaard H, Karpf DM, Hermit MB, et al. (2011) Clearance of rFVIIa and NN1731 after intravenous administration of Beagle dogs. Eur J Pharm Sci 42: 578–583.
40. Petersen LC, Karpf DM, Agerso H, Hermit MB, Pelzer H, et al. (2011) Intravascular inhibition of factor VIIa and the analogue NN1731 by antithrombin. Br J Haematol 152: 99–107.
41. Petersen LC, Elm T, Ezban M, Krogh TN, Karpf DM, et al. (2009) Plasma elimination kinetics for factor VII are independent of its activation to factor VIIa and complex formation with plasma inhibitors. Thromb Haemost 101: 818–826.
42. Hamamoto T, Foster DC, Kisiel W (1996) The inhibition of human factor VIIa-tissue factor by antithrombin III-heparin is enhanced by factor X on a human bladder carcinoma cell line. Int J Hematol 63: 51–63.
43. Gopalakrishnan R, Hedner U, Clark C, Pendurthi UR, Rao LV (2010) rFVIIa transported from the blood stream into tissues is functionally active. J Thromb Haemost 8: 2318–2321.

Seven Day Insertion Rest in Whole Body Vibration Improves Multi-Level Bone Quality in Tail Suspension Rats

Rui Zhang[1], He Gong[1]*, Dong Zhu[2]*, Jiazi Gao[1], Juan Fang[1], Yubo Fan[3]

1 Department of Engineering Mechanics, Jilin University, Changchun, Jilin, People's Republic of China, **2** Department of Orthopedic Surgery, No. 1 Hospital of Jilin University, Changchun, Jilin, People's Republic of China, **3** School of Biological Science and Medical Engineering, Beihang University, Beijing, People's Republic of China

Abstract

Objective: This study aimed to investigate the effects of low-magnitude, high-frequency vibration with rest days on bone quality at multiple levels.

Methods: Forty-nine three-month-old male Wistar rats were randomly divided into seven groups, namely, vibrational loading for *X* day followed by *X* day rest (VL*X*R, *X* = 1, 3, 5, 7), vibrational loading every day (VLNR), tail suspension (SPD), and baseline control (BCL). One week after tail suspension, rats were loaded by vibrational loading (35 Hz, 0.25 g, 15 min/day) except SPD and BCL. Fluorescence markers were used in all rats. Eight weeks later, femora were harvested to investigate macromechanical properties, and micro-computed tomography scanning and fluorescence test were used to evaluate microarchitecture and bone growth rate. Atomic force microscopy analyses and nanoindentation test were used to analyze the nanostructure and mechanical properties of bone material, respectively. Inductively coupled plasma optical emission spectroscopy was used for quantitative chemical analyses.

Results: Microarchitecture, mineral apposition rate and bone formation rate and macromechanical properties were improved in VL7R. Grain size and roughness were significantly different among all groups. No statistical difference was found for the mechanical properties of the bone material, and the chemical composition of all groups was almost similar.

Conclusions: Low-magnitude, high-frequency vibration with rest days altered bone microarchitecture and macro-biomechanical properties, and VL7R was more efficacious in improving bone loss caused by mechanical disuse, which provided theoretical basis and explored the mechanisms of vibration for improving bone quality in clinics.

Editor: João Costa-Rodrigues, Faculdade de Medicina Dentária, Universidade do Porto, Portugal

Funding: This work is supported by the National Natural Science Foundation of China (Nos. 11322223 and 11272134), the 973 Program (No. 2012CB821202), and the Program for New Century Excellent Talents in University (NCET-12-0024). The funders had no role in study design, data collection and analysis, decision to publish, or preparation of the manuscript.

Competing Interests: The authors have declared that no competing interests exist.

* E-mail: gonghe1976@yahoo.com (HG); swyxgc@126.com (DZ)

Introduction

Bone tissue is a complex composite biological material with the ability for functional adaptation. Mechanical environment is an important factor in controlling and influencing bone structure. Osteoporosis is a systemic skeletal disease characterized by low bone mass and microarchitecture deterioration of bone tissue, with a consequent increase in bone fragility and susceptibility to fracture [1]. Many factors contribute to onset of bone loss. In addition to hormone deficiency, microgravity can also lead to bone loss. For astronauts staying four to six months in space, the mineral content of lower limb bones decreases remarkably, and the rate of loss of bone mineral density (BMD) is almost 1.6% per month [2,3]. In a gravitational environment for the duration of space travel, deterioration of some bone structures is irreversible though the bone mass has started to increase [4].

Pharmacologic treatment is the most popular intervention to prevent osteoporosis, but is unsuitable for all patients because of potential side effects [5]. Thus, non-invasive and non-pharmacologic therapy is a focus of current research in osteoporosis treatment [6,7]. Low-level mechanical stimuli can improve both quantity and quality of trabecular bone in 6 to 8 years old female sheep, which (if applicable in humans) may serve as an effective intervention for osteoporosis [8]. After daily mechanical stimulation of the hindlimbs of adult sheep for a year with 20 min bursts of very-low-magnitude, high-frequency vibration, the density of trabecular bone in the proximal femur significantly increases (by 34.2%) than those in controls [6]. A pilot randomized controlled trial in disabled children demonstrated that low-magnitude, high-frequency mechanical stimuli are anabolic to trabecular bone, and may provide a non-pharmacologic treatment for bone fragility [9]. In addition, clinical studies of bone responses to exercise, bed rest, and microgravity confirmed the sensitivity of bone to physical and environmental stimuli [10]. The beneficial effects on bone mass and strength can be attributed to the sensitivity of bone cells to mechanical stimuli. However, bone cells lose mechanical sensitivity soon after stimulation, and a rest interval between each low-magnitude load cycle can create a potent anabolic stimulus [11–13]. Compared with daily loading, Ma et al. found that low-magnitude, high-frequency mechanical vibration is more effective in improving bone microarchitecture and biomechanical properties in ovariectomised rodents if the long-duration mechanical stimulus is separated by several rest days [14]. However, the influence of vibration with rest days on osteoporosis caused by mechanical disuse remains unknown. Long-term limb disuse may disorder normal bone metabolism. Bone tissue is below or next to the threshold of bone remodeling, and the amount of bone resorption in remodeling process is greater than bone formation, which results in decreased bone mass. However, this is different from osteoporosis caused by the decline of ovarian function in women after menopause, which may increase the mechanical set point of mechanostat [15]. Because of the different nature between disuse osteoporosis and estrogen-deficient osteoporosis, the bone qualities in response to this new type of low-magnitude, high-frequency intermittent mechanical intervention strategy proposed by Ma et al. [14] need to be further investigated through mechanical disuse model for the osteoporosis caused by weightlessness.

The mechanical properties of bone are determined by not only the structure and geometry, but also the tissue properties of bone material itself [16]. Considerable evidence demonstrated that bone mass and microarchitecture are sensitive to mechanical stimuli, and a feedback regulatory mechanism between external load and metabolism must exist [17]. This mechanism needs to be explored thoroughly using multi-level investigations, i.e. mechanical testing or micro-computed tomography (micro-CT) for bone qualities (e.g., elastic modulus or BMD) [18]. Atomic force microscopy (AFM) was recently used to improve our knowledge of the nanostructure of bone material because the dimensions of many microarchitecture features of interest in bone tissue are several micrometers or less [19–25]. In addition, elastic properties of bone microarchitecture components differ from the macroscopic values, and nanoindentation is a mechanical microprobe method that allows the direct simultaneous measurement of elastic modulus and hardness of the material [26–29].

The previous studies on the effects of low-magnitude, high-frequency vibration on bone quality mainly concerned one or several aspects of bone property (e.g., mechanical property, mineral content, or microarchitecture) [6–10], [14], [30], but little is known about macro-micro-nano multi-level bone quality in response to the low-magnitude, high-frequency vibration with rest days, which was essential for better understanding the underlying mechanism for this mechanical intervention strategy. Accordingly, this study aimed to explore the effects of low-magnitude, high-frequency mechanical vibration on bone quality at multiple levels when the long-duration mechanical stimulus was separated by several rest days rather than daily loading. Macro- and micro-mechanical and morphological investigations were performed in this study to determine the bone mechanical properties, nanostructure of bone material, and material properties of femora with mechanical methods separated by 1, 3, 5, and 7 d rests in the loading cycle compared with daily loading in tail suspension rodents.

Materials and Methods

Materials

This study was performed in strict accordance with the recommendations of the Laboratory Animal Standardization Committee. The protocol was approved by the Medical Ethics Committee of No. 1 Hospital of Jilin University (2013-145). All efforts were made to minimize suffering of animals.

A total of 49 three-month-old male Wistar rats were purchased from the Experimental Animal Center of Jilin University. These rats were housed as singletons, and provided with a standard rodent diet (autoclaved NIH-31 with 6% fat; 18% protein; Ca:P, 1:1; and fortified with vitamins and minerals) and tap water during the experimental period. The environmental temperature was 24±2°C in natural light condition. All rats were randomly divided into seven groups, namely, vibrational loading for X day followed by X day rest (VLXR, X = 1, 3, 5, 7), vibrational loading every day (VLNR), tail suspension (SPD), and baseline control (BCL). The temporal schematic was shown in Fig. 1A. Non-invasive tail suspension was applied on all rats except those used for baseline control (BCL, n = 7), which were fed without any treatment. One week after tail suspension, high-frequency, low-magnitude whole body vibration was performed for eight weeks, which was similar with the study of Ma et al. [14]. The animals that were loaded by whole body vibration stimuli (35 Hz, 0.25 g, 15 min/day) on the first day were given one rest day, that is, vibrational loading with 1 d rest (VL1R, n = 7). Further groups were similarly created as follows: vibrational loading for 3 d followed by 3 d rest (VL3R, n = 7), vibrational loading for 5 d followed by 5 d rest (VL5R, n = 7), vibrational loading for 7 d followed by 7 d rest (VL7R, n = 7), and no rest day or vibrational loading every day (VLNR, n = 7). The rats in the tail suspension group (SPD, n = 7) were suspended without mechanical loading during the eight-week experimental period. The equipment for vibrational loading was assembled manually with a vibrational platform and a controller whose frequency and acceleration were adjustable (Fig. 1B). The weights of rats were measured before the experiment, one week after the suspension, and per week during the experiment. At day 42 and day 43 of the experimental protocol, all rats were treated with subcutaneous injection of calcein (dose: weight, 5 mg:1 kg) and tetracycline (dose: weight, 30 mg:1 kg), respectively. At day 52 and day 53 of the experimental protocol, calcein and tetracycline were re-injected to create a fluorescence maker [31,32]. All the rats were sacrificed at eight weeks, and the femurs were prepared for tests following removal of skin, muscle, and tendons.

Micro-CT Scanning

Left femurs were initially fixed with 80% ethanol (EtOH). Then, quantitative analysis of microarchitecture of trabecular bone in the femoral head was performed with micro-CT scanning (Skyscan 1076, Skyscan, Belgium). The spatial resolution for specimen scanning was set to 18 μm. The microarchitecture parameters of trabecular bone in the femoral head, such as bone volume fraction (BV/TV), trabecular thickness (Tb.Th), trabecular number (Tb.N), trabecular separation (Tb.Sp), and BMD were calculated by CTAn (CTAn, Skyscan, Belgium) [33].

Three-point Bending Mechanical Test

After micro-CT scanning, left femurs were cleaned in normal saline and a three-point bending mechanical test was performed on each left femur using an electronic universal testing machine (AG-X plus, Shimadzu, Kyoto, Japan). The test was performed with a fulcrum span of 20 mm and an actuator speed of 1 mm/min. Failure load was recorded, and energy absorption was determined as the area under the force-deflection curve until the point of failure. The elastic modulus was calculated using the following equation:

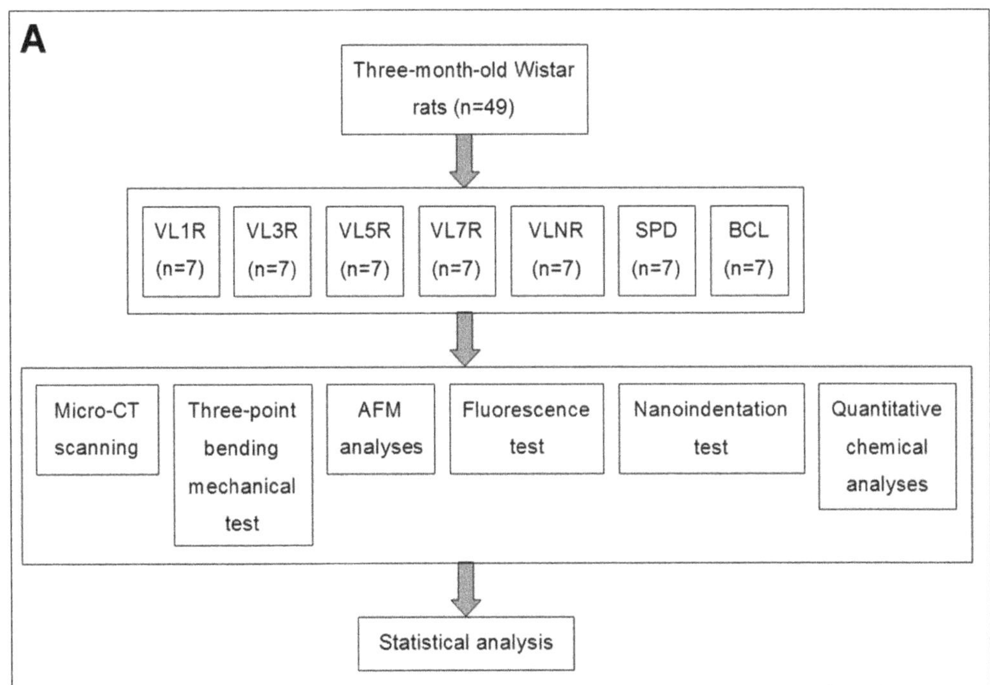

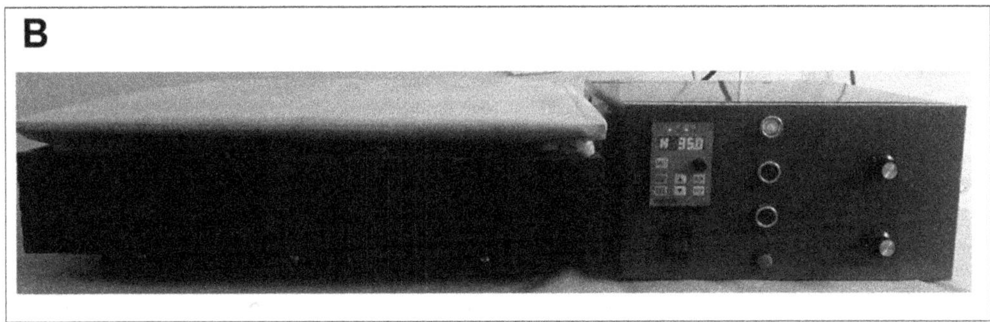

Figure 1. Temporal schematic of experiment and equipment for vibrational loading. (A) The temporal schematic; (B) The equipment for vibrational loading, which was assembled manually with a vibrational platform and a controller.

$$E = \frac{L^3}{48I}\left(\frac{\Delta F}{\Delta f}\right) \quad (1)$$

where L is the fulcrum span, $\frac{\Delta F}{\Delta f}$ is the slope of force-deflection curve, and I is the moment of inertia of an area. The cortical thickness of the fracture position was measured for calculating the elastic modulus.

AFM Analyses

After three-point bending mechanical test, sections of the left proximal femurs were cleaned in normal saline and dehydrated in increasing EtOH concentration from 85% to 100%. Longitudinal cortical bone specimens with a thickness of 2 mm were cut along the femoral shaft axis from femur shafts with a low-speed diamond saw under constant deionized water irrigation. Longitudinal trabecular bone specimens with a thickness of 1 mm to 2 mm were similarly cut from femur heads along the femoral neck axis.

Each bone sample (after 5 min of washing in ultrasonic bath, and natural drying) was placed horizontally onto the sample disk and imaged by a Multimode quadrex SPM with a Nanoscope IIIe controller (Veeco Instruments, USA). Imaging was operated under ambient conditions in standard AFM tapping mode using a commercial Silicon AFM probe (Tap300AI-G, BudgetSensors Instruments, Bulgaria) with a 125 μm cantilever length, a 40 Nm^{-1} constant force, a 300 kHz resonant frequency, and a tip radius lower than 10 nm. The size of mineral grains, i.e. the collagen bundles and the hydroxyapatite crystals, was measured using NanoScope Analysis version 1.4.0, as described by Milovanovic et al. [25].

Fluorescence Test

Right femurs were initially fixed with 80% EtOH, and dehydrated similar to left proximal femurs. Then, right femurs were embedded separately in polymethylmethacrylate (PMMA), ensuring that all bones were not demineralized. Each embedded right femur was sectioned into proximal femur and femur shaft. The right proximal femurs were cut along the coronal plane with a low-speed diamond saw under constant deionized water irrigation, which exposed the cancellous bone. Right femur shafts were then cut along the horizontal plane using a similar method, which exposed the cortical bone. Slices for fluorescence test were cut from right femur shafts. Then, the remaining parts were used for nanoindentation test. The mineral apposition rate (MAR) and bone formation rate (BFR/Tb.Ar) were calculated under fluorescence microscopy [34]. Laser scanning confocal microscopy (FV500, Olympus Corporation, Japan) was used to take pictures of analyzed fields, and one picture per right femur was obtained, and a total of 49 fluorescence images were obtained. MAR and BFR/Tb.Ar were measured by Image-Pro Plus software.

Nanoindentation Test

In this study, elastic modulus (E) and hardness (H) of longitudinal and transverse trabecular bone material, as well as those of longitudinal cortical bone material, were measured. Longitudinal trabecular bones with a thickness of 2 mm cut from left femoral heads were used for nanoindentation test in the longitudinal direction, and were also embedded separately in PMMA. Longitudinal cortical bones with a thickness of 2 mm cut from right femur shafts were used for nanoindentation test in the longitudinal direction, and transverse cancellous bones with a thickness of 2 mm of right femur heads were tested in the transverse direction. All the embedded samples were metallographically polished using silicon carbide abrasive papers of decreasing grit size (600, 800, 1500, and 2000 grit), and finally on microcloths with finer grades of diamond suspensions to the finest, 0.05 μm grit, to produce smooth surfaces for nanoindentation test. Specimens were washed in deionized water between each polishing step to remove debris. Nanoindentation tests were performed using Nano Indenter G200 (Agilent Technologies, Ltd., Santa Clara, CA, USA). A sharp Berkovich diamond indenter, a three-sided pyramid with the angle of 76°54′ between two edges, was used for all measurements. The specimens to be examined were located in the microscope and positioned beneath the indenter using the x–y table. The indenter was then slowly driven toward the surface at a constant displacement rate of 10 nm/s until surface contact was detected by the changes in the load and displacement signals. After contact, a permanent hardness impression was made by driving the indenter into the specimen to a depth of 1000 nm at a constant loading rate of 750 μN/s, holding at this load for a period of 10 s and then unloading to 15% of the peak load at a rate equal to half that used during loading. At the end of the unloading cycle, the indenter was held on the surface for a period of 100 s to establish the rate of thermal drift in the machine and specimen for correction of the data, and then completely withdrawn [35].

All indents were conducted at the similar site based on the optical microscopy observation to eliminate any local effects (Fig. 2A). Three indented areas (Fig. 2B) were selected for each trabecular specimen, and five indentations were made in each target area and 15 indentations were made in every sample, and

A

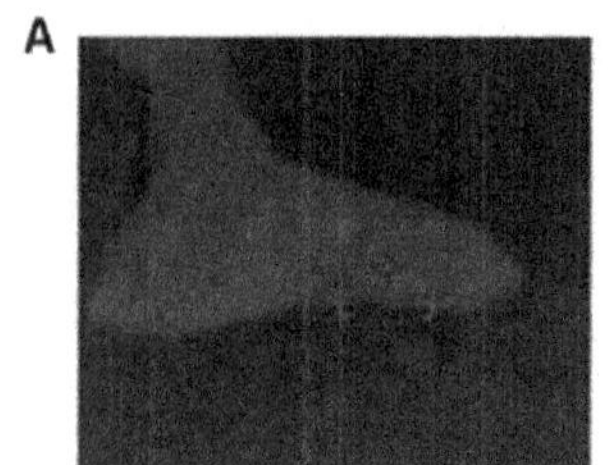

B

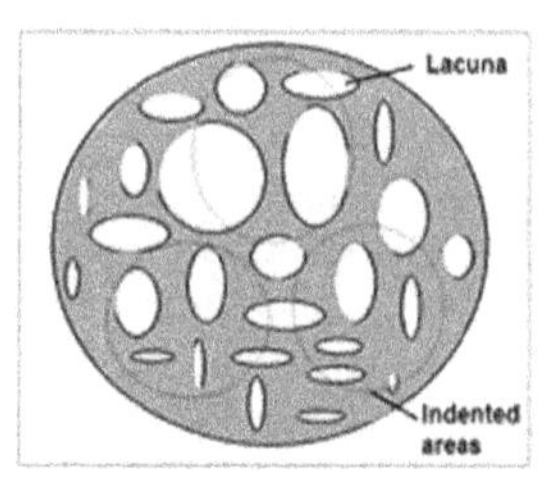

Figure 2. Indentation sites for nanoindentation test. Sample thickness is 2 mm. (A) Actual indented sites marked by red cross under optical microscopy; (B) Sketch map of indented areas marked by red circle.

the areas for each cortical specimen were similarly selected. A total of 2205 indentations were made. E and H were determined using the method of Oliver and Pharr [36]. The quantities of concern include the peak load (P_{max}), the contact area (A), and the contact stiffness (S). The equations used to calculate hardness (H) and effective indentation modulus (E_{ef}) from the measured quantities are:

$$H = \frac{P_{\max}}{A} \quad (2)$$

and

$$S = \frac{2}{\sqrt{\pi}} \beta E_{ef} \sqrt{A} \quad (3)$$

The effective modulus (E_{ef}) for the indentor-specimen combination can be derived from

$$\frac{1}{E_{ef}} = \frac{1-v_b^2}{E_b} + \frac{1-v_i^2}{E_i} \quad (4)$$

Where $v_b = 0.3$ and E_b are Poisson's ratio and elastic modulus for the bone material, respectively; $v_i = 0.07$ and $E_i = 1140$ GPa are the same quantities for the indenter, and the factor $\beta = 1.034$ is a constant for the Berkovich indenter. The basic assumption involved in this method is that the sample behaves purely elastically during unloading. Any indentation close to the mounting PMMA was removed to minimize the effects of embedding on the measurements.

Quantitative Chemical Analyses

Trabecular bones in each group were powdered to micron-sized particles using an electric grinder (Bosch Mkm 6000), and seven samples were prepared. Inductively coupled plasma optical emission spectroscopy (ICP-OES; 1.15 kW, 27 MHz; IRIS Intrepid, Thermo Electron Corporation, USA) was used for quantitative chemical analyses [37]. The user-friendly Quick Quant scan-based procedure was used to compare the intensities for measured elements in the samples with the intensities measured for standards with known concentrations. Calibration curves were calculated, and the concentrations of the measured elements in the samples were determined.

Statistical Analysis

Differences of all groups in the macro- and micromechanical and morphological properties of femurs were analyzed using Kruskal-Wallis H test of K independent sample nonparametric test. After that, Nemenyi test of two independent samples was used to determine differences of all mechanical and morphological parameters between every two groups. Data analysis was performed with SPSS 16.0 software, and the significance level was 0.05.

Results

Microarchitecture of Proximal Femurs Evaluated by Micro-CT Scanning

The region of interest (ROI) in the micro-CT image was selected one by one manually. The trabecular bones of femoral heads were included in the ROI as much as possible, and the 3D

Table 1. Microarchitecture parameters evaluated by micro-CT scanning.

	VL1R	VL3R	VL5R	VL7R	VLNR	SPD	BCL
BMD (g/cm^3)	$0.70 \pm 0.02^{a,b,c,d,e,f}$	$0.74 \pm 0.03^{a,b,c,e}$	$0.65 \pm 0.01^{a,b,c,d}$	$0.79 \pm 0.11^{a,b,c}$	$0.61 \pm 0.10^{a,b}$	$0.58 \pm 0.07^{b,c}$	$0.91 \pm 0.14^{a,c}$
BV/TV (%)	$72.06 \pm 1.26^{a,b,c,d,e,f}$	$77.41 \pm 1.47^{a,b,c,d,e}$	$83.87 \pm 2.35^{a,b,c}$	$87.04 \pm 2.84^{a,b,c}$	$62.87 \pm 1.86^{a,b}$	$50.43 \pm 2.31^{b,c}$	$89.62 \pm 2.17^{a,c}$
Tb.Th (mm)	$0.21 \pm 0.01^{a,b,c,e}$	$0.22 \pm 0.03^{a,b,c,e}$	$0.19 \pm 0.01^{a,b,c,d}$	$0.22 \pm 0.01^{a,b,c}$	$0.15 \pm 0.11^{a,b}$	$0.13 \pm 0.00^{b,c}$	$0.26 \pm 0.05^{a,c}$
Tb.N (mm^{-1})	$3.22 \pm 0.14^{a,b,c,d,f}$	$4.18 \pm 0.82^{a,b,c,d,e}$	$3.48 \pm 0.24^{a,b,c,d}$	$4.92 \pm 0.41^{a,b,c}$	$3.27 \pm 0.08^{a,b}$	$2.20 \pm 0.11^{b,c}$	$5.43 \pm 0.21^{a,c}$
Tb.Sp (mm)	$0.15 \pm 0.01^{a,b,c,d,f}$	$0.12 \pm 0.02^{a,b,c,e}$	$0.14 \pm 0.01^{a,b,c,d}$	$0.11 \pm 0.01^{a,b,c}$	$0.18 \pm 0.03^{a,b}$	$0.20 \pm 0.02^{b,c}$	$0.09 \pm 0.04^{a,c}$

n = 7 values per group. Values are shown as the median±SE. BMD - bone mineral density; BV/TV - bone volume fraction; Tb.Th - trabecular thickness; Tb.N - trabecular number; Tb.Sp - trabecular separation.
[a]Statistically different from SPD ($P<0.05$).
[b]Statistically different from BCL ($P<0.05$).
[c]Statistically different from VLNR ($P<0.05$).
[d]Statistically different from VL7R ($P<0.05$).
[e]Statistically different from VL5R ($P<0.05$).
[f]Statistically different from VL3R ($P<0.05$).

microarchitecture parameters calculated from CTAn are shown in Table 1. The three-dimensional (3D) reconstruction of micro-CT images of the trabecular bone in the femoral head is shown in Fig. 3. Compared with SPD, the trabeculae in the BCL are much denser, thicker and inseparable, whereas VL7R created a major improvement of trabecular microarchitecture compared with SPD, in which trabecular density, thickness and continuity were improved after eight weeks mechanical interventions. Table 1 shows variances in microarchitecture parameters of the different groups. BMD and BV/TV in all experimental groups were statistically higher than those in SPD ($P<0.05$), and VL7R exhibited significantly higher values than VLNR ($P<0.05$) and other vibrational loading groups ($P<0.05$), and there were statistical difference between VL1R, VL3R and VL5R ($P<0.05$). Furthermore, all these mechanical interventions with rest days displayed greater Tb.Th than daily loading ($P<0.05$), whereas VL7R showed the most obvious increase ($P = 0.006$). Dramatic increases in Tb.N of the femoral head were observed in all mechanical interventions, and the maximum was observed in VL7R than that in VLNR ($P = 0.001$). A statistically lower Tb.Sp was detected in the mechanical interventions with rest days than that in daily loading ($P<0.05$). There were improvements in all above microarchitecture parameters in VL1R, VL3R and VL5R than VLNR ($P<0.05$), but the statistical results between VL1R, VL3R and VL5R were not the same.

Failure Load, Elastic Modulus, and Energy Absorption Measured by Three-point Bending Test

The macro-biomechanical parameters measured by three-point bending test are shown in Fig. 4. BCL had the maximum failure load, elastic modulus, and energy absorption ($P<0.05$), whereas SPD had the minimum values ($P<0.05$). For failure load, a significant enhancement was observed in all experimental groups than that in SPD, and a significant increase was exclusively observed in VL7R than that in VLNR ($P = 0.006$) and other vibrational loading groups ($P<0.05$) (Fig. 4A). Dramatic increases in elastic modulus and energy absorption were observed in all experimental groups than those in SPD. Among all the vibration groups with rest days, elastic modulus and energy absorption were significantly higher in VL7R than those in VLNR ($P<0.05$) and other vibrational loading groups ($P<0.05$) (Figs. 4B and 4C), and there were no statistical difference between VL1R, VL3R and VL5R (Fig. 4).

Nanostructure of Bone Material Tested by AMF

Typical AFM topographic images and phase images of the nanostructure of trabecular bone material in the femoral head are shown in Fig. 5. Figs. 5-(T) show topographic images of VL1R, VL3R, VL5R, VL7R, VLNR, SPD and BCL. Scanning electron microscopy (SEM) (Figs. 5-(S)) revealed that bone minerals are fused together and form a sheet-like structure in a coherent manner [38]. The AFM phase Figs. 5-(P) obtained in our study show that the observed nanostructure of trabecular bone material exhibited a continuous phase, which is consistent with the SEM; nevertheless, the granular organization of the phase was evident in our sample (Figs. 5-(P)). The grain sizes of trabecular bone and cortical bone are listed in Table 2. Significant increases in grain sizes were observed in Figs. 5-(T)-SPD than those in Figs. 5-(T)-BCL, which showed a minimum grain size and a significantly narrower range (77 nm to 113 nm, Table 2). By contrast, the maximum values were detected in Figs. 5-(T)-SPD ($P<0.05$). Grain size was significantly smaller in Figs. 5-(T)-VL7R than that in Figs. 5-(T)-SPD among all the vibration groups with rest days ($P<0.05$). Grain size of Figs. 5-(T)-VL7R, Figs. 5-(T)-VL7R and

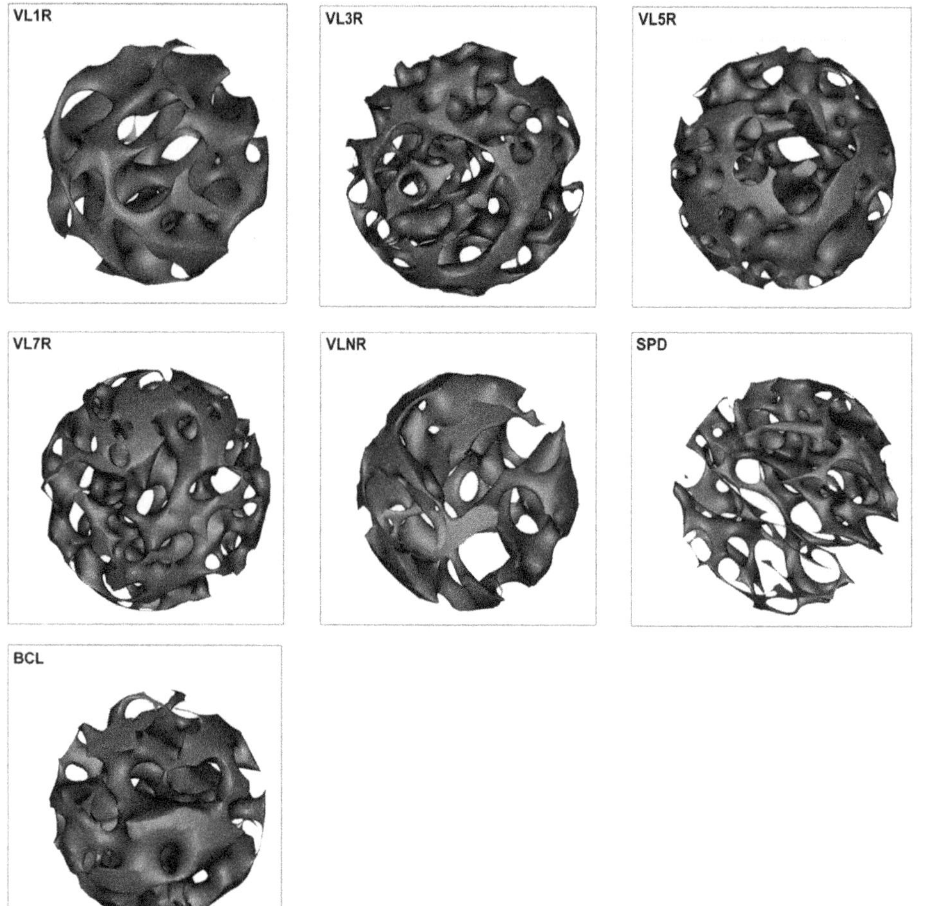

Figure 3. 3D reconstruction of micro-CT images of trabecular bone in femoral heads. VL1R: vibrational loading for 1 d followed by 1 d rest group; VL3R: vibrational loading for 3 d followed by 3 d rest group; VL5R: vibrational loading for 5 d followed by 5 d rest group; VL7R: vibrational loading for 7 d followed by 7 d rest group; VLNR: vibrational loading for no rest day or vibrational loading every day; SPD: tail suspension group; BCL: baseline control group.

Figs. 5-(T)-VL7R were improved than Figs. 5-(T)-VLNR ($P < 0.05$), and statistical difference was detected between VL1R, VL3R and VL5R ($P < 0.05$). The nanostructure of cortical bone material was similar to that of trabecular bone, and the size of grains differed among all experimental groups. Moreover, Figs. 5-(T)-SPD showed an unexpectedly low mean saturation roughness of the trabecula (approximately 70 nm, $P < 0.05$), which showed that larger grains were flattened. By contrast, the mean saturation roughness values in Figs. 5-(T)-BCL and Figs. 5-(T)-VL7R were significantly higher (approximately 110 nm to 130 nm, $P < 0.05$).

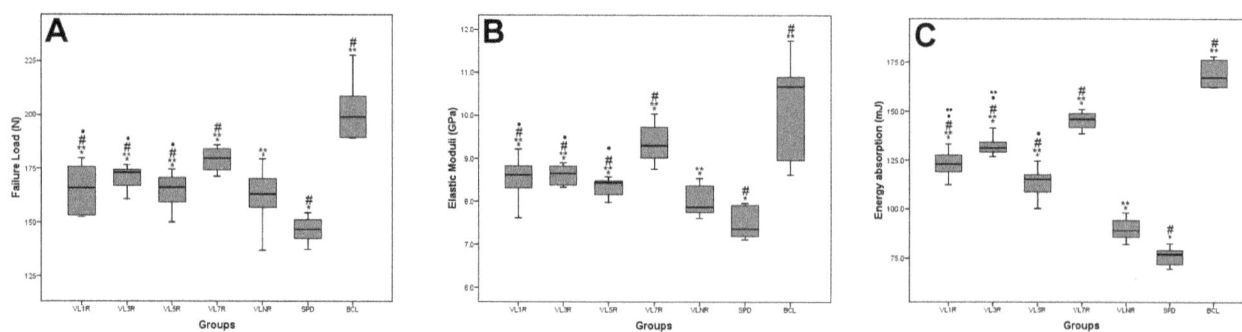

Figure 4. Macro-biomechanical parameters measured by three-point bending test. (A) Failure load; (B) Elastic modulus; (C) Energy absorption. *Statistically different from BCL ($P < 0.05$). **Statistically different from SPD ($P < 0.05$). #Statistically different from VLNR ($P < 0.05$). 'Statistically different from VL7R ($P < 0.05$). ''Statistically different from VL5R ($P < 0.05$).

Table 2. Grain size of trabecular bone and cortical bone.

	VL1R	VL3R	VL5R	VL7R	VLNR	SPD	BCL
Tb.(nm)	294±43[a,b,c,d,e,f]	347±31[a,b,c,d,e]	415±39[a,b,c,d]	220±21[a,b,c]	493±38[a,b]	684±57[b,c]	95±18[a,c]
Ct.(nm)	316±23[a,b,c,d,e,f]	359±34[a,b,c,d,e]	413±37[a,b,c,d]	197±16[a,b,c]	521±43[a,b]	659±49[b,c]	110±13[a,c]

n = 7 values per group. Sample thickness is 2 mm. Values are shown as the median±SE. Tb. - trabecular bone; Ct. - cortical bone.
[a]Statistically different from SPD (P<0.05).
[b]Statistically different from BCL (P<0.05).
[c]Statistically different from VLNR (P<0.05).
[d]Statistically different from VL7R (P<0.05).
[e]Statistically different from VL5R (P<0.05).
[f]Statistically different from VL3R (P<0.05).

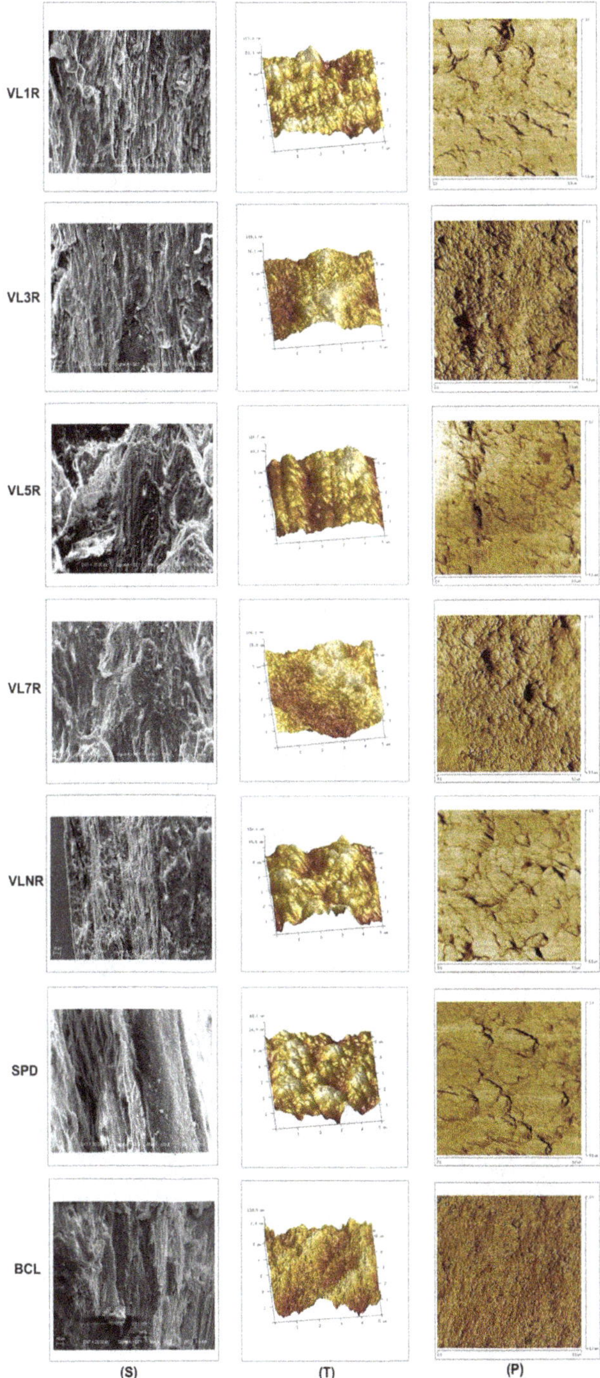

Figure 5. Scanning electron microscopy (SEM) images (Mag = 500X), AFM topographic images (5 μm×5 μm) and phase images (5 μm×5 μm) of the trabecular bone in femoral head. Sample thickness is 2 mm. Column (S): scanning electron microscopy; Column (T): AFM topographic images; Column (P): AFM phase images. Row VL1R: vibrational loading for 1 d followed by 1 d rest group; Row VL3R: vibrational loading for 3 d followed by 3 d rest group; Row VL5R: vibrational loading for 5 d followed by 5 d rest group; Row VL7R: vibrational loading for 7 d followed by 7 d rest group; Row VLNR: vibrational loading for no rest day or vibrational loading every day; Row SPD: tail suspension group; Row BCL: baseline control group.

Bone Growth Measured by Fluorescence Test

Fluorescence marker lines were clearly observed in the fluorescence graph in Fig. 6. The MAR and BFR/Tb.Ar are shown in Fig. 7. Maximum values were detected in BCL ($P<0.05$), whereas minimum values were detected in SPD ($P<0.05$). A significant increase was exclusively found in VL7R than that in VLNR ($P = 0.001$) and other vibration groups with rest days ($P< 0.05$). The MAR and BFR/Tb.Ar were increased in VL1R, VL3R and VL5R than VLNR ($P<0.05$), and there were statistical difference between VL1R, VL3R and VL5R ($P<0.05$).

E and H of Bone Material Evaluated by Nanoindentation Test

A summary of *E*, *H*, and *E*/*H* ratio of the trabecular and cortical bone sites as determined by nanoindentation is shown in Table 3. All data were obtained at an indentation depth of approximately 1000 nm [35]. *E*, *H*, and *E*/*H* ratio of longitudinal cortical bone (Ct.L) were greater than those of longitudinal trabecular bone (Tb.L), followed by transverse trabecular bone (Tb.T). No statistical difference was found in *E*, *H*, and *E*/*H* ratio for all groups ($P_{Tb.T} = 0.845$, $P_{Tb.L} = 0.172$, and $P_{Ct.L} = 0.100$ for *E*; $P_{Tb.T} = 0.707$, $P_{Tb.L} = 0.414$, and $P_{Ct.L} = 0.179$ for *H*; $P_{Tb.T} = 0.898$, $P_{Tb.L} = 0.540$, and $P_{Ct.L} = 0.231$ for *E*/*H* ratio).

Bone Composition Evaluated by Quantitative Chemical Analyses

Results of quantitative chemical analyses (Table 4) show unchanged levels of calcium and phosphorus in all groups ($P = 0.983$), and no significant difference was found in the Ca/P ratio ($P = 0.991$).

Discussion

BMD decreased when hindlimbs were suspended and high-frequency, and low-magnitude mechanical stimuli could improve the biomechanical properties and microarchitecture in various sites, including cancellous and shaft cortical bones [39–42]. Whole-body vibration mitigated the reduction of bone strength in long-term hindlimb unloading rats and the complexity of trabecular bone could be preserved [43–45]. Low-magnitude, high-frequency mechanical stimuli may provide a non-pharmacologic treatment for bone loss. But bone cells lose mechanical sensitivity soon after stimulation, and a rest interval between each low-magnitude load cycle may create a potent anabolic stimulus [11–13]. Therefore, high-frequency, low-magnitude whole body vibration with rest days was put forward. However, the most effective number of rest days for treating bone loss was still

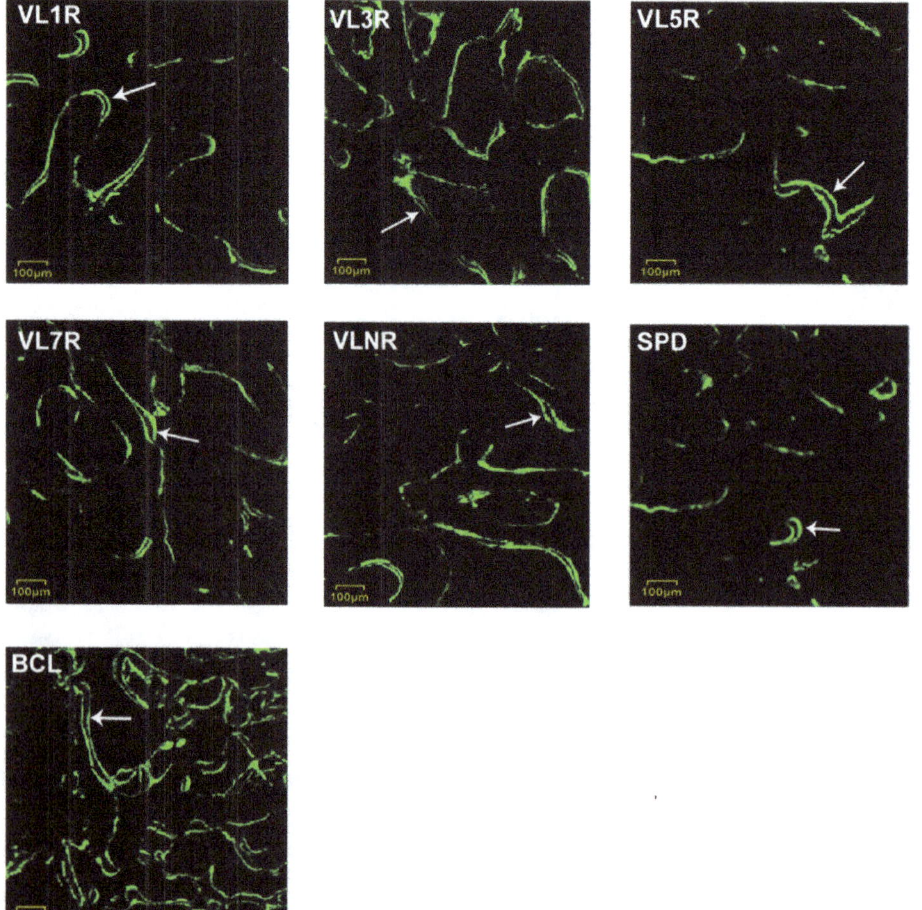

Figure 6. Fluorescence graphs of cancellous bones in proximal femurs. Arrows show the areas where the mineral apposition rate and bone formation rate were measured. VL1R: Vibrational loading for 1 d followed by 1 d rest group; VL3R: Vibrational loading for 3 d followed by 3 d rest group; VL5R: Vibrational loading for 5 d followed by 5 d rest group; VL7R: Vibrational loading for 7 d followed by 7 d rest group; VLNR: Vibrational loading for no rest day or vibrational loading every day; SPD: Tail suspension group; BCL: Baseline control group.

Table 3. *E*, *H*, and *E/H* ratio of the trabecular and cortical bone sites as determined by nanoindentation.

		VL1R	VL3R	VL5R	VL7R	VLNR	SPD	BCL
Tb.T	*E* (GPa)	14.90±1.02	15.00±1.11	15.00±1.23	15.00±0.89	14.90±0.74	14.90±1.35	15.00±1.41
	H (GPa)	0.20±0.01	0.20±0.01	0.19±0.03	0.20±0.02	0.19±0.03	0.20±0.02	0.20±0.01
	E/H	74.50±3.41	75.00±4.29	77.90±2.79	74.00±2.76	77.90±4.73	75.00±1.96	75.00±2.47
Tb.L	*E* (GPa)	23.72±2.11	23.50±2.64	23.58±1.89	23.16±2.13	23.20±2.29	23.65±3.01	23.15±1.74
	H (GPa)	1.24±0.03	1.23±0.11	1.20±0.10	1.13±0.09	1.15±0.03	1.19±0.10	1.21±0.06
	E/H	19.37±2.12	19.15±1.71	19.72±1.22	20.39±1.59	20.05±2.85	19.87±1.97	19.40±2.18
Ct.L	*E* (GPa)	30.20±2.94	30.20±3.15	30.20±2.76	30.40±2.18	30.60±3.31	30.10±2.87	30.80±2.09
	H (GPa)	1.49±0.12	1.49±0.09	1.49±0.04	1.49±0.01	1.49±0.01	1.49±0.04	1.50±0.10
	E/H	20.34±1.86	20.20±1.43	20.34±0.98	20.54±1.03	20.54±2.10	20.20±1.74	20.53±1.35

n = 7 values per group. Sample thickness is 2 mm. Values are shown as the median±SE. Tb.T - transverse trabecular bone; Tb.L - longitudinal trabecular bone; Ct.L - longitudinal cortical bone; *E* - elastic modulus; *H* - hardness; *E/H* - ratio of elastic modulus and hardness.

Table 4. Chemical composition of trabecular bone in femoral head (ICP-OES).

	VL1R	VL3R	VL5R	VL7R	VLNR	SPD	BCL
Ca [%]	24.34±2.51	24.92±1.91	24.59±2.55	24.72±3.02	24.82±2.37	24.51±2.62	24.59±2.29
P [%]	11.32±0.42	11.40±0.23	11.44±0.21	11.56±0.32	11.43±0.24	11.39±0.40	11.38±0.25
Ca/P ratio	2.15±0.19	2.19±0.21	2.15±0.23	2.14±0.17	2.18±0.21	2.15±0.19	2.16±0.23
Mg [%]	0.46±0.04	0.47±0.02	0.50±0.01	0.50±0.01	0.50±0.03	0.46±0.02	0.48±0.01
Sr [%]	0.0070±0.00	0.0069±0.00	0.0066±0.00	0.0069±0.00	0.0069±0.00	0.0067±0.00	0.0070±0.00
Fe [%]	0.015±0.00	0.016±0.00	0.013±0.00	0.015±0.00	0.012±0.00	0.013±0.00	0.023±0.00
Ba [%]	<0.005±0.00	<0.005±0.00	<0.005±0.00	<0.005±0.00	<0.005±0.00	<0.005±0.00	<0.005±0.00
K [%]	0.093±0.01	0.092±0.01	0.11±0.02	0.10±0.01	0.10±0.01	0.087±0.01	0.098±0.01
Na [%]	0.61±0.03	0.67±0.02	0.78±0.01	0.70±0.01	0.72±0.02	0.61±0.01	0.70±0.02

n = 7 values per group. Values are shown as the median±SE. ICP-OES - inductively coupled plasma optical emission spectroscopy.

unknown. Based on the 5 working days, VL5R was established in this study, and two smaller groups, i.e. VL1R and VL3R and one bigger group, i.e. VL7R were created. Groups of vibrational loading every day (VLNR), tail suspension (SPD), and baseline control (BCL) were also included for comparison to investigate multi-level mechanical properties, morphology, and chemical composition of bone to explore the effects of high-frequency, low-magnitude whole body vibration with different rest days.

In this study, macromechanical properties (i.e., failure load, elastic modulus, and energy absorption) increased in all experimental groups than those in SPD, and VL7R was significantly higher than VLNR ($P<0.05$) and other vibration groups with rest days ($P<0.05$). Similar results were detected in microarchitecture parameters, including increased BV/TV, BMD, Tb.Th, Tb.N, and lower Tb.Sp, of VL7R than those of VLNR ($P<0.05$) and other vibration groups with rest days ($P<0.05$). A 3D reconstruction of micro-CT images (Fig. 3) and fluorescence graphs (Fig. 7) showed that the trabeculae of BCL were significantly denser and thicker than SPD or vibrational loading groups, and bone growth in BCL was significantly greater than that in other groups. By contrast, significant trabecular deterioration was observed in rodents after tail suspension without mechanical intervention. Stimuli with rest days resulted in a major improvement of trabecular microarchitecture than SPD such that trabecular density, thickness, and continuity improved and bone growth rate was higher, and VL7R was more effective than VL1R, VL3R or VL5R. Whole-body vibration mitigated the reduction of bone strength in long-term hindlimb unloading rats, and mechanical stimulation in the form of whole-body vibration limited reduction of bone density when it was applied during the unloading [43,45], which was similar to the results of this study. However, our study showed that the vibrational loading for 7 d followed by 7 d rest appeared to be the optimal loading strategy for the bone loss caused by mechanical disuse, since significant differences were found in all above parameters.

The AFM phase images obtained in this study show that the observed nanostructure of the bone material exhibited a continuous phase and evident granular structure, which was consistent with the observation of Milovanovic et al. [25]. Compared with BCL, the grain sizes in all experimental groups were larger. In addition to crystal growth, two additional processes can increase mineral size, namely, crystal secondary nucleation leading to crystal proliferation and aggregation of preformed crystals [46]. Increased grain size in SPD cannot be explained by the increase in amount of minerals because our quantitative chemical analyses revealed unchanged calcium and phosphorus levels, as well as Ca/P ratio, in all experimental groups. Our findings indicate that in SPD, the existing mineral was reorganized by aggregation to larger grains, similar to the suggestion for turkey-leg tendon maturation [47,48]. Lower roughness in SPD, despite its larger grains, also supported the reorganization hypothesis, in which fused grains formed a larger flattened structure. Small mineral grain size of vibrational groups in this study was attributed to new bone formed in the remodeling process [49], and in all vibration groups with rest days, mineral grain size of VL7R was significantly smaller than VLNR ($P<0.05$) and other vibration groups with rest days ($P<0.05$), which showed that VL7R was more efficacious in improving bone loss and promoting bone formation. By contrast, large grains were possibly located in sites that have not undergone the bone remodeling process for a considerable amount of time. However, further experimental studies are needed for direct investigation of the mechanisms of grain enlargement. Nanoindentation test was used in this study to investigate the material properties of trabecular and cortical bones. Nanoindentation, which is a different method from conventional microhardness techniques, measures relatively smaller areas of bone material and provides estimates for both E and H. In this study, E and H of trabeculae and cortical bones were measured, and the average E and H of trabecular bone were considerably smaller than those of cortical bone ($P<0.05$). The E/H ratio, which represents the overall behavior of bone during the indentation process with respect to fracture toughness, was useful to describe material deformation during indentation and determine the brittleness of a material (ductile materials with higher E/H value) [50]. However, no significant difference in bone material properties was observed among all groups ($P>0.05$). Thus, the effect of disuse on the collagen bone matrix should be investigated. Other studies found that E and H of lamellae are unrelated to age, gender, and body mass index, and reductions in the mechanical integrity of whole bone must be caused by other factors, such as changes in tissue mass and organization [51,52]. Many of these changes are possibly caused by structural and histological features rather than

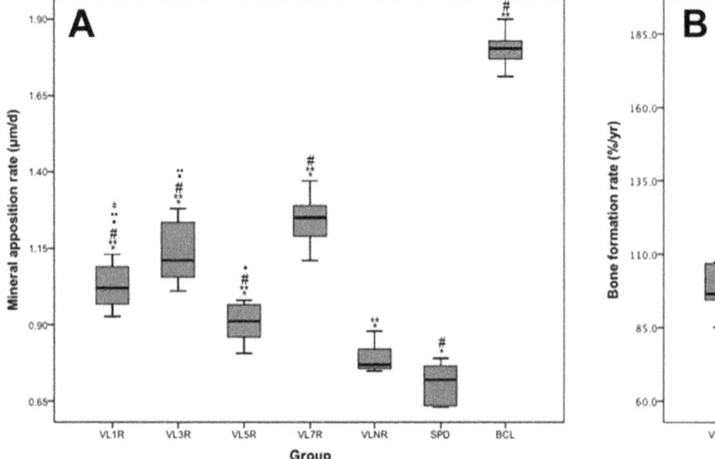

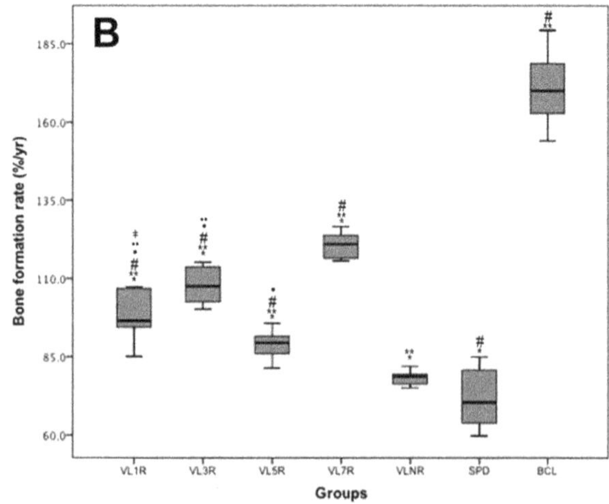

Figure 7. Mineral apposition rate and bone formation rate. *Statistically different from BCL ($P<0.05$). **Statistically different from SPD ($P<0.05$). #Statistically different from VLNR ($P<0.05$). ˙Statistically different from VL7R ($P<0.05$). ¨Statistically different from VL5R ($P<0.05$). ‡Statistically different from VL3R ($P<0.05$).

alterations in the bone matrix itself, and these changes warrant further investigation [53,54].

Some investigations suggested that high-frequency and low-magnitude mechanical signal may suppress adipose, non-esterified free fatty acid, and triglyceride contents in the liver or reduce a downstream challenge to liver morphology and function in rodents fed with a high-fat diet [55,56]. This mechanical efficacy to inhibit adipogenesis may increase with additional loading bouts if a refractory period is incorporated [57]. In this study, weights of animals sustained in tail suspension showed a similar ascending trend over seven weeks of vibration. However, animals loaded with mechanical stimuli appeared to lose weight in the last week ($P < 0.05$). The variation in weight was similar to that reported by Ma et al. [14]. At the same time, hindlimb-unloading induced loss of mass in muscles, but the response of BMD to altered loading conditions did not necessarily depend on the response of muscle mass [39]. Further studies will be performed to understand the mechanism of weight loss and the response of BMD to muscle mass affected by vibration stimuli.

This study had several limitations. First, three-month-old male rats were selected to exclude the influence of hormones with respect to osteoporosis of ovariectomised rats caused by estrogen deficiency [14]. In future studies, female rats with the same age will be investigated to determine the effect of gender. Second, though three-month-old male rats have been carefully limited in this study, body mass or size of all rats was not measured daily, which could have been responsible for the differences between individuals. Likewise, the behavioral monitoring may have been able to recognize any potential differences in activity levels between animals (those that were not undergoing tail suspension), and this study did not establish a group of tail suspension with 15 min of free activities instead of vibration stimuli, but the experimental groups only had different vibration cycles, and statistical results were unaffected by free activities during the vibration period. Further studies will record body mass or size and perform the behavioral monitoring daily, which would help eliminate those from being variables that potentially cloud the results, and an experimental group with tail suspension rodents and free activities will be included to determine the influence of free activities on bone quality. Third, bilateral femurs were used because the rat femoral heads were too small to collect all necessary specimens. In relation to the investigation on Caucasian women, which showed no significant difference in BMD of bilateral femoral necks, trochanters, and hips [58], bilateral differences were ignored in this study. Fourth, the bone turnover markers PINP and CTX-I on rat serum were not studied to quantify the difference of bone formation and bone resorption between different groups, and this will be quantified in further studies. The number of days that rats underwent vibrational loading and rest is smaller than seven. However, vibrational loading for X day followed by X day rest (VLXR, X = 1, 3, 5, 7) were studied in contrast with vibrational loading every day (VLNR), and this study showed that high-frequency, low-magnitude whole body vibration with rest days was efficacious in improving bone quality than daily loading. In future studies, the days of vibrational loading and rest will be diversified. Fifth, the samples were dehydrated before the experiment, which were different from fresh samples. Because the quantity of samples was limited, and the same sample was used for a variety of experimental study. Thus, considering the different experimental needs, all the samples were dehydrated in the same condition, which would not affect the statistical significance. The mechanical experiments on fresh samples will be carried out in the later study to make it closer to the reality.

This study showed that bone mineral reorganization and spatial arrangement were modified by high-frequency, low-magnitude whole body vibration with different rest days, which resulted in the recombination of mineral grains into different sizes and changes in mineral apposition rate and bone formation rate. The micro-architecture of bone was affected, which resulted in statistical differences in macromechanical properties. However, the mechanical properties of the bone material were not altered. This study investigated the influence of high-frequency, low-magnitude whole body vibration on bone loss caused by mechanical disuse in multiple levels, and showed that high-frequency, low-magnitude whole body vibration with 7 d rests was more efficacious in improving macro-biomechanical properties and microarchitecture than daily loading, which provided a theoretical basis for improving bone quality using this mechanical intervention in clinics.

Author Contributions

Conceived and designed the experiments: RZ HG DZ. Performed the experiments: RZ. Analyzed the data: RZ JZG JF. Contributed reagents/materials/analysis tools: HG DZ YF. Wrote the paper: RZ HG.

References

1. Lane NE (2006) Epidemiology, etiology, and diagnosis of osteoporosis. Am J Obstet Gynecol 194: S3–S11.
2. LeBlanc A, Shackelford L, Schneider V (1998) Future human bone research in space. Bone 22: S113–S6.
3. Ruff C, Beck T, Newman D, Oden M, Shaffner G, et al. (1999) Skeletal consequences of reduced gravity environments. 1st Biennial Space Biomed. Inv. Workshop 1: 86–7.
4. Lafage V, Dubousset J, Lavaste F, Skalli W (2002) Finite element simulation of various strategies for CD correction. Stud Health Technol Inform 91: 428–32.
5. Rahmani P, Morin S (2009) Prevention of osteoporosis-related fractures among postmenopausal women and older men. CMAJ 181: 815–20.
6. Rubin C, Turner AS, Bain S, Mallinckrodt C, McLeod K, et al. (2001) Low mechanical signals strengthen long bones. Nature 412: 603–4.
7. Tezval M, Biblis M, Sehmisch S, Schmelz U, Kolios L, et al. (2011) Improvement of femoral bone quality after low-magnitude, high-frequency mechanical stimulation in the ovariectomized rat as an osteopenia model. Calcif Tissue Int 88: 33–40.
8. Rubin C, Turner AS, Müller R, Mittra E, McLeod K, et al. (2002) Quantity and quality of trabecular bone in the femur are enhanced by a strongly anabolic, noninvasive mechanical intervention. J Bone Miner Res 17: 349–57.
9. Ward K, Alsop C, Caulton J, Rubin C, Adams J, et al. (2004) Low magnitude mechanical loading is osteogenic in children with disabling conditions. J Bone Miner Res 19: 360–9.
10. Rubin C, Recker R, Cullen D, Ryaby J, McCabe J, et al. (2004) Prevention of postmenopausal bone loss by a low-magnitude, high-frequency mechanical stimuli: a clinical trial assessing compliance, efficacy, and safety. J Bone Miner Res 19: 343–51.
11. Robling AG, Hinant FM, Burr DB, Turner CH (2002) Shorter, more frequent mechanical loading sessions enhance bone mass. Med Sci Sports Exerc 34: 196–202.
12. Saxon LK, Robling AG, Alam I, Turner CH (2005) Mechanosensitivity of the rat skeleton decreases after a long period of loading, but is improved with time off. Bone 36: 454–64.
13. Srinivasan S, Weimer DA, Agans SC, Bain SD, Gross TS (2002) Low-magnitude mechanical loading becomes osteogenic when rest is inserted between each load cycle. J Bone Miner Res 17: 1613–20.
14. Ma RS, Zhu D, Gong H, Gu GS, Huang X, et al. (2012) High-frequency and low-magnitude whole body vibration with rest days is more effective in improving skeletal micro-morphology and biomechanical properties in ovariectomised rodents. Hip Int 22: 218–26.
15. Gong H, Zhang M, Zhang H, Zhu D, Yang L (2006) Theoretical analysis of contributions of disuse, basic multicellular unit activation threshold, and osteoblastic formation threshold to changes in bone mineral density at menopause. J Bone Miner Metab 24: 386–94.
16. Feng L, Jasiuk I (2011) Multi-scale characterization of swine femoral cortical bone. J Biomech 44: 313–20.

17. Ruimerman R, Huiskes R, Lenthe GH, Janssen JD (2001) A computer simulation model relating bone-cell metabolism to mechanical adaptation of trabecular architecture. COMPUT METHOD BIOMEC 4: 433–448.
18. Wang LZ, Cheung JT, Pu F, Li DY, Zhang M, et al. (2011) Why do woodpeckers resist head impact injury: A Biomechanical Investigation. PLoS ONE 6(10): e26490.
19. Thurner PJ, Müller R, Kindt JH, Schitter G, Fantner GE, et al. (2005) Novel techniques for high-resolution functional imaging of trabecular bone. In: Proceedings of the SPIE, p. 515–26.
20. Thurner PJ, Oroudjev E, Jungmann R, Kreutz C, Kindt JH, et al. (2007) Imaging of bone ultrastructure using atomic force microscopy. In: Méndez-Vilas A, Díaz J, editors. Modern research and educational topics in microscopy. Badajoz: Formatex, p. 37–48.
21. Hassenkam T, Fantner GE, Cutroni JA, Weaver JC, Morse DE, et al. (2004) Highresolution AFM imaging of intact and fractured trabecular bone. Bone 35: 4–10.
22. Hassenkam T, Jøgensen HL, Lauritzen JB (2006) Mapping the imprint of bone remodeling by atomic force microscopy. Anat Rec A 288: 1087–94.
23. Hassenkam T, Jøgensen HL, Pedersen MB, Kourakis AH, Simonsen L, et al. (2005) Atomic force microscopy on human trabecular bone from an old woman with osteoporotic fractures. Micron 36: 681–7.
24. Chappard D, Legrand E, Baslé MF, Audran M (2011) New laboratory tools in the assessment of bone quality. Osteoporos Int 22: 2225–40.
25. Milovanovic P, Potocnik J, Stoiljkovic M, Djonic D, Nikolic S, et al. (2011) Nanostructure and mineral composition of trabecular bone in the lateral femoral neck: Implications for bone fragility in elderly women. Acta Biomater 7: 3446–51.
26. Pharr GM, Oliver WC (1992) Measurement of thin film mechanical properties using nanoindentation. MRS Bull 17: 28–33.
27. Doerner MF, Nix WD (1986) A method for determining the data from depth-sensing indentation instruments. J Mater Res 1: 601.
28. Ascenzi A, Baschieri P, Benvenuti A (1990) The bending properties of a single osteon. J Biomech 23, 763–71.
29. Lotz JC, Gerhart TN, Hayes WC (1991) Mechanical properties of metaphyseal bone in the proximal femur. J Biomech 24: 317–29.
30. Manske SL, Good CA, Zernicke RF, Boyd SK (2012) High-Frequency, Low-Magnitude Vibration Does Not Prevent Bone Loss Resulting from Muscle Disuse in Mice following Botulinum Toxin Injection. PLoS ONE 7(5): e36486.
31. Hembree M, Buschang PH, Carrillo R, Rossouw PE (2009) Effects of intentional damage to the roots and surrounding structures with miniscrew implants. Am J Orthod Dentofacial Orthop, 135(3): 280.e1–9.
32. Brisceno CE, Rossouw PE, Carrillo R, Spears R, Buschang H (2009) Healing of the roots and surrounding structures after intentional damage with miniscrew implants. Am J Orthod Dentofacial Orthop, 135(3): 292–301.
33. Dempster DW, Compston JE, Drezner MK, Glorieux FH, Kanis JA, et al. (2013) Standardized nomenclature, symbols, and units for bone histomorphometry: a 2012 update of the report of the ASBMR histomorphometry nomenclature committee. J Bone Miner Res 28: 1–16.
34. Li XJ, Jee WS, Chow SY, Woodbury DM (1990) Adaptation of cancellous bone to aging and immobilization in the rat: a single photon absorptiometry and histomorphometry study. The Anatomical Record 227: 12–24.
35. Rho JY, Ting Y, Tsui TY, Pharr GM (1997) Elastic properties of human corticaland trabecular lamellar bone measured by nanoindentation. Biomaterials 18: 1325–30.
36. Oliver WC, Pharr GM (1992) An improved technique for determining hardness and elastic modulus using load and displacement sensing indentation experiments. J Mater Res 7: 1564–83.
37. Rankovic D, Kuzmanovic M, Savovic J, Pavlovic M, Stoiljkovic M, et al. (2010) The effect of potassium addition on plasma parameters in argon dc plasma arc. J Phys D: Appl Phys 43: 335202.
38. Chen PY, Toroian D, Price PA, McKittrick J (2011) Minerals Form a Continuum Phase in Mature Cancellous Bone. Calcif Tissue Int 88: 351–361.
39. Yamauchi H, Mashiko S, Kimura M, Miyano S, Yonemoto K (2003) Responses of bone mineral density to isometric resistance exercise during hindlimb unloading and subsequent recovery. J Sport Med Phys Fit 52: 119–130.
40. Rubin CT, Sommerfeldt DW, Judex S, Qin YX (2001) Inhibition of osteopenia by low magnitude, high-frequency mechanical stimuli. Drug Discov Today 6: 848–58.
41. Gilsanz V, Wren TA, Sanchez M, Dorey F, Judex S, et al. (2006) Low-level, high-frequency mechanical signals enhance musculoskeletal development of young women with low BMD. J Bone Miner Res 21: 1464–74.
42. Flieger J, Karachalios T, Khaldi L, Raptou P, Lyritis G (1998) Mechanical stimulation in the form of vibration prevents postmenopausal bone loss in ovariectomized rats. Calcif Tissue Int 63: 510–4.
43. Li ZL· Tan C· Wu YH· Ding Y· Wang HJ, et al. (2012) Whole-body vibration and resistance exercise prevent long-term hindlimb unloading-induced bone loss: independent and interactive effects. Eur J Appl Physiol 112: 3743–53.
44. Matsuda J, Kurata K, Hara T, Higaki H (2009) Mechanical Vibration Applied in the Absence of Weight Bearing Suggest Improved Fragile Bone. 13th International Conference on Biomedical Engineering IFMBE Proceedings 23: 1766–8.
45. Yang PF, Jia B, Ding C, Wang Z, Qian AR, et al. (2009) Whole-Body Vibration Effects on Bone Before and After Hind-Limb Unloading in Rats. ASEM 80: 88–93.
46. Boskey AL (2001) Bone mineralization. In: Cowin SC, editor. Bone mechanics handbook. Boca Raton, FL: CRC Press: 5/1–5/33.
47. Landis WJ, Hodgens KJ, Song MJ, Arena J, Kiyonaga S, et al. (1996) Mineralization of collagen may occur on fibril surfaces: evidence from conventional and high-voltage electron microscopy and three-dimensional imaging. J Struct Biol 117: 24–35.
48. Landis WJ, Song MJ, Leith A, McEwen L, McEwen BF (1993) Mineral and organic matrix interaction in normally calcifying tendon visualized in three dimensions by high-voltage electron microscopic tomography and graphic image reconstruction. J Struct Biol 110: 39–54.
49. Su X, Sun K, Cui FZ, Landis WJ (2003) Organization of apatite crystals in human woven bone. Bone 32: 150–62.
50. Fan ZF, Smith P, Rauch F, Harris GF (2007) Nanoindentation as a means for distinguishing clinical type of osteogenesis imperfecta. Compos Part B 38: 411–5.
51. Hoffler CE, Moore KE, Kozloff K, Zysset PK, Goldstein SA (2000) Age, gender and bone lamellae elastic moduli. J Orthop Res 18: 432–7.
52. Hoffler CE, Moore KE, Kozloff K, Zysset PK, Brown MB, et al. (2000) Heterogeneity of bone lamellar-level elastic moduli. Bone 26: 603–9.
53. Rho JY, Zioupos P, Curry JD, Pharr GM (2002) Microstructural elasticity and regional heterogeneity in human femoral bone of various ages examined by nano-indentation. J Biomech 35: 189–98.
54. Sun LW, Fan YB, Li DY, Zhao F, Xie T, et al. (2009) Evaluation of the mechanical properties of rat bone under simulated microgravity using nanoindentation. Acta Biomater 5: 3506–11.
55. Rubin CT, Capilla E, Luu YK, Busa B, Crawford H, et al. (2007) Adipogenesis is inhibited by brief, daily exposure to high-frequency, extremely low magnitude mechanical signals. PNAS 104: 17879–84.
56. Luu YK, Ozcivici E, Capilla E, Adler B, Chan E, et al. (2010) Development of diet induced fatty liver disease in the aging mouse is suppressed by brief daily exposure to low-magnitude mechanical signals. Int J Obes (Lond) 34: 401–5.
57. Sen B, Xie ZH, Case N, Styner M, Rubin CT, et al. (2011) Mechanical signal influence on mesenchymal stem cell fate is enhanced by incorporation of refractory periods into the loading regimen. J Biomech 44: 593–9.
58. Faulkner KG, Genant HK, McClung M (1995) Bilateral comparison of femoral bone density and hip axis length from single and fan beam DXA scans. Calcif Tissue Int 56: 26–31.

Permissions

All chapters in this book were first published in PLOS ONE, by The Public Library of Science; hereby published with permission under the Creative Commons Attribution License or equivalent. Every chapter published in this book has been scrutinized by our experts. Their significance has been extensively debated. The topics covered herein carry significant findings which will fuel the growth of the discipline. They may even be implemented as practical applications or may be referred to as a beginning point for another development.

The contributors of this book come from diverse backgrounds, making this book a truly international effort. This book will bring forth new frontiers with its revolutionizing research information and detailed analysis of the nascent developments around the world.

We would like to thank all the contributing authors for lending their expertise to make the book truly unique. They have played a crucial role in the development of this book. Without their invaluable contributions this book wouldn't have been possible. They have made vital efforts to compile up to date information on the varied aspects of this subject to make this book a valuable addition to the collection of many professionals and students.

This book was conceptualized with the vision of imparting up-to-date information and advanced data in this field. To ensure the same, a matchless editorial board was set up. Every individual on the board went through rigorous rounds of assessment to prove their worth. After which they invested a large part of their time researching and compiling the most relevant data for our readers.

The editorial board has been involved in producing this book since its inception. They have spent rigorous hours researching and exploring the diverse topics which have resulted in the successful publishing of this book. They have passed on their knowledge of decades through this book. To expedite this challenging task, the publisher supported the team at every step. A small team of assistant editors was also appointed to further simplify the editing procedure and attain best results for the readers.

Apart from the editorial board, the designing team has also invested a significant amount of their time in understanding the subject and creating the most relevant covers. They scrutinized every image to scout for the most suitable representation of the subject and create an appropriate cover for the book.

The publishing team has been an ardent support to the editorial, designing and production team. Their endless efforts to recruit the best for this project, has resulted in the accomplishment of this book. They are a veteran in the field of academics and their pool of knowledge is as vast as their experience in printing. Their expertise and guidance has proved useful at every step. Their uncompromising quality standards have made this book an exceptional effort. Their encouragement from time to time has been an inspiration for everyone.

The publisher and the editorial board hope that this book will prove to be a valuable piece of knowledge for researchers, students, practitioners and scholars across the globe.

List of Contributors

Xiaolei Zhang, Katleen Vandamme, Ignace Naert and Joke Duyck
Department of Prosthetic Dentistry, BIOMAT Research Cluster, University of Leuven, Leuven, Belgium

Antonia Torcasio
Department of Mechanical Engineering, Division of Biomechanics and Engineering Design, University of Leuven, Leuven, Belgium

G. Harry van Lenthe
Department of Mechanical Engineering, Division of Biomechanics and Engineering Design, University of Leuven, Leuven, Belgium
Institute for Biomechanics, ETH Zurich, Zurich, Switzerland

Toru Ogawa
Division of Advanced Prosthetic Dentistry, Tohoku University Graduate School of Dentistry, Sendai, Japan

W. Joyce Tang and Sarah Zarrin
Department of Rehabilitation Research and Development, Center for Tissue Regeneration, Repair, and Restoration, Veterans Affairs Palo Alto Health Care System, Palo Alto, California, United States of America

ae-Beom Kim
Department of Surgery, Stanford University School of Medicine, Stanford, California, United States of America

Alesha B. Castillo
Department of Rehabilitation Research and Development, Center for Tissue Regeneration, Repair, and Restoration, Veterans Affairs Palo Alto Health Care System, Palo Alto, California, United States of America
Department of Surgery, Stanford University School of Medicine, Stanford, California, United States of America
Department of Mechanical Engineering, Stanford University, Stanford, California, United States of America

Jennifer T. Blundo
Department of Mechanical Engineering, Stanford University, Stanford, California, United States of America
Department of Biomedical Engineering, Columbia University, New York, New York, United States of America

Julia C. Chen, Kristen L. Lee, Nikitha Reddy Yereddi, Eugene Jang and Shefali Kumar
Department of Biomedical Engineering, Columbia University, New York, New York, United States of America

J, Christopher R. Jacobs
Department of Rehabilitation Research and Development, Center for Tissue Regeneration, Repair, and Restoration, Veterans Affairs Palo Alto Health Care System, Palo Alto, California, United States of America
Department of Mechanical Engineering, Stanford University, Stanford, California, United States of America
Department of Biomedical Engineering, Columbia University, New York, New York, United States of America

Sofia E. M. Andersson, Mattias N. D. Svensson, Malin C. Erlandsson, Mats Dehlin, Karin M. E. Andersson and Maria I. Bokarewa
Department of Rheumatology and Inflammation Research, Sahlgrenska University Hospital, University of Göteborg, Göteborg, Sweden

Qiang He, Jingjing Dong, Yang Li, Zixiang Wu and Wei Lei
Institute of Orthopaedics, Xijing Hospital, Fourth Military Medical University, Xi'an, Shaanxi, People's Republic of China

Huiling Chen
Department of Health Service, School of Public Health and Military Preventive, Fourth Military Medical University, Xi'an, Shaanxi, People's Republic of China

Li Huang
Department of General Dentistry, School of Stomatology, Fourth Military Medical University, Xi'an, Shaanxi, People's Republic of China

Dagang Guo and Mengmeng Mao
State Key Laboratory for Mechanical Behavior of Materials, School of Materials Science and Engineering, Xi'an Jiaotong University, Xi'an, Shaanxi, People's Republic of China

Liang Kong
Department of Oral and Maxillofacial Surgery, School of Stomatology, Fourth Military Medical University, Xi'an, Shaanxi, People's Republic of China

Kim E. M. Benders and Laura B. Creemers
Department of Orthopaedics, University Medical Center Utrecht, Utrecht, The Netherlands

Jos Malda
Department of Orthopaedics, University Medical Center Utrecht, Utrecht, The Netherlands,
Institute of Health and Biomedical Innovation, Queensland University of Technology, Kelvin Grove, Queensland, Australia
Department of Equine Sciences, Faculty of Veterinary Medicine, Utrecht University, Utrecht, The Netherlands

c
Department of Orthopaedics, University Medical Center Utrecht, Utrecht, The Netherlands
Department of Equine Sciences, Faculty of Veterinary Medicine, Utrecht University, Utrecht, The Netherlands

Janny C. de Grauw and P. Renévan Weeren
Department of Equine Sciences, Faculty of Veterinary Medicine, Utrecht University, Utrecht, The Netherlands

Marja J. L. Kik
Department of Pathobiology, Faculty of Veterinary Medicine, Utrecht University, Utrecht, The Netherland

Chris H. A. van de Lest
Department of Equine Sciences, Faculty of Veterinary Medicine, Utrecht University, Utrecht, The Netherlands
Department of Biochemistry and Cell Biology, Faculty of Veterinary Medicine, Utrecht University, Utrecht, The Netherlands

Jui-Ting Hsu and Michael Y. C. Chen
School of Dentistry, College of Medicine, China Medical University, Taichung, Taiwan

Ying-Ju Chen and Fu-Chou Cheng
Stem Cell Center, Department of Medical Research, Taichung Veterans General Hospital, Taichung, Taiwan

Ming-Tzu Tsai
Department of Biomedical Engineering, Hungkuang University, Taichung, Taiwan

Howard Haw-Chang Lan
Department of Radiology, Taichung Veterans General Hospital, Taichung, Taiwan
School of Radiological Technology, Central Taiwan University of Science and Technology, Taichung, Taiwan

Shun-Ping Wang
Department of Orthopaedics, Taichung Veterans General Hospital, Taichung, Taiwan
Ya-Fei Feng, Lin Wang, Zhen-Sheng Ma, Yang Zhang and Wei Lei
Department of Orthopedics, Xijing Hospital, The Fourth Military Medical University, Xi'an, China

Xiang Li
School of Mechanical Engineering, Shanghai Jiao Tong University, State Key Laboratory of Mechanical System and Vibration, Shanghai, China

Zhi-Yong Zhang
Department of Plastic and Reconstructive Surgery, Shanghai 9th People's Hospital, Shanghai Key Laboratory of Tissue Engineering, School of Medicine, Shanghai Jiao Tong University, Shanghai, China
National Tissue Engineering Center of China, Shanghai, China

Mika Yamaga, Kazumasa Miyatake, Jun Yamada, Kahaer Abula and Young-Jin Ju
Department of Joint Surgery and Sports Medicine, Tokyo Medical and Dental University, Tokyo, Japan,

Kunikazu Tsuji
International Research Center for Molecular Science in Tooth and Bone Diseases (Global Center of Excellence Program), Tokyo Medical and Dental University, Tokyo, Japan

Ichiro Sekiya
Department of Cartilage Regeneration, Tokyo Medical and Dental University, Tokyo, Japan

Takeshi Muneta
Department of Joint Surgery and Sports Medicine, Tokyo Medical and Dental University, Tokyo, Japan International Research Center for Molecular Science in Tooth and Bone Diseases (Global Center of Excellence Program), Tokyo Medical and Dental University, Tokyo, Japan

Xiao-Kang Li, Chao-Fan Yuan, Yong-Quan Zhang and Zheng Guo
Department of Orthopaedics, Xijing Hospital, Fourth Military Medical University, Xi'an, China

Jun-Lin Wang
School of Stomatology, Fourth Military Medical University, Xi'an, China

Zhi-Yong Zhang
Department of Plastic and Reconstructive Surgery, Shanghai 9th People's Hospital, Shanghai Key Laboratory of Tissue Engineering, School of Medicine, Shanghai Jiao Tong University, Shanghai, China
National Tissue Engineering Center of China, Shanghai, China

Brett Nemke
Comparative Orthopaedic Research Laboratory, School of Veterinary Medicine, University of Wisconsin-Madison, Madison, Wisconson, United States of America

Yan Lu and Mark D. Markel
Comparative Orthopaedic Research Laboratory, School of Veterinary Medicine, University of Wisconsin-Madison, Madison, Wisconson, United States of America
Orthopedics and Rehabilitation, University of Wisconsin, Madison, Wisconson, United States of America

Jae Sung Lee, Kevin Royalty and Ray Vanderby Jr.
Departments of Biomedical Engineering, University of Wisconsin, Madison, Wisconson, United States of America

Ben K. Graf and Richard Illgen III
Orthopedics and Rehabilitation, University of Wisconsin, Madison, Wisconson, United States of America

William L. Murphy
Departments of Biomedical Engineering, University of Wisconsin, Madison, Wisconson, United States of America
Pharmacology, University of Wisconsin, Madison, Wisconson, United States of America
Orthopedics and Rehabilitation, University of Wisconsin, Madison, Wisconson, United States of America

Susan K. Grimston, Marcus P. Watkins and Roberto Civitelli
Division of Bone and Mineral Diseases, Department of Internal Medicine, Washington University in St. Louis, St. Louis, Missouri, United States of America
Musculoskeletal Research Center, Washington University in St.Louis, St. Louis, Missouri, United States of America

Michael D. Brodt and Matthew J. Silva
Department of Orthopedic Surgery, Washington University in St. Louis, St. Louis, Missouri, United States of America
Musculoskeletal Research Center, Washington University in St.Louis, St. Louis, Missouri, United States of America

Katalin Sándor, István Tóth and János Szolcsá nyi
Department of Pharmacology and Pharmacotherapy, Faculty of Medicine, University of Pécs, Pécs, Hungary

Éva Borbély, Zsófia Hajna, Erika Pintér, Péter Nagy and Zsuzsanna Helyes
Department of Pharmacology and Pharmacotherapy, Faculty of Medicine, University of Pécs, Pécs, Hungary János Szentágothai Research Center, University of Pécs, Pécs, Hungary

László Kereskai
Department of Pathology, Faculty of Medicine, University of Pécs, Pécs, Hungary

John Quinn
Department of Molecular and Clinical Pharmacology, Institute of Translational Medicine Liverpool University, Liverpool, United Kingdom

Andreas Zimmer
Laboratory of Molecular Neurobiology, Department of Psychiatry, University of Bonn, Bonn, Germany

James Stewart
School of Infection and Host Defense, University of Liverpool, Liverpool, United Kingdom

Christopher Paige and Alexandra Berger
Ontario Cancer Institute, University Health Network, Toronto, Canada
Department of Immunology, University of Toronto, Toronto, Canada

Chikashi Terao
Center for Genomic Medicine, Kyoto University Graduate School of Medicine, Kyoto, Japan
Department of Rheumatology and Clinical Immunology, Kyoto University Graduate School of Medicine, Kyoto, Japan

Motomu Hashimoto, Takao Fujii and Tsuneyo Mimori
Department of Rheumatology and Clinical Immunology, Kyoto University Graduate School of Medicine, Kyoto, Japan
Department of the Control for Rheumatic Diseases, Kyoto University Graduate School of Medicine, Kyoto, Japan

Kosaku Murakami, Koichiro Ohmura, Ran Nakashima, Noriyuki Yamakawa, Hajime Yoshifuji, Naoichiro Yukawa, Daisuke Kawabata and Takashi Usui
Department of Rheumatology and Clinical Immunology, Kyoto University Graduate School of Medicine, Kyoto, Japan

Moritoshi Furu and Hiromu Ito
Department of the Control for Rheumatic Diseases, Kyoto University Graduate School of Medicine, Kyoto, Japan
Department of Orthopaedic Surgery, Kyoto University Graduate School of Medicine, Kyoto, Japan

Ryo Yamada
Center for Genomic Medicine, Kyoto University Graduate School of Medicine, Kyoto, Japan
Unit of Statistical Genetics Center for Genomic Medicine, Kyoto University Graduate School of Medicine, Kyoto, Japan

Keiichi Yamamoto
Department of Clinical Trial Design and Management, Translational Research Center, Kyoto University Hospital, Kyoto, Japan

Hiroyuki Yoshitomi
Department of Orthopaedic Surgery, Kyoto University Graduate School of Medicine, Kyoto, Japan

Fumihiko Matsuda
Center for Genomic Medicine, Kyoto University Graduate School of Medicine, Kyoto, Japan
Institut National de la Sante et de la Recherche Medicale (INSERM) Unite U852, Kyoto University Graduate School of Medicine, Kyoto, Japan
CREST Program, Japan Science and Technology Agency, Kawaguchi, Saitama, Japan

Kristian J. Carlson
Institute for Human Evolution, University of the Witwatersrand, Johannesburg, South Africa
Department of Anthropology, Indiana University, Bloomington, Indiana, United States of America

Tea Jashashvili
Institute for Human Evolution, University of the Witwatersrand, Johannesburg, South Africa
Department of Geology and Paleontology, Georgian National Museum, Tbilisi, Georgia

Kimberley Houghton
Institute for Human Evolution, University of the Witwatersrand, Johannesburg, South Africa

Michael C. Westaway
Cultures and Histories Program, Queensland Museum, Brisbane, Australia

Biren A. Patel
Department of Cell and Neurobiology, Keck School of Medicine, University of Southern California, Los Angeles, California, United States of America

Antonia Torcasio, Jos VanderSloten, Maarten Van Guyse and Pieter Spaepen
Biomechanics Section, KU Leuven, Leuven, Belgium
Katharina Jähn, Andrea E. Tamia and Martin J. Stoddart
AO Research Institute, Davos, Switzerland

G. Harry van Lenthe
Biomechanics Section, KU Leuven, Leuven, Belgium
Institute for Biomechanics, ETH Zurich, Zurich, Switzerland

Timothy M. Ryan
Department of Anthropology, Pennsylvania State University, University Park, Pennsylvania, United States of America
Center for Quantitative Imaging, EMS Energy Institute, Pennsylvania State University, University Park, Pennsylvania, United States of America

Colin N. Shaw
Department of Anthropology, Pennsylvania State University, University Park, Pennsylvania, United States of America
Center for Quantitative Imaging, EMS Energy Institute, Pennsylvania State University, University Park, Pennsylvania, United States of America
PAVE Research Group and The McDonald Institute for Archaeological Research, Department of Archaeology and Anthropology, University of Cambridge, Cambridge, United Kingdom

Peng-Fei Yang
Key Laboratory for Space Bioscience and Biotechnology, School of Life Sciences, Northwestern Polytechnical University, Xi'an, China
Division of Space Physiology, Institute of Aerospace Medicine, German Aerospace Center, Cologne, Germany
Institute of Biomechanics and Orthopaedics, German Sport University Cologne, Cologne, Germany

Bergita Ganse
Division of Space Physiology, Institute of Aerospace Medicine, German Aerospace Center, Cologne, Germany

Maximilian Sanno and Gert-Peter Brüggemann
Institute of Biomechanics and Orthopaedics, German Sport University Cologne, Cologne, Germany

Timmo Koy and Lars Peter Müller
Department of Orthopaedic and Trauma Surgery, University of Cologne, Cologne, Germany

Jörn Rittweger
Division of Space Physiology, Institute of Aerospace Medicine, German Aerospace Center, Cologne, Germany
Institute for Biomedical Research into Human Movement and Health, Manchester Metropolitan University, Manchester, United Kingdom

Lei Ren
School of Mechanical, Aerospace and Civil Engineering, University of Manchester, Manchester, United Kingdom

David Howard
School of Computing, Science and Engineering, University of Salford, Manchester, United Kingdom

Dan Hu
School of Mechanical, Aerospace and Civil Engineering, University of Manchester, Manchester, United Kingdom
State Key Laboratory of Automotive Simulation and Control, Jilin University, Changchun, P.R. China

Marie-Soleil Dubois, Samantha Morello, Kelsey Rayment, Mark D. Markel, Vicki L. Kalscheur

Zhengling Hao and Peter Muir
Comparative Orthopaedic Research Laboratory, School of Veterinary Medicine, University of Wisconsin-Madison, Madison, Wisconsin, United States of America

Ray Vanderby Jr and Ronald P. McCabe
Department of Orthopedics & Rehabilitation, School of Medicine & Public Health, University of Wisconsin-Madison, Madison, Wisconsin, United States of America

Patricia Marquis
Comparative Orthopaedic Research Laboratory, School of Veterinary Medicine, University of Wisconsin-Madison, Madison, Wisconsin, United States of America
Gulfstream Park, Hallandale Beach, Florida, United States of America

Yolande F. M. Ramos, P. Eline Slagboom, Steffan D. Bos and Ingrid Meulenbelt
Department of Molecular Epidemiology, Leiden University Medical Center, Leiden, The Netherlands
The Netherlands Genomics Initiative, sponsored by the NCHA, Leiden-Rotterdam, The Netherlands

Wouter den Hollander, Nils Bomer, Ruud van der Breggen and Nico Lakenberg
Department of Molecular Epidemiology, Leiden University Medical Center, Leiden, The Netherlands

J. Christiaan Keurentjes and Rob G. H. H. Nelissen
Department of Orthopeadics, Leiden University Medical Center, Leiden, The Netherland

Judith V. M. G. Bovée
Department of Pathology, Leiden University Medical Center, Leiden, The Netherlands

Jelle J. Goeman
Department of Biostatistics and Bioinformatics, Leiden University Medical Center, Leiden, The Netherlands

Da Jing, Juan Liu, Wei Guo, Maogang Jiang, Erping Luo, Guanghao Shen, Mingming Zhai, Shichao Tong Kangning Xie, Xiaoming Wu and Chi Tang
Department of Biomedical Engineering, Fourth Military Medical University, Xi'an, China

Jing Cai
Department of Endocrinology, Xijing hospital, Fourth Military Medical University, Xi'an, China

Yan Wu
Institute of Orthopaedics, Xijing hospital, Fourth Military Medical University, Xi'an, China

Qiaoling Xu
Department of Nursing, Fourth Military Medical University, Xi'an, China

Xinmin Xu
Department of Medical Engineering, PLA No. 323 Hospital, Xi'an, China

Rit Vatsyayan, Hema Kothari, Usha R. Pendurthi and L. Vijaya Mohan Rao
Department of Cellular and Molecular Biology, The University of Texas Health Science Center at Tyler, Tyler, Texas, United States of America

Nigel Mackman
Division of Hematology and Oncology, McAllister Heart Institute, Department of Medicine, University of North Carolina at Chapel Hill, Chapel Hill, North Carolina, United States of America

Rui Zhang, He Gong, Jiazi Gao and Juan Fang
Department of Engineering Mechanics, Jilin University, Changchun, Jilin, People's Republic of China

Dong Zhu
Department of Orthopedic Surgery, No. 1 Hospital of Jilin University, Changchun, Jilin, People's Republic of China

Yubo Fan
School of Biological Science and Medical Engineering, Beihang University, Beijing, People's Republic of China

Index

www.ingramcontent.com/pod-product-compliance
Lightning Source LLC
Chambersburg PA
CBHW061253190326
41458CB00011B/3656
9781632424907